HEALTH AND THE COMMUNITY

*Readings in the Philosophy and Sciences
of Public Health*

HEALTH AND THE COMMUNITY

READINGS *in the Philosophy and Sciences* *of Public Health*

Alfred H. Katz, D.S.W.

Associate Professor of Social Welfare in Medicine
Schools of Medicine, Public Health and Social Welfare
University of California, Los Angeles

Jean Spencer Felton, M.D.

Professor of Preventive Medicine and Public Health, School of
  Medicine
Professor of Occupational Health, School of Public Health
University of California, Los Angeles

Fp

The Free Press, New York

COLLIER-MACMILLAN LIMITED, LONDON

Garrisons pent up in a little fort
   with foes who do but wait on every side
   knowing the time soon comes when they shall ride
   triumphant over those trapped and make sport
of them: when those within know very short
   is now their hour and no aid can betide:
   such men as these not quarrel and divide
   but friend and foe are friends in their hard sort

And if these things be so oh men then what
   of these beleaguered victims this our race
   betrayed alike by Fate's gigantic plot
   here in this far-pitched perilous hostile place
   this solitary hard-assaulted spot
   fixed at the friendless outer edge of space.

R. A. K. MASON

* SONNET OF BROTHERHOOD by R. A. K. Mason is reprinted by permission from *Collected Poems,* published by the Pegasus Press Ltd., Christchurch, New Zealand, 1962. The author is Senior Lecturer in English, and holder of the Robert Burns Fellowship in English Literature at the University of Otaga, Dunedin, New Zealand.

Introduction

THIS IS A BOOK of readings in Public Health, designed to acquaint readers from many backgrounds with some of the major programs, achievements, issues, and still unsettled directions of this wide-ranging and fast-moving field.

Public Health, as a special area of practice and investigation, is hardly more than 100 years old. Yet many of its component sciences and arts go back to antiquity.

Much of the fascination and importance of Public Health derives from its steadily-enlarging scope, from the rapidity and flexibility with which its perspectives are being altered, and from its readiness to embrace new content while still retaining consistency in its goals.

In this volume we seek to give a panoramic view of the terrain now occupied by the Public Health disciplines in the United States, and to sketch in some "vistas, dimly glimpsed" toward which they may be moving.

By presenting historical, programmatic, research, and "trend-spotting" pieces under most of the headings, we have tried to make it possible for the reader to review—in limited compass—varied aspects of philosophy and practice that fall broadly within Public Health's framework.

Foreword

MOST PERIODS in history are given shorthand designations which seem
to capture something of their spirit. Often these are the merely catchy
or alliterative tags of journalists; but sometimes an historian catches
an epoch's essence more poignantly in a single phrase. Today we
appear to be in a new era which, in its physical aspects at least, might
be called the Age of Verticality. This notion is sustained by space
probes to the planets, the building of missiles, urban high rise construction, the speed and altitude of flights, and the Space Needle.

These symbols of the perpendicular might appear but slightly related to the domain of Public Health. They may seem even more
remote to the gathering between covers of a collection of individual
writings. Yet, we can draw a parallel. All of these extraordinary
ventures into space are the product and culmination of conjoined
thought. Many minds and many muscles made reality of an idea.

So it was with the assembling of these readings. They are inherently a collective product. The editors feel deep gratitude to the
many authors who gave willingly of their ideas and experiences, to the
numerous publishers and agencies that have shared the authors' cre-
ations, and to a small but able group of associates. Through a singular
alchemy the latter have converted noncalligraphic scrawls and a multiplicity of type faces into a workable manuscript. Gratefully acknowledged is the help of Martha Greiner, Harriet Tanaka, Grace Wax, and
Sylvia Steinhorn. Nor could the work have become a reality without
the patience and generous support of our respective wives and families.

The writers of the articles included have generously acceded to our
requests to reproduce their materials. The retention of original by-
lines is the form of the credit given. Publishers, however, prefer specific
wordings for the citations of permission for reprinting; hence the form
of these authorizations necessarily varies.

It must be noted that an occasional article or excerpt was written
by persons now deceased; although the editors were denied the pleasure of personal acknowledgment, our appreciation is great for their
ideas and expressions which live on.

Much that is printed in professional journals records addresses
given before a variety of societies, meetings, or task groups. Local
references and opening remarks in these presentations have mostly
been excised in the name of brevity. In other selections, we have

sought through editing to make more formal or explicit concepts or emphases which at the time of utterance were not so highlighted. Some headings have been added, and British spelling has been Americanized. We are grateful to the authors and publishers for the privilege thus afforded of slight editorial re-touching.

Where isolated paragraphs have been used, or where lengthy papers have been abbreviated, it has been the editors' wish to eliminate the duplicative and retain the fresh, original, or provocative. The cutting of many tables was necessitated by the demands of space and economy. Authors' notes or references are placed at the back of the volume to smooth the reader's path, and to provide reference for those who seek bibliographic detail.

So much for a look behind the scenes. May the view from the front be rewarding.

A H K

J S F

The Plan of the Book

TO ACCOMPLISH these purposes, this book is divided into eight sections, each having a separate emphasis.

The first, *"The Fields,"* deals broadly with historical backgrounds out of which Public Health has arisen, and with the massive social movements that shape its present concerns and changing concepts.

The second, *"The People—Target Populations for Public Health,"* provides a series of case-studies of populations of particular present interest

Section Three, *"The Settings of Public Health,"* sketches the outlines of Public Health structures, organizations, and planning processes as currently evident in the United States.

"The Sciences and Disciplines," Section Four, depicts the professional roles, the knowledge and skills brought to bear on the solution of health problems by 16 of the discrete sciences and disciplines whose contributions are integral to current Public Health investigation and practice.

"Some Changing Emphases," Section Five, illustrates a variety of major newer activities receiving present emphasis under the Public Health rubric.

Section Six, *"Some Techniques,"* considers a few of the innovative methods that have been evolved by creative practitioners and found of wide utility. Section Seven, on *"Special Studies,"* reviews for health care the implications and consequences of some recent scientific advances.

The concluding Section, *"Goals and Priorities: A Changing World,"* relates the rapidly developing sciences and programs in Public Health to philosophic and speculative views of man's nature and social change, to consideration of the place of the Public Health movement in civilization and human progress.

In each of these Sections, the Editors have been motivated to present materials which not only have intrinsic merit scientifically and as exposition, but which exemplify a broad view of practice and research. We are well aware that the pace of technologic developments may quickly make obsolete the findings of any particular research study, or programmatic statement. Our goal has been to include materials written from a viewpoint that admits of the possibility of obsolescence and change. Basic attitudes, values and goals persist, no matter how much the premises, techniques, and procedures of a particular period may alter; we have sought out materials whose authors have been aware of these immutables, and who in so doing, have exemplified and contributed to "the growing edge" of a maturing science.

Contents

FOREWORD

INTRODUCTION

PART ONE

Changing Social Conditions and Health Needs   1

1. *A Look at the Past*   3
    Social History of Medicine, *Henry E. Sigerist*   3
    The City in National Health, *Luther L. Terry*   11
    Government and Health before the New Deal,
        William G. Carleton   14

2. *Urbanization and Population Change*   23
    The Impact of Urbanization, *Jean Gottman*   23
    Family Planning in the U.S., *Ronald F. Freedman,
        Pascal K. Whelpton, and Arthur A. Cambell*   37

3. *The Rural Pattern*: Healthways on the
        Farms   45
    Occupational Health on The Farms, *H. N. Doyle*   45
    Rural Healthways in New Mexico, *Sam Schulman*   51

4. *The Metropolitan Pattern*: Healthways in
        Conurbia   62
    Health Effects from Repeated Exposure to Low
        Concentrations of Air Pollutants, *Richard A.
        Prindle and Emanuel Landau*   62
    The Epidemiology of Motor Vehicle Accidents,
        Ross A. McFarland   74
    Stream Pollution, *Rolf Eliassen*   93

5. *The International Community*   100
    Health Conditions, *United Nations*   100

PART TWO

The People: Target Populations   125

1.   *The Family in Change*   127
    The American Family Today, *Reuben Hill*   127

2.   *The Chronically Ill*   141
    The Doctor's Dilemma—Updated, *Claire F. Ryder*   141

3.   *The Aging*   149
    Housing and Social Health of Older People in the
    United States, *Wilma Donahue and E. Everett
    Ashley, 3rd*   149

4.   *The Workers*   164
    Hazards to Health in Uranium Mining and Millings,
    *Victor E. Archer, Harold J. Magnuson, Duncan
    A. Holaday, and Pope A. Lawrence*   164
    Life Stress and Industrial Absenteeism, *Lawrence E.
    Hinkle and Norman Plummer*   170
    Alcoholism in Industry, *Harry Levinson*   187

5.   *The Mothers and Their Children*   192
    Deaths Around Birth—The National Score, *Martha
    M. Eliot*   192
    Epidemiologic Investigations of Some Prenatal
    Factors in The Production of Neuropsychiatric
    Disorders, *Benjamin Pasamanick*   199

6.   *Youth and the Community*   213
    Growing Up Absurd—Jobs, *Paul Goodman*   213
    Teenagers and Venereal Disease, *Celia S. Deschin*   225

7.   *The Mentally Ill in Social Perspective*   235
    Application of Control Methods to Mental Illness,
    Ernest M. Gruenberg   235

8.   *The Mentally Retarded*   247
    Mental Retardation, *Luther W. Stringham*   247

9.   *The Migrants*   259
    Health Needs of Seasonal Farmworkers and Their
    Families, *James K. Shafer, Donald Harting, and
    Helen L. Johnston*   259

10.   *The Travellers*   268
    Satisfaction and Stress in Working Overseas, *Group
    for the Advancement of Psychiatry*   268

PART THREE

The Settings: Arenas of Health Service   273

1. *Health Administration in Federal Government*   275

Role of Public Health Service in Medical Care in the United States—Trends in Medical Care, *U.S. Public Health Service*   275

Federal Legislation Relating to Food, *Manufacturing Chemists' Association*   281

Medical Research: Past Support, Future Direction, *Dale R. Lindsay and Ernest M. Allen*   289

2. *Health Administration in Other Jurisdictions*   308

Effective Community Health Services, *George James*   308

3. *The Hospital and Regionalization*   332

Hospital Regionalization in Perspective, *Milton I. Roemer and Robert C. Morris*   332

The Hospital and Its Patients, *Richard M. Titmuss*   341

Hospitals and The Tragedy of Unused Medical Knowledge, *Leona Baumgartner*   343

Increased Expenses of American Hospitals, *American Hospital Association*   344

4. *The School*: A Primary Setting   346

School Health Programs, *Pfizer Spectrum*   346

A Study of Case-Finding Methods in Elementary Schools, *Alfred Yankauer, Jr., Ruth Frantz, Anne Drislane, and Selig Katz*   352

5. *The Armed Services*   360

Research in Preventive Medicine, *Thomas Francis, Jr.*   360

6. *The Voluntary Health Agency*   374

The Role of Voluntary Agencies in Meeting the Health Needs of Americans, *Robert H. Hamlin*   374

Conventional and "Self-Organized" Voluntary Agencies: A Comparison, *Alfred H. Katz*   384

7. *Cooperation Among Agencies*   390

Cooperation Between Departments of Health and
  Welfare, *Jonas N. Muller and Pearl Bierman*   390
Medical Care of Children in Public Programs,
  Leona Baumgartner   412

PART FOUR

The Sciences and Disciplines of Public Health   425

1. *Preventive Medicine*   428
Preventive Medicine, *Jean Spencer Felton*   428

2. *Epidemiology and Biostatistics*   431
Historical Epidemiology and Grid Analysis of
  Epidemiologic Data, *T. Ravenholt Reimert*   431
Potentialities and Limitations of Epidemiology,
  John M. Cassel   432
The City Health Department Statistician, *Howard
  West*   445

3. *Public Health Social Work*   451
Public Health Social Work, *Esther C. Spencer*   451

4. *Public Health Nursing*   466
Public Health Nursing: Definition and Process,
  Ruth B. Freeman   466

5. *Public Health Nutrition*   474
New Dimensions for Public Health Nutrition:
  The Challenge of Chronic Disease and Aging,
  Dorothy M. Youland   474

6. *Public Health Dentistry*   482
Trends in Dental Public Health in the United
  States and Canada, *Donald J. Galagan*   482

7. *Health Education*   491
Preception and Public Health, *Gordon W. Allport*   491
Posters, *Ministry of Education and Scottish Home
  and Health Department*   506

8. *Occupational Health*   508
Management and An Occupational Health Program,
  N. H. Collisson   508

9. *Space Medicine*   515
Recent Developments in Aviation and Aerospace
  Medicine, *William F. Ashe*   515

10.   *Radiologic Health*   522
Radiation Control, *Virginia Health Bulletin*   522

11.   *Genetics and Public Health*   531
Some Genetic Aspects of Public Health, *Robert W. Day*   531

12.   *Public Health Laboratories*   542
The Developing Role of Laboratories in Chronic
Disease Programs, *Wilfred D. David*   542

13.   *Public Health Psychiatry*   548
Action for Mental Health, *Joint Commission on Mental Illness and Health*   548

14.   *Behavioral Sciences in Public Health*   567
The Contributions and Limitations of Behavioral
Science in Public Health, *Lyle Saunders*   567

15.   *Administration*   583
Some Substantive Limiting Conditions in
Communication Between Health Officers and
Medical Practitioners, *George Rosen*   583

PART FIVE

The Services: Some Changing Emphases in Public
Health   599

1.   *Medical Care*   602
Medical Care Administration, *Milton I. Roemer*   602
The Medical Care Program of the United Mine
Workers of America Welfare and Retirement
Fund, *Warren F. Draper*   635

2.   *Rehabilitation*   643
The State-Federal Program of Vocational
Rehabilitation for Disabled Persons, *Mary E. Switzer*   643
Intensive Rehabilitation—Recent Experience in a
Chronic Disease Hospital, *John E. Affeldt, Vernon L. Nichel, Jacquelin Perry and Bertrand C. Kriets*   655
Alcoholics Anonymous As A Community Resource,
John Park Lee   660

3. *Poison Control*   670
    Public Health Aspects of Poisoning, *Edward Press*   670

4. *Epidemiologic Investigations*   675
    The Epidemiology of Atherosclerotic Coronary
        Heart Disease, *Jeremiah Stamler*   675
    Relationship of Amount of Cigarette Smoking to
        Coronary Heart Disease Mortality Rates in Men,
        *Robert W. Buechley, Robert M. Drake, and
        Lester Breslow*   710

5. *Nutritional Health*   715
    Malnutrition and the Health of Children, *Nevin S.
        Scrimshaw*   715
    Newer Concepts in the Management of Obesity,
        Robert W. Hillman   722

6. *Home Care*   735
    Home Care Programs, *Cecil G. Sheps and Jack
        Kasten*   735

    PART SIX
Some Technics: Innovations and Adaptations   747

1. *Multiphasic Screening*   749
    Multiple Screening in the Baltimore Study of
        Chronic Illness, *Dean W. Roberts and Charles M.
        Wylie*   749

2. *Periodic Health Examinations*   759
    The Values and Limitations of Periodic Health
        Examinations, *Norbert J. Roberts*   759

3. *Immunizations*   783
    Two Voluntary Mass Immunization Programs
        Using Sabin Oral Vaccine, *Richard B. Johns,
        Stanford Farnsworth, Hugh Thompson, and
        Frederick Brady*   783

4. *Crash Teams*   792
    Rehabilitation Operation for 10,000 Moroccan
        Paralysis Victims, *G. Gingras and M. H. L.
        Desmarais*   792

5. *Community Self-study*   799
    What Makes Communities Tick?, *Peter H. Rossi*   799

PART SEVEN

Special Studies: Resolving the Unpredictable   811

    1.   *Iatrogenic Disease*   812

       A Study of the German Outbreak of Phocomelia: The Thalidomide Syndrome, *Helen B. Taussig*   812

PART EIGHT

Goals and Priorities in a Changing World   825

    1.   *Foundations for a Social Epidemiology of Health*   827

       Man and His Changing Environment, *Edward Stainbrook*   827

    2.   *Dynamics of Planned Change*   838

       Psychodynamics of Group Opposition to Health Programs, *Judd Marmor, Viola W. Bernard, and Perry Ottenberg*   838

    3.   *The Goals of Public Health*   852

       What Sets the Goals of Public Health, *Geoffrey Vickers*   852

    4.   *After Civilization What?*

       Kenneth E. Boulding   866

       INDEX   875

PART **ONE**

Changing Social Conditions and Health Needs

1. A Look at the Past   3
2. Urbanization and Population Change   23
3. The Rural Pattern: *Healthways on the Farms*   45
4. The Metropolitan Pattern: *Healthways in
   Conurbia*   62
5. The International Community   100

1. A Look at the Past

"THERE can be no real comprehension of the history of Public Health at any period without a thorough understanding of the political, economic, and social history of that period in its relation to the contemporary Public Health situation. . . . The task of the historian must be to investigate and to demonstrate how economic, social, medical, and scientific events intertwine and interact to create specific Public Health development."

> ROSEN, G.: Economic & Social Policy in Health. *J. History of Med.*, 8:430 (Oct.), 1953.

The Social History of Medicine*

HENRY E. SIGERIST, M.D.

I

I WOULD LIKE to draw your attention to a field of studies in the history of medicine that has been greatly neglected in the past. If you open . . . any textbook of medical history, and try to find what health conditions were in rural France in the 18th century, or what disease meant to the family of an artisan at the same period, you will not find any information. We know much about the history of the great medical discoveries but little on whether they were applied, or to whom they were applied. The great achievements of the French clinic in the early 19th century are described in detail, but we do not hear that in the same period health conditions were atrocious among the industrial population of France. For a long time the biobibliographic approach was most popular in medical historiography, and the narrative boiled down to the history of the great doctors and of the books they wrote. The biographic approach was so popular because it has a strong human element and lends itself to dramatization. History thus appeared as the free play of men of genius who made their discoveries,

* Reprinted by permission from the December, 1940 issue of *The Western Journal of Surgery, Obstetrics and Gynecology*, Vol. 48, pp. 715–722. This paper was presented before a meeting of the California Academy of Medicine in San Francisco, California, on March 11, 1940. The late Dr. Sigerist was Professor of the History of Medicine, The Johns Hopkins University, Baltimore, Maryland.

being possessed by a desire to find the truth. Great interest was being shown in "firsts." Who was the first man to see a condition, who was the first to perform a given operation? I have found . . . that many great discoveries were made simultaneously by various people. Potential men of genius are present at all times. Circumstances often determine whether they may come to the fore and to what subject they may apply their genius. Pasteur was a chemist and considered it his chief task to elucidate the secret of life by studying the structure of matter. External circumstances drove him into the field of pathology where he made his most important contributions.

I have shocked medical audiences more than once by saying that medicine is not so much a natural as a social science. The goal of medicine is social. It is not only the cure of disease, the restoration of an organism. The goal is to keep man adjusted to his environment as a useful member of society or to readjust him as the case may be. In order to do this, medicine constantly applies methods of science, but the ultimate goal is social. In every medical action there are always two parties involved, the physician and the patient, or in a broader sense, the medical corps and society. Medicine is nothing else than the manifold relations between these two groups. The history of medicine, therefore, cannot limit itself to the history of the science, institutions, and characters of medicine, but must include the history of the patient in society, that of the physician and the history of the relations between physician and patient. History thus becomes social history, and I hope to show you that such an approach is promising and can contribute to a better understanding of the social problems of medicine that we are facing today.

II

The position of the sick man in society has changed a great deal in the course of time. There are still a few primitive tribes among which a man suffering from a serious disease is abandoned. Society is afraid of him, as it is of the dead, and flees from him so that he is dead socially before physical death has overcome him. In tribes of higher civilization the sick man is considered the victim of evil forces. Witchcraft, the action of evil spirits, or the wrath of a deity may be responsible for his illness. In the Semitic civilizations we find a different view. The patient is a victim, to be sure, but he suffers in atonement for sin. All suffering is inflicted as punishment for a sin committed by the man himself, or by his parents, or by his clan. The sick man is branded with the odium of sinfulness; this ancient view survived the centuries and millennia. In the Middle Ages epidemics and other natural catastrophes were frequently considered punishments inflicted by God. The days are not far remote when people believed that mental diseases were the result of a disordinate life, or that vene-real diseases were the logical punishment for sexual promiscuity.

The position of the sick man was different again in Greek an-tiquity. The Greek world was a world of the healthy and sound. The ideal man was the harmonious being, perfectly balanced mentally and bodily. Health was considered one of the highest goods, and disease a great curse because it removed man from the condition of perfection. To attend a hopeless case was regarded unethical since the end in view, the complete restoration of the patient, was unattainable. Weaklings and crippled children were destroyed. The sick man was an inferior being, and this too made his position particularly hard to bear.

Christianity gave the sick man a position in society that he had never had before, a preferential position. The new religion addressed itself to the poor, the oppressed, the sinners, and the sick. It addressed itself to suffering humanity and promised healing and redemption. All other ancient cults were for the clean and pure, excluding those who had become impure. Christianity relieved the sick man from the bur-den he had carried before. He was no longer considered an inferior being or one who was punished for sin. In suffering, man was carrying the cross of Christ, and would be rewarded in the hereafter. It was made the duty of man to attend a sick fellowman. By joining the Chris-tian community an individual became a member of the family and, just as the family was responsible for the sick children, so was the Chris-tian family for the sick brothers. When Christianity became the official religion of the Roman empire, society as such became responsible for the care of the sick.

Since the beginning of our era, the sick man has retained his pref-erential position in society. To attend him in his distress was a char-itable duty during the Middle Ages. It is more today. We know that if large sections of the population are sick this represents a menace to the whole of society. It is a matter of medical common sense to provide care for the indigent sick and to prevent serious illness and epidemics. More and more we have accepted the view that man has a right to health or, more correctly, a right to have all means that medical sci-ence can provide made available to him for the protection or restora-tion of his health. This right was justified by a German physician, S. Neumann, in 1847, who declared that the State was pledged to protect the people's property and that the only property of a poor man was his labor power which is entirely dependent upon his health. We need not look for such a justification in a state the constitution of which guar-antees life, liberty, and the pursuit of happiness. If the State is to protect these rights as inalienable, and if it is bound to promote the general welfare of the people, it seems obvious that health must be a primary concern of government.

III

The physician of primitive society was a physician, priest, and sorcerer all in one. He knew how to placate the deities, how to ward off witchcraft, and was experienced in the application of herbs. Shamanism was hereditary in certain tribes, while in others young people who had had an unusual infancy seemed to be predestined for their mission. It was the shaman's or medicine-man's function to consult the oracles to learn the nature of a man's disease and to be able to cure it.

With developing civilization, the threefold functions of the primitive medicine-man were split up. At all times there were patients who sought healing not from medicine but from religion. Every civilization developed definite forms of religious medicine, healing cults. It was in ancient Greece the cult of Asklepios, in whose temples miracle cures were performed. In the Roman period his cult was so popular that other gods entered into competition with him, and patients flocked to temples for healing all over the ancient world. In the early Christian church patients were treated with prayers. In the Middle Ages mental patients were believed to be possessed by evil spirits, and incantations and exorcism seemed the logical treatment. To our days the Catholic church and Protestant sects have practiced faith healing, so that religious medicine actually survived through the ages.

The belief in magic and witchcraft has also had a long history. What was considered a legitimate science once, was called a superstition later, but consciously or not people still wear amulets, still perform definite gestures to counteract the influence of evil signs. It is not so long since women were persecuted as witches.

The rational, empiric component of primitive medicine developed with growing civilization into a system of medicine which excluded the transcendental, and was based on observation and reason. The Hippocratic physician was no longer a priest, and anything but a sorcerer. He was a craftsman and was trained as such. He entered the services of a master as an apprentice, accompanied him to the bedside of patients, helped him in compounding drugs and performing operations, and while doing this he learned to observe the symptoms of disease, learned how to evaluate them in order to know what fate had in store for the patient, and learned treatments and cures. When he had become a master himself he practiced independently, and did it usually as an itinerant physician. Only larger cities had permanent doctors; when a town wished to secure for itself the services of a doctor, it offered him a salary raised through taxation in order to induce him to settle down. He was allowed to charge fees for his treatments, but was guaranteed a minimum income. All smaller places, however, were served by doctors who came one morning knocking at the doors offering their services, just as other craftsmen did. If there were enough sick people in the place, the doctor rented a shop, the *iatreion;* when patients were brought to him, he examined and treated them, moving on to the next town when work gave out. If two physicians entered the same city at the same time, a wild competition resulted. In a society that did not license physicians, society had no guarantee as to the knowledge of a medical man. Anybody could call himself a doctor and treat patients for fees. A physician was legitimatized by his reputation. This is why so much emphasis was laid upon *doxa,* reputation, in ancient medical ethics. Reputation was the goal of the Hippocratic oath—"and if I hold this oath and break it not, may I gain reputation among all men." Like other craftsmen, the Greek physician sold his services for money. He sold them to whomever could purchase them, and those who had no money had no medical care, a condition that was generally accepted.

Things changed with the advent of Christianity. The view became general that everybody should be attended, whether rich or poor, and should have all the care that medical science was able to give. In the early Middle Ages most physicians were clerics. They were supported by the church and could practice medicine as a charitable service. Even in the later Middle Ages, after many laymen had entered the profession, conditions remained much the same. Many doctors still had stipends from the church making them economically independent; others had salaried positions in the service of cities as municipal doctors, and still others were attached as physicians to the court of a nobleman, lay or ecclesiastic. Those who had a private practice had to follow rigid standards established by the medical faculties, which acted as the physicians' guild. There was . . . little competition. The mediaeval world was a static world in which everyone was born to a definite status and where all aspects of life were regulated by authoritative bodies.

Conditions changed again in the 16th century when a new economic order began to develop which called for free competition, free initiative, and appealed to the individual in man. A new political philosophy of liberalism was born. The traditional authorities were fought. The church, the most powerful authority of the Middle Ages, was reformed. The power of the guilds which regulated industrial life was broken. The authorities in the field of science and medicine, Aristotle, Galen, Avicenna, were opposed. The medical faculties fought a desperate battle to preserve their traditional power, . . . but in vain. Since they were not open to the new science, academies were founded and became centers of research; the medical faculties' power to regulate the practice of medicine was gradually taken over by State bodies.

This new order affected the medical profession deeply. It found itself in a competitive world in which professions were no longer divine missions, but means of making a living. Again the doctors had to sell their services to whomever could purchase them, as the Greek crafts-men-physicians had done, but at the same time the Christian view that everybody, whether rich or poor, was entitled to medical care was re-tained and even extended. Hence, a contradiction arose under which we still suffer. The medical profession for a long time refused to be dragged into the new economic order. Physicians were still eager to get salaried positions. Not only noblemen had their body physicians but middle class families as well. They paid their family doctor an annual amount which they could afford and considered fair, and if a doctor served a sufficient number of families, he was economically in-dependent and could devote much of his time to serving the poor. The doctors fought heroically against the commercialization of medicine, but in a world that was ruled by iron economic necessities, they had to sell their services in competition with each other in order to support their families. It is not by accident that the profession organized medi-cal societies and established codes of ethics and etiquette during the 19th century. It was a last desperate attempt to protect medical prac-tice from some of the worst aspects of competitive business.

IV

Let us now examine the history of the relation between physician and patient. Medicine originally was a private relationship between two persons that did not concern anyone else. Even a super-ficial glance at history reveals a strong tendency for medicine to be-come a social institution. Physician and patient are both individuals, and it is under an individual agreement that they come together. But both are members of social groups, and society at an early period of history already showed interest in the physician's actions. The pro-fession gives the doctor a great deal of power. Physical, chemical, and biologic forces are placed freely into the physician's hands. He enters all homes, and learns secrets that people would not divulge to anybody else. He is entitled to charge fees for a service, the value of which the patient cannot estimate. Ignorance, greed, all forms of misuse of the physician's power represent a serious menace to society which, there-fore, tried to protect itself by establishing standards and regulations for the physician's behavior.

As early as 2000 B.C. we find in the Code of Hammurabi a fee schedule which bases the fees on success of the treatment and social status of the patient. The Code of Hammurabi, in addition, makes the surgeon liable for his actions and punishes him severely in case of un-successful treatment. The ancient Persians submitted their surgeons to strict tests. Before being allowed to practice surgery on Persians, the candidate had to have to his credit three successful operations performed on infidels. The Greeks had no State regulations concerning the practice of medicine, but the Hippocratic oath gives evidence to the fact that there were recognized standards.

In Rome, a beginning was made in licensing doctors. Julius Caesar, in order to attract Greek physicians for the armies, gave all those who were free-born Greeks, Roman citizenship, and from then on physicians obtained ever increasing privileges. Augustus knighted his body physician. Doctors were tax exempt, free from the duty of serving in the army, of accepting lodgers, and of accepting onerous public offices. Since there was no State control of medicine, people would claim to be physicians in order to enjoy the privileges. Under Antoninus Pius, the number of privileged doctors was limited to five, seven, or ten according to the size of a community; in order to be granted the privileges, a doctor had to show his credentials.

An important step to protect society against the ignorance of doctors was taken in the 13th century in southern Italy, in the empire of Frederick II. He set definite standards for medical education, requiring three years of philosophy, five years of medicine, one practical year, whereupon the candidate was examined by the masters of Salerno in the presence of a State commissioner. No doctor was allowed to practice without a license. Pharmacies were under strict State control. Frederick II and the School of Salerno set an example that was later followed by other European countries.

The State not only protects society by requiring a definite amount of knowledge from its physicians, but also through a number of regulations that are found in the penal codes of most countries. The patient's secrets are protected by law, and the physician is made liable for his actions. He can be prosecuted if he harms his patients, which is why physicians have to carry malpractice insurance.

Society not only set standards for the physician's behavior, but took over medical functions. Many medical tasks were found to be of such magnitude that they could not be carried out by individual physicians, but required the State power. Early in antiquity, the sanitation of dwelling places and the protection of groups against epidemic diseases became administrative functions of the State. Throughout the Middle Ages Public Health was an important function of municipal administrations, and with the progress of medicine the field of Public Health broadened considerably. Whenever private medicine was unable to solve a problem, public services had to step in. This was the case in the care of tuberculous and mental patients, of indigents in public hospitals; in recent years, the fight against infant and maternal mortality and venereal diseases has become to a large extent a public function. In every country a great volume of medical work is carried out by State agencies.

The scope of medicine broadened from century to century. The physician today is the psychologic adviser of the educator, and mental hygiene is beginning to play an increasingly important part. The physician is also scientific and psychologic adviser to the court, without whose cooperation the administration of justice would not be possible. He has to determine the cause of death. He has to advise the judge as to the responsibility of a criminal, and psychiatrists are consulted more and more frequently in determining a sentence that will not merely punish but rehabilitate a criminal.

Economic developments greatly influenced medicine. The rise of industry from the end of the 18th century on created a whole set of new medical problems. The workers had to be protected against new health hazards. All civilized countries enacted workmen's compensation laws which guarantee treatment and compensation to the victim of industrial accidents and diseases, and thus force the employer to take measures in order to reduce health hazards. While industry developed, medicine progressed. Many human lives can be saved today that were irrevocably lost only 50 years ago. The progress of medicine, however, increased its cost to such an extent that large sections of the population are unable to purchase the medical services they need. A paradoxic situation has developed. We have the means of wiping out a great many diseases—which are still among us because we are not able to apply our scientific knowledge to all the people who need treatment.

While medicine progressed as a result of the great scientific development of the 19th century, the structure of society underwent basic changes following the Industrial Revolution. A hundred years ago in this country—and this applies to all industrial countries—one out of five gainfully employed persons was a wage earner, while today four out of five are wage earners or salaried employees. Where the majority of people depend for an income on the labor market and can be thrown out of a job by its every fluctuation, there is by necessity a strong feeling of insecurity and, as a result, a strong demand for schemes that will guarantee the people a certain amount of social security.

The situation became acute long ago, and in the 19th century already ways and means were sought to bring medical care to people of low income on another than a charity basis. In Russia, as early as 1864, a complete system of State medical services financed through taxation was established in the rural districts. In Germany, compulsory health insurance was introduced in 1883, and was adopted by one European country after another, and in recent years by four American republics.

Society also became increasingly aware of the economic burden of illness. Health conditions have improved tremendously but we have the knowledge enabling us to improve them still more. We still have in every country countless cases of unnecessary illness and many premature deaths. Social planning is necessary in the medical field just as much as in other human activities.

The problem is world-wide. Even this sketchy analysis will have convinced you that conditions have changed. The society in which we live is different from that of our ancestors. The physician is no longer a medicine-man, nor a craftsman, nor a priest. He has new tasks, new functions, and new weapons. A new medical science serving a new type of society necessarily requires new forms of medical service, and the sociologic approach to the history of medicine not only gives us a better understanding of the past, but can also help us in planning for the future.

The City in National Health*

SURGEON GENERAL LUTHER L. TERRY

ONCE MORE the city is in a period of change that inspires mixed emotions. Those who love her despair as they perceive new gaps in the beloved facade, a raffishness in her grooming, her growing relief rolls, another respectable old neighborhood turned honky-tonk, a sudden show of violence. Those who despise her feel vindicated as they move their homes farther from these unpleasant surroundings in which, nevertheless, they work, study, or trade.

Throughout history it has been the fate of cities to attract and repel, at times to suffer rapid change, altering their form, their contents, their functions. Now the rate of change is accelerated. For the first time since the Dark Ages the city is not growing but disintegrating into metropolitan complexes, conurbations, statistical areas, or whatever one chooses to call them.

The word "metropolis" has acquired a new meaning. The Greeks first used it to designate the mother city of a colony. Later it meant the capital city of a state or chief city of a region. Still it meant one unit of government. Today it may mean a hundred jurisdictions with no firmer governmental ties to their central city than they have with London or Tokyo.

In this time, there is the unimaginable threat of nuclear war aimed at the destruction of cities. In such a period, it is natural that the nation's city health officers once more should band together.

* Reprinted, in part, by permission from the March 1962 issue of *Public Health Reports*, Vol. 77, pp. 377–382. The address on which this paper was based was delivered at the Annual Meeting of the U.S. Conference of City Health Officers, Detroit, Michigan, November 16, 1962. The author is Surgeon General of the Public Health Service, U.S. Department of Health, Education, and Welfare, Washington, D.C.

CITIES AS INNOVATORS

The Public Health movement in the United States began in the cities. Our first National Quarantine and Sanitary Conventions were organized by city boards of health. They were held in successive years, 1857 to 1860, in Philadelphia, Baltimore, New York, and Boston. The outbreak of the Civil War thwarted Cincinnati's hope of being the hostess city in 1861. Health authorities, representatives of the city council, private physicians, and interested citizens from other walks of life made up the delegations. Although north Atlantic cities were more numerous at these conventions, cities of the south and the west sent delegations to each assembly. The concern of the cities for human health transcended, in these assemblies, the desperate issues of slavery and States' rights. The health officer of Savannah was elected chairman of the last meeting in Boston, and was given an ovation at its conclusion.

These were the first U.S. intercommunity assemblies of men active and interested in Public Health. There was to be none like them until 1872 when another city health officer, Dr. Stephen Smith of New York City, organized the American Public Health Association.

What motivated 19th century city health officers to organize the Sanitary Convention as a voluntary association? More than the obvious threat of recurrent imported epidemics was involved. City health officials were as much or more concerned about persistent local conditions: the high infant mortality rates, filth and squalor of the slums, the lack of public water supplies and sanitary facilities, the toll of endemic diseases, and the blight of crime and alcoholism.

There was, however, a bright face to this battered coin of urban life. Our cities then, as now, were centers of wealth, education, and the arts and sciences. Early, they were centers of voluntary association for reform and of action to correct or alleviate social ills that accompany city growth.

The tensions created in the cities by stimuli and capacity to respond are characteristic of a viable community. These tensions repeatedly have generated magnificent responses to human need in our cities. Often, indeed, the effort has been overwhelmed by economic and political forces beyond the control of responding groups. Yet the struggle has never been completely abandoned. Our cities have never endorsed the cynic's philosophy, "the more things change, the more they are the same." In urban life, some things get worse, but the struggle toward something better continues. Some things get better, and we never return to exactly the same lower level of achievement.

Our national health effort owes many innovations to the city, each a product of urban response to social and scientific challenge. City health administration antedates other governmental organization in this field. Baltimore, for example, possesses the longest documentary record of a permanent health organization in our country. At least as early as 1816, mortality and morbidity data were collected and reported systematically. Before 1830, the city employed medical personnel and conducted citywide vaccination campaigns.

Philadelphia built our first public general hospital. Charleston organized the first voluntary association of laywomen to visit and nurse the poor. In 1866, New York City abandoned older forms of organization and created the first metropolitan health administration, setting a mark for municipal organization: indeed, a mark for Public Health administration at all levels.

Boston gave us our first children's hospital and trained our first Nightingale nurses. Before the turn of the century New York made a world innovation by the organization of the first public bacteriologic laboratory, serving private physicians and hospitals with diagnostic tests and biologic products free of charge. Other examples could be cited, but these few will demonstrate the role of the city as innovator in health and medical affairs.

Today, the obvious threats to health in our cities differ by more than a century of scientific and social change. For bacterial invasions from overseas, we substitute chemical invasions in air pollution from local sources. For high mortality due to infectious diseases, we observe high death and disability rates due to chronic disease and mental illness. Yet the basic problems and strengths of city life remain unchanged. These, I believe, stimulate the organization of the United States Conference of City Health Officers.

City health officers have responsibilities for the health of urban populations in urban environments, both changing rapidly. Municipalities are under pressure from surrounding jurisdictions: demands for services, resistance to the city's just claims, disregard of physical and social deterioration within municipal boundaries, competition for wealth-producing industries, commerce, and trade.

Yet much of the nation's wealth and its scientific, educational, and professional resources for meeting health and medical needs are concentrated in the cities. And cities, because they are cities, have more experience in the organization and delivery of community services than do the surrounding jurisdictions.

Government and Health before the New Deal*

WILLIAM G. CARLETON

AT NO TIME in American history has any unit of government—local, State or federal—taken general responsibility for aiding nonindigent individuals in time of sickness. Until after the Civil War, even the State and local governments did relatively little in the way of sanitation and public health.

During the colonial period only alarming epidemics like smallpox and yellow fever aroused communities to take civic action. At such times a local committee would be organized to evacuate the unaffected population to the countryside or to other communities, and the members of the committee, along with others who had previously had the disease, stayed behind and waged the fight against the plague. Fires would be kept burning in the streets, and often gunpowder was exploded. Homes were "fumigated" by the burning of tar or sulfur, and often household articles and clothing were burned to prevent contamination. Frequently, neighboring communities would organize "shotgun patrols" to prevent refugees from the epidemic areas from coming near their own communities.

The earliest continuous intervention by government in the interest of Public Health was legislation by some of the colonial governments to prevent the spread of disease from "sickly vessels" arriving in port towns. Masters of ships were subjected to heavy fines for bringing such vessels into port and for failing to report sickness aboard. Coastal towns appointed quarantine officers to enforce these laws, to inspect ships and to quarantine infested ships in the roadsteads. Later, some of the colonial port towns built marine pest houses on sandy wastes of isolated islands to care for passengers and crews taken from contaminated ships. Still later, pest houses were built for local residents suffering from epidemic diseases. Sometimes the local quarantine officer became the local health officer charged with marine inspection, the marine pest house, the local pest house, and with isolating families and fumigating homes where there had been smallpox. The remuneration of the quarantine or health officer and the costs of maintaining the pest houses were borne by subsidies from the colonial governments, local private subscriptions, and local lotteries.

In colonial times there were few hospitals. For the most part these were confined to the larger port cities and ministered only to the homeless, to seamen, refugees, runaway slaves, and the destitute. Hospitals

---

* Reprinted by permission from the August 1963 issue of *Current History*, Vol. 45, pp. 71–76. The author is Professor Emeritus of History and Political Science, University of Florida, Gainesville, Florida.

were financed by private subscription, local lotteries and in a few cases, by subsidies from colonial governments. Sometimes local doctors or a religious parish would for a time maintain a local hospital for the chronically ill or the destitute. The oldest general hospital in the United States was established in Philadelphia in 1751 when the Pennsylvania Assembly agreed to "match" funds of Philadelphia citizens raised by private subscription.

Colonial governments took no responsibility for the training of physicians or even for their licensing. It is estimated that at the end of the Revolutionary War there were about 3,500 medical doctors in the United States, but less than 400 of these had received a medical degree. Most of those with a medical degree had been trained in Europe. These became preceptors for medical students. A person who wanted to become a doctor became an apprentice to an established doctor who directed the apprentice's reading and used him as a helper in his practice. Medical education was thus "in training" education. Most people never saw a doctor, and even those who did commonly relied on midwives, home remedies, family or neighbor aid, folklore, and quacks.

1789–1865

With the establishment of the federal government in 1789, matters of medical education, licensing of physicians, the building and maintenance of hospitals, care of the indigent sick, and public sanitation and Public Health were left almost entirely to State and local governments. Until after the Civil War the States and localities actually did relatively little about such matters. Reliance was placed on private enterprise, public-spirited doctors and citizens, and religious and other voluntary organizations.

During the first part of the nineteenth century the most common diseases and the great killers were not degenerative disorders but communicable diseases. The discoveries of bacteriology and epidemiology were still in the future. Only smallpox was beginning to yield to immunization. Tuberculosis, pneumonia, dysentery, diarrhea, typhoid, malaria, diphtheria, scarlet fever, venereal disease, and puerperal (childbirth) fever were common. Until about 1875, there were still some serious epidemics of smallpox, and the most devastating waves of yellow fever and Asiatic cholera occurred during the early and middle nineteenth century.

In rapidly expanding frontier America there were vast areas of freshly cleared and undrained land. Every hamlet had its stagnant millpond. In towns there were cesspools and open privies. In rural areas people often had no privies at all and used the open fields and streams. Houses were not screened from flies, mosquitoes, or fleas.

Bedbugs and body lice were common. There were few community water systems and even fewer public sanitary sewage systems. The diet in large areas of the country was predominantly salt pork and corn meal; in this pre-refrigeration age, much food was contaminated and adulterated; and people swilled vast quantities of alcohol and patent medicines. In the new mill towns, people worked long hours for low wages and lived under crowded and filthy conditions.

In the 1840's and the 1850's, immigrants poured in from Europe, and slums in the seaport cities grew. The increased mobility provided by roads, by canals, and by railroads spread communicable diseases from community to community. The increase in world trade and the larger number of ships in American ports coming from Latin America and Asia brought epidemics of yellow fever and Asiatic cholera.

Medical science was slowly making progress, but doctors still practiced blistering and bleeding and depended heavily on mercury, arsenic, opium, and other poisons and on violent purges and cathartics. Most Americans, living on isolated farmsteads and plantations, relied on home guidance medical books, midwives, roots and herbs learned from tradition and from the Indians, patent medicines, and the "wonder remedies" hawked at carnivals and fairs by colorful spielers.

The training and licensing of physicians were left largely to the local medical societies. Increasingly, during the early and middle nineteenth century, local medical societies established proprietary schools. These were in no way connected with a university or college. Little preparatory education was required; courses were inadequate; and certification from one of these schools entitled the graduate to practice medicine. Reputable medical colleges connected with universities were growing, but the vast majority of American doctors came out of the proprietary schools. Thus the State governments assumed little responsibility for training doctors, refused to regulate medical education, and allowed the licensing power to be exercised by the proprietary schools and the local medical societies, most of whose members feared that the raising of educational standards would jeopardize their own positions.

The first widespread government health measures were public regulations to rid communities of nuisances which produced bad odors. Behind this was the theory of miasmata as the cause of disease. This theory, which prevailed in the late eighteenth century and well into the nineteenth century, held that disease came from the air by way of bad odors from slaughter houses, tanneries, decaying vegetable and animal matter, privies, cesspools, duck ponds, pigsties, stagnant waters, marshes and so forth. Smallpox was realized to be a truly contagious disease, but there was little understanding of the other communicable diseases, how they were transmitted from person to person, how agents might be carried by body lice, fleas, flies, mosquitoes, or appear in water and food that looked and smelled clean. During the early and middle nineteenth century most communities passed ordinances requiring the removal of filthy and evil-smelling nuisances or action to make them less foul-smelling. These ordinances were usually enforced by the ordinary local police officials, although a few communities established a local health officer or local board of health, almost always with little or no trained personnel. Thus miasmata, a false concept, led to government measures which inadvertently struck at many of the breeding places of disease.

In 1817, there were 17 community water supply systems in the United States, and 16 of these were owned and maintained by private companies. By 1860, 148 communities had public water supply systems and around 40 per cent of these were owned by city or other local governments. Community sanitary sewage systems came somewhat later than community water supplies, but beginning around 1850 there was a noticeable increase in such systems. For the most part, the early sewage systems and disposal plants, like the community water supply systems, were owned and operated by private companies. Gradually these, like the water systems, were taken over by local governments.

A remarkable development of the 1840's was the assumption by many State governments of the care of the insane and mentally ill. Up to that time, these unfortunates were left with their families or poorly treated or mistreated in jails, prisons, and almshouses. By around 1850, 20 States had built and undertaken to maintain "asylums" for the insane. The crusade of Dorothea Dix was largely responsible for this momentous expansion of government responsibilities for the handicapped.

SANITARY CODES

During the 1850's ideas of environmental sanitation gained headway. Many more communities adopted sanitary codes, and such codes were greatly expanded in their coverage. At the same time, a strong movement was afoot to establish a national maritime and quarantine code. There were numerous State and national conferences on sanitation and quarantine. The outstanding leader in the field was Lemuel Shattuck of Massachusetts, who in turn was greatly influenced by the pioneers of Public Health in Europe. Most Public Health agitation was cut short by the Civil War, but it bore fruit afterward, and the great concentration of masses of men in the armies during the war itself added greatly to the American knowledge of sanitation, "crowd diseases," and nutritional ailments, and emphasized the need for State and local sanitary codes in civilian life.

In the first century of its existence the federal government exercised almost no function with respect to individual or Public Health. In 1796, an attempt was made to have Congress pass a law under which the federal government would make uniform national regulations covering maritime quarantine and enforce them. But States' rights forces were too strong; the bill was defeated and maritime quarantine was left primarily to the States. However, a law was passed authorizing federal revenue officers to cooperate with each State in the execution of its maritime regulations.

Another conspicuous rejection of federal activity came in President Pierce's administration when Congress, in response to Dorothea Dix's lobbying, surprisingly passed a bill to set aside federal land for grants-in-aid to the States to build and support insane asylums. Pierce vetoed the bill on the grounds that it would weaken State and local responsibilities.

However, the federal government assumed a few functions with respect to health. In 1798, Congress established the United States Marine Hospital Service for sick and disabled seamen; twenty cents a month was deducted from the wages of each seaman. This was the first example in American history of "social security." Each port of the United States had a federal director of marine hospitals, and the port's federal director of customs, under the United States Treasury, collected and administered hospital funds and supervised the director. The hospital service was usually contracted to private enterprises and was generally inefficient. Since the collectors of customs and the directors of hospitals were usually products of the political spoils system, there were all sorts of complaints of political favoritism and misuse of funds.

The federal government made a significant contribution to the understanding of general health in the nation when its 1850 Census for the first time included a breakdown of the causes of death. Subsequently each national census became more complete and accurate. Such information was indispensable to health officers and students of Public Health, and the national census stimulated cities and counties to set up registrations of births and deaths.

Early in the course of the Civil War, President Lincoln authorized the organization of the United States Sanitary Commission with limited powers to supervise the health of the Union Army. State and local chapters were set up and their volunteer members constituted a vast male and female organization to aid the army's regular medical corps. One division of the Commission gathered hospital equipment, bed-clothing, underwear, and food delicacies, even fruits and vegetables, for the soldiers. Another formed a nursing staff and worked close behind the battle lines and in the military hospitals. A third, a smaller group, composed of some of the nation's leading doctors, inspected sanitary conditions in army camps and distributed health pamphlets to soldiers.

CIVIL WAR TO NEW DEAL

Government functions in Public Health grew steadily during the 1870's, 1880's, 1890's, and during the early decades of the twentieth century. During this time, state, county and city health boards proliferated. Local sanitary codes covered street cleaning, garbage collection, sewage, housing, screening, industrial hygiene, cleanliness in food and drink, filtering and chemical purifying of water supplies, certifying and pasteurizing milk. Vital statistics were better kept. At first state and local health boards were staffed with "political doctors" and inefficient personnel, but through the years administrative and technical competence increased. Local governments assumed more responsibility for the care and hospitalization of the indigent. State governments built and maintained special schools for deaf mutes and for the blind.

The period from around 1875 to around 1920 has been called "the Age of Bacteriology." Revolutionary advances were made in discovering the specific causative agents of communicable diseases and in developing vaccines and antitoxins to immunize against them. Local health boards established laboratories to run down the sources of infection and contagion in their communities and to give vaccinations and immunizations, blood tests, and venereal disease tests. By the second and third decades of the twentieth century many communities were providing free clinics for administering vaccinations, blood tests, and venereal disease treatments. Many States and even some localities established hospitals for inexpensive or free treatment of tuberculosis.

During the early decades of the twentieth century, Public Health nursing developed. School children were required to be vaccinated against smallpox; later they were given free eye, ear, and dental examinations; and, later still, free general physical examinations. Finally, concern about malnutrition in school children led some communities to provide free milk and even free lunches in the schools.

After 1870, the States increasingly and progressively assumed control of the licensing of physicians, raised the standards for practice, and spent larger sums of money on State medical schools.

As late as 1870 the federal government's activities in health were largely limited to restricted cooperation with State officials in administering quarantine regulations at the ports; medical, nursing, and hospital treatment of sick and disabled seamen; medical care of those in the armed services and the federal prisons; and some responsibility for the health of the Indians on the reservations.

FEDERAL EXPANSION

After 1870, federal functions expanded, at first slowly, then more rapidly. In 1870, the Marine Hospital Service was drastically reorganized and its director, Dr. J. M. Woodworth, in effect became the first Surgeon General of the United States. In 1878, a devastating yellow fever epidemic swept up the Mississippi Valley from New Orleans and brought effective pressures for the establishment of a National Board of Health. This functioned from 1879 to 1883 to formulate regulations to prevent the spread of communicable diseases from State to State and to furnish federal inspectors at leading ports to check on State inspection. The Board was allowed to lapse in 1883 for a number of reasons: its inherent administrative defects (the major part of the Board consisted of seven leading physicians living in various parts of the United States and the Board was without centralized or trained staff); the antagonism of State boards of health, particularly that of Louisiana, to the National Board; and the mutual jealousies of the Marine Hospital Service and the medical departments of the Army and the Navy and the National Board. However, in 1893, the federal government finally asserted its authority over port quarantine, and the Marine Hospital Service was enjoined to maintain federal control quarantine stations at American ports.

In 1901, the federal Hygiene Laboratory was established in Washington, to conduct epidemiologic investigations and research, and in 1902 it was given the power to standardize and regulate the interstate sale of viruses, serums, toxins and other biologic products. In 1906, the Meat Inspection Act provided for federal inspection of all meat destined for interstate commerce, and that same year a Pure Food and Drug Act was passed which placed some restrictions on producers of prepared foods and patent medicines. The administration of these laws was placed in the Department of Agriculture, illustrating the tendency of the federal government at that time to scatter the administration of its Public Health measures. Under President Taft, the Bureau of Mines was set up, which among other things was to conduct industrial hygiene studies.

THE U.S. PUBLIC HEALTH SERVICE

The United States Public Health Service was established in 1912. This took over the functions of the Marine Hospital Service and most of the government's investigations and research into health matters. It was also given control over interstate sanitation and the spread of communicable diseases from State to State. Under the United States Health Service, the National Leprosarium was established in 1917 and the Division of Venereal Diseases in 1918.

In 1912, the federal Children's Bureau was set up in the Department of Labor to act as a clearing house of information about state laws on maternal and child care and on child labor. In 1921, the federal government began a program of grants-in-aid to the States for maternal and child care, and the Children's Bureau was given the administration of this program. Again this illustrated the scattered administration of the federal government's growing activities in health and welfare matters. It was not until the passage of the federal Social Security Act in 1935 that a real beginning was made in coordinating a comprehensive federal health and welfare program. This trend was accelerated in 1939 with the establishment of the Federal Security Agency.

Historically, aside from the federal government's responsibility for the medical treatment and hospitalization of disabled seamen, the entering wedge for direct individual medical help to civilians by the federal government came by way of aid to veterans of the armed services. In 1833, the federal government established a pension system for relief of veterans mentally or physically disabled while in the service. In 1865, the National Home for Disabled Volunteer Soldiers (and sailors) was set up. (By 1930, the National Home had 11 branches— "the old soldiers' homes.") In 1890, federal pensions were extended to all mentally and physically disabled veterans without regard to whether the disability was incurred in the service. In 1904, federal pensions were extended to all veterans over the age of 62, regardless of disability.

In 1917, during World War I, the Bureau of War Risk Insurance was authorized to administer the allotment program for dependent families of members of the armed services; the death and disability compensation program; the life insurance program for service men and women; the rehabilitation and vocational training for veterans; and the medical and surgical treatment of veterans. The Federal Board of Vocational Education was organized to carry into actual execution the program for rehabilitation and vocational training. To the United States Health Service was assigned the active operation of the veterans' hospitals distributed over the country with their large staffs of doctors, nurses, and technicians.

In 1921, the Veterans Bureau was established. This absorbed those functions of the Bureau of War Risk Insurance dealing with veterans, those of the Federal Board of Vocational Education, and those of the United States Health Service with respect to running the veterans' hospitals. The Veterans Administration (1930) in turn set up coordinated veterans' affairs in still more centralized fashion when it took over the functions of the Veterans Bureau, the Bureau of Pensions, and all branches of the National Home for Disabled Volunteer Soldiers.

Since 1917, hundreds of thousands of former service men and women have been treated in veterans' hospitals. This constitutes the nearest thing to "socialized medicine" in the United States. Most patients testify to satisfactory service in these institutions. Most doctors believe treatment has been competent. There are some doctors, once connected with these hospitals and later private practitioners, who insist that the cooperative practice of staff consultation is actually preferable to "the solo practice" of individual doctor and patient. However, there is a widespread belief that the veterans' hospitals represent too limited an experience from which to deduce valid conclusions about the operation of a general system of government medicine in the United States.

2. Urbanization and Population Change

MOVEMENT to the cities by the rurally born has characterized social life for centuries and contemporary Public Health planners are much concerned with effects of population growth, urban concentration, and mobility. In the developing countries, the City is an irresistible magnet attracting populations who wish to make the transition from one socio-cultural epoch to another. Population growth in relation to industrialization and the distribution of national resources becomes one of the major issues of social policy in these countries.

In more developed countries like the United States, population growth and mobility also raise pressing questions for social decision. Great numbers of workers from different social strata are constantly on the move from farm to city, from central city to suburbia, and back, carrying with them the complex consequences of urbanization. In the wake of these migrations are major, sometimes overwhelming, problems of physical, emotional, and social health. Population increases, greater longevity and technologic advances outstrip the ability of our communities to provide humanly livable environments for all their citizens.

Some of the best social thought in many disciplines seeks answers to these problems. As the selections in this Section will show, there are few solid solutions, but there are pertinent lines of inquiry and further study from which illumination of present dilemmas of policy and planning can be expected.

The Impact of Urbanization*

JEAN GOTTMANN

URBANIZATION today is a powerful trend, deeply modifying both the environmental conditions and the inner structure of modern society. Its impact on the majority of the people in Western countries cannot

* Reprinted with omission of three figures by permission of the National Committee for Children and Youth, from Volume I, *The Nation's Children*, edited by Eli Ginzberg, and published by the Columbia University Press for the Golden Anniversary Conference on Children and Youth, 1960, pp. 180–208. The author is Research Director, Study of Megalopolis, Twentieth Century Fund, and Professor, Ecole des Hautes Etudes, University of Paris, 1959–1962.

be too carefully studied. It is a particularly strong force in the United States because of the tremendous number of people involved.

The younger generation, most of whom today are born and grow up away from the farm, feels this impact in two ways: first, the environment of their childhood and adolescence is urban; second, the system to which they will eventually have to adapt their adult life is urban. This is no longer simply a steady flow from the farms to the towns. Urbanization today is one of the more striking expressions of the sweeping and profound changes now developing in the organization of society, and American-style urban growth is being reproduced increasingly in many other lands. Its impact carries the need for re-assessing many of the values held and the measures adopted for the welfare and education of children and youth.

MOMENTUM AND NEW FORMS
OF URBANIZATION

Urban growth is no more a phenomenon affecting only a small fraction of the total population and several isolated spots over a vast country. In the United States the population in urban territory rose from 45.7 per cent of the total in 1910 to 64 per cent in 1950. The farm population meanwhile declined to 15.3 per cent in 1950 and probably to 11.7 per cent by April, 1956. Farming is now the occupation of less than one out of 10 Americans; more than 90 per cent of the nation live from and by activities of an urban type. Similar percentages are being achieved or forecast for many countries in Western Europe advanced in industrialization. The trend is worldwide and appears irreversible: the progress of agricultural technics and farm mechanization make it possible to produce more agricultural goods with fewer and fewer hands. Thus a migration from farm to city goes on and must be accelerated as large numbers come of age in farming areas.

For years the terms urban and rural have represented the major dichotomy in the division of human labor and in the classification of landscapes. On one hand the green countryside was the locale of agricultural production. On the other hand the built-up, crowded, urbanized areas were the sites of manufacturing, trade, government, worship, and recreation. The rural territory extended over almost the whole land and rural life was reputed simple, natural, and healthy. Cities occupied small parcels of land surrounded with walls or boulevards, isolated spots amid rural territory, and were usually criticized as offering an artificial, unhealthy, complicated way of life. These old contrasts still exist in under-developed parts of the world. They are a tale of bygone days in the more advanced countries and especially in the United States.

Since more than 90 per cent of the population now live by pursuits other than farming, i.e., by activities within the categories of industry, trade, services, and government, usually located in cities, urban territory cannot be expected to remain limited to a few small spots on the map. Urbanization has taken on a size and a momentum that has reversed old concepts of simple contrasts between urban and rural. Cities have broken out of old bounds and scattered buildings of urban aspect and functions all over the countryside, thus coming to occupy vast regions. The U.S. Census has had a hard time trying to keep up with these trends. As suburbs mushroomed around the old urban centers defined as *cities,* the Census established first the notion of *urbanized areas,* which consisted mainly of densely built-up territory. Then, in 1940, there was introduced the *metropolitan area,* a wider concept encompassing entire counties whose economy appears tightly dependent on a central city.[1] By 1950 the area of many of these standard metropolitan areas had to be extended and the population of the 174 areas in the continental United States totalled 85.5 million or 57 per cent of the nation. In 1950 the majority of Americans lived in metropolitan regions; this does not mean they all lived in densely built-up districts, for a metropolitan area may well include green, rural looking sections, but its inhabitants engage in little agricultural activity and are primarily dependent for their livelihood on the connection with a central city of more than 50,000 people.

From 1940 to 1950, while the total population of the United States increased by 14.5 per cent, the population of metropolitan areas grew by 22.2 per cent. Since 1950 this latter rate of growth has accelerated. The Bureau of the Census estimated the growth of the country's civilian population between 1950 and 1956 to be 9.8 per cent and that of the metropolitan areas to be 14.8 per cent; but in many cases the peripheral growth has spilled over these limits into territory classified as non-metropolitan in 1950. There is no doubt that the 1960 Census will add many new counties to the list of those classified as metropolitan and it will then be recognized that the rate of increase of metropolitan population is more than 50 per cent faster than the nation's growth. Thus we see that modern urbanization takes on original forms which scatter the urban functions and population around the countryside. While the old migration from farms toward towns goes on, the towns spread out in irregular fashion back into the formerly rural countryside.

For some time now the Census has distinguished between rural farm and rural nonfarm population. In any agricultural region some nonfarm activities are needed to service the farms. In an area of large and highly mechanized farms the nonfarm population may become more numerous than the farm population which it services; in such cases however a good part of it will be concentrated in towns of some size, and counted as urban rather than rural nonfarm. In any case it seems obvious that when the rural nonfarm element of a rural territory of a small region reaches a large majority, and in some cases it goes over 75 per cent, the region depends on means of sustenance other than local agriculture.

Maps of the United States which show the proportion of rural nonfarm population in rural territory by county demonstrate such a process of gradual de-ruralization over vast stretches. This trend will undoubtedly continue in the next decades. Farming will hardly need more lands; an increased consumption of farm products may be satisfied by reducing the surpluses and increasing, if need be, the yields over much of the major agricultural regions. The "de-ruralization" ought to gain the Northeast (where it was already advanced in 1950), in the Southeast, some parts of the West, and even of the Midwest.

Modern urbanization has invaded so widely the regions formerly held as rural but without densely building them up, that the distinction between urban and rural in the old sense calls for revision. Unofficial proposals have suggested new terms such as "outer-suburbia," "ex-urbia," "interurbia," and recently sociologists offered to call these scattered populations "rurban." All such terms include some hint at the urban nature of the new areas and as they develop beside officially urban territory we may well speak of a degree of suburbanization pending new official definitions.

Urbanization has taken on a new, nebulous kind of structure.[2] This results from the scattering of residences as well as from the centering of large shopping centers or important manufacturing plants at rural crossroads and in small towns.[3] It is also due to the development of rural regions, some of which were until recently being depopulated, for recreational activities in the mountains or at the seashore. Altogether this process of urbanization causes new forms of land use and a new system of relations within a community, between communities, and between individuals and their environment.

THE REVOLUTION IN LAND USE

It would be far too simple to sum up the major effects of modern urbanization by stressing the sprawl of suburban or metro-politan patterns over vast areas against farming's retreat to more limited, specialized regions. The two trends coexist but do not conflict on a large scale. True, in some suburban areas such as central Long Island and much of New Jersey, new developments have crowded out many farms in recent years. But on the whole and for many years the abandonment of tilled land has proceeded faster than the occupation of land for urban and interurban uses. This was still true on the whole throughout the United States even in the 1950's although land has been devoured for urban use at an estimated pace of a million acres per year. Total cropland shrank from 1950 to 1954 by 10 million acres and total pasture and grazing area by 20 million acres. Woodland and forest land not used for grazing increased in the same four years by 28 million acres. The result of the present urbanization of the American population and economy is that the land is becoming greener and the country is reverting to a more natural condition.[4]

Whoever has recently traveled through or flown over the forested East has seen patches of land reoccupied by brush and young woods all over the countryside. In New England the increase of the wooded area since the beginning of the century and even in the last 10 years has been substantial. This has happened not only in Maine and Vermont but also in the "suburbanized" states of Massachusetts, Rhode Island, and Connecticut. Similar trends can be observed over much of New York, Pennsylvania, Maryland, and Virginia. It is interesting that woods are still increasing in and around the highly metropolitanized section on the northeastern seaboard which we call *Megalopolis* (from southern New Hampshire to northern Virginia). This most impressive and continued chain of metropolitan regions contains one-fifth of the population of the United States on less than 2 per cent of its land area.

Thus, even in the vicinity of the most crowded region in America, there still are more green spaces, and curiously enough more wildlife, than some 50 to 60 years ago.

The rapid shifts in land use do not affect only the rural-looking outer suburbs; they have at least as much impact on land use in the urbanized areas. In the old urban cores, the residential population is still increasing[5] but slowly, at a lower rate than in the nation as a whole, (4.7 per cent increase in the central cities of standard metropolitan areas from 1950 to 1956, while the nation's increase was estimated at 9.8 per cent); the metropolitan areas outside the central cities increased much faster (about 29.3 per cent); and within the metropolitan areas the rural parts grew fastest (55.8 per cent, adding 6 million people in six years!).

These figures concern places of residence. Much of the population in rural areas commutes to work in urban territory; and there is substantial commuting from city to city. Thus in the early 1950's close to 1,600,000 people residing elsewhere came to Manhattan to work; close to 450,000 went to Newark, N.J., to work, a figure slightly above the resident population of Newark as recorded by the Census. In most other large cities the numbers of commuters on weekdays reach hundreds of thousands. Despite endeavors at decentralization in the most crowded urban hubs, the numbers of people commuting to work have been on the increase through the 1940's and the 1950's. The Bureau of the Census, recognizing the inadequacy of recording population figures by place of residence, introduced a new question about the place of work in the 1960 count.

Urbanization, in the modern sense, creates a growing dichotomy between daytime and night-time populations in large cities. This is reinforced by the housing picture: as the trend of moving out to the periphery accelerates, the old urban core harbors age and decay. The houses emptied by middle-income occupants who prefer to move out to the suburbs or farther are taken over by tenants in the lower-income brackets who cannot afford to commute far and who often cannot for reasons of social discrimination find lodging in the highly suburban communities. Negroes and Puerto Ricans are so crowded into the large central cities that some among them commute to jobs in the suburbs. The colored population is increasing faster than the total resident population in Manhattan and Brooklyn, Washington, D.C., Baltimore, Chicago, and Philadelphia. The same trend is notable in smaller cities, especially in the highly urbanized northeast, such as Trenton or Hartford. All these cities have active business districts; but the kinds of people who walk the central city streets in daytime are increasingly different from those who are abroad at night. As urban renewal proceeds in such cities contrasts may sharpen, for some of their central districts attract only affluent residents who can afford the higher costs. Even if they do not decay as residential areas,[6] central cities become sites of great contrasts between opposite extremes of the income scale. This is especially and spectacularly so in New York City and Washington, D.C. In Washington, the urban renewal of Georgetown sharpened the contrast. These growing differences between residents and daytime population are not conducive to social happiness and relaxation of tension.

Another set of contrasting patterns has developed between the different parts of a metropolitan region: in addition to the differences between the population by night and by day and the range of income levels, the suburbs have a different set of economic activities (besides the dormitory function) and an age and educational level substantially at variance with the central cities. The suburban population today as a whole is better educated, and has better housing and more recreational facilities within easy reach than the population in the urban core. With the exception of a few large cities, the downtown areas of old urban cores are losing a good deal of their special functions as the center of the retail and entertainment trades. The present revolution in land use results from many factors, among which perfected automobile transportation, the rising standard of living for the average family, and constantly increasing specialization of labor are probably the three main agents. This revolution in land use ought to bring much improvement to American modes of living, learning, working, and relaxing.

Whether the progress of urbanization can be made to serve such improvement is a major responsibility of our time.

CHILDREN AND YOUTH IN URBANIZED ENVIRONMENT

The 1950 Census showed the suburban population to be slightly younger than the central city population. In all urbanized areas combined, the median age was 32.7 in central cities and 30.9 in the suburbs. It was observed that "the smaller the urbanized area, the greater is the difference in median age between central city and suburbs."[7] The age pyramid reveals a larger than average number of persons less than 20 years of age in the suburbs. If similar statistics were available for the rural nonfarm population living within metropolitan areas, such differences would be even sharper. The quoted remark about the size of the "urbanized area" is significant: the larger the central city the farther away extends its maximum commuting range. Many more people working in New York or Chicago can afford a residence for their families beyond the officially defined "urbanized area" than would be possible for people who work in Cincinnati or Albuquerque.

During the 1950's the migration to a metropolitan periphery of urban families with small children was probably massive, especially from the larger cities, and the suburban areas ought to be "younger than ever" in the early 1960's. The usual reason a head of household gives for moving out is: "I am doing it for the children." It is also usual that the return from the suburbs to a central city is made by parents when the children, grown up, have left home. The same move also brings back to urban cores widows and widowers and even retired couples. From 1930 to 1950, the proportion of persons aged 65 and over in the nation went up from 5.5 per cent to 8.1 per cent; but it more than doubled in New York City. Nevertheless, the great metropolis was still below the national average, with the exception of Manhattan where it stood at 8.7 per cent. Queens with 7.1 per cent, the Bronx with 7.3 per cent, and Brooklyn with 7.4 per cent already reflected semi-suburban rates. New York City was surrounded with suburban counties where the proportion of aged people was below 8 per cent, with the exception of the counties of Westchester and Rockland, N.Y. A similar situation was observed around Philadelphia, Baltimore, and Washington, but Boston, and New England as a whole, showed rather higher proportions of aged people.

The distribution of children less than 15 years old in 1950 followed a somewhat different pattern in the highly urbanized Northeastern seaboard from that in the rest of the country. On the whole New York City had a low concentration; the proportion in the various counties of the metropolitan region varied between 17 and 24 per cent, while the national average stood at 26.9 per cent. Three states of southern New England showed slightly higher figures than did New York City but the average was still below 26 per cent in all counties but one, and the same was true of rather surburbanized New Jersey and eastern Pennsylvania. The ratio of children picked up quickly in the Pennsylvanian Appalachians to the west, and south from Maryland and Virginia. The South has always had a higher birth rate than the Northeast; urbanization is not the only major factor in the distribution of children through the United States. It remains clear in Megalopolis that suburban districts have a higher ratio of children than the central urban cores. In 1950 this was the case around Manhattan, Boston, Philadelphia, Baltimore, and Washington. By 1960 the suburbs probably had a higher ratio than the nation as a whole.

The distribution of the youth, i.e., of persons aged 15 to 24 in 1950 was not different from the general pattern of children, but one significant difference may be noted. The old urban cores often showed higher rates than the outlying suburbs. This was true of Boston, Philadelphia, Baltimore, and New York City as a whole, though not of Manhattan alone. The presence of colleges in these cities and the greater opportunity offered to young job-seekers are probably the main reasons for the attraction of youngsters, especially in the ages between 19 and 24, toward the urban hubs.

The local variations of the age pyramid confirm that children are being born and reared in the United States largely away from the main urban centers but increasingly not far away. These statistics result partly from the inheritance of a traditional geographic distribution little related to modern urbanization trends, but partly also from the choice of the parents to move toward the metropolitan periphery. As the youngsters grow closer to coming of age they are increasingly drawn toward the urban centers not only by their work but also for residence. Finally, as the old urban cores have ratios of old and young people below the national average, they have a higher than average ratio of the adult and mature population (i.e., in the ages of 25 to 64). This is true even of night-time residents; the ratio is of course much higher for the daytime population as the commuters into the urban hubs are predominantly in these age brackets. Thus, although children today spend most of their time away from the cities (in the more crowded, densely occupied and built-up sense of the term "city"), they will usually spend at least part of their lives in a highly urbanized environment.

The whole evolution of the labor force indicates the growth of typically urban employment in nonagricultural and nonindustrial types of activities, or, according to a slightly different classification, the expansion of the white-collar labor force over the blue-collar. The vast majority of today's children will spend their later lives in urban or suburban work and residence. The education of most youngsters should therefore be definitely urban-oriented; it should also be more advanced for a larger proportion of the upcoming generation, as an increasing proportion of all jobs require more training, more skill, and involve more responsibility.

The isolated farm and the tightly knit and relatively isolated community of the small town in a truly rural region produce only a small minority of the younger generation. Does the present type of urban and suburban growth benefit the younger strata of the nation? For a long time it was traditionally held that boys from the farms or agricultural areas in general were a "better quality" of men, had more basic virtues—in brief were better prepared for life than city boys. This belief was not only American. It was also generally held in Europe.

Systematic sociologic studies of the early schooling and adult behavior of farm boys and city boys have exploded the old myth of the superiority of rural origin. A scholarly analysis of the records of the U.S. Armed Forces has recently shown in convincing fashion that the recruits from farming areas were on the whole less prepared for modern life than urban recruits.[8] The advantages of an urban environment for children and youth, especially in the industrialized nations of the West, were to be expected. The better organized and more strictly controlled system of supply of the large urban consuming markets has led to better nutrition. Even today in New York City it is difficult to find children (unless recently arrived there) with serious nutritional deficiencies. Water and milk have been made safer to drink in the large cities, precisely because of the dangers of infection and contamination inherent in the crowding in urban environment. Modern police forces are made necessary by the problems of crowded metropolises; and despite the merited outcry against criminality and juvenile delinquency, it ought to be recognized that people in the great urbanized areas of today are much safer by virtue of the policing and the legislation in force than their ancestors used to be in a rural environment.

The general progress of civilization has brought about improvements in nutrition, health, and security at the same time as it brought about urbanization. There is no direct relationship between, say, urban growth on one hand and better health conditions on the other. The latter could be achieved without the former and vice versa. It has happened at times. However it has been mankind's, and particularly America's experience that in the long run the two proceeded hand in hand. Similarly such modern trends as the rise of juvenile delinquency and of nervous disorders in modern society ought not to be associated too closely, as they often are, with urban growth. The latter is, like the trends, a simultaneous product of the modern evolution of society;

it does not determine them. The evil in society is of course concentrated wherever society itself is gathered. Crowding especially in its beginnings may cause the worst trends to intensify, but it also compensates this effect by working out legal and social antidotes. If it does not the people involved are at fault rather than the impersonal process. In the early nineteenth century, the first stages of the industrial revolution caused crowding of ill-paid industrial workers in slums in many cities. But social evolution has established today in American cities conditions of living and working for youngsters much different from those denounced by Charles Dickens a century ago.

Today urban areas can confidently claim better organized health and educational services than rural areas. Charities, hospitals, welfare organizations can function better in a large community than in rural areas, and the urban communities can afford these services more easily in terms of both adequate financing and competent personnel. Urbanization, properly managed, should benefit children and adolescents as well as other sections of the population needing help and care. Modern urbanization, however, with its differentiations between place of work and place of residence on one hand, between central city, suburbs, and outer suburbia on the other, requires that more thought and study be given to the new problems and opportunities it has helped to create.

ASSETS AND LIABILITIES OF URBAN AND SUBURBAN AREAS

As the central parts of cities continue to specialize in the functions traditionally concentrated in the "downtown" areas, children residing there may lose some of the advantages previously associated with cities of large size. The financial burden on the city government may become too great for it to maintain adequate services for residents who cannot offer a strong and expanding tax base. The city, having to provide adequate facilities for the noontime tide of business activities finds increasing difficulty in also meeting the welfare, health, educational, and recreation needs of a poorer resident population.

In the suburbs, meanwhile, because of the momentum of the metropolitan sprawl, local government is faced with such a rapid rise in the needs for facilities of all kinds that resources can seldom keep pace with the demand. Many suburban towns have trouble in providing adequate sewage for their rapidly expanding population. The schools are crowded and not always staffed with as qualified teaching personnel as the pupils' parents wish for.

The case of the schools is a constant issue because of the present trends of urbanization. Urban areas normally offer better schools and have a better educated population than the rural regions.

This latter proposition is true today of the suburban towns and of the daytime population of central cities rather than for the residents of old urban cores. Maps of the percentage of the adult population on the Northeastern seaboard having completed high school or more in 1950 show in clear fashion that the larger cities in Megalopolis have a lower ratio than their immediate suburbs. Otherwise the metropolitan areas show up better than the rural countryside, and that contrast is especially sharp south of Washington, D.C.

As the many stages of production, agricultural as well as industrial, are being mechanized, employers are growing more insistent on higher educational levels for the average employee. "Completing high school or more" will soon be a prerequisite for most occupations. Cities have attracted so many people for decades because they offered greater economic opportunity; to take advantage of it, educational achievement daily becomes more essential—and an education that can seldom be replaced by early occupational experience. To provide the younger generation with adequate educational opportunity is an imperative necessity for a nation which wants to maintain national progress and the processes of democracy. The difficulties of the central cities and of the expanding suburbs in providing adequate programs for their schools now become disturbing concerns.

In a report on the high schools, Dr. James B. Conant stresses the great variety of these encountered throughout the United States. He speaks for a "comprehensive high school" whose programs would correspond to "the educational needs of *all* the youth of the community." But the survey shows that there are seldom entirely comprehensive high schools and the report prefers to speak of a "degree of comprehensiveness." In some cases high schools specialize in preparing their pupils for college and higher education. "High schools whose comprehensiveness is thus limited by the nature of the community are to be found particularly in suburban areas and in high income residential sections of large cities." There are suburban high schools which may not have the same problems in supplying an adequate degree of "comprehensiveness" as the large city high school. Selective academic high schools, designed for the academically talented youth, are found "in many of the Eastern cities of considerable size and in a few of the medium-sized cities." Such specialization of one or a few high schools among many more in that city seems to favor the comprehensiveness of the system as a whole. The small high school presents more complicated problems: "The enrollment of many American public high schools is too small to allow a diversified curriculum except at exorbitant expense. The prevalence of such high schools—those with graduating classes of less than one hundred students—constitutes one of the serious obstacles to good secondary education throughout most of the United States."[9]

These remarks indicate that the long-range educational consequences of urbanization will be favorable. The report leaves aside however the question of adequate financing in the forthcoming years, when the number of high-school students in the medium-sized cities and the suburbs will rapidly swell. The conclusions concerning the small high schools make one wonder about the results of the partitioning of the mushrooming suburbs into smaller communities. Will the less affluent suburban towns find the resources for adequately comprehensive high schools? Moreover, this suburban partitioning may affect the children's education in other ways and before the high-school age.

As one reads the many volumes recently published on suburban life, one is impressed with the frequent endeavor of the new communities to remain homogeneous, tightly organized, and somewhat isolated from the surrounding areas. Such hints can easily be gathered from works such as: A. C. Spectorsky's *The Exurbanites*, John Keats' *The Crack in the Picture Window*, William H. Whyte's *The Organization Man*, etc. Such homogeneity may help solve many local problems and avoid others characteristic of more diversified groups. It may also take away from the youngsters' education and experience many valuable assets provided by the usual urban conditions, for the sheltered environment of such suburban towns does not always prepare children for real life in the outside world. The size of the town is not significant in this respect. Such closed-in communities have existed in large cities. The multiplication of such compartments in the suburbs does not necessarily entail an isolated education as the town is within easy reach of some bustling business district and of several very different towns. The fashion for such homogeneous suburbs appears indicative however of a psychologic attitude favoring social isolation which may well be going against society's present trends.

As one wishes to see today the complexities of the urbanized areas put to better use, with an aim of familiarizing youth with the variety and complexity of the world, one also wonders whether cities and suburbs take full advantage of the educational and recreational assets offered by the expanding woods in their vicinity and by the growing interpenetration of suburban residential, manufacturing, and specialized farming areas. The variety of neighborhoods within a metropolitan region is often astonishing. The proximity to existing green belts is generally greater than expected. The access to these green belts and to this wide gamut of economic institutions is worth many theoretic lessons to children reared in built-up residential neighborhoods. Such educational assets can well be used with much profit for youngsters who would otherwise have little contact with nature and with the diverse activities of modern industry—but who ought to know about it all and would love it. These contacts can well be organized in a way that would not become a nuisance to the management of the woods, farms, or plants involved.

The impact of urbanization in its present form on American society is full of opportunities which could be beneficial in terms of the education and recreation of children and youth. It is however also full of dangerous pitfalls if some of the technical consequences of urban living are allowed to run wild. The street traffic needs and gets strict regulation, especially in neighborhoods densely populated with children. A number of other safety devices and rules have to be adopted and applied since adults cannot expect from children more knowledge and responsibility than they have had the time to acquire. The time left to teen-agers for leisure has been on the increase as the school programs have been lightened in many cases and as fewer of them work full time; this leisure time needs direction and opportunity to use it properly. Failure to provide these may cause more trouble on city streets than on scattered farms. In short, urbanization may be held as one of the factors which create need for more and more care and planning by parents. Technologic progress may simplify in some ways the adults' tasks but adds new burdens to their responsibilities.

THE NEW FRONTIER

It may well be claimed that urbanization has created for today and for some time ahead a new frontier for the American people to explore and to manage. This new frontier is not simply one of civilization advancing against the wilderness, a struggle with an environment of an unknown nature, but rather the reconstruction and continuous improvement of the areas overrun by modern urban growth. It is the urban renewal in the heart of old cities, the revitalizing of the declining suburbs in the "gray zone," the building of new suburbs, the management of the green areas left in the vicinity of the metropolises. Cities age as they grow, and the task seems one of almost constantly rejuvenating the vast urban regions in which congregate most of the population. This is a frontier left by the past, which the present must not misuse; it is an essential modern aspect of the permanent struggle of mankind for a better and brighter world to live in. A nation engaged upon it can hardly stop on the way without serious prejudice to the next generation; the frontier must be pushed ahead with the needs of the younger section of the population in mind. The sooner the youth can be associated with this great task, the better it will be, for it is a consuming endeavor but one yielding great rewards.

In this great work of expanding and rejuvenating vast urban regions, the United States is today more advanced than any of the other countries in the world. All these countries, with the exception of a few backward lands, feel the impact of on-rushing urbanization. It is a major concern in the U.S.S.R. and Canada, in Britain and Germany, the Netherlands and France, Italy and Denmark, Mexico and Brazil—

even the government of Southern Rhodesia has found it necessary to appoint a Commission on Urban Affairs. Many experts and authorities throughout the world are deeply interested in this new facet of the American experiment. They may well look at the impact urban growth will have on the children and youth of America, and especially those in the large metropolitan areas of the Northeast, as a laboratory from which to learn.

Although such attention will be, and is already focused on these areas it does not follow that local solutions or experiments will be easily copied or duplicated. Every student of urban affairs knows how different is every urban area in the practical handling of its problems, and in the possible attempts at solution. Within the United States alone these differences have already proven great. What is true of New York does not necessarily apply to Philadelphia, certainly not to Washington, and even less to Los Angeles. San Francisco and New Orleans are deeply different in almost every aspect of their urban and metropolitan problems, and so are Houston and Kansas City. Each can and must learn from the experience of the others but it must always put the knowledge thus acquired into the local or regional mold before any consequences can be deduced.

Just because urban growth multiplies along a street of houses which look alike on the outside does not mean that it standardizes the people who live in them. Urbanization in fact probably brings more variety, movement, and turmoil to society than was ever expected. These processes must be recognized, their great variety respected and turned into a better system of cooperation and comfort among people. It seems important at this stage that the youth of today be given a hopeful outlook about the city of tomorrow.

1. See definitions and statistical data in *County and City Data Book* 1956 (Washington, D.C.: U.S. Bureau of the Census, 1957).

2. See Otis Dudley Duncan and Albert J. Reiss, Jr., *Social Characteristics of Urban and Rural Communities,* 1950 (New York: Wiley, 1956), especially part II, pp. 117–79.

3. The latter pattern is spreading especially in the Southeast; see, e.g., Jean Gottmann, *Virginia at Mid-Century* (New York: Holt, 1955), ch. 7.

4. The above figures are based on the *Statistical Abstract of the United States 1958* (Washington, D.C.: U.S. Bureau of the Census, 1958), Table No. 791, p. 612. See also on what follows Jean Gottmann, "The Revolution in Land Use," in *Landscape*, Santa Fe, New Mexico, Vol. 8, No. 2 (Winter, 1959), pp. 15–21.

5. No more in New York City where a 1957 census showed a decrease since 1950.

6. Raymond Vernon, *The Changing Economic Function of the Central City* (New York: Committee for Economic Development, 1959).

7. Duncan and Reiss, *Social Characteristics of Urban and Rural Communities,* p. 120.

8. Eli Ginzberg et al., *The Ineffective Soldier* (New York: Columbia University Press, 1959), 3 vols. See also to the same effect the results of an analysis of civilian statistics in Eleanor H. Bernert, *America's Children* (New York: Wiley, 1958).

9. James B. Conant, *The American High School Today: A First Report to Interested Citizens* (New York: McGraw-Hill, 1959), Section IV, pp. 77–95.

Family Planning in the U.S.*

RONALD F. FREEDMAN, PH.D., PASCAL K. WHELPTON, B.S.,

AND ARTHUR A. CAMPBELL, B.A.

BIRTH, MIGRATION AND DEATH are the key factors in the growth of a nation's population. Until about a century ago the birth rate in most countries was fairly stable at a high level; death and international migration were the changing variables, oscillating with economic conditions and the fortunes of peace and war. Today in Western nations the situation is reversed. For example, international migration now plays a minor role in U.S. population trends, and the death rate is stabilized at a low level. Successful technics of contraception, on the other hand, have made the birth rate the dynamic force in population growth. Moreover, the recent swings in the U.S. birth rate show that it is now acutely sensitive to economic and social conditions.

This vital revolution has had great impact on many aspects of the life of our society. Yet we have had little reliable information on a national scale about the extent and success of family planning. Some important facts on the whole population and on major subgroups of it are now available as a result of a national survey conducted in 1955 by the Scripps Foundation for Research in Population Problems (at Miami University in Ohio) and the Survey Research Center of the University of Michigan. Some major results of this first comprehensive study, presented in our book *Family Planning, Sterility and Population Growth* (published by the McGraw-Hill Book Company) will be reviewed in this article.

In the perspective of history it is only recently that family planning has become so widespread that it could have a major influence on population trends. In the past the number of births for the average family varied little; it tended to approach the number that the average woman was biologically capable of having. Crude methods of contraception, supplemented in some societies by infanticide and abortion, were never sufficiently widespread, effective, and flexible to cause rapid changes in the average of family size. Change in the rate of

---

* Reprinted, with omission of seven graphs, from the April 1959 issue of *Scientific American*, Vol. 200, pp. 50–55, with permission. Copyright © 1959 by Scientific American, Inc. All Rights reserved. The authors are, respectively, Professor of Sociology and Director of the Population Studies Center, University of Michigan, Ann Arbor, Michigan, and Non-resident Co-Director of the Taiwan Population Studies Center; Director, Scripps Foundation for Research in Population Problems, Research Professor, Miami University, Oxford, Ohio; and Demographer, Scripps Foundation for Research in Population Problems, Miami University, Oxford, Ohio, and Research Associate Professor, Miami University, Oxford, Ohio.

population growth thus had to be caused by other influences. Epidemic disease, famine, and war would increase the death rate; population growth would be slowed, and at times reversed. In times of peace and well-being the death rate would fall to relatively low normal levels, and the population would grow accordingly. From time to time massive migrations produced large population gains in some areas at the expense of others.

POPULATION FLUCTUATIONS

Today advances in medicine, public health, nutrition, and other fields have dramatically cut the death rate. The great 19th-century tides of international migration have been generally reduced to trickles. At the same time married couples have available to them technics that, for the first time in history, let them make effective decisions as to the number of children they will have. During the past 75 years the widespread use of these birth-control methods has begun to cause rapid changes in population trends in almost all of the Western nations.

During the depression decade, for example, the U.S. birth rate fell to an all-time low. Many population experts thought that our population would cease growing and might even decline, since the practice of family limitation was spreading to rural areas and lower-income groups. Almost no one foresaw the prolonged postwar baby boom and the accompanying population jump. Now we realize that a population that postpones marriage and childbearing in an unfavorable period may well marry younger and start childbearing earlier when conditions improve. In addition, since planned families need not be small families, the size of the average family can increase in prosperous times.

The fluctuations in the birth rate have affected capital investment, housing, recreation, education, manpower recruitment, and many other aspects of society that depend not only on the size of the population but also on the relative number of people in each age group. This in turn depends on the number of births in successive years. Our current school crisis is one painful result of the effect of postwar prosperity on the age of marriage, the size of families, and the spacing of children. The population bulge resulting from the baby boom is creating successive crises in many other social institutions as well. Starting in the crowded maternity wards, the population bulge moves inexorably up the age pyramid to the elementary schools, high schools, and colleges, then to the labor market and housing, until it finally reaches the old-age-pension system. Moreover, when one population bulge moves into the reproductive years of life, it starts another bulge that moves along 25 or 30 years later.

SURVEY

Clearly the impact of family planning requires that we learn much more about it. In the present survey our group set out to discover how couples feel about family planning and how extensively they practice it, how various groups in the population differ in their practice and how successful they are as measured by whether they have the number of children they want. To develop quantitative data on these questions, 2,713 white wives in the principal childbearing years (18 to 39) were interviewed at length. They gave detailed information on their pregnancy histories, contraception practices, and their plans for future childbearing. The wives were selected on a probability basis to give a good representation of the approximately 17 million white married couples in our population with wives 18 to 39 years old in the spring of 1955.

We secured complete interviews from 91 percent of the sample, indicating that family planning is now accepted by young married people as a topic for discussion and investigation. In most surveys on political and economic subjects, the completion of interviews from 85 per cent of the sample is considered satisfactory. Fewer than four wives in 1,000 declined to answer questions about the methods of contraception they practiced. In contrast, a larger number refused to answer questions about family income as being "too personal."

We should say a word at this point about terminology. Partly because some methods of preventing conception are morally unacceptable to certain groups, there is no general agreement on a term that applies to all methods. Here we use "family limitation" and "contraception" interchangeably and with no moral connotation for all methods (except sterilization) for avoiding conception. Included are periodic continence (the "rhythm method"), abstinence for long periods and withdrawal (coitus interruptus), as well as appliance or chemical technics, such as diaphragm, condom, douche, jelly, and the "birth-control pills" now being tested.

FINDINGS

The survey showed that in general all population groups accept the idea of couples deliberately regulating the number and spacing of their children in relation to their needs and resources. All the women were asked: "Many couples do something to limit the size of their families and to control when the children come. How do you feel about that?" Less than 5 per cent expressed unqualified disapproval of family limitation. Even among Roman Catholic wives only 13 per cent avowed such sentiments. Catholics as well as Protestants in overwhelming majorities approved family limitation in some circumstances. At the other extreme, 73 per cent of the Protestants, but only 33 per cent of the Catholics, approved limitation without qualification.

These differences reflect the doctrines of the Roman Catholic Church that forbid the use of certain methods of family limitation and restrict the extent to which other methods may be used. But there is no categoric prohibition of all methods. The late Pope Pius XII said in a 1951 address that the use of periodic continence (the rhythm method) or long-continued continence for "serious motives" is morally acceptable. One such motive is the avoidance of more children than the family can adequately care for. Catholics sometimes refer to methods forbidden by the Church as "artificial birth control." This includes coitus interruptus and the use of any chemical or mechanical agent. Since about a fourth of U.S. adults are identified with the Roman Catholic Church, its doctrines are important to national fertility trends.

As might be expected, the attitudes expressed by the wives in the sample were reflected in their accounts of their family limitation practices. The great majority of U.S. couples use some method of contraception. In our sample 83 per cent of the fecund couples (those who find that they can have children easily) had adopted contraception; 7 per cent more planned to do so after having the one or more children they still wanted. We think that the proportion may actually exceed 90 per cent, because many couples who are indifferent or opposed to contraception in early married life adopt some method when confronted with the problems of a rapidly growing family. In fact, 92 per cent of the fecund couples married more than 10 years reported efforts to control family growth.

Many couples do not practice contraception until they have had one or more children. Approximately half the couples using some method had at least one pregnancy before beginning to do so, often because they wanted to start having children soon after marriage. However, since most couples want a relatively small family, the delay before adopting control measures is usually brief. Unless in the meantime they had discovered a fecundity impairment, 89 per cent of all couples with two children had already used contraception in order to space pregnancies or restrict family size.

The majority of couples who never take control measures are those who suffer some type of physical impairment that limits their ability to bear children. Whether such impairments are discovered depends in part on whether couples dispense with contraception for extended periods. Therefore couples who do not begin contraception until they have had one or two pregnancies are more likely than others to discover physical impairments that make voluntary control unnecessary. There is evidence that poorly educated couples are more likely than others to delay taking control measures until pressed by necessity. Relatively more of them "test" their childbearing ability in this way and discover fecundity impairments that they would not otherwise know about.

Another major finding of the survey is that a majority of the fecund couples in all the major strata of the white population now practice contraception. For the purposes of the survey, strata were defined by education, income, occupation, religion, region and type of community. The widespread practice of family limitation that we found is definitely a new development. Contraception was undoubtedly taken up first by the higher-status groups: the well-educated, the professional and white-collar people, and those in upper-income brackets. As a result, family size declined more rapidly in higher-status than in lower-status groups. This led a generation or two ago to fears that the quality of the population would deteriorate as more of the nation's children came from supposedly inferior social and biologic backgrounds.

Now there are signs that eventually the historic differences among the birth rates of various population groups may be reversed. Among the wives in our survey who had been married less than five years, those with a college education expect to have more children than those with less education. Similarly, recent census figures show a lessening of birth-rate differences among socioeconomic groups, probably indicating that various segments of the population want about the same number of children. A 1940 study of Indianapolis found that among couples who planned the number and spacing of their pregnancies, those with higher incomes were having the larger families. Such couples can afford more children without sacrificing the other things Americans value as part of their standard of living, including the ability "to give the children what they should have."

Though contraception is a general practice in all strata of society, there are still significant differences among groups, particularly with respect to religion and education. Among fecund couples, 88 per cent of the Protestants, but only 70 per cent of the Catholics, reported using control measures. This divergence is not related to other non-religious differences between members of religious groups, such as education, income, occupation, or place of residence. When Catholics and Protestants who are similar in these respects are compared, the Catholics remain less likely to practice family limitation. The Catholic pattern of family limitation is also different from the Protestant. Far fewer Catholics plan their families by always practicing contraception except at the times when they want to have a child.

Interestingly enough, one factor that reduces the differences between Catholics and Protestants is whether the wife works. The differences based on religion are smallest among wives who have worked at least five years since marriage, and therefore have had extensive contacts outside the home. In these cases religion appears to have less influence on family-planning practices.

While the differences by religion are important, they should not be exaggerated. The great majority of Catholics do practice some form of family limitation. This is not necessarily a deviation from the Church's precepts, since many use only the rhythm method and for "serious motives."

Along with religion, education plays an important role in determining whether a couple adopts a family-limitation method. Presumably higher education gives a couple the wider range of contacts and information likely to make them analyze their family situation more self-consciously. It may cause them to want a style of life that requires careful planning, including the planning of family growth. In any case, the more education couples have, the more likely they are to use contraception and to avoid unwanted pregnancies.

Education is also important in explaining the relationships of other characteristics, such as income, to family-limitation practices. For example, lower-income couples are less likely than others to practice contraception. But when couples with similar educational backgrounds are considered, differences by income become much smaller. In the same way, farm-city differences almost vanish when couples with similar educational backgrounds are compared. The fact that farm couples in general are somewhat less likely than urban couples to try to restrict family size reflects their lesser educational attainments.

So far as we know, contraception was formerly less widely practiced in the country and the small town than in the metropolis. Our study shows, however, that the distinction has been disappearing. This represents a marked change in a generation or two, and is probably the result of a double process. On the one hand, the tremendous mobility of Americans has thoroughly mixed people of different backgrounds in communities of different sizes and types. On the other hand, the influence of the metropolis has been reaching out to every section of the country, spreading common standards and aspirations that affect not only what people consume and produce, but also how many children couples want and how couples plan family growth. The educational attainments of farm and small-town couples are becoming more like those of urban couples, and so are their family-planning practices.

Just as the family-planning practices are becoming more uniform, so are the goals. Most couples, the survey revealed, want a small or moderate-sized family. Each woman in the sample was asked a variety of questions to discover what family size was her objective. At various points in the course of the interview she was asked how many children she expected, how many she wanted and how many she considered ideal. These questions elicited slightly different answers, but there was a remarkable consensus on no less than two and no more than four children. If all couples have the number of births they are expecting, the average will be about three. Catholics expect an average of 3.4 births per couple, and Protestants expect 2.9. While it is probably biologically possible for U.S. couples to have an average of eight births, most of them are likely to come close to achieving their more moderate plans because they will use family-limitation methods fairly successfully.

Although a large majority of couples will come close to their goals, many will not be so successful. About one family in six may be "underplanned" because physiologic conditions prevent the bearing of as many children as are wanted. For some couples inability to have any children is a major tragedy, and for others their failure to have an additional child or children causes serious distress.

At the other extreme, are those who have more children than they want. In the case of approximately one couple out of seven in our sample the last pregnancy was not wanted by one or both parents. This is a common situation among larger families. More than half the wives who had borne more than four children said they or their husbands did not want the last pregnancy. Such unwanted pregnancies are much more frequent among couples with little education than among the better educated; in fact, they are about four times as frequent among those with a grade-school education as among those with a college education. Here is another indication that family planning is more extensive and effective among the better-educated couples. It is also likely that unwanted pregnancies are relatively frequent among Negro families, not included in this study. Negroes are presently concentrated in the lower educational and income groups in which accidental and unwanted pregnancies are most prevalent.

"ACCIDENTAL PREGNANCIES"

Another measure of success in family planning is the incidence of "accidental" pregnancies—those that begin when the couple is using some method to try to avoid conception. The wives in the sample reported that about 12 per cent of all their pregnancies were "accidents." However, a more meaningful "accident" rate is based on pregnancies that occur after use of contraception is begun. On this basis about one pregnancy in four occurred when the couples were using some method of contraception. Accidental pregnancies do not necessarily result in unwanted children, because in many cases the couples have merely been seeking to postpone a child they had planned to have later. Only about 24 per cent of all pregnancies begin after the deliberate discontinuance of contraception in order to have a child.

Nevertheless, most couples are successful in having the small number of children they want. Even the significant minority of couples who miss their goal do so by no more than one or two children in most cases.

Since Americans have adopted reasonably effective means to control the size of their families, an understanding of the goals of their planning is of great importance in predicting population trends. Because the goals are likely to change with social and economic conditions, they should be studied from time to time along with changes in the effectiveness of family planning. The Office of Population Research at Princeton University is now following a sample of couples who had a second child in 1956, in order to learn what factors will determine which of them will have a third child. Such studies of particular stages in the family life-cycle are important because many families do not grow according to a plan envisioned at marriage. There is interaction between the plans of the parents and their changing situation in the 10 to 20 years most of them have for childbearing.

This first study of a representative national sample of young married couples can only serve as an introduction to a complex subject. It shows that family planning of the U.S. population can be investigated with significant results.

3. The Rural Pattern: Healthways on the Farms

ALTHOUGH technologic advances are swiftly reducing the numbers of those needed as food producers, the rural sector is still an important one in our economy. In the United States the health needs of the farm population have been overlooked, in a relative sense; medical care has lagged; even Public Health services have failed to reach much of the rural population because of distance and obsolescent jurisdictional boundaries based on political subdivisions.

The articles to follow document this lag. They bring evidence, however, of growing recognition of these rural health problems and illustrate some new means for dealing with them.

Occupational Health on Farms*

H. N. DOYLE

HEALTH AGENCIES have many undischarged responsibilities toward rural Americans. To comprehend the responsibilities of official agencies for occupational health on farms, it is useful to grasp the extent of industrialization of American agriculture.

The population of the United States in 1910 was 92 million. Today, it is 166 million, an increase of 80 percent. In 1910 there were 322 million acres of cropland. Today there are 350 million acres of cropland, an increase of only 9 percent. Yet, this acreage produces more than enough food for our expanded population. It is estimated that 310 million acres will supply our 1960 population, thanks to the increase in productivity per acre. Improved soil management, such as erosion control and the use of fertilizers and other agricultural chemicals, including pesticides and weedkillers, have contributed part of this gain. Power machinery has increased the farmer's capacity to plow, sow, harvest, and manage livestock. Furthermore, market crops now grow on about 75 million acres formerly used to grow feed for the horses and mules which have been replaced by power machines.

* Reprinted by permission from the February, 1957 issue of *Public Health Reports*, Vol. 72, pp. 145–148. The paper is based on a talk delivered to the American Conference of Governmental Industrial Hygienists, Philadelphia, April 1956. The author is Chief of the State Services Branch of the Division of Occupational Health, U.S. Public Health Service, and currently is on an assignment at the U.S. Mission in Geneva, Switzerland.

Mechanization has made it possible for farms to produce more than enough for our present needs through the efforts of only 6,500,000 farm workers, or 11 percent of our working population, whereas in 1910, 11,600,000, or 31 percent, were employed in agriculture.

The number of American farms in 1954 was 5,425,000, as compared with about 6,600,000 in 1910. More important, half of our present farms produce nine-tenths of the crops. This concentration offers a striking parallel to many industries in which a small number of large companies account for a high percentage of the total production.

Even as large manufacturing concerns tend, with large-scale operations, to employ the latest advances in mechanization, so, and frequently to a greater degree, large farms tend to employ mechanical equipment. The capital investment associated with many of the new mechanical farm devices often runs to a sum which is not economic for a single-family farm.

Some idea of how mechanization has progressed in farming may be obtained from United States Department of Agriculture statistics which reveal that between 1941 and 1952 the number of tractors increased from 1.7 million to 4.4 million (159 percent), the number of grain combines from 225,000 to 940,000 (318 percent), and the number of mechanical corn-pickers from 120,000 to 635,000 (429 percent). The increase of total power on American farms during that period exceeded 70 percent. Farm output per man now has approximately doubled in the 15 years since Pearl Harbor.

Agricultural changes during the past generation, therefore, have come to create new working conditions even as industrialization changed working conditions in mines and mills.

How do these new conditions affect the health and safety of farm workers? Farming is intrinsically hazardous. Injuries have always been frequent on farms. Although statistical evidence is lacking, experience has led us to expect many injuries from the handling of farm horses. A limited survey in one county within the past 6 months showed that 8 out of 29 recent accidents were associated with horses. Even with mechanization, farmers tend to keep a few horses. Of 44 farms visited in this survey, 36 had at least one horse, and the total was 182.

Other farm animals also, particularly bulls, present hazards to farm hands. Injuries from the use of sharp or heavy tools or the stress of heavy lifting also are common farm afflictions, frequently resulting in chronic conditions, herniation, paraplegia, or impairment of vision.

The danger of infections from injuries incurred on the farm must be considered much greater than that in industry. The danger is heightened by the nature of the working environment, the inaccessibility of first-aid facilities, and the absence of interest in giving prompt care to minor wounds and other dermatologic conditions. The prevalence of the tetanus hazard on farms is well recognized by physicians, but other organisms also must be considered.

A number of bacterial diseases are associated with agricultural work. Brucellosis, or undulant fever, is thought to be the most common one, but reliable statistics are lacking. It is not likely that all brucellosis is correctly diagnosed or that all diagnosed cases are reported. One factor contributing to the incidence of brucellosis is that rather than call upon a veterinarian, many farmers themselves vaccinate cattle and thereby risk accidental infection. Other diseases of significance on farms include anthrax, erysipeloid, leptospirosis, tularemia, bovine tuberculosis, and various forms of salmonellosis.

By occupation, the farmer is exposed also to viral and rickettsial diseases, including equine encephalomyelitis, psittacosis, Q fever, and Rocky Mountain spotted fever. There is a long list of mycotic diseases, of which actinomycosis and histoplasmosis are examples. A number of parasitic diseases also are potential farm hazards.

Moving from these biologic hazards to physical agents, we find that farm work involves exposure to extremes of temperature, both high and low. Heat exhaustion and heat stroke undoubtedly affect many farm workers. Another condition of possible significance is skin cancer, produced by prolonged exposure to the sun's rays.

The increased use of machines has brought a whole group of hazards new to agriculture. Noise exposures, for example, may now be sufficient to affect the hearing of farmhands who operate machines for extended periods. When more is learned about the problem of vibration, it may also be found to have adverse health effects on agricultural workers. Maintenance and repair work on farm machinery introduce hazards associated with welding.

Accidents incurred in the use of farm machinery represent one of the major categories of farm hazards. Accident rates in agriculture are far above industry as a whole. In 1954 only the mining and construction industries had higher death rates: Agriculture had 60 fatal work accidents per 100,000 (a total of 3,800) as compared with a rate of 25 per 100,000 for all industries. The injury rate, according to the National Safety Council, was 4,930 per 100,000 as compared with 3,240 per 100,000 for all industries.

HAZARD FROM CHEMICALS

In addition to biologic and physical hazards, the industrial hygienist who looks at present-day farming is struck by the number of toxic chemicals in use. Although many of these are soil conditioners and fertilizers involving little hazard, the majority are insecticides, fungicides, rodenticides, nemotocides, and weedkillers which are employed specifically because of their toxic properties. While some are comparatively safe, nearly all present a degree of danger, and some must be classified as extremely hazardous. In particular, the heavy metals, such as lead, arsenic, and mercury, the halogenated hydrocarbons, and the organic phosphates present serious potential dangers to the people using them, and sometimes to others working or living in the vicinity.

In dealing with industrial exposure to hazardous materials, we frequently express the view that any material, regardless of toxicity, can be used safely provided that proper control measures are employed. The same philosophy might be applied to agriculture, but assurance of proper control measures is harder to obtain, at least at the present time. The reasons are apparent. Industrial operations are usually peformed in a fixed location where exhaust ventilation or other suitable control methods are feasible. Industry has been subjected to fairly extensive and intensive educational programs on health and safety for at least a generation. Large companies usually have full-time safety and medical departments alert to potential dangers. Furthermore, personnel of insurance carriers and official agencies make frequent visits to industrial plants to check for possible hazards.

On the other hand, agricultural workers generally have little idea of the hazards of handling and applying powerful chemicals. Although most chemicals of this type carry warnings on the container labels, the tendency is to pay little or no attention to the labels, particularly if a material has been used previously without untoward incident.

Moreover, the methods of application are almost as varied as the materials used. Many of these methods present dangers that would not be tolerated in manufacturing establishments. For example, the application of fumigants such as carbon tetrachloride in connection with grain storage may employ techniques that would horrify an industrial hygienist. A recent farm survey observed workers tying handkerchiefs over their faces to protect themselves from heavy concentrations of carbon tetrachloride.

The hazards of farm life are not to be ignored. And they are not ignored although much remains to be done to protect the farmer's health.

HEALTH SERVICES FOR FARM WORKERS

Occupational health programs are conducted in official agencies either because of laws specifically concerning industrial working conditions or because of broad powers regarding the protection of health. Virtually all such programs were introduced to cope primarily with problems associated with manufacturing, and, sometimes, also mining. Few of them gave much thought initially to the farm worker. In recent years, certain State officials have devoted attention to specific farm problems brought to their attention. For example, in Florida, in 1952 there were 46 claims for parathion poisoning filed; in 1953, there were 45. The Florida State Division of Industrial Hygiene has since conducted an educational campaign among citrus grove and truck garden owners on the hazards of insecticides and preventive measures.

Also, California has conducted investigations of the high incidence of occupational disease among its agricultural workers. In 1954, of 23,101 reports of occupational disease in California, 3,143 (13.6 percent) were for agricultural workers.

In addition to purely occupational influences, the health of many farm workers is affected by environmental factors that are much less significant among present-day urban workers. Farm laborers, especially migrant workers, sometimes must live where housing and sanitation levels are far below those now considered acceptable or safe. Large numbers of workers move from one State to another in pursuit of peak season farm work, and they stop at places where waste disposal is primitive, where water supplies are of questionable quality, where food spoilage is difficult to prevent, and where protection against flies and other disease carriers is absent. With this mobile population, numbering more than the citizens of several States, public health considerations demand far more than control of the traditional occupational diseases. In addition to basic sanitation, there must be answers to knotty questions of medical care for persons not eligible for service available to permanent residents. Otherwise, it is reasonable to expect that transient workers will be permitted to carry communicable disease to every community that summons their services.

While rural health services can use all available community resources, occupational health personnel must not overlook their special responsibility. Industrial hygienists, in checking the working environment in factories and mines, are also concerned with the water supply, washing facilities, waste disposal, and food sanitation. Nor should they neglect these points with respect to farm work, or, for that matter, in other situations where rural workers are housed temporarily, as in construction camps. Since such responsibilities also rest upon other personnel in State and local health agencies, policies for the best utilization of available man-hours must be developed to meet the individual situation. It is important, however, to recognize the place of environmental and medical care services in the occupational conditions of agricultural workers.

SOUTH DAKOTA AND IOWA PROGRAMS

As stated before, a number of State occupational health officials have concerned themselves, to a limited extent, with specific or selected health needs of agricultural workers. To our knowledge, however, no agency has ever considered the total need, with the objective of ascertaining the extent and severity of health problems on the farms of its State. This approach, which has been applied effectively by the States in planning logical and sustained programs for the improvement of worker health in industry, must now be used in agriculture if we are successfully to protect and improve the health of the farm family and its helpers.

The first stirring of activity in this direction came in 1955, when the South Dakota Department of Public Health requested assistance in planning an occupational health program for the State. In response to this request, the Public Health Service suggested that the program be developed to give industry and agriculture equal consideration from the start. To help develop such a program, the Occupational Health Program of the Public Health Service assigned a veterinarian to South Dakota in September 1955. Through this project it is hoped to evaluate the effectiveness of certain survey techniques and to develop useful information regarding occupational health problems and methods for their attack.

Coincidentally, during 1955 the State University of Iowa Medical School established an Institute of Agricultural Health which will study similar questions in Iowa.

It is significant, we believe, that these related projects were independently conceived and started at this time. Although the existence of health and safety hazards on the farm has been recognized by public health authorities for some years, the South Dakota and Iowa programs represent the first positive steps taken toward a comprehensive approach to the problem.

While some findings from these two States may become available relatively soon, other States need not wait for them before taking stock of the adequacy of their activities with respect to this particular segment of the employed population. Indeed, because of variations in crops, climate, soil, and other factors, problems will be found to differ in each locality, and all States can contribute appreciably to scientific knowledge while carrying out a public health activity of real merit.

The subjects which need exploration are numerous. Study needs to be made of the toxicology and proper application of chemicals, of the safe use of mechanized equipment, of the general health status of agricultural workers as compared with the rest of the population, of the effectiveness of educational measures, and of the availability of health resources.

This is a new and complex field confronting the industrial hygienist. Occupational health needs on the farm may not be readily anticipated, but in every State where agriculture is a significant industry,
an earnest beginning should be made to meet this public health
responsibility.

Rural Healthways in New Mexico*

SAM SCHULMAN, PH.D.

THE HEALTHWAYS PATTERN described in this paper is not particular to
any specific village, although it is basically a village pattern. It is that
of a village invented for our purpose. In the northern counties of New
Mexico, and in the Conejos and San Luis Valleys of southernmost
Colorado, a rural neighborhood—a village—is called a *placita*, and
that is the name of this invented village, La Placita. La Placita is
hopefully a modal prototype representative of a larger population of
such villages. The pattern of health-disease related traits described for
La Placita will be found with greater or lesser similarity in the geographic area described above. There is no such place as La Placita:
there are no such people as *placiteños,* but there are many places with
people like them.[1]

The composite La Placita is based on an examination of source
materials[2-20] and on a one-and-one-half-year's recent exploratory field
work.[21]

La Placita is within easy driving distance of Espanola, N. Mex., an
old cluster of villages now grown to town status, and of Santa Fe, the
New Mexico state capital. Most of the way to either place is over a
paved highway, but the approach to the village is on a graded but un-
paved road sometimes difficult or impossible to traverse after a heavy
snow or a flash springtime deluge that occasionally is experienced in

* Reprinted, by permission, from *Culture, Society, and Health* (proceed-
ings of a conference held and sponsored for the study of man, New York,
New York, on June 1, 2, and 3, 1960), in the *Annals of the New York
Academy of Sciences*, Vol. 84, Article 17, 1960, pp. 950–958. The investi-
gation reported in this paper was supported in part by research grant
RG 5615 from the Division of General Medical Sciences, Public Health
Service, Bethesda, Maryland. The author is Associate Professor in Nurs-
ing and Psychiatry in the College of Nursing, University of Florida,
Gainesville, Florida, formerly with the New Mexico Department of Public
Health, Santa Fe, New Mexico.

this area. It had been traditionally an agricultural community (but now most of the able-bodied men and even some of the women do wage work in nearby towns and cities or bordering states). It was settled shortly after the American Revolutionary War. The irrigation system of its founders—including several hand-hewn flumes of wood— is still in use.

"Old-timers" in the village say that there has been no major change in either its appearance or in the composition of its families during their lifetimes. In fact some of them remember their fathers saying the same thing. A glance at the colonial Spanish and Mexican archives in Santa Fe show property transactions, petitions of various sorts, old maps; and the names and places on these documents are familiar today.

La Placita is one of a group of villages in the Rio Grande watershed tenaciously held for centuries by Hispanic colonists and their descendants in spite of great human and natural obstacles. These were the last outposts of colonial Spain in the wilderness, virtually without communication with the outside world and visited only occasionally by trade and military caravans from Mexico. The threat of annihilation from hostile Indians and even from quiescent Pueblos was constant. In 1786 Bernardo de Galvez, considering the defensibility of his most northern ward, noted that ". . . the province is very distant and surrounded in all directions by different enemies."[22]

From its founding, La Placita has been a poor village, its inhabitants existing at a marginal level. Class distinctions have always been few. There have been a couple of families who were thought of as *ricos*, but they lived in homes like those of everyone else, perhaps a bit larger, perhaps with less crudely made furniture. *Placiteños* have usually asked little beyond existence from the land; the land has given them little more. In spite of being cut off from others, of the threat of savage extermination, of minimal productivity of the land, La Placita and *placiteños* have continued to exist over the generations.

Of such villages Saunders[15a] wrote: "The rhythm of life was slow. The pattern of activity was governed by seasonal rather than daily changes. Nothing in the daily routine was very compelling as long as the seasonal activities of planting, crop-tending, and harvesting were carried on. The rate of social change was also slow. One year was much like another year, and there was no need to be much concerned about time. The focus of attention was the present. There was nothing very memorable in the past to be recalled. There was no particular expectation of the future. Villagers lived in the present and did what needed to be done or what was pleasant to do at the time they were necessary or pleasant."

In virtual isolation, with a high degree of interpersonal and intra-familial dependence, and with the maintaining of a system of continuously reinforcing norms of behavior, La Placita—along with its sister villages—developed a distinguishable and specific subculture, "folk" in nature.

In the *placiteño* subculture its institutional or sociocultural complexes were related directly to analogous complexes of Mexico or of the larger Hispanic world; in addition it possessed peculiarities and modifications of its own. This is seen in institutional complexes such as those of church or home, or in sociocultural complexes such as those of property and inheritance, language and communication, health and disease.

The health-disease complex of La Placita has its roots in medieval Spain and precolonial America, and it is closely related to those of other areas of the Hispanic New World where similar admixtures have been made. Belief in the harmful power of *ojo* ("the eye") is common to all southern Europe and Hispanic America; belief in the protective power of the *oshá* root is probably restricted to the high areas of New Mexico and southern Colorado (with some diffusion along the present United States-Mexico border); belief that the water of the Rito de la Placita, taken with wine early in the morning, will lessen the joint pains of *rumos* is probably restricted to La Placita and one or two neighboring villages.

Factors contributing to major cultural change were limited during the entire Spanish and Mexican periods in La Placita. With the introduction of "American" ways after the acquisition of New Mexico by the United States in 1846 the factors affecting change increased geometrically. Until about 30 years ago the *placiteño's* medical system was relatively static and traditional. In recent decades the traditional system has been challenged, at times invaded, by segments of the modern medical community. On the other hand, the traditional system has been stubbornly retained by some *placiteños:* even when there has been a surface acceptance of the tenets of scientific medicine, under that surface there remains a core content of traditional beliefs and behaviors. There are a few *placiteños* who accept modern medicine completely, or as completely as village culture will permit, although any degree of sophistication regarding its true nature is either lacking or minimal. These few accept and defend modern medicine because they have seen it work.

With some broad strokes of the brush I shall try to delineate some of the major facets of the health-disease complex of La Placita.

In this village there are about 100 nuclear families, almost all living close to or sharing a common yard and well with their neighbors, related by blood or marriage. They live in homes of adobe, sun-dried mud-straw bricks. Most houses have flat roofs with a thick layer of adobe to hold them down; a few have pitched roofs of corrugated iron. Rooms are few. Beds are shared: by a conjugal pair, or by such a pair plus an infant, or by siblings, or by grandparents and grand-children. In some homes the children sleep on individual soft sheep-skins on the hard-packed mud floors. Heat is supplied by a small cast-iron stove and, perhaps, by a corner fireplace. In many homes cooking is still done on a large kitchen wood stove. Here the fuel is wood: chiefly dead *piñon* gathered in the local national forest. A few homes have stoves that burn propane or butane. Windows and doors are few; they are left open during the day, closed tightly at night.

Placiteños like to keep their homes neat and orderly. Furnishings, curtains, pictures, and portraits have their specified places and are carefully rearranged if disturbed. The women of the village frown on a poor housekeeper. Not one house in La Placita has a porcelain bath-tub, but periodic bathing by bucket is required of all family members. To be clean is a mark of propriety, especially on social occasions such as visiting, receiving visitors, or going to church. It is also considered proper esthetically. A flimsy wooden "privy" behind or at the side of every home in the village is the only means of serving its members' evacuation needs; it is generally unscreened. Most homes have elec-tricity, used chiefly for illumination. Water for drinking is obtained from the family shallow well. There are a few families in La Placita who still get their water for potable purposes from the irrigation ditch that circles the village, but this is considered "less convenient" than a well. For more than 40 years villagers have talked about a community water supply system. Such talk has been revived recently. The village may cooperate with the State's department of public health in the dig-ging of a community deep well and the construction of a water supply system attached to it. Many of the village's housewives approve such a move. With electricity and piped water, a washing machine may be more than just a dream.

Placiteños eat simply but well. Meat is not a frequent item on the family's table, but many foods are liberally laced with lard. Sun-dried strips of beef or mutton (or even of venison) are occasionally cooked into more routine table fare. Tinned foods or "store-bought" foods are now used often, but the bulk of any meal is likely to consist of locally grown and preserved products: corn, beans, fruits. An almost indis-pensable food, grown locally and eaten in large amounts, is chili. Some *placiteños* have taken to certain *gringo* foods and have them meal after meal: coffee, fried potatoes, packaged desserts. Candy and soft drinks are markedly popular with children in the village (who typically have considerable dental caries).

Neighboring villages think that La Placita is a quiet place, not given to exuberant or loud affairs. One may hear at a local dance in one of the villages a young man say to his date, "*No seas placiteña*" (roughly translating: "Don't be a stick-in-the-mud, like those from La Placita. Perk up, now."). Interestingly enough, *placiteños* say similar things about people from neighboring villages. Excessive emotionalism is frowned upon, but the sometimes unusual behavior of a *loco* is tolerated. Mental illness as understood by the modern medical community is poorly understood by *placiteños*, although they may believe that a wide spectrum of illnesses has its origin in psychic or emotional stress, or "fright." One may be "outside of his mind" if he is constantly deviant in behavior or if he is markedly retarded but, unless such behavior is antisocially directed, sanctions, coercions, and treatment are not used. (If, however, witchcraft is suspected of bringing about aberrant mental states, highly specialized treatment may be sought.) The mentally retarded and the mentally ill who from time to time are found in La Placita are usually enveloped and protected by their families. Institutionalization of a mentally afflicted family member is an alternative rarely sought. There is presently only one child who comes from La Placita in the state home for retarded children, and he was not entered until he was 16, when his family thought he was physically unmanageable. However, there are several *locos* (wild or bizarre ones) in the village; they do not do anything of consequence, but they do not usually hurt anyone either.

It is deemed necessary in La Placita to take precautions in daily life to avoid sickness and harm, but there is no well-constructed system of preventive medicine. Precautions may be generalized (that is, "Don't go out into the night air because you will get sick") or highly specific (such as, "You should carry a small bit of dried *oshá* root with you, and rattlesnakes will not strike you"). Children in La Placita go to a consolidated school in a neighboring village, and the county health nurse comes around periodically to give them "shots" to keep away diseases. Some of the old-timers have never liked the idea of these young women coming around with their needles and puncturing the skin. It is not a natural thing to do, but most *placiteños* offer no such objection. Some understand that the "law" demands that "shots" be given. Some others have observed within their own families that since the shots there have been definitely fewer deaths from whooping cough, diphtheria, and other diseases among the children.

A healthy person in La Placita is one who looks healthy and acts healthy. A healthy child, hence, is one who is plump and rosy; he should also be physically active and eat well. A healthy adult is one who is well proportioned, well muscled, well colored, and who does a good day's work. *Placiteños* are seldom obese, but the occasional heavy-set person is considered to have decided health advantages over the more thinly put together person. A few families are firm believers in vitamins and tonics, but most others see little use in such preventive medications.

A sick person in La Placita is one who is unable to perform the routine functions of daily life. If, furthermore, he loses color and strength and goes to bed, sickness is even more definite. Typically the *placiteño* tries to ascribe a name to an illness so that he may take the necessary steps to minister to the afflicted. It is only a rare case when an affliction is seen as incurable; in the vast majority of cases an illness has a cure. It is a basic assumption among *placiteños* that something, however minimal, must be done to cure an illness that is curable.

There are two essential steps in the curative process: (1) naming or identifying the disease entity, and (2) treating it. Although the process may not be fully conscious or deliberate, the *placiteño* will seek to resolve certain key questions about an illness.

What kind of illness is this? Although the lines of division among causative and symptomologic patterns are indeed hazy, an initial attempt is made to classify an illness into some part of what seems to be a threefold typology: physical, emotional, magico-religious.[23] The therapies and therapists could differ markedly, depending on the disease type. An illness caused by overeating of green fruit can more than likely be handled by the administration of one of several empirically proven *remedios mejicanos* (a folk or home remedy); an illness caused by the unwitting magical power of a stranger over a child can be treated only by essentially magical procedure (that is, recovering the stranger and having him pass water to the afflicted child, mouth to mouth).

Is this an illness that is caused by an internal predisposition, or is the cause external to the afflicted? An internal cause of disease might include familial tendency, or heredity, or it might be something associated with such factors as age, sex, and stature. If it is external to the afflicted, it is self-engendered (that is, did he make himself susceptible by exposing himself to disease situations), or is it other-engendered (that is, was he "attacked" by an external agent)? If an external agent is responsible for the disease, what kind of agent is it: animate, inanimate, spiritual; base animal, human, spirit, God? If the agent is animate or spiritual, did it really intend harm? Is this possibly one of those rare diseases that have no known cause and hence have no known cure?

The *placiteño* will rapidly sift and sort the answers to these questions and to others like them and we will select a name. It is quite possible that another *placiteño*, sifting and sorting the same responses, will come up with another name. Whatever the name or names, therapeutic procedures depend upon them. Associated with naming a disease is estimating its exigency: How important is it? How a disease is treated and how others relate to the afflicted will depend upon "how important" the malady is. (It is conceivably possible to arrange all possible afflictions as named by *placiteños* on a continuum of exigency from "slight" to "high," and a disease's location on that continuum would provide an accurate indication of the intensity and immediacy of treatment that it would be afforded.)

Placiteños rarely find that the etiology of an affliction belongs to any one single slot in their system of classification. Any single individual in the village may be "certain" that his evaluation is correct, but a collective view of all evaluations would probably show that only the relatively simple afflictions (such as overindulgence, skin abrasions, muscle soreness) show a high degree of agreement. More difficult afflictions (such as chronic disease, pain in nonobservable body parts, slowly progressive disease) would show greater variety in naming. In this village therapeutic procedures for minor ailments are usually simple, but for difficult ailments therapy may be complex and varied.

Almost every home in La Placita has a spot where herbs are kept.[24] These are usually gathered, dried, and stored by the woman of the house. In the old days the supplies were more varied than they are now, but even today the stocks of herbs may be considerable. Today both drugstore and grocery also have made noticeable additions to the folk pharmacopoeia, such as oils, linaments, patent medicines, and aspirins. Collectively the herbs and the medicine-cabinet items are the bases for innumerable *remedios*. In the case where an affliction is evaluated as minor, or where a *remedio* can be self-administered, the afflicted *placiteño* himself will prepare the brew, the infusion, the poultice, or the salve. He may ask others for their "pet" cures, prepare, and try them. Often the mother, grandmother, or grandfather may be referred to since one of these may have assumed the intrafamilial role of repository of herbal information. Within the family too, there may be a member who is well versed in the technics or "has the touch" naturally of massage. In La Placita massage is more than a device for relaxation; it is a therapeutic technic. *Sobando* and *traqueando* (massaging and bone "cracking") are resorted to in most illnesses, from the simple to the highly complex.

If self- or other-administered *remedios* within the family do not suffice to treat an ailment, the afflicted may turn to special therapists. Within the folk culture there are several; within the modern medical community there are others. In La Placita there are two young wives and one old man who are known as *sobadores*, outstanding therapeutic massagers. They will visit homes, or receive patients in their own homes, and perform required tasks. These may be done for a fee. Within the village there is another woman, a native midwife (*partera*), who is called upon for her special services by most of the expectant mothers.

In a neighboring village there is a woman who specializes in the preparation of herbal decoctions for sale or for a fee. In La Placita she is called a *médica;* further down the Rio Grande valley she might be

termed a *curandera*. She is an herbal folk specialist. In other villages
close by there are other women who are *parteras-sobadoras-médicas*,
expert in all of the usual folk-curing arts. Almost all folk curers are
women in these villages. An exception is an old man who lives "way
over the mountain" from La Placita who is an *albolario* (or *arbolario*).
He is an antiwitch. Not only can he use herbal arts well, but he has
the power to say and do things that dispel the curses of witches or
evildoers. He would be called upon only if bewitchment were suspected as the cause of illness. Sometimes even a *brujo* (witch) may be
sought out to break a spell he has created. Interestingly enough, everybody in La Placita will talk about witches, but no one knows where to
find one.[25]

There are those in the village, of course, who will go to a physician
when they suspect that they are ill or when they experience no success
with home remedies. Most *placiteños*, however, are reluctant to seek
out physicians. In several nearby towns and cities there are practitioners of "modern" medicine ranging from chiropractors and naturopaths, through osteopaths, to medical doctors. When it is necessary to
see a "doctor" most *placiteños* do not discriminate by title among
these town branches of the healing arts. There is, however, a noted
preference for chiropractors and osteopaths since both will manipu-
late muscles; moreover these practitioners seem to establish more
friendly relations with *placiteños*. Medical doctors use strange equipment, speak strange words, "look at you and write prescriptions, and
charge heavily for services," avow the *placiteños*. Their methods and
tactics are the most alien to *placiteño* culture of all the "doctors."

Placiteños as a rule do not like to go to hospitals for any reason.
The regimen of life is strange in a hospital. The food is too bland. The
nurses and doctors see you only as a "case" and only spasmodically.
Most important of all, a hospitalized patient is cut off from his family.
To "Anglo" hospital workers it does not seem to make much sense, but
patients from La Placita like to have their families nearby, even if they
just stand silently in the hospital corridors. This kind of visiting is
frowned on by hospital authorities. Then too, as everyone in the village knows, a hospital is meant for those who are seriously ill; to go to
a hospital admits of the utter exigency of an illness and of the inability
of the folk culture to cope with it. A few in La Placita have been to
hospitals, and they have verified all the bad things the villagers already
knew about hospitals. The high cost of inpatient treatment also deters
favorable attitudes toward hospitals.

Within driving distance of La Placita is the shrine of Our Lord of
Esquipula in Chimayo, N. Mex.[26,27] Here in his small church the Black
Christ is revered. In a wide hole in the ground of a tiny room off the
church proper is the earth "which heals by faith." Every once in a
while a small group will go down to the sanctuary, offer their prayers,

and return with the holy earth. For some ailments it is taken in a draught, for others it is made into mud and plastered over an afflicted organ. There have been no miraculous cures among the afflicted in La Placita, but a cripple in a nearby village was so cured that he hung his crutches along with hundreds of others on the wall of the shrine, and now walks upright. A few *placiteños* say that the sanctuary earth has helped their chronic illnesses.

Once a month in the rural schoolhouse in La Placita (now unused because of a school consolidation program), a room is cleared, and a team of nurses and a doctor come up from the health department to examine babies. Mothers from about six other villages join the women of La Placita when clinic day comes. They sit in large and small groups and exchange gossip, family news, and recipes. The women and their children dress as well as they can. For some it is an important social occasion. Although this is definitely a woman's affair many men come along; they drive the family automobile or pickup truck. The men gather in little knots outside the schoolhouse; some go down the road for a beer. Many of the women are proud of their children as they display them, plump and clean, to the medical people. The doctor says a child has fine muscles, and the mother beams. These "well-child" clinics are well attended, and there is not a baby in the entire village who has not been taken to the clinics at least occasionally.

A few of the people in the village go down to other clinics in the cities; chest clinics, clinics for "private" diseases. They do not enjoy these clinic visits as social functions. Some in fact try to delay going until there is no other alternative.

Two of the men in the village work for employers who insist that their employees subscribe to health insurance plans. The families of these workers are the only ones in the village who are covered by such plans. Some families on "welfare" have minimal medical coverage. The others prefer to pay for illness when it occurs and can see little benefit in health insurance that is "paying for illness before it ever comes."[28]

The only community health "programs" in La Placita are provided by two men's organizations (other than the irrigation ditch association): they are the local *morada* ("house") of the *Hermandad de Nuestro Padre Jesús* (the "Penitentes") and the *Mutua* (a mutual protective association of farmers). In the event of sickness, "brothers" of both organizations will aid their stricken members in any way they can. They can do least in the way of monetary contributions, since they are poor, but they can till a man's fields and harvest his crops, gather and split firewood for his family, share their own families' food. Should the afflicted "brother" die both groups are pledged to supply his widow and children with food, kindling, and clothing until they can be reabsorbed by their own families.

SUMMARY

A hypothetic village in northern New Mexico—La Placita —has been used to evaluate descriptively the healthways of village-dwelling, rural Spanish-Americans. Through isolation a distinguishable folk culture, inclusive of a health-disease complex, has developed in this village and in others like it. Major aspects of the health-disease complex of this village mentioned here have been: hygienic aspects of home life, eating habits and diet, mental health, precautionary aspects of health, identification and treatment of disease, folk medicine, medical practitioners, and community health. Stressed has been the concept of multicausal factors in illness and of a corresponding multiphasic and possibly highly varied therapy.

Noted is the trend to include parts of the modern medical system as acceptable alternatives in therapy.

ACKNOWLEDGMENTS

Instrumental in the field work that provided the data upon which much of the paper is based were Julian Samora, Frances Fell, Serafin Vigil, Carmen Trujillo, and Thomas Weaver. Marion Hotopp, Lyle Saunders, and Anne M. Smith read and criticized an earlier draft. To all the foregoing the writer is appreciative, but he accepts responsibility for what is said here.

1. In an area such as that of Hispanic New Mexico, where almost all geographic and population entities have names, the term placita is encountered at every hand as a rural neighborhood name (such is also the case with llano, rancho, valle, vega, arroyo, and other ubiquitous designations). As postal or railroad services were extended to many of these population clusters, local designations gained official legitimacy. Thus there are actually several villages with the term placita (or a variant of the term) as their legitimate names or as part of such names. The village described in this paper is not one of these: it is a fictional entity.

2. Bunker, R. & J. Adair. 1959. *The First Look At Strangers.* Rutgers Univ. Press. New Brunswick, N.J.

3. Burma, J. H. 1949. Present status of the Spanish-Americans of New Mexico. *Social Forces.* 28:133–138.

4. Clark, M. M. 1959. *Health in the Mexican-American Culture.* Univ. Calif. Press. Berkeley, Calif.

5. CORNELL UNIV. SOUTHWESTERN SEMINAR FIELD NOTES. 1951–1953.

6. Edmondson, M. S. 1957. *Los Manitos: A Study of Institutional Change.* Middle American Research Institute, Tulane University. New Orleans, La.

7. Francis, E. K. 1956. Multiple intergroup relations in the upper Rio Grande region. *Am. Sociol. Rev.* 21:84–87.

8. Gourley, G. 1960. Reinforcement of family ties. *Public Health Rpts.* (U.S.) Washington, D.C. 75(1):65–68.

9. Hacker, D. B., M. S. Franks, V. Fesker, R. J. Grass, M. Hotopp & E. M. Lantz. 1954. *A Study of Food Habits in New Mexico.* Bull. 384. Agric. Exptl. Sta., N. Mex. Coll. Agric. and Mech. Arts. State College, N. Mex.

10. Lantz, E. M. & P. Woods. 1958. Nutrition of New Mexican Spanish-

American and "Anglo" adolescents. *J. Am. Dietetic Assoc.* 34(2):138–153.

11. Leonard, O. & C. P. Loomis. 1941. *Culture of a Contemporary Rural Community—El Cerrito, N. Mex.* U.S. Dept. Agric., Bureau of Agricultural Economics. Government Printing Office. Washington, D.C.

12. Mead, M. 1953. *Cultural Patterns and Technical Change.* UNESCO. Paris, France.

13. Samora, J. 1959. The conception of health among Spanish-Americans: a working paper. Rural Health Survey report. Santa Fe, N. Mex.

14. Saunders, L. 1944. *A Guide to Materials Bearing on Cultural Relations in New Mexico.* Univ. N. Mex. Press. Albuquerque, N. Mex.

15. Saunders, L. 1954. *Cultural Difference and Medical Care.* Russell Sage Foundation. New York, N.Y.

15a. *Ibid.* 51.

16. Saunders, L. 1958. Healing ways in the Spanish southwest. In *Patients, Physicians, Illness.*: 189–206, 567–569. E. G. Jaco, Ed. Free Press. Glencoe, Ill.

17. TEWA BASIN STUDY. c. 1935. *The Spanish-American Villages.* Vol. II. (Albuquerque, N. Mex.)

18. Ulibarri, H. 1958. *The Effect of Cultural Difference in the Education of Spanish Americans.* Coll. Education, Univ. N. Mex. Albuquerque, N. Mex.

19. Van Der Eerden, M. L. 1948. *Maternity Care in a Spanish-American Community of New Mexico.* Catholic Univ. Am., Anthropological Series, No. 13. Washington, D.C.

20. Winnie, W. W. 1957. *The Spanish-speaking population of New Mexico.*

21. This presentation is not meant to be a synthesis or evaluation of data gathered during the course of a field project. At this writing data-gathering is still the project's most important activity. This paper represents a "skimming" of the coded data, and elaboration is perforce descriptive and tentative. A more complete report is planned for 1960 or 1961.

22. De Galvez, B. 1951. *Instructions for Governing the Interior Provinces of New Spain.* 1786. :72. The Quivira Society. Berkeley, Calif.

23. Foster, G. 1951. *A Cross-Cultural Anthropological Analysis of a Technical Aid Program.* :47–54. Smithsonian Institution. Washington, D.C.

24. Curtin, L. S. 1947. *Healing Herbs of the Upper Rio Grande.* Laboratory of Anthropology. Santa Fe, N. Mex.

25. Weaver, T. 1960. A comparative study in witchcraft: Pueblo Indian and Spanish American. Univ. N. Mex. Albuquerque, N. Mex. (Unpublished M.A. thesis.)

26. Borhegyi, S. F. 1953. The miraculous shrines of Our Lord of Esquipulas in Guatemala and Chimayo, New Mexico. *El Palacio.* 60(3):83–111.

27. Borhegyi, S. F. 1954. The Cult of Our Lord of Esquipulas in Middle America and New Mexico. *El Palacio.* 61(12):387–401.

28. Saunders, L. & J. Samora. 1955. A medical care program in a Colorado county. In *Health, Culture, and Community: Case Studies of Public Reactions to Health Programs.* :395. B. D. Paul, Ed. Russell Sage Foundation. New York, N.Y.

4. The Metropolitan Pattern: Healthways in Conurbia

Health Effects From Repeated Exposures to Low Concentrations of Air Pollutants*

RICHARD A. PRINDLE, M.D., M.P.H., AND EMANUEL LANDAU

ONE OF THE BEST documented facts in the whole complex field of air pollution is that it can, in certain circumstances, result in acute illness and sudden death. Everyone knows about the disasters in Belgium's Meuse Valley, in Donora, Pa., and in London. Continuing research is uncovering other such episodes, long after they have occurred. In the United States we plan to continue our search for further evidence from the past. We hope to develop eventually a warning system that will predict the weather and other conditions which made possible such abnormally high concentrations of air pollutants and thereby mitigate, or even eliminate, future air pollution disasters.

Nevertheless, although more Americans than ever before are doing research today in air pollution, an increasing proportion of this effort is devoted to the long-term effects of exposure to low pollutant levels.

Our approaches to the determination of chronic effects of pollution have been of two major kinds: (a) the repeated laboratory exposure of human and animal subjects to specific pollutants or mixtures; and (b) the epidemiologic approach, using the community as a field laboratory.

LABORATORY RESEARCH

In pursuing the first kind of research, the Division of Air Pollution, Public Health Service, has encouraged attempts to develop technics capable of measuring minute changes in physiology to supplement new knowledge of pollutant concentrations at levels which cause marked pathologic variations or death. Accordingly, we have recently

* Reprinted by permission from the October 1962 issue of *Public Health Reports*, Vol. 77, pp. 901–909. This paper was presented before the Verein Deutscher Ingenieure (DI) Kommission (Commission for Clean Air) June 20, 1962, at Düsseldorf, Germany. The authors are, respectively, Chief, Division of Public Health Methods, Office of the Surgeon General, Public Health Service, U.S. Department of Health, Education, and Welfare, Washington, D.C., formerly Deputy Chief of the Division of Air Pollution, Public Health Service, Washington, D.C.; and Chief of the Biometrics Section, Field Studies Branch, Division of Air Pollution, Public Health Service, Washington, D.C.

undertaken studies of physiologic and metabolic activities. Unfortunately, because of lack of knowledge about the physiologic effects of pollutants, the choice of metabolic activity to be studied must often be based on trial and error. In some cases, a chance observation by other investigators, discovered in a search of the literature or through personal communication, offers a clue which seems worth pursuing. In one such instance, because of the similarity of certain toxicologic effects of ozone to those produced by ionizing radiation, our researchers are following, in rats exposed to ozone, the urinary excretion pattern of creatine and creatinine, known to be affected by radiation. Possible alternations in protein and purine metabolism after exposure to various pollutants are being sought by analyses of the urinary excretion of uric acid and amino acid nitrogen. Measurements of oxygen consumption, also in progress, may yield useful information during long-term inhalation exposures. These approaches are then coupled with studies of pulmonary function for comparison with human disease states.

The following examples illustrate some of the various approaches in the study of the long-term effects of air pollution on animals and man. In a study using classic laboratory techniques, repeated inhalation of ozone at a concentration of 1 ppm (2.6 mg./m.^{3}), only slightly greater than that existing in some urban atmospheres, produced chronic bronchitis and bronchiolitis in small animals.[1] The smaller bronchioles were partly occluded by hyperplastic or sloughed epithelium mixed with acute inflammatory exudate in guinea pigs which survived the experiments and were sacrificed at the end of more than 400 days of exposure. The bronchiolar walls displayed fibrosis extending into the alveolar ducts and alveoli. A mild degree of emphysema was considered to be secondary to the bronchial occlusion. The changes were less marked in rats and hamsters and inconsistent in three mice examined. No evidence of intrapulmonary injury was detected in two dogs whose lungs were examined microscopically, but the trachea and major bronchi showed slight epithelial injury. Rats and guinea pigs which died during the course of the exposure exhibited massive pneumonia; slight fibrosis was noted as early as the 25th day of exposure.

Groups of nine-month-old rats were exposed continuously up to two years to one, two, four, eight, 16, and 32 ppm of sulfur dioxide to determine the long-term effects as manifested by survival, hematologic response, and clinical symptoms.[2] Exposed rats exhibited changes in skin, fur, and conjunctiva and respiratory distress of increasing severity with increasing concentrations of the gas. A marked difference in the death rate of the group exposed to the 32 ppm concentration (84 mg./m.^{3}) was observed, as compared with controls, and groups exposed to lesser concentrations of sulfur dioxide also began to die before the control group. All control animals survived the first nine months. By 18 months and until the end of the experiment, the survival rate of rats at all exposures to SO_2 except 32 ppm was similar but distinctly different from that of control animals. The earlier age at death of exposed animals was considered compatible with a process of accelerated aging, possibly resulting from the stress of such exposure.

It is becoming increasingly evident that oxides of sulfur, in concentrations attainable in community air, may affect the human respiratory tract. A research team at the Harvard School of Public Health has shown that the acute response in human beings resembles that in guinea pigs. Normals persons who inhaled either sulfuric acid mist or sulfur dioxide for brief periods exhibited markedly shallower, more rapid breathing.[3,4] More recently another team of investigators at Harvard measured pulmonary function in healthy volunteers exposed to controlled levels of sulfur dioxide.[5] During administration of the gas, all measurements of resistance showed an increase, greatest for pulmonary flow resistance (PFR) on quiet breathing, intermediate for PFR on panting and for airway resistance, and smallest for total respiratory resistance. Pulmonary flow resistance showed no change at 1 to 2 ppm of sulfur dioxide; it increased an average of 19 per cent above control levels at 4 to 5 ppm and 49 per cent at 8 to 19 ppm; and when sulfur dioxide was combined with aerosol, the increase was 72 per cent. However, investigators at St. Luke's Hospital in Cleveland observed no changes in resistance in normal subjects exposed briefly to sulfur dioxide in concentrations of 2.5 to 23 ppm, combined with particulates and aerosols, whereas emphysematous subjects exhibited a decrease in airway resistance.[5]

Although the acute effects of exposure to high concentrations of carbon monoxide are well documented, the chronic effects from long-term subtoxic doses are controversial. Recent findings suggests that, besides its known effects upon hemoglobin, carbon monoxide exposure may affect the eye and nervous system adversely. Since 1955, carbon monoxide levels in the Los Angeles atmosphere have been increasing by about 1 ppm (0.0012 mg./m.^{3}) per year. It is estimated that gasoline engine exhaust is the source of about 75 per cent of the total carbon monoxide content of Los Angeles air, with significant contributions also from metallurgic and oil-refining operations.

Research workers[6,7] have found an average blood carboxyhemoglobin of 3.8 per cent, not markedly different from average levels in groups with lesser degrees of exposure, in subjects exposed to carbon monoxide in their working environment, from smoking, or while commuting to work in private automobiles. The carbon monoxide concentration in a garage and automobile inspection center where the exposed group worked ranged from 10 to 150 ppm, (0.06 mg./m.^{3}); in the working environment of the control group, the ambient carbon monoxide level was less than 10 ppm (0.012 mg./m.³). Although 17 of 68 exposed subjects, compared with three of 25 controls, complained of headache, dizziness, or unusual fatigue at the end of the workday, no relationship could be found between carboxyhemoglobin levels and occurrence of those symptoms.

In a preliminary study performed by Public Health Service scientists at Cincinnati, Ohio,[8] the levels of carbon monoxide in the passenger compartment of stationary vehicles in heavy traffic were greatly increased, reaching a maximum of 370 ppm (0.44 mg./m.³). Investigators at the University of Michigan[9a,10] sought to determine whether atmospheric carbon monoxide levels in urban areas might interfere with the driver's ability to operate his vehicle. Data collected from appropriate sites in Detroit for one year showed that median daily values of atmospheric carbon monoxide ranged between 0 and 20 ppm. During periods of high atmospheric stability and heavy traffic, concentrations reached 100 ppm at some sampling sites and persisted at this level for several hours. In homes several hundred feet from street sampling sites, concentrations approximated those in the street. Analysis of reports of more than 4,000 consecutive accidents involving almost 5,000 persons failed to reveal a higher accident rate associated with occupations in which high carbon monoxide exposure would be expected. In an attempt to relate the carbon monoxide content of the blood to air levels, a cigar smoker and a nonsmoker traveled in a police scout car for eight hours for a distance of 130 miles. The carbon monoxide in the vehicular air, monitored continuously—reflecting outside traffic conditions and not influenced by any tobacco smoke in the car—average 17 ppm with a peak of 120 ppm when the engine was idling. The smoker's blood carboxyhemoglobin rose from 3.1 to 3.9 per cent, the nonsmoker's from 0.8 to 1.2 per cent.

In a study of 237 persons involved in traffic accidents (including both drivers and pedestrians) and brought to the hospital for treatment, 50 per cent of the drivers had less than 3 per cent carboxyhemoglobin, 50 per cent of the pedestrians had less than 2 per cent, and only three persons had levels of 10 per cent or more; in one of these the carboxyhemoglobin was 31.5 per cent. It was concluded by the investigators that carbon monoxide concentrations in the general atmosphere of Detroit do not impair driving ability,[10] but further work is now underway to substantiate or amend these findings.

Studies undertaken on animals have demonstrated that guinea pigs exposed to automobile exhaust, at a concentration several times normal, for 1, 2, and 4 weeks, were especially susceptible to severe pulmonary disease.[9b] This came to light accidentally following an epidemic which produced pneumonia in the test animals. Significantly higher mortality occurred in the animals exposed to irradiated exhaust, comparable to heavy photochemical smog, than in animals exposed to nonirradiated exhaust or in control animals, which also experienced the epidemic but were exposed only to pure air. This finding parallels the results of another study in which animals exposed for only two hours to pure nitrogen dioxide at levels similar to those occasionally found in community atmospheres were much more susceptible to infection by certain pneumonia organisms (personal communication, Richard Ehrlich, Armour Research Institute, Chicago). More serious illnesses and more deaths occurred in this group than in the control animals, which were exposed to the same organisms but otherwise breathed only pure air.

Irradiated exhaust, that is, automobile exhaust which has been diluted with air and then exposed either to sunlight or to artificial light with ultraviolet components, is chemically different from exhaust which has not been irradiated. It has been shown that this irradiated gas is chemically similar to the so-called "photochemical smog" so notorious on our west coast. It also causes the same types of damage to vegetation as the "smog" found in California. Constituents include ozone, "oxidants" (oxygen-containing compounds of high reactivity), other hydrocarbons, and oxides of nitrogen.

These ingredients appear to result from complex interactions due to photochemical action on the unburned hydrocarbons and oxides of nitrogen found in exhaust gases. Merely mixing ozone with hydrocarbons, such as gasoline vapors, can stimulate this process to some degree. Because these ingredients appear to be more biologically potent, causing damage to plants and eye irritation in people, our recent studies have been focused on them to a large extent.

Physiologic experimentation in which measures were made of respiratory function of guinea pigs, including pulmonary resistance, respiratory rate, and minute volume, has shown that the greatest changes occurred in those animals exposed to irradiated exhaust. In general, these changes have occurred when the animals have been exposed to concentrations two or more times the usual ambient levels. However, some physiologic changes have occurred in animals at "community" levels, and certain specific pollutants have been observed to produce effects at or near these concentrations. This would appear to indicate that the observed maximum levels present in communities at this time are borderline with respect to causing immediate effects such as changes in pulmonary function and may be highly significant in their long-term effects.

Last year workers at the University of Southern California were able to produce true squamous cancers in the lungs of mice, similar in type to those found in human beings, by exposing the animals first to infection, then to air containing ozonized gasoline. In this experiment, one group of animals was exposed to a virus type of influenza and another was unexposed. Each of these groups was divided after recovery into two further groups, one exposed to purified air and the other to ozonized gasoline. In the animals receiving the infection alone, approximately 8 per cent showed squamous changes in the bronchi consistent with healing processes after infection and occasionally demonstrated metaplastic changes. In the animals exposed to ozonized gasoline alone, there were no significant findings. In the uninfected animals exposed to pure air, the findings were negative. A striking 30 per cent of the animals which had been infected and subsequently exposed to ozonized gasoline demonstrated the presence of squamous carcinoma. Interestingly enough, the male-female ratio was approximately 3 to 1, similar, in fact, to that found in humans and obviously not associated with smoking habits or occupation.[11,12]

EPIDEMIOLOGIC RESEARCH

Considerable epidemiologic research has also been undertaken with the community used as a laboratory. While increasing effort has been devoted to the chronic effects of normal low levels of community pollutants, the Public Health Service has continued to support research into the extent of previously unreported air pollution disasters.

The literature of air pollution disasters was enriched recently by the publication of a paper reporting excess mortality, presumably due to elevated levels of pollutants resulting from an extended temperature inversion in New York City as long ago as November 1953. This excess mortality in the largest metropolis in the United States was determined retrospectively by an examination of death records.[13] It parallels in that respect the experience of the 1952 disaster in London, the largest metropolitan area in Great Britain. However, while the London episode was studied almost concurrently, the study in the United States was made more than five years after the event.

In the 1953 incident, 220 excess deaths were attributed to cardiac and respiratory diseases, again paralleling the London episodes. These deaths must have been accompanied by increased morbidity. Unfortunately, the precise magnitude of this morbidity is uncertain, since it is extremely difficult to obtain reliable morbidity data for past years.

There are some possible sources of illness data, such as hospital admissions, physician visits, group medical practice usage, health surveys, and the like. It is obvious that it is no easy matter to collect such data after the lapse of nearly a decade. The less current the records, the greater is the danger that they may no longer exist. Therefore, it was gratifying to find that an examination of the records on emergency room visits to the largest New York City hospitals for November 15–24, 1953, undertaken recently by the same group which reported on mortality in New York City, revealed about twice the expected number of visits by patients with respiratory and cardiac conditions.[14]

The line of demarcation between an acute air pollution episode and the chronic long-term effects of low levels of air pollution can become quite blurred. This difficulty is exemplified when we looked for causes of the large number of asthmatic responses to sublethal levels of pollutants which have been observed in New Orleans, Pasadena, and Nashville.

In New Orleans, it was demonstrated that there had been sharp periodic increases in emergency clinic visits to Charity Hospital by nonwhite asthmatics. This has occurred often enough so that adequate documentation is now possible.[9c] The usual number of visits to Charity Hospital by asthmatics was 25 per day for the period 1953 to 1961.

Frequently, however, outbreaks of asthmatic attacks have seriously strained the facilities of the hospital. In August 1958, for example, an outbreak of asthma involved 100 people, with 3 deaths. There have been instances of daily admissions of 150 and even 200 Negro adult patients. Asthma outbreaks have been accurately predicted in advance on at least two occasions; the predictions were made on the basis of meteorologic data which had shown that the outbreaks were associated with particular wind movements.

We are now able to report that these asthma outbreaks are thought to be related to particles of a silicon-containing compound emitted into the atmosphere as a result of poor combustion of garbage and refuse in the New Orleans City dumps. This could possibly be an instance of an air pollutant acting as an allergen and creating an allergic response in certain susceptible individuals. Obviously, testing of skin and pulmonary sensitivity and further research are indicated to verify or disprove this hypothesis.

How are we to consider the response of asthmatics to insults to the respiratory tract in such diverse air pollution areas as Los Angeles and Nashville? Are these responses the product of acute or chronic insults? In the Los Angeles area a study was conducted from September 3 to December 9, 1946, of 137 bronchial asthma patients of 5 practicing physicians.[15] The study revealed that the average number of patients afflicted on days when oxidant values were above a level that caused eye irritation was significantly greater than the average number on days when oxidant values were below this level. Similarly, the number of persons who had attacks on days when plants showed damage from air pollutants, a biologic indicator, was significantly greater than the number on other days.

In Nashville, also, it was found that attack rates were significantly different when comparison was made of days with the highest and the lowest sulfur dioxide levels.[16] The statistical significance was even greater when the daily data on asthma attacks were lagged one day to take account of possible delayed reactions to sulfur dioxide. A possibly corroborative finding was that the pattern of attacks for adult asthmatics reflected differences in air pollution levels in different sections of the city. Thus, the attack rate was three times as high in an area of high pollution as it was in a low-pollution area. It is particularly noteworthy that the sulfur dioxide levels in Nashville are not high even at their worst.

Evidence from episodes in the Orient which afflicted American servicemen and their dependents also shows that air pollution appears to be an etiologic agent for a condition that was originally called "Yokohama asthma."[17] This is now referred to as "air pollution asthma." Some of the servicemen and their dependents were relieved of asthmatic attacks when they were moved out of affected areas in Japan and Okinawa. Conversely, some persons who were not evacuated quickly from the areas continued to manifest asthmatic symptoms. Accordingly, it appears that for some susceptible individuals this kind of asthmatic response may be truly a chronic effect of air pollution.

A further bit of evidence is based on recent data on illnesses of employee groups. These data indicate a high degree of relationship between respiratory illnesses lasting eight days or more and levels of sulfates in selected cities in the United States.[18] If this relationship were to be more completely documented, it might explain some of the striking rise in the prevalence of chronic respiratory diseases which has been observed recently.

The best indication of all of the chronic effects of air pollution is undoubtedly provided by the statistics on chronic bronchitis in Great Britain.[19] There, the disease is the third leading cause of death and the leading cause of disability.

In the United States there has been increasing acceptance of the view that a group of chronic respiratory diseases in this country, comprising emphysema, chronic bronchitis, bronchiectasis, and "other chronic interstitial pneumonia," is similar to the chronic bronchitis syndrome observed in Great Britain and that the apparent differences reported in the two countries may merely reflect differences in medical diagnostic criteria and terminology in patients with cases of differing severity and degree of infection.

We are aware that in the United States no evidence has been produced to demonstrate that air pollution is an etiologic agent for the emphysema syndrome. Nonetheless, there is an ever-mounting accumulation of evidence linking the two. Well known is the phenomenal rise of deaths from emphysema in the American population as a whole since 1950.[20] One may, with considerable certainty, ascribe part of the increase to the increasing acceptance of this classification as a cause of death, which in turn is due to the increasing discussion of chronic respiratory disease in the medical literature. Nevertheless, we have no reservation in stating that part, perhaps most, of the seven-fold increase in the frequency of this diagnosis as a cause of death is due to the greater prevalence of the disease.

One reason for assuming an air pollution factor as a cause of emphysema is the urban-rural comparison of mortality in the United States. Certainly, when the age-adjusted urban rates are double the rural rates, there would appear to be some factor which is directly related to residence in cities. Attention has been drawn previously to the fact that smoking differences among males, by residence, are relatively small and presumably do not account for the urban-rural ratio found for emphysema.[21] The well-documented greater pollution of urban atmospheres as compared with rural points to a possible causal relationship.

It is recognized, of course, that there may also be an occupational exposure factor. The records of the Social Security Administration show that emphysema is the second leading cause of disability among male workers 50 years of age and older.[22] It is clear that the evaluation of the role of air pollution in the increase in mortality from emphysema will have to take account of the occupational history of the decedent as well as his smoking habits.

Because of the increased interest in chronic respiratory diseases there has been a growing awareness of the need to inform people of the importance of certain symptoms. Accordingly, the National Tuberculosis Association has announced its intention of conducting a campaign during the spring of 1963 to alert people to the significance of "shortness of breath" and "chronic cough."[23] It is quite possible that people became so accustomed to these symptoms that they pay little attention or attach no importance to them. An increasing amount of data on the prevalence of emphysema and chronic bronchitis should be forthcoming as this educational campaign progresses.

In order to learn more about the long-term effects of air pollution, it was found necessary to conduct extensive field studies on selected populations. In 1959 the Division of Air Pollution of the Public Health Service, in cooperation with the Pennsylvania Department of Health, the Pennsylvania Electric Co., and others, undertook a study of two small communities in Pennsylvania, Seward and New Florence.[24] The study had the elements of a natural laboratory setting inasmuch as the towns were virtually identical demographically. These towns, inhabited by about 1,000 persons each, are approximately 4 miles apart, with a soft-coal-burning electric power plant between them. The prevailing wind pattern was such that the town of Seward was subject to much higher levels of air pollution than New Florence. Thus, for the period of the study, the level of dustfall in Seward was three times that of New Florence, the level of sulfation was seven times as high, and the level of SO_2 was at last nine times as high. Nevertheless, the SO_2 level in Seward was below that generally found in London.[25]

The purpose of the study was to determine the long-term effects of low concentrations of air pollutants. An attempt was made to include the entire adult population of both sexes 30 years old and over. In addition to X-rays, the study used the long Medical Research Council questionnaire, with slight revisions, chiefly in terms of a much more detailed work-experience history. A battery of pulmonary function tests, including the body plethysmograph, was administered to the study group. The analysis, which was scheduled for completion in the summer of 1962, takes into account such variables as smoking and occupational and residence exposure of the townspeople.

In the preliminary report, one significant finding was that the average airway resistance (measured by the body plethysmograph) was higher in Seward than in New Florence even after differences in height and age were taken into account.

A curious finding was that the male population of the polluted area was almost one inch shorter than that of New Florence. One would rightfully hesitate to attribute this difference in height to the difference in the environment. Yet this possibility should not be dismissed arbitrarily because of its apparent implausibility. One may only say that differences of this sort would have to be documented in many other communities before we could accept the hypothesis that the stature of the inhabitants was related to exposure to air pollutants rather than to ethnic or socioeconomic differences.

Since this study was completed, considerable effort has been made by the industry to reduce the pollution in the area. A restudy some time in the future might prove of considerable interest in evaluating the possible benefits of such reduction in pollutant levels as may have been achieved.

The long-term effects of the Donora disaster have also been studied in the United States.[26] The resurvey of Donora 10 years after the disastrous smog of 1948 has shown that the persons who became ill during the outbreak have had a less favorable morbidity and mortality experience than the persons who were not affected in 1948. While it is true that those who became ill were probably less healthy to begin with than who did not, it is likely that chronic effects due to unusually high levels of air pollution have been manifested in the affected group. Further, it is possible that repeated exposure to air pollution, even at very low levels, may have contributed to the long-term unfavorable experience.

The responsibility of air pollutants for the increasing frequency of lung cancer in the United States is at the moment a matter of some disagreement. Authoritative quantitative estimates of the role of air pollution as an etiologic agent do not exist, and only informed guesses can be made. Nevertheless, it is our thesis that, without decrying the importance of cigarette smoking as a factor, air pollution is also an important etiologic agent. This is not a novel idea. The World Health Organization report on lung cancer mentioned a number of possible etiologic agents and noted the prominence of air pollution in the list.[27] Once again the sharp urban-rural differential in mortality rates for this disease is manifested. Also, lung cancer mortality rates appear to be related to the size of the urban area, the larger areas having the higher age-standardized mortality ratios.

The studies by Dean[28] and Eastcott[29] on migrants from Britain to South Africa and New Zealand suggest the role of air pollution as a causative factor in lung cancer. Unfortunately, there is no completed comparable study as yet in the United States. A study of British and Scandinavian migrants to the United States is underway, but we will have to wait several years for the results.

CONCLUSIONS

The great volume and variety of air pollutants in the United States offer unparalleled opportunities to study the chronic effects of low-level air pollution on health. In what other country is there amassed the concentration of automobiles found in Los Angeles with its resultant oxidant type of smog? The lethal concentration of pollutants in Donora in 1948 created a far different air pollution problem than is found currently on the west coast. In the United States, air pollution arises from many and varied sources in every category, industrial, residential, municipal, and automotive, and makes necessary a wider range of research activities than in many other countries.

In summary, we in the United States are devoting considerable time and effort to this important question: Does longtime exposure to low concentrations of air pollution result in adverse health effects? Our preliminary answer, based on both laboratory and epidemiologic studies, is yes. The evidence as yet is only qualitative; much more will have to be done before the necessary quantitative answers are found on which to base rational control standards. Hopefully, with the data the Public Health Service is able to collect and that amassed by researchers in Europe and throughout the world, this goal can be attained.

1. Stokinger, H. E., Wagner, W. D., and Dobrogorski, O. J.: Ozone toxicity studies. III. Chronic injury to lungs of animals following exposure at a low level. *A.M.A. Arch. Indust. H.* 16:514–522, December 1957.

2. Ball, C. O. T., et al.: Survival of rats chronically exposed to sulfur dioxide. *Physiologist* 3:15, August 1960.

3. Amdur, M. O., Silverman, L., and Drinker, P.: Inhalation of sulfuric acid mist by human subjects. *A.M.A. Arch. Indust. Hyg. & Occup. Med.* 6:305–313, October 1952.

4. Amdur, M. O., Melvin, W. W., Jr., and Drinker, P.: Effects of inhalation of sulfur dioxide by man. *Lancet* 2:758–759, October 10, 1953.

5. Research in air pollution; conference report. *Pub. Health Rep.* 75: 1173–1189, December 1960.

6. Hofreuter, D. H.: The automotive exhaust problem. *A.M.A. Arch. Environ. H.* 2:559–563, May 1961.

7. Hofreuter, D. H., Catcott, E. J., and Xintaras, C.: Carboxyhemoglobin in men exposed to carbon monoxide, *A.M.A. Arch. Environ. H.* 4:81–85, January 1962.

8. Rose, A. H., Jr., Stahman, R. C., and Stevenson, H. J. R.: *Exhaust contamination in passenger cars.* Technical Report A61–2. Robert A. Taft Sanitary Engineering Center, Public Health Service, Cincinnati, Ohio, February 1961.

9. U.S. Public Health Service: *Six years of research in air pollution, July 1, 1955, to June 30, 1961.* Washington, D.C., 1961 (*a*) p. 196, (*b*) pp. 204–208, (*c*) p. 137.

10. Clayton, G. D., Cook, W. A., and Frederick, W. G.: A study of the relationship of street level carbon monoxide concentrations to traffic accidents. *Am. Indust. Hyg. A. J.* 21: 46–54, February 1960.

11. Wiseley, D. V., Kotin, P., Fowler, P. R., and Trivedi, J.: The combined effect of repeated viral infection on pulmonary tumor induction in C57 black mice. *Proc. Am. A. Cancer Res.* 3:278 (1961).

12. Kotin, P.: *Combination of stimuli in experimental lung cancer.* Presented at the Fifth Air Pollution Medical Research Conference, Los Angeles, Calif., December 4–7, 1961.

13. Greenburg, L., et al.: Report of an air pollution incident in New York City, November 1953. *Pub. Health Rep.* 77:7–16, January 1962.

14. Greenburg, L., Field, F., Reed, J. I., and Erhardt, C. L.: Air pollution and morbidity in New York City. *J.A.M.A.* In press.

15. Schoettlin, C. E., and Landau, E.: Air pollution and asthmatic attacks in the Los Angeles area. *Pub. Health Rep.* 76:545–548, June 1961.

16. Zeidberg, L. D., Prindle, R. A., and Landau, E.: The Nashville air pollution study: I. Sulfur dioxide and bronchial asthma; a preliminary report. *Am. Rev. Resp. Dis.* 84:489–503, October 1961.

17. Phelps, H. W., Sobel, G. W., and Fisher, N. E.: Air pollution asthma among military personnel in Japan. *J.A.M.A.* 175:990–993, March 18, 1961.

18. Dohan, F. C.: Air pollutants and incidence of respiratory disease. *A.M.A. Arch. Environ. H.* 3:387–395, October 1961.

19. Ogilvie, A. G., and Newell, D. J.: *Chronic bronchitis in Newcastle-Upon-Tyne.* Livingstone, Ltd., Edinburgh and London, 1957, p. 2.

20. U.S. National Office of Vital Statistics: *Vital Statistics of the United States:* 1950, 1959. U.S. Government Printing Office, Washington, D.C., 1952, 1961.

21. Prindle, R. A.: Some considerations in the interpretation of air pollution health effects data. *J. Air Pollut. Control A.* 9:12–19 (1959).

22. U.S. Social Security Administration: *Disability applicants under the Old-Age Survivors and Disability Insurance Program, 1960.* Social Security Administration, Washington, D.C., January 1962, tables 10 and 11.

23. Williams, G.: *Program possibilities in respiratory diseases.* Presented at the 58th annual meeting of the National Tuberculosis Association, Miami Beach, Fla., May 20–23, 1962.

24. Prindle, R. A., et al.: Comparison of pulmonary function and other parameters in two communities with widely different air pollution levels. *Am. J. Pub. Health.* In press.

25. World Health Organization: *Air pollution.* WHO Monograph Series No. 46, Geneva, 1961.

26. Ciocco, A., and Thompson, D. J.: A follow-up of Donora ten years after: methodology and findings. *Am. J. Pub. Health* 51:155–164, February 1961.

27. World Health Organization: *Epidemiology of cancer of the lung; report of a study group.* WHO Technical Report Series No. 192, Geneva, 1960, pp. 5–6.

28. Dean, G.: Lung cancer among white South Africans. Report on a further study. *Brit. M.J.* 16:1599–1605, December 16, 1961.

29. Eastcott, D. F.: The epidemiology of lung cancer in New Zealand. *Lancet* 1:37–39, January 7, 1956.

The Epidemiology of Motor Vehicle Accidents*

ROSS A. MACFARLAND, PH.D.

ACCIDENTS constitute a greater threat to many segments of our population than does disease. Incapacity and loss of life resulting from accidents have increased extensively, and accidental deaths now exceed the combined deaths from all infectious and communicable diseases (excluding chronic diseases). Year after year, the National Safety Council has been reporting more than 90,000 persons killed in accidents, about 400,000 permanently disabled, and almost 10 million injured severely enough to disable them for more than one day.[1] Using the criterion of injuries requiring the attention of a physician or one or more days of inactivity, the National Health Survey, conducted in 1957, suggests that accidental injuries are even more prevalent. On this basis, the total number of persons receiving nonfatal injuries is approximately 49 million in a single year.[2]

Of special importance is the fact that accidents now rank first as a cause of death between the ages of one and 35 years and are outranked in the older age groups chiefly by cancer, heart disorders, and the so-called degenerative diseases. The fact that most accident victims are in the younger age groups implies an enormous cost to the productive resources of our country.

The accidents which result in injury or death take place on the highway, at home, at work or school, in recreational activities, and in many other places. Motor vehicle accidents over the past few years have been responsible for about 38,000 deaths annually, or about 40 per cent of the total for all kinds of accidents. It should be of special interest to physicians that, while mileage death rates have shown an improvement over the years, the motor vehicle fatality rates based on the total population of the United States have remained at essentially the same level for the past decade. Apparently one may expect to drive farther in a given year without being killed but still be as likely to be killed within that time as previously.

Measurement of the fact that a death has occurred is less meaningful than the measurement of how much lifetime has been lost prematurely. If one takes the average life expectancy tables from the vital statistics reports of the United States and multiplies these figures at

* Reprinted, with omission of four figures and one table, by permission from the April 28th 1962 issue of the *Journal of American Medical Ass'n.*, Volume 180, pp. 289–300. This paper was presented at the session on Medical Aspects of Automobile Injuries and Deaths, at the 110th Annual Meeting of the American Medical Association, New York, New York, June 27, 1961. The author is the Daniel and Florence Guggenheim Professor of Aerospace Health and Safety at the Harvard School of Public Health, formerly Professor of Environmental Health and Safety, Boston, Massachusetts.

each level by the number of motor vehicle accident deaths, one can estimate the years of expected life lost. In 1957, this figure amounted to approximately 1.5 million years. The highest concentration of life years lost was between 15 and 25 years of age, and approximately one-half of the total occurred between 15 and 30 years of age.

The number of males killed on the highway exceeds the number of females killed by almost 3 to 1, and the disproportion is marked in the age range from 20 to 40 years, in which men outnumber women about 6 to 1. It is also noteworthy that about one-fourth of the pedestrian fatalities are men over 65 years old.[3]

Nonfatal injury from motor vehicle accidents also predominates in young men. Of the 4.7 millions estimated to be injured annually, according to the National Health Survey, more than one-fourth are in the 15 to 24 year range. More than one-half of all persons requiring hospitalization for injuries received the injuries in motor vehicle accidents.

It is important to question what is actually known about the various causes of motor vehicle accidents and injuries, and what is their relative prominence. The data in routine accident reports have not been revealing in this regard. Except in limited areas, little information is available concerning the basic causes of accidents. Alcohol is beginning to emerge as a major factor, but what is known of the relative frequency of mechanical malfunction, inadequate design from the standpoint of human engineering, or particular medical disorders as causes of accidents? What do we know of the effectiveness of any of the accident-prevention remedies which have been applied?

A great deal of research has been carried out in the field of highway accidents, but our knowledge and methods of control are limited. A critical analysis reveals a great many shortcomings which pertain to the studies which have been attempted. These are: (1) inadequate time sampling and criteria of accidents; (2) studies of single variables out of context; (3) poor sampling techniques, especially lack of control groups; (4) lack of appropriate statistical procedures; and (5) conclusions based on intuitive, rather empiric information. There is urgent need for careful, well-designed, and relevant research in the field of highway safety.[4]

In many areas in the deficiencies of our knowledge of the causes of motor vehicle accidents and injuries, physicians, by nature of their training and capabilities, can make significant contributions. A recent survey among the medical profession indicated that a great majority of physicians believe they have a responsibility in accident prevention. The major need appeared to be a more definite blueprint of what to do and how to do it.

In recent years, the traditional function of medicine, to treat disease and injury, has been broadened to include the prevention of disease. Extending responsibility to include the prevention of injury and disease is logical, not only because physicians and surgeons must care for the injured, but also because their broad training in the biologic sciences and their role in teaching and advising patients places them in a favorable position to make significant contributions. This is particularly true, since human factors play such a predominant role in the causation of most accidents. Furthermore, the most effective kind of teaching may be carried out under conditions which have an emotional background, to reinforce the ideas involved.

More specifically, the responsibility of the physician for reducing motor vehicle injuries and deaths would include: (1) measures insuring the existence of effective emergency services for accident victims, and (2) measures directed towards the prevention of the accidents. Some examples of the latter would be: (1) cooperating with authorities to remove hazardous drivers from the road, by, for instance, the determination of blood alcohol levels of individuals apprehended for driving under its influence, (2) assisting State motor vehicle departments in establishing sound policies formed on a basis of scientific fact, in regard to medical problem drivers, (3) participating in research programs directed to the acquisition of basic knowledge of accident causes, and (4) the indoctrination of individual patients in regard to medical fitness in order to drive with safety.[5,6]

EPIDEMIOLOGIC APPROACH TO
ACCIDENT PREVENTION

THE EPIDEMIOLOGIC METHOD. One of the greatest difficulties in understanding the basic causes of accidents has been the lack of an over-all conceptional framework within which the results of different approaches and different kinds of data might be integrated. In recent years it has been demonstrated that accidental injuries on the highway are amenable to study by methods evolved for the investigation of contagious and epidemic diseases. Thus, the epidemiologic approach offers one of the most promising methods for overcoming the difficulties which have retarded effective study in the accident field.

EXTENSION OF THE EPIDEMIOLOGIC METHOD TO ACCIDENTS. It is not generally appreciated that accidents exhibit some of the same biologic and physical interrelationships as do disease processes. When the prevalance and incidence of accidental injuries have been analyzed in a standard epidemiologic manner, it has been shown that accident distributions, like disease, show characteristic variations. They occur at different rates and in regard to different agents and circumstances among different groups of the population.

It is clear that there are specific variables which can be isolated and that the pathogenesis of accidental injury, as in the case of disease, arises in the presence of a susceptible host, a predisposing environment, and an inciting agent. Thus, the etiology of such events involves a study of the interrelationships between the host, the agent, and the environment, as they combine together in producing an accident.

The first step is an epidemiologic approach to accidents involves a study of their distribution in terms of who had the accidents, when, where, and how they occurred, with regard to different classes of accidents or agents and mechanisms of injury.[8] This step represents the descriptive phase of epidemiology and is usually carried out in terms of data available from existing sources, such as vital statistics, official reports, and various public records. It is important, in assessing the magnitude and scope of the over-all problem, to consider the relative significance of various classes or circumstances of accidents in contributing to the total. Furthermore, this aids in the identification of segments of the population for which accidental injury is disproportionately high or in which specific types of accidents are frequent. This step also serves as a starting point for the development of causal hypotheses to explain associations apparent in the data, and for more analytic, detailed studies to test these hypotheses. When the basic physical, physiologic, and psychologic characteristics of the host are associated with the agent, i.e., the vehicle, under any given set of environmental conditions, information can be obtained which will aid in the understanding and prevention of accidents. Factual information of this kind can be discovered only by carefully controlled experimental studies, epidemiological surveys, and statistical analyses.

ILLUSTRATION OF THE EPIDEMIOLOGIC APPROACH TO THE ANALYSIS AND CONTROL OF MOTOR VEHICLE ACCIDENTS. In the Armed Services the off-duty motor vehicle accident has been a particularly vexing problem, ranking ahead of diseases and all other types of accidents in causing death, disability, and noneffectiveness.[9] Attempted preventive measures center about the control of weekend passes to lessen the mileage driven at these times. An epidemiologic analysis carried out at a large military base revealed that the chief problem was not the week-end, long-distance trip but the late at night and early morning driving relatively close to the base, throughout the week as well as on weekends. Approximately 70 per cent of the accidents occurred within 10 miles of the base, and over 90 per cent within 50 miles. Several sections of highway were especially involved. One segment of the driving population of the base was identified as having a disproportionately high frequency of accidents and as one which should be the object of preventive measures. This group comprised the younger, unmarried, enlisted men living on base in government quarters. Their accidents occurred chiefly during the late night and early morning hours in connection with the search for recreational activities (especially tavern-hopping).[10]

Recommendations for several specific control measures were made on the basis of the findings, and it was possible to carry out an evaluation of the effectiveness of one of the proposed procedures. For a period of 10 weeks, military police patrolled five high-accident sections of the highway in accordance with a predetermined schedule during off-duty hours. These patrols stopped at random private cars bearing the base tag and secured from each driver information about himself, the origin and destination of his trip, and a number of other items. They also took into protective custody those drivers who appeared excessively fatigued or under the influence of alcohol. After the patrol countermeasure was introduced, the accident rate dropped 42 per cent and remained at a lower rate for 9 weeks after the experiment was terminated. A comparison of the rates with those of the corresponding period for the previous year confirmed the improvement.[10]

APPLICATION OF EPIDEMIOLOGIC PRINCIPLES FOR THE PREVENTION OF MOTOR VEHICLE ACCIDENTS

The general epidemiologic principles of control involve, either singly or in combination, (1) reducing the susceptibility of the host, (2) making the agent less hazardous, and (3) modifying the environment to lessen the possibility of adverse host-agent interactions. While much of the essential information in the field of highway accidents remains to be derived, some factual data have been obtained in regard to each of these areas.

Thus far, appreciable associations between the characteristics of persons and accident frequencies have been found for only a limited number of factors, including those which are of a relatively temporary nature. Some of the important general characteristics which will be discussed are: youth and sex; lack of training; history of repeated accidents; inferior personal-social adjustments; certain attitudes and values; and skill changes in elderly drivers.

CHARACTERISTICS OF PERSONS ASSOCIATED WITH HIGHER ACCIDENT RATES. The evidence of the past few years indicates that youthful drivers, as a group, are more frequently involved in accidents and show higher accident rates than would be expected on the basis of their numbers in the driving population. For example, two recent studies, in Connecticut and Massachusetts, indicate that the rates are highest for the youngest drivers, those of age 16, which in these two states is the minimum age for licensing. The rate decreases with succeeding years of age, so that at about age 25 to 30 the involvement rate becomes lower than would be expected if age were of no significance.

The question of whether there is a difference between youthful males and females in regard to motor vehicles accident rates is difficult to answer because of variation in the amounts and kinds of driving. Based only on the number of drivers, without reference to how much they drive—i.e., exposure to the possibility of accidents—it appears that female drivers are far less frequently involved in accidents than males. As far as the question of the relative safety of driving by girls and boys or young women and young men is concerned, however, these figures are not helpful, because they do not take into account the fact that youthful males drive a great deal more than females. If boys and young men drive three times more than equal-aged members of the opposite sex, they acquire three times as much exposure to the possibility of accidents; on that basis, there would be very little difference, if any, between the safety records of the two sexes. Moreover, it is known that the peak of annual driving mileage occurs later for females, at the ages at which they are driving to supermarkets, to bridge clubs, and chauffeuring children. Accident rates for women are highest at these later ages.[11]

The evidence that accident rates among young drivers are disproportionately high presents the paradox that the driver is most susceptible to accidents at the time of his greatest potential operating skill, in terms of such factors as reaction times and physical coordination. Hence youthfulness, rather than age, per se, has been cited as the important factor. The factors underlying this youthfulness have usually been interpreted as inexperience, various factors of immaturity, and attitudes particularly characteristic of youth.

Accidents are characteristically most frequent during the early phases of learning a new job or skill and decrease with increasing time on the job. It would be reasonable to assume that the same situation would prevail on the highway. In the process of learning to drive, there are many accident-potential situations which are never encountered, and practice in handling such situations is not gained except during the course of acquiring further experience. The judgment of traffic situations is perhaps the most important factor in whether an accident occurs, and developing this judgment depends on actual experience on the road.[11] The driver may often operate with insufficient margins of safety, simply because his experience has not yet been sufficient to enable him to appreciate completely the speeds with which emergency situations develop and his own limitations in regard to the time relationships and physical forces involved.

Closely allied to the factor of experience is that of training. Adequate training has been shown to be a very important method of keeping accidents low in many types of activity. In regard to highway safety, many studies have been made of the effectiveness of driver training. The results are in fairly good agreement that drivers who have taken formal driver training tend to have fewer accidents and violations than those who learned to drive in other ways.

Although it is clear that trained drivers initially have better records than the untrained, the studies made thus far do not conclusively indicate that the better record is solely the effect of the training. The studies do not eliminate the possibility that those electing to take driver training may be those who would have better attitudes toward safety and be safer drivers in any event. Experimental evidence on this point has been limited until recently. One study of teen-age drivers who were given psychologic tests prior to their being old enough to learn to drive has indicated that those who later elected to take driver training were indeed different in several personality traits and adjustment tendencies from those who later rejected driver training and learned to drive in other ways.[9]

The latter point does not imply that driver training has no beneficial effect. The control it can provide the driver and the development of attitudes favorable to safe driving are in themselves justification for driver training programs.

One concept which has been prominent is that certain persons suffer accidents repeatedly on the basis of their inherent and persistent behavior tendencies and that the identification and treatment of such individuals would prevent many accidents. However, thus far, these tendencies have not been precisely defined or identified by research. Moreover, the statistical evidence is convincing that the influence of a proneness factor, where it can be detected in the accidents occuring within large groups, is limited. Furthermore, the small group of accident repeaters is a constantly shifting one over a period of time, persons dropping out of the group and new persons coming in continually.[12]

A clinical theory of accident proneness has been developed on the basis of detailed psychiatric and psychologic studies of patients who have sustained injuries.[13] In this view, a high frequency of accidents in certain individuals may be explained by abnormal characteristics of personality through which accidents serve certain emotional needs. This concept postulates a personality type or syndrome which is predisposed toward having repeated accidents. However, objective methods suitable for predictive studies are greatly needed for verification of this concept. . . .

It is questionable whether the accident proneness concept could explain an appreciable number of the cases of high frequency of accidents. Proneness would be but one of many factors influencing the frequency. Some persons are accident repeaters on the basis of chance alone; others have more accidents than their fellows because they are more frequently exposed to risk. It would be more profitable in accident research to concentrate on the specific causes of repeated accidents and to try to identify those specific personality character-istics that are associated with repeated accidents for which the in-dividual is primarily responsible.

A promising concept is that frequent accidents in an individual represent one manifestation of a poor adjustment in meeting the social and personal demands of life. That is, if a person repeatedly makes mistakes in meeting his personal and social obligations, he is also likely to make errors in other activities while at work, at play, or driving. This concept implies that a man works or drives as he lives. It was developed by comparing the frequencies of various kinds of antisocial behavior or inadequate personal adjustments in the accident repeaters and accident-free individuals in groups of industrial workers and taxi drivers.[14] Objective support has been given to this concept. Several studies have now demonstrated that accident repeaters are far more likely to be known to such agencies as the courts, collection and credit organizations, Public Health and venereal disease clinics, and social welfare agencies than are accident-free subjects matched to them with respect of age, experience, and exposure to risk.

The attempt was made in one study at Harvard University to use the number of contacts with agencies of the foregoing types as a score to predict the accident repeaters in a group of truck drivers. The im-portance of a number of items from public and social agency records in distinguishing between accident-free and accident-repeater drivers in a large group of truck drivers was determined statistically. When the chi-square values for the most discriminating items were applied as weights to similar items in a score for drivers in a new group, it was possible to classify the accident-repeater drivers with an accuracy of over 80 per cent.[15]

The identification of the attitudes underlying unsafe behavior has been difficult, partly because of the unreliability of measuring atti-tudes and basic personality traits. However, attitudes are regarded by many as a host characteristic of the greatest importance, and most safety education and propaganda is directed toward establishing safe attitudes.

The role of traits of personality and attitudes has received a great deal of attention in the field of highway safety. It seems quite logical that risk-taking behavior would be influenced by such factors as atti-tudes towards speed, traffic regulations, competing traffic, the actions of other drivers, and the social and legal restraints. However, there is little evidence of what the attitudes of safe versus unsafe drivers may be. One extensive study among military personnel has indicated that the two groups differ in regard to the personal values they hold.

Accident-prone drivers, as compared to those having few accidents, consistently scored higher on the "theoretical" and "esthetic" scales of the Allport-Vernon test of values, while scoring low on the "religious" scale. From a psychodynamic point of view, drivers with high accident rates tended to find the social environment barren and unrewarding, did not identify themselves with parents, regarded authority figures as unpleasant, and showed regressive, masochistic trends in their phantasies.[17]

Another study was specifically directed toward the teen-age driver. Of two groups of students from various high schools in Pennsylvania,[18] drivers in the first group had had two or more traffic accidents. Those in the second group were chosen to match the individuals in the first group, with respect to geographic location and length of driving experience, but had had no accidents. It was found that the youthful drivers having accidents tended to score high, and those free of accidents tended to score low with regard to each or a combination of the following attitudes toward driving: (1) as activity which relieves psychic tension; (2) as a form of behavior by which youthfulness may be compensated for and the role of an adult may be assumed; (3) as a form of behavior in which confidence in one's ability may be manifested; (4) which does not consider speed as an element of danger, but, if it is considered dangerous, as an attitude manifesting desire for danger; and (5) which places greater emphasis on the power of a vehicle than on its style or utility.

On the personality tests it was found that the youths who had had accidents showed more disregard of social mores, more defiance of authority, and more of a tendency to excessive activity and enthusiasm. On the basis of items in the various scales, it was concluded that persons who have had the following experiences are more likely to manifest the kind of behavior which results in accidents: (1) a drive to leave home, (2) an urge to do something harmful or shocking, (3) a tendency to be influenced by people about them, (4) association with peers to whom parents object, (5) a desire to frighten other individuals for the fun of it, (6) a tendency to become readily impatient with people, (7) a tendency to be somewhat suspicious of overfriendly people, and (8) a possibility of having been in trouble with the law.

Factors which are characteristic of older persons are also reflected in the accident statistics. Several recent studies have indicated an upturn in accident rates for older drivers beyond about age 60. Apparently there is also an increased frequency of older drivers being judged at fault in the accidents in which they are involved. Such driving errors leading to accidents as failing to grant right of way, improper turning, and driving in the wrong lane or on the wrong side of the road appear to be particularly characteristic of the older driver.[19-21]

Slow reaction times and sensory deterioration have been proposed as important causes of motor vehicle accidents among the elderly. Experimental studies on aging suggest, however, that changes in simple reaction times and sensory measures are of less importance than central nervous system changes which relate to the organization of perceptions. In older persons the mechanisms concerned with organizing incoming stimuli are less efficient, and more time or stronger signals are required to assess the meaning of new situations. The delay in response due to this factor is appreciably greater than the slowing of specific movements. Older persons are apt to become muddled when they have to organize changing patterns of stimuli and carry out a sequence of responses within a short period of time.

TEMPORARY CONDITIONS IN DRIVERS RELATED TO THE RISK OF ACCIDENTS. A number of specific variables having a temporary influence on safe driving are relevant to the control of host factors. Some of the areas of greatest importance are (1) deterioration of skill with fatigue; (2) disorganization of skill by emotional states; (3) effects of alcohol on driving; (4) the role of disease processes; and (5) the influence of drugs and medications.

Statistics from various fields have often been cited to show that as persons become tired they are more likely to experience accidents. On the highway, the effects of fatigue are most obvious in "driver-asleep" accidents. In many others, however, it is difficult to determine the influence of fatigue. It has been demonstrated that subjects do less well on a variety of psychologic and psychomotor tasks after prolonged driving. This fact has been interpreted to indicate reduced efficiency and hence increased liability to accidents. Such findings provide some basis for the regulations governing hours of driving and intervening rest periods which have been adopted for commercial drivers by the Interstate Commerce Commission.[12]

The role of fatigue in highway safety, however, involves more than the hours of driving. Actually, in the case of truck drivers, the greatest frequency of accidents (about 60 per cent) has been found within the first three hours of driving rather than near the end of the day's run. The amount and quality of previous rest, length of time since last rest, nature of activities prior to driving, and concurrent emotional stress are some of the numerous complicating factors.

Confidential interviews with professional long-haul truck drivers have revealed that under conditions of extreme fatigue, hallucinations and illusions of obstacles on the highway may be experienced. Experiences of this kind were reported by 37 of a sample of 53 drivers. Some accidents have occurred as a result of efforts to avoid the hallucinated animals or objects on the roadway. The following report is an example:

> The operator of a semitrailer, traveling on a flat, straight stretch of roadway during the middle of the night, in clear weather, suddenly "saw" a calf standing in the road ahead. He swerved his vehicle sharply to the left and it overturned in the roadway. A second vehicle belonging to the same company was following close behind. Separate reports were made by each driver, but the second driver denied the presence of the calf. An interview with the first driver revealed that, while extremely sleepy, he had frequently seen "things that are not there." On repeated occasions he had "seen" herds of mules in bright, shining harness crossing the roadway in front of him. After an emergency stop he would realize that the mules were really nonexistent and that he had been "dreaming."[16]

Some accidents on the highway have been traced to preoccupation with anxieties or carrying over emotional states, such as anger, into the manner of driving. However, the usual investigation of accidents does not often include an evaluation of such factors. It is well known that when people are emotionally upset or preoccupied, some disorganization of behavior is likely to occur. Under such circumstances, one may misinterpret the meaning of a situation or ignore important stimuli. Thus, inappropriate responses may be made. For example, under stress, it is quite common for a previously established response to break through, in place of one more recently learned and more appropriate.

Alcohol is frequently cited as a cause of motor vehicle accidents, but precise appraisal of the problem has been difficult. Complete and accurate determinations of alcohol in the body fluids of drivers and pedestrians have rarely been available. The National Safety Council has indicated that in 1959 one of every five drivers involved in a fatal motor vehicle accident and one of four adult pedestrians killed had been drinking.[1] These figures are believed to be conservative in the light of recent evidence.[23]

Many statistical studies indicate that large numbers of drivers become involved in accidents after drinking, but very few yield information on what the risk of an accident may be or on the association between accident likelihood and the amount of drinking. Data from one controlled study suggest that the risk of becoming involved in an accident when the blood alcohol level is 0.10 per cent is more than twice that when the blood alcohol level is 0.05 per cent. It becomes approximately 10-fold at levels of 0.15 per cent and above. Additional data also show that as the level of blood alcohol increases, there is an increase in driving errors leading directly to accidents.[24]

One of the implications of such studies is that the risk of accidents is not only greater after alcohol ingestion, but also that an increase in risk appears at relatively low levels of alcohol in the blood. This is also borne out by direct experiments on the effect of alcohol on driving skill and performance. For example, the scores of 160 drivers on an extensive operational driving test averaged 25 per cent to 35 per cent poorer at blood alcohol levels of 0.40 per cent to 0.06 per cent compared to their scores before drinking. An increase in errors was apparent in some when the blood alcohol level was only 0.032 per cent.

Physicians should indoctrinate their patients regarding the effects of alcohol. For example, it is not realized generally by the layman that, after being absorbed, alcohol is eliminated from the blood stream and tissues of every person at a rate of only about 10 ml. (one-third ounce) per hour, and that common procedures such as exercise and drinking of black coffee do not affect this rate. As a result, blood alcohol levels may remain significantly elevated for an appreciable period after drinking. In one experiment, a subject consumed the alcohol equivalent of eight highballs over a period of four hours. The blood alcohol level reached 0.15 per cent in slightly more than two hours from the beginning of the period and remained above this level for nine hours; 14 hours after the last drink was finished the blood alcohol level was still 0.09 per cent. Such data are in part the basis for the regulation adopted by the airlines and supported by the pilots' union that pilots abstain from alcohol for 18 hours before flying. Medical departments in highway transportation industries might consider the advisability of a similar practice for commercial drivers.[5]

The role of various disease processes and physical defects as a predisposing factor in accidents is of special concern. It is reasonable to assume that reduced alertness, faulty sensorium, impaired coordination, disturbed balance, and the like may contribute to an accident when a person thus afflicted encounters a hazardous situation.

Dramatic accounts occasionally appear in the newspapers of drivers who have experienced serious accidents because of advanced physical disabilities, such as heart failure, diabetes, and epilepsy. Only limited information is available, however, on the frequency of such occurrences or for the development of criteria for advising patients or establishing standards of physical fitness for driving.

One of the most important medical considerations relates to the likelihood of a sudden impairment or loss of consciousness in the driver. Interesting data on this subject have come from an analysis of the medical and accident records of the London Transport Executive in England. This public transportation agency has on the average about 20,000 bus drivers in its employ. During the 11-year period from 1949 through 1959, there were 46 instances of a driver losing consciousness while operating a bus. Accidents resulted in 26 of the 46 cases. In view of the approximately 220,000 driver-years during this period, loss of consciousness seems a relatively infrequent happening. However, in an operation of the size of the London Transport Executive, one such instance occurs every 10 months.[25]

In the cited study, myocardial infarction was found in 14 of the 46 drivers losing consciousness while at the controls of a bus. Two of the vehicles were stationary at the time of the attack. In the 12 cases when the bus was in motion, seven of the drivers had sufficient warning to be able to stop without accident. Collisions resulted in the other five.[25]

The opinion has been expressed that heart disease, leading to sudden collapse, is probably of less importance in the total number of accidents than cerebral arteriosclerosis present in the older segment of the driving population. Some medical authorities believe that epilepsy and diabetes, when undiagnosed or improperly managed, may account for the great majority of blackouts. Thus, these diseases may constitute the greatest hazard among the various conditions involved in impaired consciousness while driving.[6]

The objection has been raised that an arbitrary prohibition of driving by all persons afflicted with certain conditions would be needlessly restrictive and unfair to many persons who are capable of driving responsibly and safely. In some States the cooperation of the medical profession has been enlisted to help the motor vehicle administrator handle these problems on an individual basis, to allow driving by persons in cases in which safety would not be jeopardized. In Massachusetts, for example, certain special-risk drivers may obtain licenses and drive under a program of continuing medical surveillance. This policy covers persons with such diagnoses as epilepsy, diabetes, and multiple sclerosis, as well as those with amputations, hemiplegias, and paraplegias. Thus far, the safety record of this group has been satisfactory.

The American public is reluctant to accept limitations on personal freedom, especially regarding the privilege to drive. For example, most authorities agree that a diabetic patient who requires insulin should not drive a school bus or a public conveyance. However, if the problem of medical fitness to drive is to be satisfactorily worked out, there must be large-scale and long-range studies of patients with these diseases. No one has yet carried out a scientifically controlled study showing that drivers with any disease, including deafness, epilepsy, color-blindness, diabetes, cardiac disease, or musculoskeletal handicaps, have a higher accident rate than otherwise comparable groups.

Physicians are aware of the possible influence on safety of the principal action or side effects of medications and drugs prescribed and those available over the counter for self-prescription. Unless patients are instructed, they may not realize that the effects of a sedative persist up to 24 hours after the ingestion of some preparations in the dosages ordinarily prescribed for relaxation and sleep. A dangerous attitude of overconfidence is reported to be produced in some persons by certain energizing or tranquilizing agents, and slowed reaction times are said to result from certain of the tranquilizing drugs.[6] After self-medication with proprietary preparations to relieve pain or the symptoms of a cold, disturbances of vision and equilibrium and episodes of drowsiness have been reported in some persons. Preliminary findings from research on the effect of various drugs on human behavior and efficiency suggest that attitudes and motivation may be influenced by relatively small doses of a large number of substances. If the changes observed after the ingestion of certain of these compounds were carried over into driving practices, safety would be compromised.[6]

THE VEHICLE WITH REGARD TO HIGHWAY SAFETY. In various fields of medicine it has been possible to control a disease once the agent has been clearly identified. In the field of highway safety, the agent is the automobile and its various components. It would be possible to reduce injuries and fatalities if the driver and passengers could be adequately protected during a crash either by restraining devices or by vehicles so designed that severe injuries would not be produced.

The automobile manufacturers have developed many new features in their equipment which have contributed to safety, for example, improved braking and steering systems, lighting, tires, and many other items. The power and performance of engines have also been improved, but this variable does not always contribute to safety unless wisely controlled by the driver. All of the manufacturers have contributed safety features in recent years, such as stronger door locks. Other items are being developed, and the biologic and medical scientist should be able to contribute more precise criteria on the tolerances and limitations of the human body. Such information should aid the engineer in designing to these requirements.

It is obvious that basic research on the human factors in automotive safety should be expanded so as to provide convincing evidence for additional safety considerations in design. The Cornell Crash Injury Project is identifying some of the relevant items. Also, the precise measurement of impact forces in motor vehicle crashes, both in regard to the equipment itself and to the occupants, is being carried out experimentally. Additional design criteria should result from these studies.

It is of interest that the automobile manufacturing companies are developing human engineering programs, and this trend should be encouraged. Some of the principal areas involved in this concept are: (1) adequate dimensioning and adjustability of seats; (2) location and design of controls for safe and efficient operation; (3) windshield and window design for maximum visibility; (4) design of instruments to give essential information rapidly; and (5) design for crash protection of occupants.

Many accidents occur because the physical dimensions and abilities of the users of equipment and their sensory and psychologic capacities and limitations have not been adequately considered in the original design of the equipment. Considerations which are important in regard to efficiency and safety in the design of equipment for human use are as follows: (1) Difficulties may result from neglect of consideration of variations in body size and biomechanics. (2) Errors frequently occur in the use of equipment which interferes with established habit patterns. (3) Errors are likely when excessive or inappropriate demands are made upon perceptual capacities. (4) Mistakes in the use of equipment may be due to poor arrangement or design of the operating controls.

In the automotive field, examples of faulty design in modern vehicles may be found from the standpoint of the range in body size of the drivers, the biomechanics of human movements and postures, and the characteristics and limits of human perception. A few illustrations are taken from an evaluation of recent model trucks.[9,16]

A common defect is insufficient range of adjustability in the seat, either horizontally or vertically. Again, important controls are often placed too far away. For example, in one model only 5 per cent of the drivers could reach and operate the handbrake from the normal driving position. Clearances are frequently inadequate; in one model only the shortest 40 per cent of drivers could get the knee under the steering wheel when raising the foot to the brake pedal. Within the car or truck, instruments are frequently designed or placed so that they cannot be read accurately and rapidly. Knobs and switches are sometimes identical in design and cannot be distinguished from each other readily. Often they are located so that they can be operated inadvertently or by mistake.

The advance analysis of equipment in the interests of safety requires an operational analysis of the task, including a survey of the responses to be performed, the layout of the working area, the location of controls and instruments, and the way the operator carries out his reactions. A functional concept of accidents is a basic consideration. That is, the errors and accidents which may occur during operation should be anticipated. Human limitations also must be considered. If the duties are too complex, the operator may be forced beyond his limits of attention and ability. Finally, a wide margin of safety should be provided to prevent situations which place the operator near his maximum aptitude or effort, especially as adverse factors such as fatigue or physiologic stress are encountered.

If the viewpoint of human engineering, or biotechnology, is carried out in practice, fewer errors and accidents in the operation of equipment should result.

ENVIRONMENTAL INFLUENCES ON SAFE DRIVING. In many instances the control of accidents depends on the identification of specific char-acteristics in the environment and some means of regulating the inter-action between the driver (host factors), his vehicle (the agent), and the environment. A number of the more important environmental in-fluences on safe driving are: (1) extremes in the physical environ-ment, e.g., temperature and toxic agents; (2) low levels of illumination and efficiency of vision; (3) adverse road conditions and driving practices; (4) poor design of highways as sources of error; and (5) the psychosocial environment and control measures.

Certain atmospheric or climatic variables may affect the frequency of accidents by influencing human behavior as well as by creating specific environmental hazards. Cold temperatures, for example, pro-duce risks such as slippery roads and frosted windshields. Cold also results in impaired dexterity and muscular control in persons with chilled extremities, enhancing accidents. Although no data are avail-able for the analysis of the effects of temperature upon driver safety, an increase in accident rates among industrial workers is well docu-mented for low and high temperatures. Also, laboratory studies have demonstrated deterioration in a variety of tasks requiring psycho-motor coordination and vigilance as temperatures rise toward 90°F., (32.2°C.). This effect is accentuated if the humidity is extremely high.[16, 28]

Toxic substances in the atmosphere are other possible sources of highway accidents. Human performance may be impaired from ex-posures to less than those amounts which produce clinical symptoms of toxicity. Carbon monoxide provides a good example. The possibility of being poisoned from this gas has been greatly reduced in the opera-tion of motor vehicles. However, small amounts will be rapidly ab-sorbed in the blood, resulting in an oxygen deficiency that is not likely to be noticed by the driver. The initial reaction consists primarily of lowered attention, difficulty in concentration, slight muscular inco-ordination, sleepiness, and mental lethargy. A marked impairment of night vision also occurs. These first symptoms are not permanently injurious but, owing to their nature, could easily involve a driver in hazardous situations.[6]

In motor vehicles, carbon monoxide usually comes from leaks in the exhaust system, but the exhaust of preceding vehicles may also be drawn in through ventilation systems. An additional amount of carbon monoxide may also be present from other sources, increasing the total effects. For example, the blood of a person who has been inhaling cigaret smoke may already contain from 5 per cent to 8 per cent carboxyhemoglobin from the tobacco smoke. This results in sufficient anoxia to reduce night vision in degree roughly comparable to the effects of an altitude of about 8,000 feet. Furthermore, any factors influencing the supply, transport, or utilization of oxygen may be additive in their effects, resulting in a state of oxygen deficiency having serious implications for safety. Alcohol, carbon monoxide, certain drugs, and high altitude provide a few samples.[5, 6]

Many examples might be given from the experimental studies in the field of the effect of low levels of illumination on visual efficiency. For example, a significant factor in host-environment relationships is efficiency of vision. In the United States, accident rates per unit of travel are three times higher at night than during the day.[1] Presumably, this is due partly to the lower visibility provided by nighttime illumination, a contention supported by lower accident rates on lighted highways and by the reduction in rates following improvement of illumination on particular highways.

Obviously any adverse influence upon the efficiency of vision at low levels of illumination would place a driver at a disadvantage. Older drivers are especially vulnerable in this connection, since the ability to see at low levels of illumination decreases regularly with increasing age. This effect is noticeable by middle age and becomes marked in the elderly. It has been calculated that for a dim light or object to be just seen by an eye in the dark, the illumination must be doubled for every increase of 13 years in age.[29] Furthermore, it has been demonstrated that recovery from glare is highly correlated with age, so that older drivers would be at a distinct disadvantage in night driving.[30]

In the field of highway safety, the use of tinted windshields by older drivers may present special hazards at night, since the glass further reduces visibility by reducing the intensity of light reaching the eye. For this reason, the denser tinting should be above the eye level of the driver. The increase in light required for threshold perception is marked as age increases. Slightly more intensity is needed at all ages when test lights are seen through ordinary clear windshield glass. When tinted glass is used, a larger increase in intensity is required.[31] This fact illustrates in quantitative terms the importance of the interrelationship between factors relating to the host, the agent, and the environment.

The atmospheric conditions outside the vehicle also have an influence upon highway safety. Rain and snow tend to be accompanied by a lower volume of traffic but with increased accident rates per unit of travel. It has been reported that accident rates on wet roads may be 20 per cent higher than on dry roads. Reduced visibility due to lower illumination or obstruction to vision is one human-related variable. Snow, rain, or sleet on the windshield has been given as a contributory cause in about one-half of the cases reported for obstructed vision. The reduction in visibility possible from rain on the windshield was found in an Air Force study to have the effect of reducing visual acuity to as low as 20/360.

Another effect of wet weather on visibility relates to changes in the reflectance characteristics of road surfaces. Seeing objects on the roadway by silhouette at night becomes more difficult, and the glare effects of extraneous lights are increased by the added specular reflection from the road surface.

Other human variables include the driving practices in relation to the reduced traction of wet, icy, or certain other types of road surfaces. For example, when skidding accidents on the Pennsylvania Turnpike were analyzed, it was apparent that the particular practices carried out by the drivers often precipitated or prolonged the skidding. It was concluded that a lack of training in proper methods of operating on slippery roads was an important causal factor in these incidents. These observations emphasize the importance of including training under various adverse conditions and in specific emergency practices. The value of such training has been well demonstrated in the field of aviation.[6, 12]

Analyses of accidents by location, and comparisons between the accident rates on highways of different types, have indicated that many hazardous features can be eliminated through traffic engineering and the design of highways.[32] As yet, only a few studies have been made to provide human engineering data relevant to the design of highways. Observation of passing maneuvers, for example, has led to criteria for the width of lanes. The determination of sight distances for no-passing zones affords another example of the necessity to consider data on human capabilities, such as the time required in making a decision to carry out a given maneuver.

Perhaps the area in which there has been greatest emphasis on the role of human factors relates to criteria for highway signs and markers. There is now a substantial body of experimental data on the basis of which the visibility of directional, informational, and warning signs is directly related to the visual capacities of the driver population.

Accident frequencies may also be influenced by factors of a psychosocial or sociologic nature. On the highway, traffic may be considered a social aggregate of drivers, and driving a form of social behavior carried out according to specific codes. Within this context, the motor vehicle may represent not only a means of transportation, but also variations in the meanings which automobiles may have for drivers in terms of the extrinsic motivations they have come to embody; for example, power, prestige, and many others. Such factors may influence risk-taking behavior. Also, the relative anonymity of the drivers in their interactions with others on the highway and the limitations upon intercommunication appear to enhance risk-taking and unsafe practices which in other contexts would be considered antisocial behavior.[4]

Although the areas cited offer promising fields for further study, limited experimental data have been accumulated. Also, there is little factual information on the effectiveness of educational programs, propaganda, and enforcement activities on accident rates. Controlled research programs are urgently needed in these important areas.[9]

1. *Accident Facts,* Chicago: National Safety Council, 1960.

2. Persons Injured by Class of Accident, United States, July 1957–June 1958 National Health Survey, Series B-8, U.S. Department of Health, Education and Welfare, February, 1959.

3. Accidental Injury Statistics, Selected Data, May 1960, U.S. Department of Health, Education and Welfare, United States Public Health Service, 1960.

4. McFarland, R. A., and Moore, R. C.: Epidemiology of Accidents, in Halsey, M. N. (Ed.): *Accident Prevention: Role of Physicians and Public Health Workers,* New York: McGraw-Hill Book Company, Inc., 1961.

5. McFarland, R. A.: Role of Preventive Medicine in Highway Safety, *Amer J Public Health* 47:288–296 (March) 1957.

6. McFarland, R. A., and Moore, R. C.: Human Factors in Highway Safety: Review and Evaluation, *New Engl J Med* 256:792–798 (April 25); 837–845 (May 2); 890–897 (May 9) 1957.

7. Francis, T., Jr.: Teaching of Epidemiology, in World Medical Association, *Proceedings of First World Conference on Medical Education,* London, 1953, Oxford, England: Oxford University Press, 1954.

8. MacMahon, B.; Pugh, T. F.; and Ipsen, J.: *Epidemiological Methods,* Boston: Little, Brown & Company, 1960.

9. Commission on Accidental Trauma: Annual Report to the Armed Forces Epidemological Board, Department of Defense, Reports 1959 and 1960.

10. Dunlap, J. et al.: Development and Evaluation of Countermeasures for Reduction of POV Accidents to Service Personnel, Stamford, Conn.: Dunlap and Associates, 1959.

11. McFarland, R. A., and Moore, R. C.: Youth and the Automobile, in Ginzberg, E. (Ed.): *Values and Ideals of American Youth,* New York: Columbia University Press, 1960.

12. McFarland, R. A.; Moore, R. C.; and Warren, A. B.: *Human Variables in Motor Vehicle Accidents: Review of Literature,* Boston: Harvard School of Public Health, 1955.

13. Dunbar, H. F.: *Psychosomatic Diagnosis,* New York: Paul B. Hoeber, Inc., 1943.

15. Tillmann, W. A., and Hobbs, G. E.: Accident Prone Automobile Driver: Study of Psychiatric and Social Background, *Amer J. Psychiat* 106:321–331 (Nov.) 1949.

16. McFarland, R. A., and Moseley, A. L.: *Human Factors in Highway Transport Safety,* Boston: Harvard School of Public Health, 1954.

17. Conger, J. J. et al.: Personal and Interpersonal Factors in Motor Vehicle Accidents, *Amer J Psychiat* 114:1069, 1957.

18. Rommel, R. C. S.: Personality Characteristics and Attitudes of Youthful Accident-Repeater Drivers, *Traffic Safety Res Rev* 3:14–14, 1959.

19. Welford, A. T.: *Skill and Age,* London: Oxford University Press, 1959.

20. McFarland, R. A., and O'Doherty, B. M.: Work and Occupational Skills, chap. 14, pp. 452–502, in *Handbook of Aging—Individual, Psychological and Biological Aspects,* Chicago: University of Chicago Press, 1959.

21. Marsh, B.: Aging and Driving. Paper presented on Receipt of Annual Award of Theodore M. Matson Memorial Fund, 1960.

22. Bartlett, F.: Bearing of Experimental Psychology upon Human Skilled Performance, *Brit J Industr Med* 8:209–217, 1951.

23. Haddon, W., Jr., and Bradess, V. A.: Alcohol in Single Vehicle Fatal Accident: Experience of Westchester County, New York, *JAMA* 169:1587–1593, 1959.

24. Smith, H. W., and Popham, R. E.: Blood Alcohol Levels in Relation to Driving, *Canad Med Ass J* 65:325–328, 1951.

25. Norman, L. G.: Medical Aspects of Road Safety, *Lancet* 1:1039–1045 (May 14) 1960.

26. Uhr, L., and Miller, J. G.: *Drugs and Behavior*, New York: J. Wiley & Sons, 1960.

27. McFarland, R. A.: Human Limitations and Vehicle Design, *Ergonomics* 1:3–20, 1957.

28. McFarland, R. A.: Machine Design and Human Engineering, chap. 16, in *Modern Trends in Occupational Health*, Schilling, R. S. F.: London: Butterworths, Ltd., 1960.

29. McFarland, R. A. et al.: Dark Adaptation as Function of Age. I. Statistical Analysis, *J Geront* 15:149–154 (April) 1960.

30. Wolf, E.: Glare and Age, *Arch Ophthal* 64:502–514, 1960.

31. U.S. Congress: *Federal Role in Highway Safety*, 8th Congress, 1st Session, House Document no. 93, Washington, D.C.: U.S. Government Printing Office, 1959.

Stream Pollution*

ROLF ELIASSEN

POLLUTION of the surface waters of the U.S. threatens one of the nation's most valuable natural resources. It menaces not only the water supplies of many of our cities, which consume over 15 billion gallons of water per day, but also recreational fishing, boating and bathing, commercial fishing, agricultural irrigation and even the very industries that produce much of the pollution. It must be remembered that the industries themselves require billions of gallons of water daily for processing and cooling purposes, and the pollution of river water may destroy its usefulness to them. Each river is a natural resource which one must expect to use and re-use from source to mouth.

The social and economic costs of pollution are beyond computation; they include such diverse items as effects on the health of our people, the expense of water purification, limitation of industrial expansion, loss of revenue to fishermen and recreational interests, decline of real-estate values.

* Reprinted, with omission of five illustrations, from the March 1952 issue of *Scientific American*, Vol. 186, pp. 17–21, with permission. Copyright © 1952 by Scientific American, Inc. All rights reserved. The author is Professor of Civil Engineering, Stanford University, Stanford, California, and formerly was Professor of Sanitary Engineering, Massachusetts Institute of Technology, Cambridge, Massachusetts.

There are approximately 20,000 significant sources of stream pollution in the nation; about 10,000 of them are municipal sewage systems and the other 10,000 are industrial plants. A single river such as the Delaware is estimated to receive each day 500 million gallons of domestic sewage and hundreds of millions of gallons of industrial wastes. The industrial needs for water are staggering: according to a recent survey by the National Association of Manufacturers, the manufacture of viscose rayon requires an average of 180,000 to 200,000 gallons of water for each ton of product; rayon yarns, 250,000 to 404,000 gallons per ton; woolens and worsteds, 140,000 gallons per ton; rolled steel, 110,000 gallons per ton; whiskey, 80,000 gallons of water per 1,000 gallons of whiskey; synthetic gasoline, 15,800,000 gallons per 1,000 barrels, and aviation gasoline, 1,050,000 gallons per 1,000 barrels.

There are three categories of pollution—chemical, physical and biologic. The chemical pollutants include such toxic substances as cyanides, acids, chromates, copper, zinc, arsenic and mercury, which kill fish and other life and render water unfit to drink. Among them also are organic chemicals which, though not toxic themselves, serve as food for bacteria. The physical agents of pollution are often overlooked, but they, too, are important. For example, heat, which not many people would consider a form of pollution, has become a major problem; after being used and re-used many times by industries for cooling purposes, the water of a stream sometimes is raised by as much as 50 degrees above its natural temperature, and it loses its cooling value. Another physical contaminant, which will give increasing trouble, is radioactive waste. In addition there are physical agents, such as clay particles, that make waters colored or turbid. The third type of contaminant—biologic—of course is familiar to everyone; responsible for typhoid fever, dysentery, gastroenteritis and a host of other diseases, it has been the concern of health authorities for centuries.

Before discussing methods of reducing stream pollution, it would be well to consider the characteristics of streams and their ability to absorb pollution. Water is not dead—it is alive with flora and fauna, with energy and movement, with all sorts of matter. One of its most important assets is its content of dissolved oxygen. If the oxygen content falls to less than four parts per million, the water becomes unsuitable for game fish. When it drops to zero, as has happened in a good many streams in this country, the stream becomes septic, generates foul odors and is a serious nuisance to the nearby population. But most important is the fact that oxygen helps give a stream the power to purify itself.

Organisms in a stream use the dissolved oxygen in their metabolic processes as they consume organic matter. Their oxidation of this material, plus coagulation and settling, reduces the concentration of polluting organic matter in the stream. By this self-purification a stream into which a city pours its wastes may regain its original purity many miles downstream from the source of the pollution.

There is a limit, however, to this capacity. The stream loses its ability to absorb organic pollution and purify itself if its microorganisms use up the dissolved oxygen faster than it can be replenished from the atmosphere. The rate at which the microbe population uses up oxygen depends primarily on the amount of organic matter in the water. This establishes what is known as the biochemical oxygen demand (B.O.D.) of the stream. In the unending struggle of a river for self-purification, the B.O.D. must never be allowed to get out of hand and reduce the oxygen balance below a certain level. This minimum is generally considered to be four parts of oxygen per million parts of water.

The problem, then, is to reduce the amount of organic matter to the stream's capacity to absorb it, and to get rid of toxic materials. Sanitary engineers and scientists have developed many ways to do this. One of them is the settling tank, where sewage and industrial waste is held for a short time (usually about two hours) until enough of the solid material settles to the bottom so the liquids can be discharged into the stream. On the average, settling will remove about 55 per cent of the suspended solids and 35 per cent of the organic matter that would exert an oxygen demand in the stream. By chemical treatment still more of the pollutants can be precipitated. Iron or aluminum salts, particularly sulfates and chlorides, are added to the liquid, and by reaction with the water they form particles which serve as nuclei to adsorb and coagulate colloidal and suspended material. This method is widely used to precipitate inorganic and organic matter in industrial wastes, particularly toxic substances such as come from metal-finishing plants using chrome-plating processes.

There are a great many other treatments, but we shall consider in detail only a few of the important biochemical ones. Essentially these are based on the same natural processes by which a stream purifies itself; that is, they use microorganisms to break down the organic matter.

One device is the trickling filter. This consists of a large bed of crushed rock or gravel, from 10 to 200 feet in diameter and 3 to 8 feet deep, with microorganisms growing in the bed so they cover the stones with a coat of slime. The population of organisms in this slime is very complex, and the myriads of different kinds of bacteria and multi-celled animals, acting together, can break down many varieties of organic material—cellulose, fats, greases, proteins, and so on.

The sewage to be treated is trickled through the rock bed, and the bacterial slime goes to work on its solids. With the aid of their enzymes the bacteria consume soluble organic matter directly as food. Material that is in colloidal form may be adsorbed on the surface of the slime; it is then ingested directly by protozoa or may be hydrolyzed and become soluble food for bacteria. If necessary, the sewage or waste is recirculated through the bed several times—as much as 30 times in the case of some industrial wastes. The trickling filter can remove from 60 to 95 per cent of organic matter from liquid wastes. It has proved to be the answer to many of the pollution problems of industries and of small and moderate-sized cities.

Some of the largest cities have resorted to a more economic method, called the activated sludge process. Activated sludge is a mass of gelatinous material consisting of fuzzy particles about one milli-meter in diameter. It is generated from microorganisms that occur naturally in sewage, and it is built up by letting the organisms "brew" for several months until they attain the proper balance of population. Once the sludge is formed, it purifies sewage in much the same way as the trickling filter, except that the operation takes place in a large tank instead of a bed of rock. Fine air bubbles are blown through the liquid in the tank to furnish dissolved oxygen for the organisms as they work on the sewage. The mixture then flows to settling tanks where the sludge, carrying the converted organic matter, is deposited. This process removes 90 to 95 per cent of the organic matter from sewage and usually yields clear water as the effluent. The sludge, after settling, can be used again.

After the organic matter has been removed—by the trickling filter, by activated sludge or by some other process—the water often needs to be treated further to kill disease-producing bacteria before it is discharged to the stream. The most commonly used disinfectant is chlorine. By adding from five to 15 parts of chlorine per million to the effluent and keeping the liquid in a tank for about 15 minutes, it is possible to destroy more than 99 per cent of the bacteria.

The sludge removed from the sewage also must be treated. Much of its material is putrescible, and it is about 100 times more concentrated in the sludge than in sewage. The most common method of handling sludge is anaerobic fermentation, that is, breakdown of the material in the absence of dissolved oxygen. This is done in large "digestion" tanks. In these tanks, where the sludge is kept anywhere from two to 100 days, bacteria and other microorganisms decompose most of the putrescible organic matter into simpler compounds of carbon, oxygen, hydrogen, nitrogen, sulfur and phosphorus. Some of the end products are discharged as gases, mainly methane, carbon dioxide and hydrogen sulfide. The gas mixture, about 65 per cent methane, has a heating value of 600 British thermal units per cubic foot (better than manufactured cooking gas). It can be used to heat the digestion tanks and furnish power for pumping and other equipment in the disposal plant.

The solid residue from the digestion of sludge is a humuslike material which makes a good fertilizer; it may contain from one to five per cent nitrogen and some phosphorus and potash. Some large activated sludge plants dry the sludge without digesting it first, and sell the dried sludge as a fertilizer base. Dried sludge from the sewage plants of Milwaukee is marketed and known throughout the country as Milorganite.

New York City, Chicago, Los Angeles, Philadelphia, Cleveland and London all have large activated sludge plants; Chicago's, the largest, treats an average of 1.1 billion gallons of sewage per day. Not all make use of the sludge products; for example, New York City dumps its liquid sludge into the Atlantic Ocean, because this is more economic at present than processing the sludge into organic fertilizers. The need for such fertilizers is great, however, and one day New York's sludge will be used.

It will cost substantial amounts of money, of course, to make the streams and other waters of the U.S. reasonably free of pollution. The construction costs of municipal sewage treatment plants such as have been described in this article run from $10 to $50 per person served by the sewerage system. Added to this are operating costs, which range from $10 to $40 per million gallons of sewage treated.

Los Angeles has just spent $42 million for a treatment plant to protect the Santa Monica bathing beaches; New York City is spending $200 million for treatment plants; Pittsburgh and neighboring towns in Allegheny County will spend about $80 million; Miami is completing a $10 million project. Since 1915 municipalities in this country have spent about $10 billion for sewers and sewage-treatment plants, and it is estimated that they will have to spend another $10 billion in the next 20 years to build enough plants to handle their sewage.

In addition, U.S. industries will probably have to spend about $10 billion more to change processes and build plants to dispose of their wastes. Management realizes that public opinion is gradually forcing industry to shoulder its part of the burden of alleviating stream pollution, and that waste treatment must be considered an integral part of invested capital and production costs. Operating, maintenance and financing costs for these plants will eventually amount to a quarter of a billion dollars yearly, the cost of which can only be passed on to the consumers of the industries' products. If the public wants stream-pollution control, it must be willing to pay in terms of increased taxes and increased costs of consumer goods.

To control pollution intelligently we need standards for the discharge of wastes and the degree of purity we want in our streams. The standards of course will depend on the priorities to be given the various possible uses of the available water—domestic and industrial water supply, bathing and other recreation, fishing, the transport of wastes. To develop water standards for each of these uses and for regulating them, we shall need surveys. Very little has yet been accomplished in this direction, nor have many states passed enabling legislation for pollution control.

Every State has an agency in which this function may be vested, whether it is the Department of Public Health, as in Massachusetts, or a specific Water Pollution Board, as in California. Primarily stream pollution is a State problem. But where a stream runs through more than one State, regional authorities are needed, and several have already been formed, including the Ohio River Valley Water Sanitation Commission, the Interstate Commission on the Delaware Basin, the New England Interstate Water Pollution Control Commission and agencies for the drainage basins of the Hudson and Potomac Rivers. The States have also found that they need the cooperation of the Federal government. The Taft-Barkley Act of 1948 authorized the U.S. Public Health Service to assist the States in developing pollution-control programs.

The Public Health Service, with the aid of States, regional agencies and industries, has collected and analyzed some data on the needs for waste-treatment facilities in the major drainage basins in the country. These studies have helped citizens to realize that their pollution problems may originate far upstream, even in another State. Industry is cooperating extensively in these surveys, particularly through the National Task Committee on Industrial Wastes sponsored by 22 of the nation's leading industries and the Public Health Service.

There are still many unsolved problems in the treatment of wastes. It should be possible to develop more economic processes than those now used. Moreover, for some of the organic pollutants no effective treatment has yet been found. The hope for solution of these problems lies in further research.

Microbiologists and sanitary chemists have made great strides in the treatment of toxic wastes such as phenol and formaldehyde. Studies are currently in progress in the Sedgwick Laboratories of Sanitary Science at the Massachusetts Institute of Technology on the fermentation of a number of concentrated organic wastes from the chemical, paper and cotton textile industries. Experiments are being conducted on the effectiveness of various microorganisms, combinations of nutrients, temperatures and degrees of acidity. These studies are making available new processes which can handle a greater variety of organic industrial wastes.

Radioactive wastes have created a serious problem for the sanitary engineer. With the growth of the nuclear industry in such fields as atomic power and tracer research, to say nothing of nuclear weapons, stream-pollution control is becoming a matter of primary concern. The processing of radioactive wastes is being studied intensively in many laboratories.

Under the sponsorship of the Atomic Energy Commission, the author and his colleagues have been investigating the removal of low concentrations of radioisotopes from liquid wastes by chemical coagulation, sedimentation and filtration. Evaporation is effective in separating radioactive material from liquids, but it is too expensive. The M.I.T. studies have disclosed that coagulation is a good and economical method of removing radioactive substances when they are in colloidal form or suspended as solids. Dissolved substances present a more complex problem, but it has been partly solved; certain special coagulants that precipitate ions can remove more than 90 per cent of the radioactive material. Research is also in progress on the possible toxic effects of beta and gamma radiation from substances such as radiophosphorous and radioiodine wastes on microorganisms that help a stream to purify itself.

We can clean up our streams to almost any degree we like by spending enough money. To restore our heavily populated rivers to their pristine purity would be much too costly, but sound engineering and the expenditure of about $20 billion by municipalities and industries could reduce the pollution of the streams of the U.S. to a reasonable level.

5.   The International Community

Health Conditions*

UNITED NATIONS

THE GENERAL STATE OF HEALTH

The measurement of levels of health as a component of levels of living for the purposes of international comparison has been considered by experts.[1] It was found that it is difficult to design suitable indicators of health from the knowledge at present available. Among the statistical data commonly used to designate the state of health of a country or population, the experts found that general mortality, expectation of life, and infant mortality rates are relatively better indicators of health than other types of information. For example, the ratios of physicians and hospital beds per unit of population are considered unsuitable because they give no indication of the distribution and utilization of these facilities and therefore do not necessarily reflect the state of health of the population.[2]

Tables giving the general mortality, expectation of life, and infant mortality rates show a continuing decline of the general and infant mortality rates in practically all the countries listed. Also, the expectation of life at birth, on which data are available only in a limited number of countries, is increasing.

From these and other data, it is evident that conditions of physical health have been steadily improving throughout the world in recent years, although there is no informational basis for drawing such a conclusion in regard to mental health. The most rapid progress—indicated by the largest drops in mortality rates—has taken place in economically less developed areas where mass diseases such as malaria have been brought under control. While significant progress has also been made in developed areas, the fight against cancer and heart disease, disorders which tend to dominate the medical picture in these areas, has not yet produced such striking results in mortality reduction as have been obtained in the fight against communicable diseases. Thus, the developed countries, having brought the major commu-

---

* Reprinted by permission, with omission of 12 tables, from *Report on the World Social Situation*—including studies of urbanization in underdeveloped areas prepared by the Bureau of Social Affairs, United Nations Secretariat, in cooperation with the International Labor Office, the Food and Agriculture Organization, the United Nations Educational, Scientific and Cultural Organization and the World Health Organization, published by the United Nations, New York, 1957, Chap. 3, pp. 28–48.

nicable diseases increasingly under control, are now temporarily slowed in their health progress by the recalcitrant character of the degenerative diseases—and, one might add, of senility itself—while the less developed countries are reaping the benefits of modern medicine in fields where specific causes, cures and preventives have become fairly well known.

CONTROL AND PREVENTION OF DISEASES

In many countries, particularly in economically underdeveloped regions, certain communicable diseases either in epidemic or endemic form are still a serious health problem, and constitute the main causes of mortality and morbidity among the population. In these countries, however, statistics on communicable diseases are seldom available or reliable. Morbidity statistics in particular on the diseases in question are usually lacking, even in countries with more advanced statistical services.

In studying the mortality rates of a group of communicable diseases in a number of countries, it is found that, with the exception of Egypt where the information comes from limited areas and is probably incomplete, the rates seem to have continued to decline; they are lowest in Denmark and the Netherlands in 1955. It should, however, be pointed out that most of the countries reviewed are economically and technically advanced, and that communicable diseases in general are therefore not a major health problem.

Infective and parasitic diseases

MAJOR EPIDEMIC DISEASES. A concerted effort has been made by many Governments to ensure (with the minimum interference in international traffic) the maximum security against the spread of the major epidemic diseases (smallpox, plague, cholera, yellow fever, typhus and relapsing fever) from one country to another. A set of international regulations on these diseases, which consolidated and brought up to date some thirteen international agreements dating back to 1903, has been adopted as the International Sanitary Regulations (WHO Regulations No. 2), and by the end of 1954, 61 States and 73 Trust and Non-Self-Governing Territories had agreed to carry out the provisions of these Regulations without reservation, while eight States and two Territories accepted them with certain reservations.[3]

Except for smallpox, there have been no recent serious outbreaks of the major epidemic diseases in any part of the world; large numbers of people living in areas where smallpox and cholera are endemic, however, are still threatened by these diseases. There have been comparatively few human cases of plague, except in India, Burma, and

Indonesia; it has not invaded fresh areas. Yellow fever has been mainly confined to the countries where it is endemic, and there the disease has appeared to be generally under control. However, the appearance in 1954 of yellow fever in Trinidad (where there had been no known cases of this disease for the previous 40 years), and its northward spread in Central America, reaffirmed the need for continuous vigilance. Typhus and relapsing fever have been reported in certain countries, mostly as sporadic cases with few more important outbreaks.

It should be noted that certain of these communicable diseases, such as plague and yellow fever, appear to exist more or less permanently in wildlife, which provides a reservoir of infection that may suddenly start to spread the disease among domestic animals and humans. Thus, the sporadic, although strictly limited, outbreaks of plague are apparently due to the prevalence of that disease among wild rodents in certain parts of Africa, the Americas, and Asia.[4] The recent reappearance of yellow fever in the Americas may be due to the perpetuation of the disease by the continuing infection of monkeys in jungle areas and its outbreak from the jungle into inhabited areas. In the case of outbreaks both in Trinidad (1954) and in continental Central America (1950–54), the origin was traced to infection by jungle mosquitoes of a species other than the traditional carrier, Aedes Aegypti, which had been exterminated in inhabited areas (infected jungle mosquitoes have recently been discovered north of the Rio Grande). The Central American outbreak was preceded by an epidemic among jungle monkeys which was accompanied by a high mortality of these animals.[5] There are vast areas in South America and Africa where yellow fever is known to be endemic.[6]

VIRUS DISEASES. During the period under study, epidemics of influenza have been widely reported. Among countries reporting the greatest prevalence were Austria, Denmark, Finland, Greece, Italy, Spain, Sweden, Switzerland and the United Kingdom in the European area; Canada, Guatemala, Uruguay and Venezuela in the Americas; Ethiopia and Madagascar in Africa; Hawaii, Japan and the Philippines in the Pacific area.

In some of the virus infections the symptoms vary in nature and severity in different epidemics. Close study of the symptoms and careful research on the nature of the virus causing a particular outbreak must therefore be continued in order to devise effective precautionary measures. Fortunately, specific control measures are now available for some of these diseases. To be effective, however, the virus strains used in the vaccine must be related to the epidemic strains, and the vaccine administered at the appropriate moment. A number of Governments have therefore set up special centers which keep in close touch with each other and report observations on the early development of the disease to the World Health Organization. There are at present 57 influenza centers. The World Health Organization has also designed six regional centers to assist and co-ordinate similar studies on poliomyelitis.[7]

Until the recent introduction of vaccination, poliomyelitis—especially in its paralytic form—has been practically the only major contagious disease with an increasing rate of incidence.[8] It has been affecting hitherto relatively immune groups of the population. Forty of 50 years ago the maximum attack-rates were nearly always recorded in the 0–4 years age-group, but have since shifted to higher age-groups. In Sweden, for example, the children most affected by poliomyelitis are now in the 7–15 age-group, and, in some yearly records, even the 15–25 age-group.[9] Poliomyelitis has not only been affecting a wider range of the population in countries where the disease has long been recognized,[10] but it has also been appearing in epidemic form for the first time in more and more countries, including economically less developed countries.[11] There has been a recent intensive outbreak of poliomyelitis in Argentina and an unusually high incidence in certain parts of Serbia (in Yugoslavia).

Considerable progress has been made in recent years, however, toward control of poliomyelitis through vaccination. Campaigns have been especially successful where the series of injections necessary for immunization has been completed before the start of the annual poliomyelitis season.[12]

As poliomyelitis has come under increasing study, another but similar virus disease, meningoencephalitis, has been recognized in areas formerly believed free from infection. Several outbreaks of this disease have occurred in Central European countries since 1952; its clinical and pathologic similarity to poliomyelitis may have prevented a proper diagnosis of possible earlier outbreaks.[13]

TUBERCULOSIS. In the case of pulmonary tuberculosis, the death-rate seems to have continued to fall—in some cases dramatically—during the last few years in those parts of the world where reliable statistics are available.

When considering the mortality from this disease, it should be remembered that the introduction of chemotherapy during recent years, while not achieving a complete cure, may have prevented many people from dying of tuberculosis. The reduction of the mortality rate, therefore does not always mean that the prevalence of the disease has decreased. In many countries tuberculosis morbidity has not decreased so much as mortality. Where the death-rates have dropped by about half, the number of reported cases has dropped little, and the number of known infectious cases has sometimes even increased.[14]

Adding to this the fact that the extent and behavior of tuberculosis among the great majority of the world's population is at present unknown, the goal of control of this disease may still be far off, but scientifically planned surveys are now being undertaken in parts of Africa and Asia which will provide further valuable information on which sound tuberculosis control programs may be based. In some of these countries the disease seems to be less common in rural and more common in industrial areas than was thought.

The management of pulmonary tuberculosis is rapidly changing from a clinical to a Public Health approach. The use of BCG vaccination as a protective measure against tuberculosis is becoming more and more widespread. For instance, in India an annual average of 25 million people are tuberculin-tested, of whom approximately 10 million receive BCG vaccination. The use of drugs in ambulant patients for therapeutic or prophylactic purposes, as a public health control measure, depends on the wide-spread availability of an effective, nontoxic drug that will be cheap and easy to produce, to distribute, and to take. New drugs are bringing such an approach to tuberculosis control within sight.

PNEUMONIA. There has been a striking decline in the number of deaths from pneumonia since penicillin and other antibiotics have become available, as given evidence by a recent WHO survey.[15] Nevertheless, pneumonia still ranks among the diseases causing the greatest number of deaths even in the developed countries where antibiotics are widely used, and in particular is a leading cause of death among infants and among the aged.

Figures comparing 1936–38 and the more recent rates of pneumonia deaths in 20 countries show that the decrease has been moderate among infants under one year of age, extremely important among children and adults, and much less marked among the aged. Among people over 80 in a few countries, such as France, Finland, the United Kingdom and Portugal, an increase in pneumonia deaths is recorded for certain years.

Of the different forms of pneumonia, the one responsible today for the greatest mortality is bronchopneumonia in the majority of the reporting countries, including Canada, Finland, Denmark, the United States, Ireland, Italy, Norway, the Netherlands, the United Kingdom, Sweden, Switzerland, Australia and New Zealand. In Japan, however, lobar pneumonia causes most deaths.

MALARIA. The extensive DDT-residual spray work carried out in many countries has greatly increased the number of people protected against this disease. For example, in six countries of Asia (Afghanistan, Burma, Ceylon, India, Indonesia and Thailand), recent estimates[16] indicate that the malaria control programs have already directly protected 121 million people out of 250 million living in malarious areas. In a few countries and territories of Africa (such as French West Africa, French Cameroons, Liberia, Nigeria and Tanganyika), pilot projects have been initiated in order to collect essential information for planning large-scale anti-malaria programs.

The methods of preventing malaria have had to be modified recently because, as noted in previous reports,[17] it has been discovered that some anopheles mosquitoes—known as carriers of the disease—in certain areas are developing a resistance to insecticides. This has resulted in a change of approach to malaria control. The practice now aims at stopping the transmission of the disease during three of four consecutive years by intensive DDT-residual-spraying, and then discontinuing the spraying completely in order to prevent the development of resistant anopheles mosquitoes. The new approach is based on recognition of the fact that "Malaria eradication does not mean or require eradication of the anopheline species that carry the disease in a given area. It only means eradication of the malaria parasites."[18] Malaria, when it does not kill, is spontaneously self-curing. Inasmuch as infection lasts generally no longer than three or four years, at the most, except in certain rare forms, the effort is made to establish complete control of the mosquitoes for that period of time through intensive DDT-residual-spraying. If the life-and-infection cycle in the "parasite to mosquito to human being" circuit is thus interrupted and the human population ridden of malaria parasites, mosquitoes may well remain or reappear in the inhabited areas after residual-spraying is discontinued, but they will not be disease carriers, because they will find no parasite-infected human beings to bite. Thus, eradication of the disease has practically been achieved throughout, or in large areas of, British and French Guiana, Italy, the United States, Argentina, Ceylon, Thailand and Venezuela. For the success of this procedure, it is essential that complete malaria control be achieved during the three or four-year period during which previously infected human beings still carry the malaria parasites; this implies the necessity of regularly spraying even remote villages, including those where malaria rates have been low. Moreover, the controlled areas should be as large as possible, so as to minimize the possibility of the reintroduction of malaria parasites through the movements of infected human beings or mosquitoes.

In the remaining parts of the world, malaria control or eradication work has been initiated, or the disease has already become insignificant as a public health problem.

YAWS AND SYPHILIS. It is estimated that there are today some 50,000,000 cases of yaws, one of the treponematoses caused by a spirochete similar to that of syphilis. The eradication of yaws and endemic syphilis has been a major target in many projects organized by national health administrations, assisted by the World Health Organization and other international organizations, particularly UNICEF. In the Cameroons, the Gold Coast, Haiti, India, Indonesia, Laos, Liberia, Malaya, Nigeria, the Pacific Islands, Sierra Leone and Thailand, yaws control programs are now being carried out and are in various stages of completion. Control of endemic syphilis is in progress in Bechuanaland and Iraq, and the eradication of the disease is being achieved in Yugoslavia. By the end of 1955, by means of internationally assisted campaigns, no less than 50,000,000 persons had been examined and 15,000,000 treated with penicillin. By eliminating yaws, the well-being of the afflicted people is improved and at the same time their potential for productive work is increased. However, concerted and persistent action by national bodies and community effort still needs to be encouraged. In developed countries the prevalence of venereal syphilis has fallen dramatically since penicillin was introduced.

BILHARZIASIS. Because of the intensity of its morbid symptoms, its socio-economic aspects and its wide distribution throughout the world, bilharziasis is one of the most important helminthiases (diseases caused by worms in blood vessels). It is estimated that there are about 150,000,000 infested people in the world suffering from this disease, in the transmission of which certain snails act as intermediate hosts. The infestation rate is in fact a reliable indicator of poor environmental sanitation in any area. In many countries where bilharziasis is a problem, special efforts have been made with WHO assistance on the distribution and importance of bilharziasis in Africa, in the Eastern Mediterranean Region, and in certain regions of the Western Pacific. For example, the classification of snail vectors, the intermediary hosts of the bilharziasis parasites, and the study of their ecology have been added to the understanding of the epidemiology of the disease and the selection of control methods. The discovery of new molluscides with a residual effect is necessary.

FILARIASIS. Considerable progress has been made in the control of onchocerciasis,[19] the blinding filariasis. This disease, which affects nearly 20 million people in tropical Africa, as well as in Central and South America, is spread by several species of tiny flies, belonging to the genus *Simulium*, which carry the microscopic young forms (microfilariae) of the worm, *Onchocerca volvulus*, known to cause the disease. When the infected *Simulium* fly bites human beings, it transmits the microfilariae which reach adult stage in the human host. They produce subcutaneous nodules, generally attached to bones in several parts of the body. The adult worms produce hundreds of thousands of new microfilariae in the nodules, which invade the tissues of the skin and the eyes through lymphatic circulation, producing characteristic lesions. If the disease is not halted it may in time so damage the eye that vision is seriously impaired and total blindness may result.

Because of the high incidence of blindness in villages in river valleys of the Sudan, East Africa, Nigeria and the Gold Coast, the disease has become known there as "river blindness." Similar conditions exist in other African territories; the association of onchocerciasis with rivers is due to the fact that *Simulium* develops in quick-running waters, where the adults deposit their eggs and the young forms live attached to submerged vegetation and stones. One species of *Simulium* deposits its eggs on crabs of a certain kind which act as host to the larvae and pupae.

The control of onchocerciasis is now possible, since there are effective and practical methods of fighting both the parasite worm and its vectors.[20] In Guatemala and Mexico, successful campaigns have been conducted to reduce the incidence of onchocercal blindness and other disabling eye lesions by surgical removal of the nodules; the use of new drugs in mass campaigns in endemic areas of Africa and the Americas has also made considerable progress in the treatment and control of this disease. A successful campaign through the extermination of *Simulium* with insecticides (DDT) has been carried out in certain districts of Kenya: while in 1945 a survey carried out among children below the age of six years showed an infection rate of 36 per cent, re-examination in 1953, following successful control of the vector, showed that not a single child in this age-group had contracted the disease.[21] Similar campaigns are being started in the Belgian Congo, French West and Equatorial Africa.

It is estimated that more than 250,000,000 people are affected by the other filariases—including infections which can produce elephantiases—in the tropical areas of the world. The results of treatment by piperazine derivative drugs promise new possibilities for the control of the parasites, if the treatment campaigns can be organized on a mass scale. Successful experiments have already been carried out in the Pacific area. Vector control measures have been sucessfully employed in certain areas of endemicity and against certain species of vectors, but no generalization of the techniques used is yet possible, owing to the different biology of the many species of vectors involved.

TRACHOMA. Trachoma and infectious conjunctivitis affect no less than 400,000,000 people all over the world. These diseases present a vast social problem, because of the high percentage of blindness or disabling eye lesions they produce.

Trachoma, in particular, may reach extremely high percentages of infection among children in many of the areas where it is prevalent. In various territories of North Africa, where practically all the adult population was found to be suffering from the disease or from its sequelae, the percentage of infection among children of pre-school age has been found to be as high as 70 to 90 per cent. In India, 78 per cent of rural school children in selected villages were found infected in Uttar Pradesh and 48 per cent in East Punjab; in Taiwan, in a pilot project area, 48 out of every 100 children were found to be trachoma sufferers. New areas of endemicity of this disease have been detected in the course of surveys carried out in South Africa and Western Australian territory. Satisfactory results obtained in the treatment of trachoma and infectious conjunctivitis by some sulfonamides and antibiotics, the latter being especially effective, have encouraged mass campaigns on a national scale. Successful initial results have been obtained in Morocco, Taiwan, and Tunisia, and new campaigns of this type have been started in Egypt, Indonesia, Spain, and Yugoslavia.

LEPROSY. The effectiveness of sulfones in the treatment of leprosy, together with the recognition that this disease is not, in most cases, so highly infectious as was formerly believed, has led to revolutionary changes in the measures used for its control. The old policy of compulsory life-long segregation of all recognized patients has been replaced in most countries by one which aims at the early detection of the disease, temporary isolation of selected infectious patients, and ambulatory or domiciliary treatment of most of the others.

The progress in the treatment of leprosy has led to an increase in the number of leprosy sufferers seeking such treatment; this is due to the enhanced confidence in new methods of treatment and the disappearance of the fear that application for medical assistance would result in confinement in leproseries. Most of these institutions are, however, still in operation because of the necessity to continue the segregation of advanced cases, including those discovered too late for successful treatment by new methods. It has also been found that leprosy patients cured after many years of confinement are often unable to shift for themselves and have to be kept in the leproseries.[22] In a number of countries today, the patients are no longer isolated, but reside in relative liberty in the proximity of the place where they are registered for treatment, reporting for treatment at appropriate times.[23]

In spite of the progress already achieved, leprosy remains an important health problem in many countries of Africa[24] and other underdeveloped areas. Now that there is less concealment of the disease, the total number of patients throughout the world has had to be revised upwards, from a WHO estimate of between two and seven million in 1952, to a total of 10 to 12 million today.

Leprosy control measures have been carried out by a number of

Governments, sometimes in combined efforts—for example, in Brazil, Burma, Ceylon, Ethiopia, French Equatorial and West Africa, India, Indonesia, Nigeria, the Philippines, Thailand, and Venezuela. The rehabilitation problems of the cured patient are also attracting a great deal of attention. In particular, the social problems caused by the fear and social stigma attached to this disease have to be tackled, and the public educated to accept the cured patient as a full member of society.

TRYPANOSOMIASIS. Most of Africa south of the Sahara (except the southern part of the Union of South Africa) is affected by diseases known as trypanosomiases which are transmitted by tse-tse flies. Trypanosomiases are caused by several species of minute protozoa, called trypanosomes. There are two of these species that cause somewhat different forms of sleeping disease in human beings, and that also affect domestic animals, primarily cattle (other species affect animals only). Many wild animals may carry in their blood parastic trypanosomes which are harmless to these animals but dangerous to man. The wild animals therefore serve as a reservoir of infection, since the tse-tse fly transmits the trypanosomes from them to man or to domestic animals. The tendency of human populations to migrate into the relatively small areas that are free of the disease-carrying tse-tse flies has caused these areas to be overcrowded, in view of the type of agriculture practice, and low in per capita agricultural yield. Other areas are infected by trypanosomes which, while relatively harmless to human beings, are fatal to cattle; in these areas, the human population, although not exposed to sleeping disease, is apt to be deprived of animal protein in the diet, of draught animals for work and of fertilizer needed to cultivate the fields. In short, the tse-tse fly, directly through the debilitation it causes, or indirectly, has a serious effect upon the productivity of the African rural population and presents one of the greatest barriers to African progress.[25]

Until recently, there were only two basic methods of eliminating tse-tse flies. These were either to kill off the wild animals which provided the tse-tse fly with its food, or to cut down the forests, woodland, or bush which provided its home. The application of the first of these methods resulted in a serious depletion of African wildlife, but did not lead to satisfactory control of the tse-tse fly; nor has the second of these methods proved successful. In recent years, more efficient methods of dealing with this disease have been employed.

The incidence of trypanosomiasis or sleeping sickness has declined in many endemic areas in Africa, thanks to chemo-prophylaxis and the public health measures adopted. In other more limited regions, the use of residual insecticides has reduced or sometimes eradicated the tse-tse fly. Nevertheless, numerous endemic foci and reservoirs of infection continue to exist and impel health authorities to persevere in their control measures.

The administration of chemical drugs to human beings who have incurred sleeping sickness has also become more general in recent years. While, prior to the introduction of these drugs, sleeping sickness was almost inevitably fatal, it may now be cured by use of the drugs at an early stage of the disease; some of these same drugs may also be administered prophylactically against one of the forms of the disease.

DEGENERATIVE DISEASES. Most of the infectious diseases considered in the preceding paragraphs are health problems today primarily in the economically less developed countries. In the more developed countries where the communicable diseases that were major health problems 50 years ago are no longer prevalent, the chronic degenerative and malignant diseases have become important causes of mortality and morbidity. As the life span extends, these diseases and the care of aged persons become the main preoccupation of most of the national health authorities. During recent years, in many of the technologically advanced countries, increasing efforts have been directed to research on the etiology and prevention of the degenerative and malignant diseases such as cancer and atherosclerosis. So far, no practical solution has been found to the problem of the prevention of these diseases. A number of countries, principally the United States, have advocated the "multiple screening" process as a means to detect early, and therefore treat more effectively, some of the degenerative and malignant diseases.

In the consideration of this group of diseases, special attention should be called to the fact that statistics which are cited refer almost exclusively to the economically and technologically advanced countries, and therefore do not have world-wide coverage.

HEART DISEASE. It should be kept in mind that cardiovascular diseases, like cancer affect mainly middle-aged and older persons; their incidence and the resulting mortality rates in particular countries are, therefore, to a considerable extent affected by the age distribution of the population. There may be relatively low over-all mortality from cardiovascular diseases in a country with a high birthrate and therefore a high percentage of young people in its population, while at the same time age-specific death rates from these diseases show them to be important causes of death. Thus, over-all mortality from heart disease is much lower in the Netherlands than in Norway (male rates per 100,000 of total male population are 306.0 and 358.8, respectively), but mortality for men above 40 is approximately the same in both countries (932 in the Netherlands and 936 in Norway);

this apparent discrepancy is due to the fact that young people and children constitute a much higher percentage of the population in the Netherlands than in Norway.

In almost every country for which data are available, and for all age-groups, male mortality from cardiovascular diseases is higher, sometimes much higher, than female mortality, although the differential declines at the oldest age levels. Mortality from these diseases for both sexes increases rapidly with advancing age.

Even within specific countries, a wide range in mortality rates according to the type of locality may be found, with female mortality generally lower in each locality than male. Thus, according to a survey made by the United States Public Health Service, in New York State male mortality from heart disease for the 45–64 years age group during 1949–1951 was 653.4 per 100,000 inhabitants, while in New Mexico it was 309.0; female mortality from heart disease was 223.2 in New York and 79.2 in New Mexico.[26]

Degenerative heart disease is now the most frequent cause of death in Northern America, in most of Europe, and among the more prosperous segments of the population in many other parts of the world. The increasing dominance of degenerative heart diseases in these areas can not be explained solely as the result of reduction of other causes of mortality or of the changing age structure of the population. The mode of life appears to be involved, and there is increasing evidence that the type of diet consumed in industrially advanced, high-income areas may play an important role in the development of degenerative heart diseases.[27]

CANCER. The increased incidence of certain forms of cancer, especially cancers of the respiratory system, has been remarkable in recent years and has given rise to much apprehension. This development is most striking in countries with relatively high levels of industrialization and income. A WHO study of the increase over recent years in deaths from cancers of the respiratory system has shown increases ranging from 21 to 50 per cent in men. Among women in almost all countries, mortality from cancer of the respiratory system has been found to be not only much lower than among men, but also to be increasing less rapidly, so that the male-female differential is growing. With improved diagnosis and treatment, some forms of cancer peculiar to women (in particular, cancer of the uterus) have been declining or stationary as causes of death in a number of countries.

In spite of the rapid increase in cancers of the respiratory system, cancers of the digestive organs, which are increasing more slowly, still appear to take more lives than any other type of malignancy. In Japan, cancers of the digestive organs account for 73.6 per cent of all cancer deaths; in 18 other countries, this percentage, while lower, still shows that more cancer patients die from cancer of the digestive organs than from any other type of cancer and often from all other types together.

As in the case of mortality from cancer of the respiratory organs, mortality from cancer of the digestive organs is higher—in some cases, strikingly so—among men than among women.[29] Mortality from such cancers increases from the age of 40 and becomes extremely important after 60.

Much study is now being devoted to the causes of increased cancer mortality. Improvements in diagnostic methods, aging of the population, and decrease of deaths from other causes undoubtedly account for much of the rise, yet it would appear that these factors cannot explain its whole extent, in particular the rapid rise in male cancer of the lungs and other cancers of the respiratory system. Thus, improvement in diagnostic techniques cannot explain the more rapid rise in mortality from such cancers among males than among females. Extensive research is being conducted on the significance of the statistical correlations that have been found to exist between heavy cigarette smoking and frequency of cancer of the respiratory organs. The possibility that exhaust fumes and other types of air pollution in urban industrial areas may contribute to the frequency of respiratory cancer is also being investigated.

Accidents

The increasing use of machinery, and in particular, the expansion of motorized traffic in many parts of the world have been accompanied by constantly increasing accident rates. Special attention is therefore being given in many countries to the study of the physical and psychologic problems involved in the causation of accidents.

In countries covered by a recent WHO study of the problem,[30] accidents of all kinds were responsible for between 2.4 and almost 7 per cent of all deaths, with rates running considerably higher for men than for women.

Transport fatalities—most of them resulting from motorcar accidents—appear to be the major form of accidental deaths in these countries and are increasing in absolute figures as well as in relation to other forms of accidental death. In a number of countries, such as Australia, Canada, Germany (Federal Republic), Italy, Sweden and the United States, transport fatalities now account for one half or nearly one half of the total number of such deaths, this ratio being much higher among men than among women.

Apart from transport fatalities, the major causes of accidental deaths are as follows: falls, which in certain countries are responsible for up to two-thirds of all accidental deaths; drowning, which may account for up to one-third; fire and explosions, which sometimes cause up to one quarter; and poisoning, accounting in some places for nearly one-fifth of all accident victims.

In economically developed countries, mortality from accidents has now become a major cause of death among children, particularly among boys. In fact, it appears that in these countries more children now die from accidents than from all infective and parasitic diseases put together.[31] In 1954, deaths from accidents accounted for 58 per cent of all deaths among boys 5–19 years of age in Canada, 45 per cent in the Netherlands, and 38 per cent in England and Wales. Next to transport fatalities, drowning tends to account for the largest number of accidental deaths among children, particularly in the younger age-groups (in the Netherlands drowning accounts for more deaths in the 1–5 year age-group than do transport fatalities). In Finland more than half of the accidental deaths other than transport fatalities are caused by drowning; in Iceland, however, where swimming lessons are compulsory, drownings have been decreasing as a cause of death. Among infants up to one year, suffocation is the most common cause of accidental death in the countries under consideration.

Male-Female Differences in Mortality Trends

It will be noted from the above discussion that in the case of the degenerative diseases that are increasing as causes of death in modern industrial societies—especially heart diseases and cancers of the respiratory organs and the digestive system—the male rates have, as a rule, risen to significantly higher levels than have the female rates. The same is true of deaths from accidents. One result is that the female life expectancy has lengthened more than that of the males in these countries.

A considerable sex differential is also found in certain other diseases that are believed to be more common in highly urbanized and industrialized societies than elsewhere. This includes ulcers of the stomach and duodenum, which are generally not, however, major causes of death and for which the mortality rates have not been increasing during the period under review.[32]

A similar picture of sex differences holds in regard to suicide rates, which would also appear to be higher in the more urbanized and industrialized countries.[33]

HEALTH PROMOTION AND PROTECTION

Progress in health is not to be judged merely by the reduction of mortality rates or the control or prevention of specified diseases. Good health is a positive concept which involves general protection of the individual against sickness and the promotion of a general state of well-being. This is recognized in the growing emphasis that is being given by national health administrations to the healthy development of children, the health education and health conscious-ness of the public, to mental health and to environmental sanitation. The recent development in the use of atomic energy has also brought to attention the health problems involved and the need for protective measures against exposure to excessive radiation.

A balanced picture of the world health situation must, therefore, take into account those aspects that are related to the promotion and protection of the health of populations. There are, however, extremely few statistics of a reliable and comparable nature bearing on such matters. Perhaps the salient fact to be recorded is the growing recog-nition of their importance.[34]

It does appear, however, from scattered data on infant mortality and from other sources, that the state of health of children in many parts of the world has been improving, partly as a result of the atten-tion given to maternal care and child health services; efforts have been made in many countries to extend these services to rural areas and to link the preventive and curative aspects. Nevertheless, children in many countries still suffer from undernutrition (which may have serious implications for subsequent adult health), and this is fre-quently aggravated by heavy helminthic infestations. The diet of children in most of the under-developed areas is deficient in animal protein. Skimmed milk powder is at present being widely distributed and used for feeding the weaned child, or in school feeding schemes, but a lasting solution to the problem of child malnutrition is still being sought. Research into the ways and means of using locally available sources of protein for child feeding is being carried out in Africa, Central America, and India.

Mental Health

The need to safeguard mental health has become obvious in countries where mental health disorders constitute a serious Public Health problem—leading, in some of the more developed countries, to the occupancy of approximately one half of the existing hospital beds by the mentally ill. Such figures do not refer to the patients treated in general hospitals whose diseases are wholly or partly of psychologic origin.

The reasons for this situation are complex. On the one hand, where people are living longer, problems of old age increase, and more cases of mental disorders, such as the arteriosclerotic or senile psy-choses, occur and require special care. Psychoses due to such causes accounted for about 40 per cent of the first admissions to New York

State mental hospitals in 1953 and 1954. On the other hand, it is also believed that psychologic stress or conflict in connection with changing social conditions may cause psychoneurotic and psychosomatic diseases and other mental health problems, including those associated with juvenile delinquency. Finally, there is good reason to believe that the number of patients who seek help in the mental field has a tendency to increase as soon as attention is called to the fact that adequate medical care is available for them.

The assessment of mental health conditions is, however, complicated by the fact that few countries have reliable statistics on the subject, and even within a given country, concepts and definitions may vary widely. The extent to which existing mental disorders receive professional treatment or result in hospitalization may also vary widely. In Japan, according to a recent survey, less than 10 per cent of all the cases of mental disorder found in a given region received some form of care by physicians or psychiatrists—90 per cent had no professional guidance at all. Statistics on, say, hospital admissions for mental illness—which are sometimes used as an indication of rates of mental illness—are usually not comparable from country to country, and particularly cannot be used to compare industrialized and non-industrialized countries. Thus, while it is commonly believed that different types of society and culture produce differing amounts of mental illness (as well as differing forms), there is insufficient statistical information to permit firm conclusions on this subject at present.

Studies in mental health have shown that the causes of mental derangement often occur in infancy or early childhood and that the normal development of the child in relation to his parents, family, or society is of vital importance. Increasing attention is, therefore, being given to mental health activities in all health services—especially maternal and child health services—and to the adoption of preventive measures.

In the field of therapy, greater attention is now being given to the need for treating patients with a view toward their maintaining, or at least recuperating at an early date, their integration with society. More and more use is therefore made of outpatient departments and of day hospitals, particularly in the United Kingdom, Canada, and the United States, while in ordinary hospital work the need for creating a therapeutic community is being stressed. In this context mention should also be made of the increasing interest in the use of group psychotherapeutic technics. As to drug therapy, there has been an important development in recent years, consisting of the introduction of substances such as chlorpromazine and reserpine which have a "tranquilizing" effect upon the nervous system. By controlled use of these drugs, it has been possible to improve the psychotherapeutic and sociotherapeutic accessibility of mental patients and thereby to cut down the average length of hospitalization in many establishments.

Environmental Sanitation, and Environmental Hazards from Industrial Development

In the economically less developed countries, the major problems of environmental sanitation relate to the transmission of disease, and the principal efforts during the period under review have been directed toward the improvement of water supply and excreta disposal and the control of insects. Particular attention has been given by many countries to the adequate provision of water to the rural population.

In the more industrially advanced countries, improved environmental sanitation has greatly reduced the transmission of disease. The activities of health departments include continuing supervision of water supplies, sewage collection and disposal, and food hygiene programs. In addition to such continuing action against the dangers of biologic contamination or pollution, however, the health authorities in these countries must also deal with dangers from the presence in the environment of certain chemical or physical substances or processes.

While industrialization has helped provide the technical means and material resources for considerable advances in health, it has also brought new hazards to health. Reference has already been made to the increases in accidents directly associated with expansion of motor transport, as well as to increases in degenerative diseases which may be to some extent associated with certain modes of living and habits of consumption in a high-income industrialized society. The toxic effects of insecticides (traces of which remain on food that reaches the table), of certain food additives and other chemical products ingested into the body[35] are further examples of dangers that may accompany technologic advancement. So also are certain hazards to health deriving from environmental contamination.

Countries now highly industrialized, or undergoing extensive industrialization, are faced with new factors which already exercise a detrimental effect on sanitary conditions, even in areas considered to have achieved high standards of sanitation. Pollution of waters by industrial wastes is one important new factor. Toxic wastes from several types of industry, particularly such metal-processing wastes as cyanide and chromium, make water totally unfit for human consumption; organic wastes from such industries as pulp and paper mills or food processing plants, although not specifically toxic, by fouling streams make water so unpalatable as to be unsuitable for water supply; acid wastes from mining operations or from other industrial processes render the water so corrosive and so difficult to purify that its value for general purposes is greatly reduced. Pollution by industrial wastes may affect the recreational use of interior and coastal waters; it may exterminate fish and shellfish and thus affect food and nutrition; and it may also render water unusable for agricultural purposes. Air pollution attributable to industrial gases, fumes and smoke, including exhaust gases from internal combustion engines, has already become a serious matter in many industrial areas. The notorious "smogs" of London, Los Angeles, and the Ruhr are good examples of this hazard.

Aside from these specific conditions, industrialization, when associated with over-rapid urbanization, may lead to a number of other problems in community sanitation. Among them are problems associated with deterioration of housing, over-taxing of water and sewage systems, and the breakdown of services relating to public cleansing, food and restaurant sanitation.

Radiation[36]

Atomic radiation presents a health problem that is associated with some of the most important of modern scientific and technologic developments. It is a problem that has come to public attention particularly in connection with the testing of atomic and thermonuclear bombs and the industrial use of atomic energy, but recently interest has been directed to the total picture of the radiation received by populations in a modern technologic society.

Humanity has always been exposed to a certain amount of atomic radiation, coming from cosmic sources and from the naturally radioactive elements (uranium, radium, potassium 40, carbon 14, etc.) that are found locally in the earth or are incorporated in the body. It has been estimated that the background gamma radiations from the earth usually produce about 45 per cent of the total of natural irradiation, cosmic rays (at sea level) about 30 per cent.[37] The amount of radiation from natural sources is variable, because radioactive minerals are not equally distributed throughout the inhabited world, and because the intensity with which cosmic rays hit the earth at any point of its surface depends on several factors, including altitude.

Artificial irradiation is derived from:[38]

(1) The contamination of the environment, the atmosphere, or water by radioactive waste from atomic industries or from users of radioelements;

(2) The radioactive fallout, at greater or lesser distances from the source, or radioactivity resulting from the explosion of nuclear devices;

(3) The occupational exposure of certain groups of workers: medical practitioners, radiologists, dentists, nurses, atomic energy

workers, uranium or thorium miners, and the industrial or scientific users of radiation generators or radioisotopes;

(4) The medical use of X-rays, other ionizing radiations and radioelements in the detection, diagnosis, investigation, and treatment of human diseases;

(5) The use of certain devices which emit radiation, such as television receivers, watches with luminous dials, and the X-ray generators used for the purpose of fitting shoes.

The amount of artificial radiation must vary considerably in different countries, and there is inadequate information as to the overall significance of these factors. In certain countries where estimates have been made, it appears that the greatest gonad irradiation of the population is due to diagnostic radiologic procedures, the amount from this source about equalling that from all natural sources in certain instances. The total present contribution from occupational exposure, from the products of atomic industries, from radiotherapy, and from the miscellaneous radiating devices mentioned above is likely to be considerably smaller. That from radioactive fallout appears at present to be in the region of 1 per cent of the natural gonad irradiation in most areas.[39]

Radiation may have effects on the individual, or through him on his descendants. The former effects, called "somatic," occur primarily in those persons who are themselves exposed to occupational or other hazards, or to accidents. These include such effects as chronic or acute injuries to the hands suffered by radiologists, bone conditions sometimes leading to cancer in radium workers, forms of anemia, such as leukemia and aplastic anemia, and a variety of other effects.

The health problem associated with the genetic effects of radiation is different in nature from the problem of direct bodily injury. When radiation affects the germinal tissues of the productive organs of a wide range of organisms from lower creatures to mammals, it has been shown to produce mutations in their offspring although these effects may not appear under natural conditions of breeding for many generations. It should be stressed that mutations of a similar kind occur spontaneously, and one is not dealing with a mysterious injury of an entirely new type: radiation may merely influence the rate of production of such alterations in heredity. The great majority of mutations from both sources are thought to be harmful and also "genetic effects of radiation are characterized by the fact that no threshold is known or substantially suspected to exist."[40] Moreover, the genetic damage done by radiation is thought to be irreversible and cumulative. In other words, what counts from the point of view of genetic change is not the amount of radiation time, but the total accumulated dose of radiation to all members of the population from the beginning of each individual's life to the time that the offspring are conceived. No precise correlation between the amount of accumulated radiation and the genetic effect has been calculated, but available scientific information leads to the conclusion that the greater the total dose of radiation received, the greater the likelihood of genetic defects in the total off-spring over many generations. All sources of radiation, natural and artificial, contribute to this total.

Because of the complex character of radiation hazards and the length of time needed to observe their effects on individual human beings and on populations, relevant factual information is at the present time inadequate. Vast quantities of data are needed before final conclusions can be reached as to the levels of radiation danger, both somatic and genetic.

Provision of Health Services

As the concept of health has undergone considerable evolutionary change during recent years, the scope of health services has been greatly broadened.[41] Many countries are now undertaking to provide a more comprehensive health service, and to make the service available, as far as possible, to all sections of the population. Perhaps the most important and significant recent feature in the provision of health services is the development of local health units through a system of decentralized integrated health services. This involves the creation of local health units in which both curative and preventive services are provided by teams of medical and health auxiliary workers (medical assistants, sanitary overseers, dispensers, nurses, midwives, etc.) under the direction of physicians or medical officers.[42] In an increasing number of countries, such units are being integrated into decentralized national systems of health protection, and in some cases they are also co-ordinated with over-all economic and social development programs. They are particularly important in the rural areas of the less developed countries, where they are beginning to compensate for the concentration of health facilities in the cities.

To the extent that a general promotion of health is indicated by the improvement in health services and facilities, such recent developments in the establishment of local health centers, clinics, dispensaries, etc., should be taken into account.

Available statistics bearing on the extent of health services are largely limited, however, to numbers of hospital beds. The demands for hospital beds are increasing in many countries, and the provision for hospital service is, as a rule, taking priority over that of an integrated local health service. According to the information made available by Governments, the increase in hospital beds in a great number of countries has been considerable during the past few years. In considering the need for hospital beds in a country, the mere ratio of inhabitants per hospital bed is not adequate to indicate the extent of fulfilment of such a need without further analysis of the distribution and use of the hospital service in connection with the total health service and the requirements of the country. Hospitals are often concentrated in large cities and inaccessible to many of the inhabitants of the hinterland. Experts have considered that the number of hospital beds in relation to population has only a potential significance as regards "treatment" given to the population[43] and it cannot be considered as fully representing a decisive factor for determining health levels.[44]

Availability of Trained Health Personnel

In many countries, the provision of health services is limited by a shortage of health personnel. During recent years, both medical educators and Public Health administrators have been aware of this problem and have pointed out the need for close and frequent consultations between the teaching institutions in the medical and allied fields and the health authorities in order to secure effective co-ordination of teaching schedules as well as the supply of different types of personnel to meet the needs of health services.[45]

This involves both qualitative and quantitative adjustments in the education and training of health personnel. The aim of medical education to prepare physicians of the future has been set[46] and the team concept of health workers has been defined.[47] These changes are particularly important today when the social legislator looks more and more to the medical scientist for advice on how best to apply knowledge in medical sciences for the well-being of the community as a whole.

In a number of countries, opportunities have been provided for the study of "social" or "comprehensive" medicine, by the creation of Chairs or Departments of Social Medicine in universities or Schools of Public Health, and the teaching of preventive and social medicine in undergraduate medical education has been intensified. Recent alterations in the teaching of medical students have taken the form of revision of the pre-clinical courses to allow an earlier introduction of the student to the patient in his family environment—the allocation of a student to a family which he follows under guidance for a certain period. The psychologic aspects of medical care are, rather belatedly, being given increased attention in some of the more advanced medical schools.

The quantitative aspects of the supply of physicians have been the subject of a recent study.[48] As in the case of the index of hospital beds, "the population per physician" ratio is considered to have limited significance because of difficulties in ascertaining the distribution and utilization of this service. The gross insufficiency of physicians is, however, evident in the less developed areas, where, in some cases, there is only one physician for every 50,000 or more inhabitants, as compared with one doctor for about every 900 inhabitants in the more highly developed countries. In the great majority of the countries for which data are available, there has been some improvement in the ratio during the period under review, 1948–1954.

The question of the availability of medical personnel concerns not only physicians, but also a variety of auxiliary personnel. The Governments of a number of countries, in addition to planning and readjusting of professional education for medical and allied personnel, have made use of the team concept of health workers by training and utilizing auxiliary medical and health workers to solve the problem of shortage of fully qualified medical personnel. In South East Asian and African countries and territories, "medical assistants" or "health assistants" have been widely used to carry out some of the functions of fully qualified doctors.

The use of various categories of health auxiliary workers—including auxiliaries in nursing, midwifery, environmental sanitation and dental work—has enabled many countries to extend health services to larger sections of their populations. Health progress indicated in the rates for specific regions or localities, no doubt reflected to an important degree this extension of services, particularly to rural areas.

1. *Report on International Definition and Measurement of Standards and Levels of Living* (United Nations publication, Sales No.: 1954.IV.5) and World Health Organization, *Expert Committee on Health Statistics*, Fourth Report, WHO/HS/56, 1954.

2. World Health Organization, *Report of the Study Group on the Measurement of Levels of Health*, WHO/PHA/25, 1955, p. 13.

3. World Health Organization, *Annual Report of the Director-General for 1954*, Official Records of the World Health Organization, No. 59, p. 41.

4. R. Pollitzer, *History and Present Distribution of Plague*, World Health Organization Monograph Series No. 22, 1954.

5. J. Austin Kerr: "The Last Refuge of Yellow Fever," *Courier*, vol. VIII, No. 12 (Paris, UNESCO, 1956), p. 26.

6. *Epidemic Diseases* (Memorandum by the World Health Organization), United Nations, A/AC.35/L.88, para. 21.

7. World Health Organization, *Annual Report of the Director-General for 1954, op. cit.*, p. 14.

8. J. M. S. de Gear, *Poliomyelitis in Underdeveloped Countries*, World Health Organization Monograph Series No. 26, 1955, p. 31.

9. John R. Paul, *Epidemiology of Poliomyelitis, ibid.*, p. 12.

10. M. J. Freyche and J. Nelson, *Incidence of Poliomyelitis since 1920, ibid.*, pp. 59–106.

11. J. M. S. de Gear, *op. cit.*, pp. 34–38.

12. *Poliomyelitis Vaccination: A Preliminary Review*, a report prepared by a World Health Organization Expert Committee on Poliomyelitis (Geneva 1956).

13. "Virus Meningo-Encephalitis and Poliomyelitis," *Bulletin of the World Health Organization*, vol. 12, No. 4, 1955.

14. World Health Organization, *Annual Report of the Director-General for 1954, op. cit.*, p. 7.

15. See "Mortality from Pneumonia," World Health Organization *Epidemiological and Vital Statistics Report*, vol. 9, No. 9, 1956.

16. Documents presented to the ninth session of the Regional Com-

mittee for South East Asia, World Health Organization, August 1956.

17. *International Survey of Programs of Social Development* (United Nations publication, Sales No.:1955.-IV.8) p. 28.

18. E. J. Pampana, "Changing Strategy in Malaria Control," *Bulletin of the World Health Organization*, vol. 11, No. 4–5, 1954, p. 514.

19. "Onchocerciasis, A New Field of World Health Organization Activities," *Journal of the American Medical Association*, vol. 10, No. 7, July 1955, pp. 226–230.

20. World Health Organization, *Report of Expert Committee on Onchocerciasis*, World Health Organization Technical Report Series No. 87, Geneva, 1954.

21. Anthony Levers, "In the Valley of the Blind," *Courier*, vol. VIII, No. 12 (Paris, UNESCO, June 1956), p. 10.

22. *Social Conditions in Non-Self-Governing Territories: Public Health. Communicable Diseases* (Memorandum by the World Health Organization), United Nations, A/AC.35/L.205, paras. 10 and 11.

23. *Ibid.*, para. 12.

24. *Ibid.*, paras. 8 and 9.

25. J. Ford (Director, East Africa Tse-Tse and Trypanosomiasis Research and Reclamation Organization) "The Sleep that Kills," *Courier*, vol. VIII, No. 12 (Paris, UNESCO, 1956), pp. 12–14.

26. Philip E. Enterline and William A. Stewart, "Geographic Patterns in Death from Coronary Heart Disease," *Public Health Reports*, vol. 71, No. 9, September 1956.

27. World Health Organization, *Joint FAO–WHO Expert Committee on Nutrition*, Fourth Report, World Health Organization Technical Report Series No. 97, Geneva 1955, p. 42.

28. Omitted.

29. "Mortality from Malignant Neoplasms of Digestive Organs and Peritoneum," World Health Organization, *Epidemiological and Vital Statistics Report*, vol. 9, No. 5, 1956.

30. "Mortality from Accidents," World Health Organization, *Epidemiological and Vital Statistics Report*, vol. 9, No. 1, 1956.

31. *Ibid.*, p. 123.

32. See "Death from Ulcers of Stomach and of the Duodenum in Selected Countries," World Health Organization, *Epidemiological and Vital Statistics Report*, vol. 8, No. 9, 1955, pp. 361–365. Stationary or declining mortality trends do not, of course, imply that morbidity trends may not have been rising.

33. See "Mortality from Suicide," World Health Organization, *Epidemiological and Vital Statistics Report*, vol. 9, No. 4, 1956. It should be noted that there are few data for less developed countries; that the reliability and comparability of suicide rates are open to considerable question; that some of the more developed countries have rates as low as under-developed countries; and that, in general, published suicide rates have not shown any broad upward tendency in the more developed countries during the last 50 years or so, in spite of rapid urbanization and industrialization during that period.

34. Relevant programs have been treated in some detail in *International Survey of Programs of Social Development, op. cit.*

35. World Health Organization, *Joint FAO/WHO Expert Committee on Nutrition*, Fourth Report, World Health Organization Technical Report Series No. 97, Geneva, 1955.

36. Many of the statements contained in this section are drawn from reports on the Proceedings of the International Conference on the Peaceful Use of Atomic Energy, held in Geneva, August 1955; *The Biological Effects of Atomic Radiation*, a collection of reports made by expert committees on this subject to the National Academy of Sciences of the U.S.A. and published by the latter in 1956; and *The Hazards to Man of Nuclear and Allied Radiations*, a report of the Expert Committee appointed by the United Kingdom Medical Research Council.

37. *The Responsibilities of the Medical Profession in the Use of X-Rays and Other Ionizing Radiation*, forthcoming Statement by the United Nations Scientific Committee on the Effects of Atomic Radiation.

38. The following information on the sources and amounts of artificial irradiation is taken from the Statement of the United Nations Scientific Com-

mittee on the Effects of Atomic Radiation, cited above.

39. According to the reports sent to the United Nations Scientific Committee on the Effects of Atomic Radiation by the United Kingdom and the United States of America.

40. Austin M. Brues, "Commentary on the Modes of Radiation Injury," in *Peaceful Uses of Atomic Energy—Proceedings of the International Conference in Geneva*, August 1955, vol. 11 (New York, 1956), p. 73.

41. See the discussion of health services in the *International Survey of Programs of Social Development*, pp. 11–17.

42. In the Soviet Union, for example, a widely distributed network of health establishments provides both curative and preventive services for the rural population. Every rural district varying from 50,000 to 100,000 population has one district hospital with about 100 to 150 beds, two to five rural medical centers and a number of health stations, nursing homes, and temporary or permanent nurseries.

43. *Report of the Study Group on the Measurement of Levels of Health*, op. cit.

44. *Expert Committee on Health Statistics*, Fourth Report, *op. cit.*, p. 22.

45. World Health Organization Technical Report Series No. 55, p. 17.

46. World Health Organization Technical Report Series No. 69, pp. 4–5.

47. WHO/Educ/44.

48. J. L. Troupin, "Medical Schools and Physicians—Quantitative Aspects," *Bulletin of the World Health Organization*, vol. 13, No. 2, 1955, pp. 357–361. National ratios of physicians to population are also given in the United Nations *Statistical Yearbook*.

PART TWO

The People: Target Populations

    1. The Family in Change   127

    2. The Chronically Ill   141

    3. The Aging   149

    4. The Workers   164

    5. The Mothers and their Children   192

    6. Youth and the Community   213

    7. The Mentally Ill in Social Perspective   235

    8. The Mentally Retarded   247

    9. The Migrants   259

   10. The Travelers   268

"A NEW approach to health itself is being fostered by professional groups as well as in the popular mind. Health is now being thought of, not in terms of disease or mortality figures, but in a positive way, in terms of physical fitness, mental and emotional adjustment, and social satisfaction and usefulness. In other words, health is no longer considered solely as an end, but also as a means. The Public Health responsibility cannot be considered liquidated once we have reduced infant mortality to the vanishing point, or conquered malaria or syphilis, or even cancer and heart disease. It must be geared to promoting ever higher standards of human efficiency and satisfaction.

As an important corollary of this approach, Public Health workers are obliged to take a new look at the origins of social pathology. Health problems cannot be isolated from the environment—both physical and social—in which they exist. Such factors as the individual's job, his family life, his housing, his recreation must all be assayed for their impact on health and disease. In other words, we must now not only put emphasis on the individual and his needs, but also consider him in relation to his whole complex socio-economic environment."

Joseph W. Mountin, M.D., "The Health Department's Dilemma," *Public Health Reports* (March) 1952.

1.   The Family in Change

A BASIC social institution, the nuclear family, is a major determinant of personality and behavior, and thereby an important factor in the maintenance of illness or health. To endure as an institution, the family has shown amazing flexibility in the variety of socio-cultural forms in which it expresses biologic and psychologic drives. Dr. Hill, a sociologist, charts some ways in which the American family has been adapting to broad changes in our society.

If the family is a nuclear unit of social life, and a matrix of social growth, it is also a major instrument for transmitting the technical advances of a culture. Hence, to effectuate their programs, workers in the health professions need full awareness of the impact and circumstances of family life in each culture or subculture with which they deal. Illness as well as health is transmitted via the family— as Dr. Dingle and his collaborators demonstrate in their studies of family life—and the Public Health approach is increasingly a family-centered one.

The American Family Today*

REUBEN HILL, PH.D.

AT THE TURN of the century, most people had the greatest respect for the institution called the family, yet they were loath to learn much about it. The family was taken for granted, ignored, shunted aside, and expected to do the nation's patching and mending without reward or attention. According to the cherished beliefs of the period, all husbands and wives lived together in perfect amity, and all children loved their parents, to whom they were indebted for the gift of life. Moreover, even if one knew that these things were not true, he ought not to mention it!

Today much of that has been changed. Gone is the concealment of the way in which life begins, gone the irrational sanctity of the home. The aura of sentiment which once protected the family from discussion

* Reprinted, in part, by permission of the National Committee for Children and Youth, from Volume I, *The Nation's Children*, edited by Eli Ginzberg and published by the Columbia University Press for the Golden Anniversary White House Conference on Children and Youth, pp. 76–107, 1960. The author is Director of the Minnesota Family Study Center and Professor of Sociology at the University of Minnesota, Minneapolis, Minnesota.

clings to it no more. It is no longer considered a virtue to be naive or ignorant about the family. We want to learn as much about it as we can and to understand it as thoroughly as possible, for there is a rising recognition in America that vast numbers of its families are in trouble —sick from internal frustrations and from external pressures in a society which expects the individual family to act as buffer between a poorly integrated social order and the country's children. If fiscal policies are bungled and inflation results, the family purse strings are tightened; if real estate and building interests fail to provide housing, families must adapt themselves to obsolete dwellings or be shoehorned into quarters shared with other families.

The now famous Bill of Rights for Children of the 1930 White House Conference would be no more than a list of platitudes if individual families did not secure these rights for their children. Alas, this is too much to expect of economically and educationally marginal families. This is one reason subsequent White House Conferences have included analysis of the optimum relationship between the family and government, and between the family and community planning. We are engaged in the process of reconstructing our family institutions in these conferences through criticism and discussion.

As the ban on discussion of the family has been lifted, many have assumed expertness in diagnosing the American family's ills—and their approach usually begins "What's Wrong with the Family?" A wide variety of writers have addressed themselves to this theme recently, and the range of national magazines carrying their articles suggests the high readership provoked by problems of courtship, marriage, and the family. *Life, Look, McCall's, Ladies Home Journal, Better Homes and Gardens, Harper's,* and *The Atlantic* have featured the family and its problems in recent months. College presidents, psychiatrists, ministers, social workers, and judges appear frequently, but included among the authors can be found a labor leader, a motion picture arbiter, an anthropologist, a political commentator, and the American Mother of the Year. Each touches the ailing body of the American family in a different place, but all agree she is ailing. They point to the high divorce rate, to the changes in our sex morality, to juvenile delinquency, and to the rise in forced marriages of teenagers as proof of the breakdown of the family. The causes they list are most varied:

It's the breakdown of character.

It's modern women—they ought to stay home and take care of their children.

It's the search for happiness—we need to return to the old-fashioned virtues of responsibility and adherence to duty.

Alcohol is the key to it all.

There aren't enough parks and playgrounds.

It's poor sex adjustment—what people need are the facts of life.

The trouble is easy divorce—people know they can get out of marriage if it doesn't work.

It's dissimilarity of family backgrounds and temperament.

I regard much of this hue and cry in the public press as useful and healthy, but I do not have too much confidence in the diagnoses advanced by America's self-styled family experts. My approach is that of a family sociologist who has been greatly impressed by the universality of the family as an institution in all countries and in all times, and by its great capacity for adaptation and survival. The social scientist studying the family takes the comparative approach, and asks what troubles experienced by the American family are also reported for families in industrializing and urbanizing societies in other parts of the world. From this vantage point it is possible to conclude that many of the disorders of the American family appear to be "growing pains," discomforts incident to adaptive change, normal symptoms of reorganization following adjustment to a new and baffling industrial urban society. Let us examine these changes in some detail, remembering that there is still much to be learned about the 40-odd million American families in this country and that research is just beginning to answer some of our questions.

A major shortcoming of the diagnoses formulated by writers in the mass media is the fact that they have been based on a limited number of observations. The psychiatrists drew primarily from the biased sample of cases they observed in clinical practice. Judges are prone to write from the distorted view of marriage sick enough for couples to seek adjudication of their troubles through divorce. Other writers relied heavily on the accumulated personal contacts of a lifetime of shrewd observations, often involving no more than a hundred families all told. I hope to improve on this by turning to the several research studies and surveys by social scientists in recent years, covering several thousand families, and the findings of the censuses and sample surveys of the Bureau of the Census which cover the country as a whole.

In a quick review I hope to answer three major questions: (1) What long-term and what short-term changes are occurring in marriage and family patterns in America? (2) Is the family any less important to its members and to American society today than formerly? and (3) What are some implications for conference discussion and for social action of these changes in family patterns?

CHANGES IN MARRIAGE AND
FAMILY PATTERNS

A number of changes in the family tend to be tied to the highly interrelated phenomena of industrialization, urbanization, secularization, and democratization. These we term long-run trends, since they have been more or less continuous and cumulative in their impact on family patterns since well before the Civil War. Another set of changes should be designated as short-term because they tend to be relatively temporary fluctuations around a long-term trend line. They may occur as a consequence of changes in the age and sex composition of the population, or may flow from the vacillations of the country's economy and polity best seen in the cycles of depression and prosperity, of inflation and deflation, and hot wars and cold wars.

As a backdrop for discussing long-term trends let us identify the typical family pattern of a century ago when we were largely a rural frontier society. There were, to be sure, several coexisting minority family patterns which differed in some respects, the colorful but numerically insignificant plantation family of the Southern upper class to mention only one. John Sirjamaki is our source:

> The majority family of the nineteenth century tended to be typically of large size because, although the matter was never put so crassly, many persons were needed for the ceaseless, backbreaking labor of the farms. In 1790, the median family had 5.4 children, and the birth rate which sustained it, 55 per 1,000 population. This high fertility resulted in such volume of children that the median age of the population in 1790, the first year in which a federal census was taken, was 16 years. Relatives of course multiplied in consequence, and the social obligations of kinship were well observed. Kinship was traced bilaterally, that is, on both the male and the female sides of the family, although the former may have been of slightly greater social significance in that it was better supported by the patriarchal practices of the society.
>
> Authority in the majority family was lodged in its male head. European practice and law alike fostered such patriarchy, and American experience appeared to justify it. At any rate, the concentration of power in one person who could organize family members in common enterprise and safeguard their welfare was genuinely necessary in farm life, and this command seemed to rest naturally with the husband and father. His rule was, however, considerably tempered by the fact that women did not always bend easily in obedience to their mates. The rugged frontier existence developed competence and self-reliance in them, and from an early time they had high prestige in frontier society.
>
> The custom of separate domicile by newly wedded couples was adapted to the rural economy of family-sized farmsteads. Such farms were frequently too small to support the related families of two generations, and children upon marriage therefore established themselves apart from parents, often on land or with funds or tools partly provided by them.
>
> Another majority family pattern was the comparative freedom young people exercised in their choice of marriage partners. For a while this was hindered by the requirement that a bride bring

a dowry in money, goods, or estate to her husband in marriage. But this custom did not long persist because women, often in short supply, were gladly taken in wedlock without the added lure of a dowry, and many families had little enough property to bestow anyway. Moreover, because the bringing of a dowry was based upon arranged marriages and necessitated haggling over property settlements, it came to seem excessively gauche and unsentimental.

Of the quality of family living in the nineteenth century it is difficult to generalize, since Americans were of many conditions and domestic felicity is never constant or universal. More was then required than now of the family as an institution in the struggle for existence; hence, successful marriages were judged by their permanence, or fertility, or affluence, and less by the private happiness of the mates. Parent-child relationships were amiable, but often, because mothers were kept busy with household chores, older children were required to take charge of the younger ones. . . . But the hardships of frontier existence often reached into family living, constraining it and removing its joy. The struggle to survive was so relentless that family members had to labor ceaselessly. Houses were often meanly built and small, and the standard of living within them low. Loneliness was frequently the fate of many families, especially those on farm and frontier. Many mothers, worn out by excessive childbearing, died in early middle age, average life expectancy was below 40 years in the first half of the nineteenth century. Amelioration of many of these hardships eventually arrived with the industrial development of the country, but for some families it was slow in coming and for others it did not come at all.[1]

LONG-TERM TRENDS.   One can recognize in this majority family pattern of the nineteenth century many characteristics which have survived into the twentieth century: freedom of mate selection, separate domicile for newlyweds (although one couple in five begin marriage even today in the home of one of the parental families), parental subsidy of marriage (although the support today may need to be more subtle and less openly admitted). In other respects there have been tremendous changes as America has industrialized and urbanized, changes which we identify as long-term trends: changed ways of making a living, decreased self-sufficiency of families, smaller households, increased mobility of families, changed authority patterns, and changed age and sex roles within the family, to mention only a few. Activities once centered in the home, such as production of food and clothing, family recreation, vocational apprenticing, and religious instruction, have been shifted to canneries, factories, recreation centers, vocational schools, and Sunday Schools.

From 1890 to 1960 the proportion of American families subsisting from farming changed from almost half to less than one-tenth. With this changed mode of making a living, the authoritarian, economically integrated, self-sufficient form of family which for centuries had been functionally adapted to rural living has become obsolete. As the family ceased to be a producer of goods and services, the need for an authoritarian foreman in the family disappeared. But as the family ceased to make its own living, and the father left the home to earn money to buy the goods the family once produced, the self-sufficiency of the family also disappeared. The rugged familism which extended the frontier and gave the tenor of individualism to America has disappeared, except as it is found in isolated rural and mountain areas.

The family became dependent upon the availability of jobs, on continued prosperity, and on the productivity of the wage earner. Where the father's productivity was not great enough, mothers left the home to supplement the father's pay check. Children, once viewed as potential added hands who soon could earn their keep, have become in the industrial age mouths to feed, bodies to clothe, and minds to educate. Today children are financial liabilities from birth through their schooling. Conservative estimates place the cost of rearing a child to age 18 at $20,000, and there is still his college education ahead of him.

In order to get ahead in the world, young families have become mobile, migrating for added education, better jobs, and in response to the demands of military service. Compared with other countries of the world we are a people on wheels—one family in five moves annually, and one in three of these crosses county lines every year.

In the course of these long-term shifts in the economy and the larger society, the family has given up many services it once provided its members: schooling, religious instruction, recreation, medical care, and job placement. Many see in these changes evidences of family decay and disorganization, but I find abundant proof that there is no repudiation of the basic business of families; namely, reproduction, housing, feeding, socializing, and guiding children from infancy to adulthood. Indeed, the family is now more of a specialized agency concentrating on personality development of its members, providing warmth, love, and sanctuary from the anonymity of urban existence, services no other agency in society is prepared to offer.

SHORT-RUN CHANGES. Let us turn now for a moment to the examination of some short-run changes which have occurred in recent years. Family behavior has become increasingly subject to short-run fluctuations integrally related to the economic and political shifts in our highly interdependent type of society. Individuals are increasingly making their marital and reproductive decisions deliberately, taking into account their personal outlook of the moment. The result is often that millions make the same kind of decision at the same time. If conditions are bad, as they were during the depression of the '30s, for example, people postpone marriage or if married put off childbearing. At that time, hundreds of thousands of young women, after waiting for several years to marry, had to face the specter of spinsterhood because the men, when they did marry, turned to a younger age group for their brides. Later, when conditions improved, young people who might have waited decided to marry, or if married decided to have children, and the marriage rates and birth rates responded violently.

The propensity to marry has been so affected by the prosperity of the past decade and a half that a greater increase in the proportion of the population married has occurred than in the previous half century. Among men 20 to 24 years of age, the proportion married nearly doubled from 1940 to 1955, from 27 per cent to 51 per cent. Among women of the same ages, the percentage married also increased sharply, from 51 per cent to 70 per cent. The number of marriages in America during the war and postwar years has been increasing rapidly, only divorce among the vital statistics being more volatile.

Divorce has been subject both to long-term and short-term changes. The long-term trend has been on the increase since the first census covering divorce in 1870, reflecting among other things the emancipation of women through education and industrialization. As a short-term phenomenon, the divorce rate follows the marriage rate, which in turn reflects so closely the fluctuations of the business cycle. A cynic once said the basic cause of divorce is marriage! It is true that when marriage rates are low, as in a depression, so is divorce, and when marriage rates go up, so does divorce, for most divorces occur in the early years of marriage. Henry Bowman has used the analogy of a great throng of people on an open drawbridge. As more crowd to get on, others fall off the open end into the water below.

Divorce reached a high of one divorce for every two and one-half marriages in 1946, and has since declined to one in five marriages (the lowest figure since 1941), in line with the more recent decline in the marriage rate. Most vulnerable to divorce during this period have been the childless, the teen-age couples, veterans, the grammar-school educated, and low income groups. Not only are grammar-school educated persons more likely to become divorced (the rate is twice that of persons with a college education), but they end their marriages on the average nine years earlier than college people who do divorce.

A corollary trend which is noteworthy is the high rate of remarriage of the divorced, three-fourths of whom marry again within five years, and 87 per cent of whom eventually remarry. Most likely to remarry are divorcees whose first marriage occured before the age of 18. We are in effect operating a type of trial marriage system in this country in which the first marriage breaks in and domesticates the parties, and the second marriage reaps the benefits.[2] The remarriage rate is good evidence that the high rate of divorce in our society constitutes no repudiation of marriage itself. Marriage has never been more popular; about 70 per cent of the population between the ages of 14 to 90 were married in 1958. Eighteen per cent were single, and most of them will eventually marry. Eight per cent were widowed, 3 per cent separated, and only 2 per cent were in divorced status.

A British social scientist commented on these statistics: "You Americans talk a lot about divorce, but in Europe we worry about the fact that people don't bother to marry. Over 90 per cent eventually marry in America, but only 70 per cent do in Sweden and Switzerland, and fewer yet in Ireland. The age at first marriage of men in rural Ireland is almost 40, more than 10 years later than in America." Americans have indeed been legal in their channeling of the sex drive in wedlock. They have had low rates of illegal cohabitation, concubinage is unheard of, and common law unions are rare. Yet we have one of the highest rates of change of married partners of any Western civilization. Paul Landis has called our form of marriage serial polygyny! You may wish to reverse it and call it brittle monogamy.

Let us turn to another trend which like divorce looks different when viewed as a long-term, than when viewed as a short-run, phenomenon—namely, the size of completed families. Since frontier days the size of households has been shrinking steadily. In 1700, 7.4 children had been born to the average mother 45 years of age and over. By 1910 the number had dropped to 4.7, by 1940 to 2.9, and by 1950 to 2.5 children.

A reversal of this long-term trend is in the making as a consequence of the prolongation of the baby boom of the 1940's and '50's. When a boom continues beyond 10 years, it begins to look like a trend. The increase in the birth rate was a direct result of the rapid increases in marriages of the war and postwar years, beginning first with many more first babies, later with more second and third babies, and now fourth babies. Since 1950, the number of first babies has declined sharply just as the marriage rate has, both examples of short-run changes, but the number of second babies has held up, and third and fourth babies continue to increase. Comparing 1940–41 with 1954–55 the birth rate of third and fourth babies is up 70 per cent.

The shift in family size, however, is not to large families of seven or more children, which have continued to decline from 15 per cent of completed families in 1910, to less than 4 per cent of completed families in 1957. Childlessness, at the other extreme, is also in decline, having dropped from 20 per cent in 1940, to less than 10 per cent in 1957. A recent nation-wide study[3] could uncover no interest in childless or one-child families, and found the most favored family size to be between three and four children. In successive polls the proportion favoring the four-child family has increased from 20 per cent in 1941, to 41 per cent in 1955, while the proportion favoring two children has declined from 40 to 19 per cent over the same period. This same study provides evidence that the higher birth rates of the last 15 years and the prevailing favorable climate for medium-size families will soon affect complete family size in the United States. Asking women not yet 45 years of age how many more children they expect to have, the researchers found women born 1916–20 (who reach the end of child-bearing in 1960–64) have had or expect to have 2.9 children, women born 1921–25 expect 3.0 children, and women born 1931–37 expect 3.2 children, which is substantially more than the 2.4 children pro-duced by mothers who had completed their childbearing by 1950. It is rather exciting to see a long-term trend change directions.

Closely related to the trend of number of children is the pattern of spacing children, which has undergone some changes with the wide-spread use of birth control. There is now a tendency to bunch all the children in the early years of marriage, so that women complete child-bearing in their late twenties and early thirties. The average mother in the United States in 1950 had her last child at age 26. Coupled with an earlier age at marriage for husbands, which has dropped in 60 years from 26.1 to 22.6, and for women from 22.0 to 20.4, husband and wife have a much longer period of companionship together than their parents enjoyed. With her children in school by the time she is in her early thirties, the wife is freer to re-enter the labor force—40 per cent of wives aged 30 to 40 with children in school are gainfully employed. Indeed, there has been a 77 per cent increase in married women ages 35 to 44 in the labor force in the last decade.

Needless to say, this shortening of the period in which the husband must be the sole breadwinner makes marriage less of a financial com-mitment for men, and brings to the relation a more companionate quality. The traditional sentiment that a new husband must support his wife as her father did has now been attenuated in nearly all strata of our society by the growing desire of wives to share in their husband's financial struggles.

CHANGES IN SEX ROLES. As a consequence of these many changes —younger age at marriage, changes in child spacing, as well as changed ways of making a living and the changed emphasis on serv-ices performed in the family—the relationships between husband and wife, and between children and parents have changed sharply with respect to the locus of power, and in the division of duties and re-sponsibilities in the family. Wives and children are becoming economic partners with the husband-father in spending, as well as in earning, the family income. The family is becoming democratized in the process.

Participation by wives in family decision-making extends beyond financial matters, and is concurrently being strengthened by their higher education, wider contact outside the home, exercise of responsibility in civic associations, activities in professional organizations, and by explicit encouragement by experts. Male pretensions to superior authority are widely ridiculed in contemporary comedy, cartoons, children's literature, and other forms of popular art. Moreover, when family decision-making is viewed as a symbol of power, the superiority of shared power in creating and maintaining warmth and affection becomes evident. It is easier to love a reasonable, companionable man, and harder to love an authoritarian husband and father today.

Equally striking in the blurring of sex lines are the changes in the division of tasks and responsibilities in the home. Here the middle classes lead the way, according to a recent study covering hundreds of Omaha families at various educational and occupational status levels. The investigator asked who was primarily responsible for the performance of each of a hundred homely tasks that must be performed to keep a family going. His findings may be stated briefly:

1. The middle classes have gone farthest in bringing the husband into taking responsibility for family tasks, and also designate more tasks as the *joint responsibility* of husband and wife.

2. The lower classes placed more of the burdens on the mother and the children, while the upper classes were the only group to turn to outside help for any substantial proportion of family jobs.

3. For all classes, to be sure, the majority pattern is for the wife to assume responsibility for the greatest number of tasks (40–50 per cent). Second most popular pattern is that of *joint responsibility* (25–28 per cent); third in line is the husband assuming chief responsibility for 20–23 per cent of tasks, followed by children with 6–10 per cent, and outside help 1–14 per cent of tasks.

4. Joint responsibility was the majority pattern for certain types of tasks involving especially control and decision-making, such as disciplining children, training in manners, supervising school work, deciding when to buy a new car, planning the budget, and so on.

There remain today only two or three tasks securely monopolized by one sex: childbearing and sewing by the wife, and the most arduous physical maintenance chores by the husband. Painting, repairing, fueling, and car-washing are increasingly taken on by the wife, sometimes alone, often with the husband. Her dress on these occasions will be male work clothes, and her language will also often be appropriate to the task!

The same crossing of ancient boundaries by the husband is also fast becoming commonplace—diaper-changing, dish-washing, cooking, house-cleaning, laundering, and shopping are duties shared with the wife, especially if she is gainfully employed—and he has learned to wear an apron, a butcher's apron, to be sure, but an apron! Such sharing of tasks fluctuates, rotates, and changes unevenly, frequently provoking conflict, but the net effect is greater companionship between husband and wife, and more freedom for later leisure time pursuits together. Some women and men resent this as a usurpation of their prerogatives, indeed some feel bereaved of function, but most welcome it.

Still another source of marital integration is the trend in America to undertake leisure-time pursuits together. Except in family enterprises like farming, or small family retail enterprises, few couples have been able to coordinate their work lives at the same vocation, but the decline of segregated amusements, "for men only" and "for women only," in favor of recreation for couples, more than offsets this handicap. It has become impolite to invite husbands only, or wives only, to most social functions; today, as a consequence, agreement upon friends and outside interests now appears as important in predicting marital adjustment as approval by the parental families once did. It appears probable that the urban husband spends more hours per week in the company of his wife than in any decade since factories removed manufacturing of goods from the home. Recreation and social activities now integrate the sexes.

But companionship in marriage is more than sharing common tasks in the home and participating in common leisure time activities. Nelson Foote has advanced the concept of "matching careers" to describe the phenomenon of mutual stimulation to development which occurs in a highly companionable marriage.

To expect a marriage to last indefinitely under modern conditions is to expect a lot. The conception of marriage as continually requiring the incitement of new episodes of shared activity will have more consequences than can be foreseen, but a few implications can perhaps be inferred. Happiness as a criterion of success, for instance, is inherently unstable over time. And even at a given time, the prospect of future achievement of aims may have more effect on the judgment of a marriage by its partners than their current state of gratification. Certainly marriage counselors report many cases of mates who disclose no specific cause of dissatisfaction yet complain that they have lost interest in their marriages. Successful marriage may thus come to be defined, both by married people and by students of marriage, in terms of its potential for continued development, rather than in terms of momentary assessments of adjustment. . . .

In particular the notion of matching careers need not imply that husband and wife pursue identical professional careers outside the home. . . . Though their careers be differentiated both in and out of the home, the point that seems decisive in understanding the quality of their marriages appears to remain in the degree of matching in their phases of distinct but comparable development. A simple test may be this, how much do they have to communicate when they are together?[4]

How is this self-conscious appetite for a marriage that will lead to further development of the partners distributed within the occupational classes? Our information on this question is inadequate, but it would appear that it is primarily in the professional classes that companionship and mutual development are sought. In rural and working classes, the relative prominence of functional economic interdependence as the basis for family stability seems much greater than in the more leisured white-collar, business, and professional levels. Moreover, the trend is for more and more of the working force to move from agriculture and manufacturing into the services. If in turn they shift in their interests in marriage to the focus of the professional classes, the implications for family stability are provocative, for repeated studies show that the professional classes are the least vulnerable to divorce of all occupational strata.[5]

The standard view that industrialization and urbanization are inexorably destructive of family stability and solidarity is thus contradicted by the fact that the professional group, which has a low divorce rate, is also the fullest beneficiary of such aspects of industrialism and urbanism as the reliance on science, spatial and social mobility, and emphasis on the welfare and freedom of the individual. The professional group is most liberal in its views about divorce, and is most egalitarian in its views on the propriety of employment of married women, and in espousing the notion of equal authority for husband and wife within the family. It appears to be the most cosmopolitan in the range of its choice of marriage mates; most heterogamous in crossing ethnic, class, and religious lines; least affected by propinquity and closest in ages at marriage. It would seem that voluntary commitments emphasized by the professional groups may be stronger bonds for marriage than the economic and legal sanctions which held together traditional families. To adapt an old saying, what is poison to the rural, traditional family may be meat to the urban, professional family.[6]

PROFESSIONALIZATION OF FAMILY ROLES. What do these trends I have cited add up to? Increasing specialization by the family in services performed for its members, increased emphasis on quality of performance, shift in focus from production of goods to interest in personality development of children, and high affirmation of companionship in marriage and parent-child relations. Possibly Nelson Foote's term, "The Professionalization of Marital and Family Roles," describes best what is taking place in America today.

Marriage is increasingly viewed as a kind of joint career for which preparation can provide the skills and insights to achieve success.

Miller and Swanson have been tempted to call the emerging family the "colleague" family. "As specialists at work may find in each other skills they lack, but skills they equally need, and as they defer to one another's judgment on the grounds of different competence without feeling that they have personally lost in prestige, so husband and wife may now relate in this way."[7] They see this trend toward specialization leading to the professionalization of the wife's functions. She can no longer learn them satisfactorily from her mother's tutelage and example; they must be rationalized. Intuitive processes give way to formal rules and special technical knowledge. Moreover, the skills employed are subject to improvement as they are submitted to critical appraisal and functional selection. In career terms, the women's magazines provide a kind of in-service training, supplemented with the postgraduate work of the mother study clubs, the meetings with the specialists at the nursery school, the cooking classes, and the growing number of handbooks for preparing unfamiliar or exotic foods.[8] The rise of college and high-school courses in preparation for marriage and parenthood attended by men as well as women, and the development of counseling services further affirm this desire on the part of young people to get professional training for their marital and parental roles.

Planning for parenthood today actually goes beyond planning for the control of conception, although a recent nationwide study reveals that children born today are more likely than ever to be wanted, planned children. They are more likely to be seen as a fulfillment rather than a frustration of marriage goals today than in the depression and post-depression period. Planning for parenthood today includes programs of education for parenthood to facilitate the understanding of children in general and one's own children in particular, and thereby to help parents contribute to the maximum development of their personalities. This is a trend of vast significance for personality development and mental health.

Not only are parents professionalizing their marital and parental roles, they are undertaking once again training of the child for the job world, not by providing technical skills, but by helping him in human relations. The child must learn the nuances of interpersonal relations to function in the large and complex organizations of industry, business, and government. The child must study his own relations to others and gain better control over himself and his associates. Parents in the professions today do have relevant, hard-bought skills to make the critical judgments of social situations that their children will need. Miller and Swanson expect, moreover, a reappearance of the parent as the counselor and aid of his children after they have become adults and parents in their own right, thus enabling children to serve as a means of self-continuity and companionship as well as fulfillment.[9] In sum, parents have learned that in the contemporary world, a parent is far better advised to endow his child with competence in interpersonal relations than to leave him with "a competence" in the old sense of the word.

1. John Sirjamaki, *The American Family in the 20th Century* (Cambridge: Harvard University Press, 1953), pp. 38–42. Copyright 1953 by the President and Fellows of Harvard College.

2. A highly reliable serious study of second and third marriages of the divorced and widowed is Jessie Bernard's *Remarriage* (New York: Dryden Press, 1956).

3. Ronald Freedman, Pascal K. Whelpton, and Arthur A. Campbell, *Family Planning, Sterility, and Population Growth* (New York: McGraw-Hill, 1959).

4. Nelson N. Foote, "Matching of Husband and Wife in Phases of Development," in *Transactions of the Third World Congress of Sociology*

(London: International Sociological Association, 1956), IV, 29 (2nd re-printing by permission).

5. W. J. Goode, *After Divorce* (New York: The Free Press, 1956), see especially Chapters IV and V, which summarize these studies, pp. 43–67.

6. Foote, in *Transactions of the Third World Congress of Sociology*, IV, 30.

7. Daniel R. Miller and Guy E. Swanson, *The Changing American Parent* (New York: Wiley, 1958), pp. 200–1.

8. Miller and Swanson, *The Changing American Parent*, p. 201.

9. Miller and Swanson, *The Changing American Parent*, p. 204.

2. The Chronically Ill

The Doctor's Dilemma—Updated*

CLAIRE F. RYDER, M.D.

WHAT IS the real "doctor's dilemma" today? What will *your* role be as physicians in this rapidly changing world of ours? Let us first recognize that medicine today is different from what it was a decade ago, and even more dramatically different from what it was two decades ago.

The population explosion we are experiencing in the United States means that there are increasing numbers of persons to be served. But of even greater significance is the marked alteration in the age composition of our population, showing a sharp increase in the number of older persons. Unfortunately, the manpower and womanpower in the professions are not keeping pace with the steadily increasing need for services.

Currently there are over 16 million Americans who are 65 and older. A dramatic index of the sharp rise in the number of our senior citizens is the fact that this represents a 236 per cent increase over the number of older persons in our population just 40 years ago. To make a further comparison with the year 1920, life expectancy for a person born then was 54.1 years; life expectancy for the person born in 1959 (the latest year for which estimates are available) rose to 69.7 years.

As members of the medical profession, we can take justifiable pride in the fact that increasing numbers of Americans are living into the so-called golden years. Coupled with the notable advances in medical care that have taken place in recent years is our great success in the primary prevention of infectious diseases. Public Health applications of medical research triumphs have drastically reduced, and in some cases eliminated, the great toll that these diseases used to take of infants and children.

* Reprinted, in part, by permission from the December, 1961 issue of *The Journal of the American Medical Women's Association*, Vol. 16, pp. 933–938. This paper was delivered as the Commencement address at the Woman's Medical College of Pennsylvania, Philadelphia, June 13, 1961. The author is Associate Chief for Care Services, Division of Chronic Diseases, Bureau of State Services, Public Health Service, U.S. Department of Health, Education, and Welfare, Washington, D.C., and formerly Chief, Long Term Illness Program, Division of Chronic Diseases.

CHRONIC DISABILITY

Progress in preventive measures against infectious diseases has sparked what might be termed a revolution in disease, and has resulted in a significant shift to chronic ailments in the health profile of the American population. It now appears that for the privilege of living longer we have to pay in the coin of the degenerative diseases. Those prevented from dying of typhoid fever, smallpox, pneumonia, and other diseases with high mortality rates a generation ago are now living on to die of cardiovascular disease, cancer, diabetes, or another chronic disease with high prevalence among older people.

National Health Survey data show that three-fourths of all aged persons have one or more chronic conditions. In comparison with the rest of the population, the over-65 age group suffers two to three times as much from chronic illness. And although the aged represent less than 9 per cent of the population, they constitute over 55 per cent of all persons with limitations in mobility due to chronic illness.

These are the over-all dimensions of the doctor's dilemma. It is no exaggeration to say that the health and medical professions have found their tasks remade for them by the increasing number and proportion of older persons in the population. As physicians we must appreciate the effect of these changes on our clinical practice and research. Furthermore, since we are basically responsible for the increase in the aged population, we must do something about meeting the health needs of this group.

TIME LAGS

The challenge to the medical profession is magnified by the time lag that now exists between progress in research and application of findings at the grass roots level. Our government invests millions of dollars annually in medical research. Recent discoveries have given us the potential of substantially reducing deaths from cancer, preventing some heart diseases, reducing mental illness, lessening physical handicaps, saving eyesight, eradicating tuberculosis, preventing poliomyelitis, and drastically reducing the incidence of tooth decay. But the fact is that unnecessary deaths and handicaps continue to occur because vital break-throughs in research are not being applied at the grass roots level. I should like to cite a few examples of how this time lag adversely affects the health of our people.

The first example concerns cancer of the cervix which can be detected in its earliest asymptomatic stage by an easy screening device—the Papanicolaou examination of cells. If all cervical cancers could be discovered in this way before they become invasive, it is predicted that cancer of this site would be 100 per cent curable. But the tragic fact is that more than 10,000 women die each year of cancer of the cervix. Other types of cancer are not so easily detected or controlled. Nevertheless, it is estimated that if all current knowledge of control, detection, and treatment of cancer were fully applied, at least 85,000 cancer deaths a year would be avoided.

Next to cataracts, the two leading causes of blindness are glaucoma and diabetes. Yet, about 1 million persons who have glaucoma and 1.5 million persons who have diabetes are receiving no treatment because they do not even know they have the disease! In countless thousands of these undetected cases, a simple screening test today followed by prompt diagnosis and treatment could prevent blindness in future years.

A great research triumph just a little over a decade ago was the demonstration that recurrent attacks of rheumatic fever can be prevented through continuous prophylaxis with antibiotics. But this knowledge—a vital tool against rheumatic heart disease—is still not applied generally. Currently, rheumatic fever and rheumatic heart diseases take 20,000 lives each year in this country. Illustrating the lack of application of this therapy are the findings of a recent study of 1,000 persons hospitalized because of recurrent attacks of rheumatic fever. Ninety per cent of those affected—some 900 persons—could have avoided a second attack if they had been placed on a continuous schedule of antibiotics at the time of the first attack, and if they had conscientiously followed this regime.

Too often we tend to lose sight of the fact that a research discovery in the laboratory, until it is applied, saves mice not men. It is up to us, the members of the medical profession, to see that vital breakthroughs in research do not break down at the delivery-of-services level.

Of course, the perfect solution to the problem of chronic illness would be total prevention. Hopefully, we look to the day when this will be a reality. But for the present, we must face up to the fact that we have no equivalent of Salk vaccine or smallpox inoculation for the degenerative diseases. However, despite the lack of definitive answers, it is a serious mistake to assume that nothing can be done with regard to primary prevention.

We would be remiss if we did not keep in mind the various guidelines provided by research. For example, we should give consideration to studies that would determine to what degree weight control is beneficial in heart disease and diabetes. We should be alert to research findings that suggest that the use of a fat-controlled diet and polyunsaturated fatty acid may be of value to some individuals as a means of lowering serum cholesterol. In these and many other research areas, sufficient evidence has accumulated to guide us in measures we can recommend for health maintenance.

Because of the great gaps in knowledge, reduction of the impact of chronic illness for the most part pertains not so much to the prevention of the occurrence of the disease as it does to the prevention of disabling aftereffects. In this regard, our mightiest weapon is early detection—before complications have set in.

DISEASE DETECTION

Screening for hidden disease has been successfully used as a casefinding tool for many of the serious disabling diseases: notably diabetes, glaucoma, tuberculosis, heart disease, cancer of the uterus, hypertension, and kidney disease. In those instances where tests indicate suspicious results, it is the prompt follow-through by the physician that makes the health-saving or even the life-saving difference.

How ironic that this valuable means of preventing so much unnecessary suffering is not fully utilized. How does one persuade the people to avail themselves of detection programs? Many chronic diseases have an insidious onset, with no obvious symptoms. When pain and discomfort compel the patient to seek medical attention, the disease, unfortunately, has already had a running start. This is but another aspect of the doctor's dilemma.

More than ever before, change is the keynote in medical practice, with the rate of change ever-increasing. In the past two decades the development of new diagnostic technics, the discovery of new drugs that are dramatically effective in combating disease, and the change in the basic concept of the etiology and treatment of certain diseases have literally revolutionized the practice of medicine. Furthermore, it is not being overly optimistic to anticipate that additional breakthroughs will continue to make existing knowledge obsolete. All of these factors provide the backdrop to another dilemma of the modern physician—the need for continuous education and training.

CURRENCY IN LEARNING

Let us consider the effect of future change. A few years hence, when you are engaged in day-to-day activities, you will face the dilemma common to all physicians—how to find the time to keep abreast with medical progress. You must, for your effectiveness as physicians will be at stake. Increasingly, the application of new knowledge with regard to early detection or treatment of disease can spell the difference between life and death or between the limitation of functional impairment and extreme disability. And it goes without saying that you must possess the knowledge before you can apply it.

Many conscientious physicians make an effort to keep up with current progress on a do-it-yourself basis. This is in the right direction, but even more effective is attendance at intensive refresher courses, workshops, or institutes, particularly with regard to restorative services for the chronically ill. To put it bluntly, graduation from medical school can no longer be considered the pinnacle of learning, but instead must be regarded as a foundation on which to build. To function at maximum efficiency the modern physician must be a perpetual student.

But let me add a note of cheer—push-button progress may one day ease the lot of the physician in an unexpected manner. The British now manufacture a slide rule on which the physician records the patient's symptoms; once set in this way, the slide rule reveals a list of possible diagnoses for the consideration of the physician. Development of an elaboration of the diagnostic slide rule has been predicted. This would be a machine into which the physician would feed information gained from the bedside findings. A push of a button and a perfect diagnosis and therapy regime would emerge. Although this machine has yet to be invented, perhaps we should not be too skeptical.

IMMOBILIZATION

But back to the realities of the present. In discussing the changes which have taken place, I have alluded to new concepts on medical care. In this regard, we have done a complete about-face with respect to our ideas on immobilization, particularly in therapy for chronic illness, which is usually associated with protracted confinement to bed. Formerly, attention was focused only on the treatment of the disease. What once was considered a therapeutic measure—bedrest—is now viewed differently. We know that immobilization will produce irreversible impairments more damaging than the disease itself. Immobilization has led to atrophy of muscles, contractures, stiffness and soreness of joints, incontinence, bedsores, and metabolic as well as psychologic changes.

It is most pertinent at this point to pass along a maxim dating back to 42 B.C. According to the sage Publius Syrus: *Graviora quaedam sunt remedia periculis.* "There are some remedies worse than the disease."

The findings on the adverse effects of immobilization do not reflect upon the skills and effectiveness of physician services involved. What they do point up is the need for comprehensive care, including those many services needed to supplement and support physician care. This is at the core of the doctor's dilemma—updated: the need to integrate his services with the many paramedical services required in the treatment of the chronically ill.

DEPENDENCY

Another aspect of today's dilemma is that dependency is no longer regarded as a measure of economic status only. As physicians we have become aware of the effect of physical, social, and emotional dependency upon the health of the individual. We have ample evidence of the extent to which dependency in one category tends to encourage dependency in other categories; and conversely, we have been encouraged by cases that clearly demonstrate that the achievement of independence in one sphere paves the way to independence in other spheres.

The shift to chronic ailments in the health profile of the American population means that the modern physician will be increasingly involved in measures to eliminate or minimize dependency through restorative medical services. Where older individuals are involved, we must lower our rehabilitation goals to make them more reasonable and practical than they are at the present time. Rehabilitation to make the individual physically capable for re-employment is an admirable goal, but not feasible for the majority of older persons. However, we must keep in mind that responsibility in medical care includes the development of the maximum potential of the individual. When we rehabilitate the elderly, bedfast individual to the point of independent living—even if this can be only to permit him to care for his own personal needs—we restore to him a large measure of human dignity and self-respect.

FROM TRADITION TO TEAM

A few decades ago the practice of medicine was relatively uncomplicated, consisting of a direct and close patient-physician relationship with little or no involvement of ancillary personnel. Today, medicine is multifaceted and complex, and the changing role of the physician stems from the technologic advances in medicine, the growing trend to specialization, the role of clinics, and the tendency toward combined practice.

To meet the complicated needs of long-term patients, the physician can no longer serve as a self-sufficient entity. He must have the help of paramedical personnel: nurses to serve in the home, physical therapists, speech therapists, social workers, homemakers, and others. Moreover, the modern physician now finds that he must call upon community resources to provide the essential supportive services and personnel. To an increasing extent, the physician must become a counselor to his patients, serving as liaison between them and community resources.

For the old-time family physician, who has devoted a lifetime of practice based on a close doctor-patient relationship and sole management of his patient, comprehensive medical care calls for a breaking away from the traditional approach. Now he must supervise and consult with nurses, therapists, and medical specialists. However, such shared responsibility should in no way detract from his basic relationship to the patient.

How well the practicing physician can function on a team depends to a large extent on the services and facilities available within the community. Many problems of integration and co-ordination of services must be resolved on the community level. Furthermore, the physician must be adaptable to working with the team in a variety of settings—the hospital, the nursing home, or the patient's own home.

In those communities in which the vital ancillary services are not available, the physician is obviously handicapped. In many communities, however, there exists not a dearth but a plethora of services with duplication and overlapping of some services, and lack of coverage in other vital areas. For example, in one community of 100,000 population, a recent survey showed that there were over 200 agencies, programs, and services provided for the chronically ill and older individuals.

Consider the dilemma of a physician in such a community when he attempts to find the answers he must have. Which agency can provide the services needed for his patient? If institutionalization is required, which is the proper facility? If social services are needed, where can the necessary resources be found? The physician in his search for the appropriate solution must often use—and indeed waste—much of his valuable time in making numerous calls or contacts.

In an effort to resolve this problem, an increasing number of communities are marshalling their resources, creating programs which enable agencies, facilities, and services to function in a combined or correlated action. This has taken many forms—ranging from the simple roster of resources to the creation of complex central information, referral, and counseling services. These measures are designed to assist the physician in his search for the appropriate, comprehensive, and continuous care needed by his patients.

SUMMARY

It is thus clear than an updated version of the doctor's dilemma has many dimensions. First the practicing physician of today must become oriented to the changing population pattern and the corresponding changes in medical needs. In a real sense, he must also be a perpetual student in order to keep up with the constant advances in medical technology. Then, modern physicians should become acclimated to the team approach, working with others in the health and social welfare fields. And, finally, the physician has a responsibility to participate in the development and operation of essential health services within the community.

As researchers uncover new knowledge and develop new technics for the primary or secondary prevention of chronic diseases, the physician must use his talents in the Public Health effort to translate these findings into action programs. In this regard, Thomas Huxley's comment is most pertinent: "Knowledge is meaningless unless it leads to action."

This, then, is medicine today. A dilemma, true, and one that is challenging, demanding, complex—and wonderful. Now indeed is an exciting time to start.

3. The Aging

CONSTITUTING less than 4 per cent of the total in 1900, but nearly 8 per cent in 1960—such is the rapidity of change found in the ratio of persons over 65 to the United States population. This increase in relative and absolute numbers is the product of many brilliant medical discoveries, of material improvements in the standard of living, and of the growth—although inadequate and uneven—in the provision and utilization of medical services for the aged. In the broad social progress that increased longevity represents, clinical medicine and social welfare provisions have made the salient contributions, but Public Health increasingly cooperates in the tasks of prevention, screening, and the provision of care for one of the foremost "target populations."

Implicit in the medical advances that increase longevity is the intensification of the social and psychologic problems of the elderly. Drs. Donahue and Ashley consider the relationship of housing and social life to health status.

Housing and the Social Health of Older People in the United States*

WILMA DONAHUE, PH.D., AND E. EVERETT ASHLEY, 3rd, M.B.A.

SOCIAL CHANGE AND THE PROBLEM OF HOUSING

Nearly all social institutions in the United States are undergoing marked if not revolutionary alterations in response to the rapid social, economic, and technologic changes which have come to characterize western culture. Corollary to the underlying industrialization of the economy, the population has become largely urbanized, the

* Reprinted with permission from *Aging and Social Health in the United States and Europe*, report on a seminar of the Fourth International Gerontological Congress held at Merano, Italy, July, 1957, published by the University of Michigan, Ann Arbor, Michigan, 1959. The authors are, respectively, Chairman of the Division of Gerontology, The University of Michigan, Ann Arbor, Michigan; Director, Division of Program Evaluation and Statistics, Office of Program Policy, Housing and Home Finance Agency, Washington, D.C., formerly Chief, Reports and Statistics, Division of Plans and Programs, Housing and Home Finance Agency, Washington, D.C.

kinship household has dissolved into its components of one- and two-generation families, geographic mobility has become commonplace, suburban areas have extended far from the central sources of community facilities and services, and the principle that only youth has the attributes required by a competitive machine society is tacitly accepted.

These changes in social and economic conditions are having discernible effects on the housing needs of older people and on their ability to satisfy them. The continual outward growth of cities, and the tendency of young families to congregate and segregate in the newer suburban areas leave a relatively large proportion of the older generation to occupy the dilapidated dwellings of the inner residential rings surrounding crowded business and industrial districts.[1, 2] Age-discriminatory hiring and retirement practices, which reduce their income level, force many older persons to seek cheap slum housing incompatible with healthful and useful living. The disappearance of the household economy deprives the elderly of the security of continued occupational roles within the family. The fragmentation of the extended family also denies parents the shelter, care, and emotional relationships the older generations of the past could expect and demand from their grown children. Thus, although many older people are well housed, a significant proportion is being forced by circumstances inherent in modern society to occupy unsatisfactory dwellings in unhealthful neighborhoods, or to seek a substitute for the protective care or benevolent oversight of their children.

Inadequate housing and living arrangements which any population group experiences constitute a threat to social health. A number of ecologic studies[3, 4, 5] have shown that social morbidities, such as disease, extended illness, suicide, accidents, mental illness, and isolation, occur in high proportion among populations living in deteriorated housing and disorganized neighborhoods. Poor housing and these social morbidities have not been demonstrated to have a causal relationship, but appear, like poverty, unemployment, and social and educational status, to be associated factors and, like the others, interfere with the attainment of good social health by the community. Thus it may be assumed that the good housing of older people will assist in reducing the incidence of illness, disability, and mental and social breakdown among the elderly, who, because of the nature of the aging process, are especially vulnerable.

Housing and living arrangements can be considered to have good social efficiency when they are of such nature as to facilitate the personal adjustment of the members of the group. This implies the need for determining the factors in housing related to the adjustment of older householders and for applying these criteria in the measurement of the suitability of their housing.

Unfortunately, the determinants of good adjustment in the later years have not yet been clearly established. Only a few controlled studies[6, 7, 8] have been made; but on the basis of these and of the reports of experienced observers, it appears that good adjustment of older individuals depends to a significant degree upon the maintenance of 1) health and personal security, 2) independent action, 3) social experience and group membership, and 4) useful activity. Thus, housing and living arrangements, if adapted to meet these needs, would provide for the practice of good health measures, continued integration with the community, socialization of the individual, protection of privacy and of maximum independence compatible with physical and mental health status, and for the continued stimulation of the growth of the personality.

In this paper it is proposed to examine these criteria as they apply to various housing practices for older people, to report on how well the criteria are being met in housing older people in the United States today, and to outline some of the practical areas for housing research.

CRITERIA FOR THE SOCIAL EFFICIENCY OF HOUSING OF OLDER PEOPLE

Of the 15 million persons aged 65 years and over in the United States, approximately 95 per cent are living in households—70 per cent in their own, and 25 per cent in the households of others—and 5 per cent are living in institutions or some other type of quasi-household.[9] Although data are not available, it is assumed that a significant proportion of the 30 per cent living in the households of others or quasi-households could live independently "through the proper control and manipulation of their environment or by the provision of a more suitable environment."[10] It is obvious, however, that there will always be a residual percentage in need of institutional or sheltered care, especially as advanced age is attained.

Although the kind and number of needs of those living independently and those housed communally may be considered to be basically the same, the patterns, in terms of strengths and weaknesses, may vary for different groups. For example, useful activity and continued contact and interchange with the environment may be important to able-bodied or even frail persons, but they are probably relatively insignificant to the sick whose life-space has necessarily shrunk to the size of their own beings in the battle to maintain the integrity of the physical self. To the sick, the paramount needs may be for security, for the supporting figures of doctor and nurse, and for medical service. The criteria used to evaluate the efficiency of housing in promoting the adjustment of the aging must then be thought of and treated as flexible variables, depending upon whether they are being applied to individual dwelling units or communal arrangements for the able-bodied, to facilities housing the sick and senile, or to some intermixture of the two.

The criteria, further, can have no fixed value applicable to all members of any one population group of older people, because, as at any other age, there are wide individual differences in desires and tastes. One important area needing systematic investigation is that of the personal and social characteristics related to good and bad adjustment in various types of accommodations and to the tolerable range of individual differences in each instance.

1. Health and Physical Care

While people over 65 years of age account for only about 8 per cent of the population, they comprise almost 40 per cent of the chronically ill. Roughly, from 15 to 20 per cent of the noninstitutionalized members of this age group report long-term illnesses. This propensity toward illness and disability is the basis of the consciousness which older people have with regard to the need for health care. In a study of 100 randomly selected older people living normally in the community, Tibbitts, Hunter, and Coons[11] found that health and physical care were their prime needs, and that the absence of a means of satisfying these needs provoked considerable anxiety.

In individual dwellings, healthful housing for older people, as for those of any other age, is dependent largely upon design features which minimize accident hazards, permit easy care of the household, and provide proper size and space arrangements. Standards for these and other environmental features have been published[12, 13, 14] and are being incorporated in housing especially designed for occupancy by older people. The value of these design features recommended and used has not yet been tested experimentally, and since their inclusion increases construction costs, it seems that they are appropriate subjects for investigation.

The provision of well designed housing, however, is not an assurance of good adjustment of the occupants; because, in addition to the need for a good housing environment, they also have the need for the psychologic security of knowing that health care is available in times of illness or when frailty becomes advanced. This raises the questions of the relation between housing and health care, and of whose responsibility it is to provide and staff health facilities. In the United States today this is the most pressing policy problem facing the Federal Housing agencies. What is needed is research.

Do older people want health care facilities incorporated into housing projects designed for them, or do they prefer to use the regular community health care facilities where they have been accustomed to receive care as younger people? What effect does a pre-arranged health care plan have upon personal adjustment of older people living in a housing project? What is the effect upon physically and mentally able old people of living in close proximity with the sick, disturbed, and senile? Is there an optimum proportion between the able and the sick which can be tolerated without adverse effects upon the adjustment of the well? Is the presence of healthy older persons conducive to a better adjustment of the mentally confused or ill?[15]

If older people are found to prefer the inclusion of health facilities in housing projects, and if they are not adversely affected by the close proximity of illness and death, is there sufficient medical personnel, or is there likely to be enough in the foreseeable future to provide a dynamic health care and rehabilitation program in each housing development? What is the quality of health care now being provided in housing plans currently offering life care to residents?

2. Integration with the Community

In the past in the United States, it was assumed that the health and happiness of old people depended upon peace and quiet, and that these were best provided in the remote countryside. Today, the point of view is almost reversed with the result that it is now thought that one good test of the adequacy of housing is the degree to which people find opportunity for participation in formal and informal organizations in the community.[16] It is now commonly recommended that special housing (independent and communal) for older people be sited in the hearts of cities, often in slum clearance areas, in renovated hotels or old mansions, or in "close in" residential areas. The shifting point of view is not the result of careful measurements of the physical and mental health and participation of an older age group living under crowded urban conditions as compared with a group living in suburban or rural settings. It is rather the wholehearted acceptance of the hypothesis that the old want and need to live in close proximity to community facilities and services, and that it is better and cheaper for the community to have them do so. Objective studies which would permit a comparison of the adjustment of older people living in the more rural or developed suburban areas with that of older people living in central residential districts are needed to verify or disavow the present trend of thought and action.

Do older people have fewer visits from friends and relatives when housed in the more rural areas, or do they have more visitors because parking is easy and the prospect of a special trip out of the city is pleasing? Do older people living outside the central residential districts necessarily participate in community functions less frequently than those living in the community? If elderly people have strong preferences for living outside of urban areas, is it detrimental or beneficial to personal adjustment for them to do so? What is the optimum siting of a housing project for the elderly to bring about maximum integration in community life?

A related question is that of the effect upon integration with the community when the housing project or the communal home provides practically all the services needed—health, shopping, church, library, social, and educational? The trend toward the development of retirement villages in large housing tracts including all community services makes this an especially important current problem for investigation. As Kutner[17] observes in his study of *Five Hundred Over Sixty*, such villages tend to segregate and isolate the aged from younger contemporaries; and it is yet to be demonstrated that age separation is sufficiently acceptable to older people themselves to warrant promulgation of retirement cities. There are available in the United States some retirement communities where all households are occupied by elderly residents, and others where 5 to 20 per cent are occupied by younger families. A comparative study of the adjustment of the old age group in each type population structure would yield evidence on the relative merits of the two plans.

3. Socialization

The need for social experience and interpersonal relationships does not appear to abate with age.[18] Psychiatrists[19] point out that the need for security offered by close ties and group membership may actually increase as the individual grows older and is less capable of managing his own environment. Although investigations of older groups are lacking, there are some provocative studies of the social life of residents of housing projects occupied by young families which suggest that homogeneity of the social structure of the population fosters good adjustment of the group and of its members. In one project,[20] where the dwelling units were poorly built and inconvenient, all occupants were veterans' families of about the same age and financial status, with the common goal of obtaining a college education for at least one member of each family. In spite of the many inconveniences of the dwellings, 90 per cent of the residents felt that the social life in the project was so satisfactory that they would not consider living any other place. They summed up their feelings about membership in the group with the statement, "We're all in the same boat." In contrast, Festinger also studied a government housing project. Here the resident population was much more heterogeneous, being made up in part of families forced to live in the development because of an acute housing shortage, and, in part, by workers left over in the project after the war. Members of both groups felt that only "low class" people, with whom they would not associate, would live in a government project. The consequences of this feeling were that most residents lived in a state of self-imposed isolation, made no more than one or two friends in the project, and made almost no attempt to make friends outside, for they felt others looked down on the project families. They also found the physical inconveniences of the dwellings a major source of irritation, and were eager to move away into other residential areas.

Taietz[21] reports one of the few studies of the personal adjustment of the residents of old age homes. He concluded that homogeneity (economic, occupational, and educational) fosters the formation of primary friendship and interest groups, which in turn facilitate good personal adjustment within the home.

In a study of a university student village owned and operated by the University of Minnesota, Caplow and Forman[22] found that homogeneity is of crucial importance in group formation and that only powerful inhibiting factors can prevent intensive and intimate interaction among persons of similar status whenever opportunity affords.

Socialization of the elderly living in private houses constitutes a special problem, but opportunity for interpersonal relationship is as important to the good adjustment of the isolated as for those living within a housing development or communal home. In a study of a group of older women[23] each member of which was essentially homebound by a physical disability, it was found that a companionship program, utilizing the technics of friendly visiting and group identification, resulted in the improvement of the personal adjustment of the women. Without change in kind or extent of medical treatment, all the women showed improvement in health to the point where they no longer allowed their disabilities to keep them at home. They were again able to take part in social activities with other people and to participate in community life.

When it is not feasible for older people to achieve their own personal relationships within their homes or neighborhoods, it is necessary that provisions be made to supplement their inadequate housing arrangements with special accommodations and services. Kubie and Landau,[24] in a report based on detailed case studies, point out that participation in a day center situated in close proximity to their homes helps elderly people living in the densely crowded areas of New York City to preserve their mental health and to overcome loneliness.

Spatial relationships and architectural features also have an influence on the socialization and group membership of individual householders and group residents. Festinger[25] showed that for younger people the site plan affected the number and nature of social contacts within a housing development. The sheer distance between houses was a deterrent to socialization of adjacent householders. The direction in which a house faced as related to others in the vicinity determined what families would become friends. For example, on a half-moon court, those people living in adjacent houses and in the ones facing each other made the most friends. The occupants of houses in the court which faced outward on the street and had only one-half as many friends as those facing the court. In another study of two-story dwellings, Festinger found that practically no friendships were formed between the residents of the two floors, while most friendships occurred among those living in adjacent apartments. He also determined that living close to staircases or near the mail box added much to the social contacts of the individual.

4. Privacy and Independence

A current policy affecting the housing of the older age group is that of providing living arrangements and community service to enable older persons to live independently in their own homes, or if they are residents in communal homes, to help them preserve their privacy and dignity as human beings.

Chapin[26] believes good mental hygiene is dependent upon freedom to be by oneself, and "that hindrances to its realization lead to frustrations, irritations, and resentments. . . . The respect of self as an individual with status can hardly thrive when the person is continuously open to pressures of the presence of many others . . . privacy is needed for thinking, reflection, reading, and study, and for esthetic enjoyment and contemplation. Intrusions on the fulfillment of personal desires need to be shut off in order to avoid the internal tensions that are built up from the frustrations, resentments, and irritations of continual multiple contacts with others."

But objective evidence, as Chapin points out, is not conclusive regarding the value of privacy. Pan,[27] in a study of institutionalized and non-institutionalized older people where there was an obvious difference in the availability of privacy, found that the institutionalized older people gave more evidence of poor adjustment than did the non-institutionalized. On the other hand, Leprowski,[28] in a similar study, found that there was no significant difference when levels of adjustment of institutionalized and non-institutionalized groups of older people were compared on the basis of health, friends, work, economic security, religion, usefulness, happiness, and family.

Cottman[29] in a study of rural and small town residents found a direct relationship between the degree of satisfaction with housing and the amount of space providing greater privacy within the house; the most satisfied occupied the most space, and the least satisfied had the least space. Chapin[30] studied non-crowded as distinct from space-crowded households, and found some evidence of lower morale and poorer adjustment among the space-crowded.

Such studies give only indirect evidence that absence of privacy may have some detrimental effects. More definitive studies are needed, however, to measure the effects of loss of different degrees of privacy and independence before firm conclusions can be drawn regarding housing design, spatial requirements, and administrative policies. There is reason to assume that there may be wide individual differences in attitudes toward privacy, and that, for some people, good adjustment may be promoted through close association affording little or no privacy.

Controlled studies of the same persons living under different conditions of privacy and independence should not be too difficult to establish. Many homes for the aging offer facilities ranging from private rooms through double or triple rooms to large ward accommodations. Thus, a selected population could be housed under the several conditions successively and measurements made of health, personal adjustment, and satisfaction with the living arrangements in each situation.

Studies of groups housed in companion-type apartments (private sleeping rooms with common sitting, dining, and kitchen) which provide both privacy and companionship opportunities in a family-like setting are needed to determine personal satisfaction, happiness, and health. How many people, what degree of homogeneity—socioeconomic, age, physical status—results in the best adjustment of residents of companion apartments?

5. Personality Growth

Surveying the increasing rate at which elderly persons are being admitted to State mental institutions, Busse[31] asks why there should be a growing proportion of the aged population unable to remain adjusted in the community. No doubt the answer to Busse's question is a complex one; but if, as Chapin[32] assumes, healthful living may be achieved by the creation of physical conditions in a dwelling which promote "the normal growth of personality that is flexible, tolerant, and capable of mature integration," then housing may be an important component of the answer.

There are practically no systematic factual data on any age group of the influence of physical factors in housing upon the personality and behavior of the occupants. Chapin[33] reasons, however, that ease of circulation of residents within the dwelling and the provision for privacy reduce irritations and resentments and thus contribute to a sound emotional and mental life. For the elderly, one might add such other physical factors as ease of housekeeping, reduction of strain in reaching and stooping, and the environmental compensation for reduced sensory acuity.

Investigations of the extent of the effect of these various physical factors upon the behavior and emotional adjustment of elderly householders would be most useful in the planning of special housing for this age group. For example, in one housing development, no partitions were included in the one-story dwellings in order to increase the ease with which the older people could circulate within the house.[34] It is expected, in this instance, that privacy will be obtained by pulling curtains around beds, kitchen, and other areas. Obviously, such a design is based on the assumption that visual privacy is all that is required by the occupants. One may, however, raise the question for study of what constitutes psychologic privacy, and whether there is a difference in the quality of privacy when it is auditory as well as visual in nature. Basically, the question is that of what physical circumstances of housing promote growth and maintain the integration of the personality of the elderly.

Within communal type dwellings, architectural provision is usually made for common sitting room space; and in some of the homes of more recent design, space for group activity, such as occupational therapy, social gatherings, etc., is also included. It is assumed that the residents want and use this type of common space to the same extent and in the same way they would use sitting rooms and recreational space in their own private homes. Observation casts doubt upon this assumption and indicates the need for a careful study of the use and psychologic meaning of shared space. Such an investigation should also include study of the utilization and meaning of the space when the home provides a planned activity program designed to stimulate mental and emotional growth. For example, in one home for the aged in which a large recreational room had been provided, the residents rejected its use because of its location under the chapel. After the introduction of an activity program which was carried out largely in the recreation room, attitudes changed, and it was no longer considered irreligious to use this space for play and work.[35]

It seems apparent that almost every phase of housing as it relates to the social well-being of the older segment of the population is in need of systematic study and evaluation. In the meantime, the number of older people is increasing rapidly, and they must be and are being housed without the benefit of objective criteria. Following is an appraisal of how needs of older people are being met currently in the United States, and of the methods by which various developments are being financed.

THE LIVING ENVIRONMENT OF OLDER PEOPLE
IN THE UNITED STATES

By all odds, the most striking characteristic of the living arrangements of older people in the United States is the high concentration of one- and two-person families. The United States Bureau of the Census in the 1950 Decennial Census of Housing[36] found that over 68 per cent of the persons 65 years of age or older in April, 1950 consisted of either single individuals or couples. Some 25 per cent were single individuals, the remaining 43 per cent couples. In absolute numbers there were, in what are known as non-farm areas, 1,405,000 single individuals 65 years or older maintaining their own separate houses or apartments. Of these 985,000 were women, 420,000 were men. Couples in the older age groups totaled 2,402,000.

Bureau of the Census figures disclosed that going hand-in-hand with the smallness of the family groups among the elderly was a notable underconsumption of housing. Thus, over 80 per cent of the householders in the 65-and-older categories lived in dwellings in which there were fewer than ¾ persons per room. Among younger families, in contrast, only about 56 per cent had little congestion in their living quarters.

At the end of the spectrum, only 2 per cent of the older households were seriously overcrowded, i.e., had an average of more than 1½ persons per room. This contrasts with the more than 6 per cent of younger families whose homes were unhealthfully congested.

Much of the lack of crowding in the homes of older householders results in large measure from the fact that they do not contract the size of their quarters as rapidly as their families diminish. Houses bought to meet the needs of families with several children are all too commonly retained even after all the children have married and established homes of their own. A significant number of the single individuals who maintain separate households are the surviving members of married couples who continue to occupy the same quarters even after the demise of their husbands or wives.

Many of those who were 65 or older in 1950 acquired their present living quarters at a time when building costs were substantially lower and when larger houses constituted a bigger share of the annual output of new accommodations. It is not surprising, therefore, to find that households headed by a person 65 years of age or older tended, in 1950, to have larger quarters than those of the younger segment of the population. Nearly three-fifths of the older group had quarters containing five or more rooms, whereas less than half of the families with household heads under 65 had dwellings that large.

That older householders do not more readily readjust their living arrangements to suit their curtailed space requirements is a reflection, in large measure, of the fact that 68 per cent of the nonfarm families in the United States, where the heads were over 65 years of age, own their own homes. The proportion of home ownership among these age groups exceeds that of any other in the population.

This high percentage of home ownership among the aging is a reflection of one of the social mores of the United States, that home ownership is a desirable attainment. A home owner achieves, thereby, economic status in the community. In addition, it affords him a sense of security which dates back to the period in our culture before the Social Security program and pension plans began to help provide some measure of economic security for old age. The gradual acquisition over the years of an equity in and ultimately outright title to a house was one of the most effective ways many families had of building up some protection for themselves in their later years.

Except for their size and sometimes their location, these owned homes do provide many older householders with suitable shelter, at least as long as they are ambulatory. One evidence of this fact is that the Bureau of the Census found that some 75 per cent of the homes owned and occupied by household heads 65 years of age or older were in satisfactory physical condition.

For an indeterminant proportion of this group living in sound and fully equipped dwellings, however, home ownership is becoming a progressively greater burden as the years go by. Large houses become increasingly difficult to operate. Because of sentiment, inertia, or economic necessity, some older householders continue to live in houses which are beyond their physical and economic capacity to cope with. Undoubtedly this contributes to the fact that a somewhat larger share of the older families in the United States live in substandard housing than is true of their younger counterparts. With failing strength and diminished incomes, some older household heads find the problem of proper house maintenance and yard care more than they can handle. As a result their homes gradually deteriorate to the point where they have to be considered substandard. Still others become adversely affected by the impact of urban blight and neighborhood decay. Hence, the Bureau of the Census found that in 1950 nearly twice as many houses owned and occupied by older persons were in poor physical condition as was true of the residences of younger home owners.

All of the poor quality of housing occupied by the aging cannot, however, be attributed to the senility of its occupants. Actually, the character of the quarters occupied by renters among the older age groups was far worse in 1950 than that of the home owner. In contrast with 7 per cent of dwellings in poor condition occupied by home owners, close to 12 per cent of the dwellings rented by persons 65 years of age or older were found by the Bureau of the Census to be in bad physical repair.

This heavier concentration of low quality units among renters is reflected in the comparative figures on rents and values. Thus, in contrast with the rest of the population there was a heavier concentration of older families (40 per cent vs 21 per cent for younger families) who were renting quarters in 1950 for less than $30 a month. Whereas rents of older householders tend to concentrate at the lower end of the rent scale, the values of homes owned by householders with heads 65 or older, while not so high as those of their younger counterparts, were nonetheless better distributed in the middle and upper value ranges.

NEED FOR CROSS-NATIONAL HOUSING RESEARCH

Europe and some other areas experienced the aging of the population more than a generation earlier than the United States, with the consequence that many countries have already had years of experience in providing housing for large numbers of old people. The United States, while younger in experience, has built a wide variety of housing, as already described in a previous section of this paper, which is now available for comparison with foreign developments.

Cross-national studies of the adjustment of residents in matched types of dwellings in different countries would assist in determining the universality of the needs each type is meeting.

Surveys could be made to indicate the numbers, types, costs, and financing of the housing in various countries. The relative responsibility of government, the church, and other voluntary agencies in providing housing would also make an interesting and worthwhile study.

The question of provision of medical care as an integral part of housing schemes as compared to its provision by the community should be studied from the point of view of quality, efficiency, cost, and psychologic effects of different arrangements upon residents.

A study of the responsibilities assumed by families for their older members in various countries and the effects of different national family practices upon the amount, type, and financing of special housing for the elderly would have important implications for further planning of housing in many countries.

Finally, it is suggested that the attitudes of older people toward different aspects of housing be investigated. What is their preference with regard to: 1) private dwellings as opposed to communal residences, 2) size of special housing developments, 3) location of project with reference to community and family, and 4) number to be housed under a single roof. Another, although somewhat different, study of the attitudes of older persons would be that of their self-image and sense of personal status as independent householders, compared with that as residents of various types of group-living facilities.

1. Cogwill, D. C., "Trends in the Ecology of the Aged in American Cities, 1940–1950," *Journal of Gerontology*, 12 (1957), pp. 75–80.

2. Ashley, E., "Where and How Older People Live Today," in W. Donahue (ed.), *Housing the Aging* (Ann Arbor: University of Michigan Press, 1954), pp. 13–20.

3. Faris, R. E. L. and Dunham, H. W., *Mental Disorders in Urban Areas* (Chicago: University of Chicago Press, 1939).

4. Schroeder, C. W., "Mental Disorders in Cities," *American Journal of Sociology*, 48 (1942), pp. 40–47.

5. Britton, R. H. and Altman, I., "Illness and Accidents Among Persons Living Under Different Housing Conditions," *Public Health Reports, 56* (1941).

6. Morgan, C. M. "The Attitudes and Adjustments of Recipients of Old Age Assistance in Upstate and Metropolitan New York," *Archives of Psychology, 214* (1937).

7. Landis, J. T., "Attitudes and Adjustments of Aged Rural People in Iowa," unpublished doctoral dissertation, Louisiana State University, 1940.

8. Cavan, R., Burgess, E., Havighurst, R., and Goldhamer, H., *Personal Adjustment in Old Age* (Chicago: Science Research Associates, Inc., 1949).

9. U.S. Census.

10. Vivrett, W. K., "An Environment for Living Independently," *Geriatrics, 12* (1957), pp. 209–251.

11. "The Needs of the Aging," unpublished Ms., Division of Gerontology, University of Michigan, 1948.

12. Massachusetts State Housing Board, *Standards of Design for Housing the Elderly* (Boston: The Board, 1954).

13. Committee on Hygiene of Housing, *Housing an Aging Population* (New York: The Committee, American Public Health Association, 1953).

14. Kleemeier, R., "Environmental Settings and the Aging Process," in J. Anderson (ed.), *Psychological Aspects of Aging* (Washington: American Psychological Association, 1956).

15. Dr. A. Berggren of the Royal Social Board of Sweden reports that the housing of sick older people in the same facility with the able-bodied resulted in an increase in the incidence of reported illness among the healthy persons.

16. Wirth, L., "Housing as a Field of Sociological Research," *American Sociological Review*, 15 (1950), pp. 50–60.

17. Kutner, B., Fanshel, D., Togo, Alice M., and Langner, T. S., *Five Hundred Over Sixty* (New York: Russell Sage Foundation, 1956).

18. Tibbitts, C. (ed.), *Living Through the Older Years* (Ann Arbor: University of Michigan Press, 1949).

19. Greenleigh, L. F., *Psychological Problems of Our Aging Population*, (Bethesda, Md.: U.S. Public Health Service, 1952), (mimeographed).

20. Festinger, L., "Architecture and Group Membership," in R. K. Merton, *et al.*, (eds.), *Social Policy and Social Research in Housing* (New York: Association Press, 1951).

21. Taietz, P., *Administrative Practices and Personal Adjustment in Homes for the Aged.* Bulletin 899 (Ithaca, N.Y.: Cornell University Agricultural Experimental Station, 1953).

22. Caplow, T. and Forman, R. "Neighborhood Interactions in the Homogeneous Community," *American Sociological Review*, 15 (1950), pp. 357–366.

23. Coons, D. and Donahue, W. *A Group Program for Shut-ins* (Ann Arbor: Division of Gerontology, University of Michigan, 1955), (mimeographed).

24. Kubie, S. H. and Landau, G. *Group Work with the Aged* (New York: International Universities Press, 1953).

25. Festinger, L., *op. cit.*

26. Chapin, F. S., "Some Housing Factors Related to Mental Hygiene," *Journal of Social Issues*, 7 (1951), pp. 164–170.

27. Pan, J. S., "Personal Adjustment of Old People," *Sociology and Social Research*, 35 (1950), pp. 3–11.

28. Leprowski, J. R., "The Atti-

tudes and Adjustments of Institutionalized and Non-institutionalized Catholic Aged," *Journal of Gerontology, 11*
(1956), pp. 185–191.

29. Cottman, H. R., *Housing and
Attitudes Toward Housing in Rural
Pennsylvania,* (State College: Pennsylvania Agricultural Experiment Station, 1942).

30. Chapin, F. S., *op. cit.*

31. Busse, E. W., "Mental Health
in Advanced Maturity," in W. Donahue and C. Tibbitts (eds.), *The New
Frontiers of Aging,* (Ann Arbor: University of Michigan, 1957), p. 144.

32. Chapin, F. S., *op. cit.*

33. *Ibid.*

34. Pan, J. S., *op. cit.*

35. Donahue, W., Hunter, W., and
Coons, D. "A Study of the Socialization
of Old People," *Geriatrics, 8* (1953),
pp. 656–666.

36. U.S. Bureau of the Census,
Census of Housing: 1950 (Washington: U.S. Government Printing Office,
1954).

37. Ashley, E. E., "Proceedings of
a Workshop on the Design and Financing of Housing for Older People," unpublished Ms., Eighth Annual Conference on Aging, University of
Michigan, Ann Arbor, 1955.

4. The Workers

WITH the age of controlled nuclear power, a new industry—the mining and milling of uranium—has been added to the lengthening list of hazardous work exposures. As described by Archer and his co-workers, epidemiologic scrutiny has uncovered significant findings in the areas of lung cancer, heart disease, and motor vehicle accident fatalities for uranium workers, emphasizing again the continuous need for worker and worksite surveillance in new dangerous trades.

There has long been agreement among enlightened leaders of industry and labor that the human problems of work need solutions based on study and rational action. Withdrawal from work, seen in excessive industrial absenteeism, is one of the foremost problems and has been carefully studied by Hinkle and Plummer for more than a decade. Their paper documents the finding that much absenteeism is concentrated in a group of workers who are reacting to on-the-job dissatisfactions and other stressful life situations.

For some workers, the stresses of living result in disabling addictive behavior, such as chronic alcoholism. Levinson reviews problem drinking in the industrial setting, outlining some effective remedial approaches.

Hazards to Health in Uranium Mining and Milling*

VICTOR E. ARCHER, M.D., HAROLD J. MAGNUSON, M.D.,
DUNCAN A. HOLADAY, M.A., AND POPE A. LAWRENCE, M.S.

LARGE-SCALE mining and milling of uranium ores started in the United States during World War II as a result of the demand for raw material for nuclear weapons. The number of workers involved was at first only

* Reprinted with omission of three tables and three illustrations, by permission from the February 1962 issue of the *Journal of Occupational Medicine*, Vol. 4, pp. 55–60. This paper was presented at the Forty-sixth Annual Meeting of the Industrial Medical Association, held in Los Angeles on April 13, 1961. The authors are, respectively, Field Investigator with the National Cancer Institute, U.S. Public Health Service, assigned to the Occupational Health Field Station, Salt Lake City, Utah; Director, Institute of Industrial Health, University of Michigan, Ann Arbor, Michigan, formerly Chief of the Division of Occupational Health, Bureau of State Services, Public Health Service, U.S. Department of Health, Education, and Welfare, Washington, D.C.; Chief of the Occupational Health Field Station, Public Health Service, Salt Lake City, Utah; and Assistant Chief for Operations, Epidemiology Branch, National Cancer Institute, Public Health Service, Bethesda, Maryland.

a few hundred. Nevertheless, several facts suggested that this new industry be watched carefully for adverse effects on the health of its workers; these were: (1) uranium is toxic in its own right; (2) uranium and its decay products emit considerable ionizing radiation of three types; and (3) there is considerable documentation in the literature that between 30 and 70 per cent of the miners in the uranium-containing mines of the Schneeberg and Joachimsthal areas in Europe died of lung cancer.[1, 2]

In response to a request from health officers concerned with the potential hazard, the U.S. Public Health Service, in cooperation with the Atomic Energy Commission and the State Health Departments of Colorado, Utah, Arizona, and New Mexico, in 1949 began environmental studies in uranium mines, and in 1950 initiated medical studies. There was exemplary cooperation from the uranium mining and milling industry.

Progress reports have been made periodically to the industry and to agencies responsible for enforcing control measures. This paper summarizes the envionmental and medical findings, with emphasis on the medical aspects.

The major deposits of uranium ore developed commercially in the United States since World War II have been in the Colorado Plateau, with Colorado, Utah, Arizona, and New Mexico having the major production. More recently, South Dakota, Wyoming, and Washington also have begun to develop sizeable production. Estimates of the numbers of miners and mill workers are as follows: In 1945 there were 350 miners and 600 mill workers; in 1950, 550 and 800; in 1955, 2157 and 1800; and in 1960, 5760 and 3000.

SUMMARY OF ENVIRONMENTAL FINDINGS

Environmental surveys have shown potential hazards from silica dust, and from radon and radon decay products in the atmosphere of most of the uranium mines in the Colorado Plateau.[3] In the mills, the major potential hazards have been identified as airborne silica, uranium, vanadium, acids, and alkalis. Build-up of radium in pipes or tanks might produce localized areas of high gamma radiation.

By the use of air measurements of radon and reasonable assumptions as to radon-radon daughter equilibrium, ventilation rates, relative biologic efficiency of alpha particles, and retention and localization of dust, it has been possible to calculate what the radiation dose to the lungs or bronchi of an underground uranium miner might be.[4] If one assumes an average concentration of radon of about 3000 $\mu\mu c/L$. in mine air,[5] such calculations would indicate that the average American uranium miner prior to 1953 may have received 2000–3000 rem as an average dose to his lungs during 10 years of work. Variations in mine atmospheres are such that in an individual miner the dose might have been higher or lower by a factor of 20. Nonuniform distribution of the radiation delivered, as well as other variable factors, could alter these doses for parts of the lung by a factor of 10 or more. Although far from precise, these calculations have led to the conclusion that there is a greater potential radiation hazard in underground uranium mines than in uranium mills.

Early in the surveillance of the mines, agreement was reached on a recommended working level of radon and radon products of 300 μμc/L., equivalent to 1.3×10^5 Mev of potential alpha energy per liter. Holaday and associates[3] have shown that adequate ventilation, combined with other dust control measures, is capable of substantially reducing or eliminating both radioactive dust and other dust hazards. There has been considerable progress in improving conditions, especially in the newer and larger mines. Nevertheless, surveys continue to show that conditions in many mines do not meet the recommended levels.

MEDICAL STUDIES

Medical observations of workers in the uranium mines began in 1950, and are now in their 12th year. They have consisted essentially of periodic physical examinations by mobile examining teams, and systematic follow-up of individuals during and after significant mining experience. Annual censuses of all uranium miners, combined with systematic follow-up, have permitted determination of mortality rates and causes of death. Uranium miners have been examined during the summers of 1950, 1951, 1953, 1954, 1957, and 1960. In 1954 and 1957 an effort was made to examine all uranium miners in the Colorado Plateau area; in 1960 it was not possible to include miners in the new and rapidly expanding Grants, N.M., area.

Each examination consisted of (1) taking of an occupational history; (2) collection of social data for follow-up purposes; (3) physical examination; and (4) 10–15 different laboratory procedures, including 14×17-in. chest roentgenograms. In 1957 and 1960 cytologic examinations of sputum were important additions.

All the findings reported in the periodic physical examinations in the miners have not been completely analyzed and no detailed report can be made now. There are a number of laboratory findings of considerable interest, one being the prevalence of roentgenographic changes consistent with silicosis. In 1960, 3.1 per cent of 1589 workers had X-ray evidence of silicosis; most of these had had over 20 years of mining experience. Only four cases of silicosis were found in men who had worked only in uranium mining, whereas 46 were found in those who had had both uranium and other mining experience. Another important finding in 1960 has been an unusually high prevalence, in some of the mining areas, of sputum samples showing abnormal cells. Although reports and analyses are incomplete, and we do not yet have data for strict comparisons between 1957 and 1960, the sharp upward trend of suspicious findings in sputum specimens examined thus far is cause for concern. This important lead is being intensively pursued to determine its significance, both to the individual miners involved and in relation to mining and exposures.

Uranium mill workers were examined during the summers of 1950, 1951, and 1953, but have not been included in later studies. In the approximately 800 uranium mill workers examined between 1950 and 1953, a number of cases of silicosis were found, possibly due to previous mining. Also, effects attributed to vanadium were found, notably chronic cough, upper respiratory irritation, and green coating of the mucous membranes of the mouth and pharynx. A trace of vanadium was occasionally found in urine. Eight mill workers who had worked in a crushing department from two to six years each were checked for radium body burden in the Los Alamos whole-body counter. Each had a body burden less than 0.005 µg. of radium, the lower limit of the measurement.

Uranium miners examined in one or more of the years when field examinations were conducted constitute the study group for epidemiologic purposes. In this time, 3,306 different miners from about 400 mines were examined at least once. The number of individuals in the study group by year of first examination is as follows: 1950, 147 miners were examined; in 1951, 177; in 1953, 147; in 1954, 974; and 1861 in 1957.

Because of the high mobility of these miners, only about 800 have been examined more than once. This group of 3306 has been followed by a variety of technics so that contact at least annually has been maintained. As of April 1959 we had lost touch with only 2 per cent of the study group. When deaths are reported, death certificates and other medical data are collected.

An analysis of the mortality of the study group through 1959 has just been completed by the life table technic. The uranium miners were first grouped as white or nonwhite, the latter being largely Indian. Within each of these racial groupings three cohorts were established, according to length of underground uranium mining experience as of 1957 (cohort 1—open pit experience, surface experience, occasional; cohort 2—less than 3.0 years; and cohort 3—3.0 years or more). There were 2,666 white miners, and 640 nonwhite, representing 11,060 total white person-years, and 2,210 total nonwhite person-years.

Expected numbers of deaths from the principal causes were calculated, using age-specific mortality rates for the general population of white males in Arizona, Colorado, New Mexico, and Utah. These rates were weighted according to the numbers of miners in each of the States.

Observed and expected numbers of deaths were found to be significantly different for only four causes of death: (1) "other heart disease," where the excess is due primarily to cor pulmonale among uranium miners; (2) "other cardiovascular disease," where there is a deficit; (3) "other accidents," where the excess mortality is due mainly to accidents in mines; and (4) "all other causes." Respiratory cancer was over twice as high as expected, but the difference was too small to be significant at the 95 per cent confidence level.

The total white uranium miner study group is heavily weighted in favor of men who have worked underground in uranium mines only a short time. It is well known that in man there is a latent period of at least several years between exposure to radiation and diagnosable neoplasm. One would therefore expect that the longer the time a man had spent underground, the greater would be his risk.

In Cohort 1, only two deaths occurred among the 263 miners, whereas approximately 7 were expected. These numbers are too small to permit any valid interpretation.

The white Cohorts 2 and 3, however, containing 1496 and 907 men, respectively, are sufficiently large to justify examination for significant differences among the causes of death. In Cohort 2, for example, one finds that the 43 deaths from "all causes" are significantly higher than the 29.7 deaths expected ($P < 0.05$). The 24 deaths due to accidents from "all causes" other than motor vehicles is significantly greater than the 5.6 deaths expected ($P < 0.01$).

In white Cohort 3, significant differences between observed and expected deaths are found in major cardiovascular-renal diseases ($P < 0.05$); heart disease other than arteriosclerotic ($P < 0.01$); respiratory cancer ($P < 0.05$), and accidents other than motor vehicle ($P < 0.01$).

Mining accidents and cor pulmonale stand out in the total study group and in both white Cohorts 2 and 3. Both cor pulmonale and respiratory cancer stand out more sharply in white Cohort 3 than in the total study group. The use of 3 or more years underground as the criterion for grouping the data available for this analysis would seem actually to minimize the importance of prolonged underground uranium mining experience because it includes so many with relatively brief exposures. It is noteworthy that the 6 lung cancer deaths occurring in the period covered by this analysis had uranium mining histories of 1, 7, 8, 9, 10 and 12 years.

The total autopsy rate was only 27 per cent, but five of the six lung cancers were proved by autopsy while the sixth had a firm clinical diagnosis based on chest films and bronchoscopic examination. Most of the heart disease deaths were clinical diagnoses.

The results of the life-table analysis presented above have dealt exclusively with the white component of the uranium miner study group because the nonwhite component is too small for valid statistical treatment.

The total number of deaths observed through 1959 in the nonwhite group is 11, of which 9 were due to motor vehicle accidents, one to infection, and one to suicide.

DISCUSSION

Studying the incidence of lung cancer in the uranium mining population of our western States has been difficult for more reasons than the relative isolation of widely scattered mines and the independence and mobility of the miners. More serious obstacles have been the relatively small population at risk in the early days of mining operations and the long period of exposure and observation required for abnormalities to become evident. Because of these facts, it was early realized that conclusive results would be obtained slowly, and that recommendations for environmental controls could not wait for medical findings which might portend a disastrous situation.

While the occurrence of only six deaths from lung cancer in 13,270 man-years of risk may seem too little evidence for serious discussion, nevertheless the odds are less than 1 in 20 that five of these would occur by chance among the 907 miners who had worked underground for three years or longer. Implication of elevated lung cancer risk is supported by suggestive trends in the prevalence of abnormal sputum samples collected in 1960. Furthermore, since the close of the latest life-table analysis there have been four more confirmed lung cancer deaths and one additional case diagnosed.

Thus, although it is still too early to define with precision the health status of uranium miners, there are enough disturbing implications in present trends to warrant intensified efforts to lower their environmental exposures to radioactive dust and gas and to silica dust. Plans for an accelerated program to this end are already under way.

SUMMARY

1. Uranium miners in the Colorado Plateau have been under epidemiologic surveillance since 1950; during this time the working population has increased from approximately 350 to nearly 6000.

2. Deaths in a study group of 3,317 miners, followed two to nine years between 1950 and 1959, with 13,270 person-years of observation, have been analyzed by the life-table technic.

3. Preliminary calculations applied to a cohort of 907 white miners with three years or more of uranium mining experience show five lung cancer deaths to have occurred where 1.1 was expected; eight deaths from heart disease other than arteriosclerotic where 0.4 was expected;

and 10 deaths from non–motor-vehicle accidents where 2.5 were expected. All of these differences are interpreted as significant at the 95 per cent confidence level.

4. Concurrent environmental surveys of uranium mines have shown a high proportion of operating mines with concentrations of radon daughter products above the recommended working level of 1.3×10^5 Mev of potential alpha energy per liter of air.

5. A continuing program of education and promotion of improved environmental control is being accelerated.

1. Hueper, W. C. *Occupational Tumors and Allied Diseases.* Thomas, Springfield, 1942, pp. 435–456.

2. Lorenz, E. Radioactivity and Lung Cancer: A critical review of Lung Cancer in the Miners of Schneeburg and Joachimsthal. *J. Nat. Cancer Inst.* 5:1, 1944.

3. Holaday, D. A., *et al. Control of Radon and Daughters in Uranium Mines and Calculations on Biologic Effects.* Public Health Service Publication No. 494. Washington, D.C., U.S. Government Printing Office, 1957.

4. Bale, W. F., and Shapiro, J. V. *Radiation Dosage to Lungs from Radon and Its Daughter Products. Peaceful Uses of Atomic Energy.* Proceedings of the International Conference in Geneva, Aug. 1955. New York, United Nations, 1956, pp. 233–236.

5. Holaday, Duncan A. Radiation exposure in uranium mines and mills. *Hearings on Employee Radiation Hazards and Workmen's Compensation before the Subcommittee on Research and Development of the Joint Committee on Atomic Energy, Eighty-Sixth Congress, March 10–19, 1959.* U.S. Government Printing Office, Washington, 1959, p. 198.

Life Stress and Industrial Absenteeism—The Concentration of Illness and Absenteeism in One Segment of a Working Population*

LAWRENCE E. HINKLE, JR., M.D. AND NORMAN PLUMMER, M.D.

PAST STUDIES have revealed much about the causes of absence from work among industrial employees. It is known, for example, that the curve of absence rises and falls with the curve of the business cycle. It

* Reprinted by permission, with omission of ten illustrations and seven tables, from the August 1952 issue of *Industrial Medicine and Surgery*, Vol. 21, pp. 365–375. This paper was presented at a Joint Meeting of the Industrial Medical Association, the American Association of Industrial Dentists, and the American Association of Industrial Nurses in Cincinnati, Ohio, April 23, 1952. The authors are, respectively, Director of the Human Ecology Study Program of the Departments of Medicine and Psychiatry, Clinical Associate Professor of Medicine and Medicine in Psychiatry, Cornell University Medical College, New York, N.Y., formerly Assistant Professor of Clinical Medicine, Cornell University Medical College; General Medical Director, The New York Telephone Company, New York, N.Y., formerly Medical Director, The New York Telephone Company.

is known that absence is affected by such factors as the age of employees, their length of service, the type of sick benefit plan in the industry in which they work, the compensability of their ailments, and the administrative practices of those in supervision over them. It is known that in all industries the absence rate for women is far greater than that for men.[1] It is known that 90 per cent or more of absence is caused by nonoccupational illnesses, of which the respiratory diseases greatly predominate while the digestive disorders run a close second. It has been recognized that especially among women employees the so-called "nervous ailments," although few in number, contribute a disproportionate amount of time lost. But absenteeism in industry is a problem of increasing magnitude for which we have no adequate answer. In these present days of full employment, time lost because of absence has risen to as high as 10 per cent of total working time in some industries.

Some studies of the past decade have suggested that a relatively small proportion of the employees may contribute a disproportionate amount of the total absence. Fulton[2] stated that 68 per cent of the minor sick absenteeism is produced by only 20 per cent of the plant population. Johnson[3] estimated 55 per cent to 60 per cent of lost time as being attributable to 12 per cent or 15 per cent of the employees. Gafafer[4] reported that 27 per cent of the female workers of a public utility contributed 63 per cent of the disabilities over a six-year period. It has also been suggested that a small group of employees are responsible for the majority of accidents,[5] and there has been some evidence to indicate that those who are frequently ill have a higher accident rate than others.[6, 7] Experience in working with female employees of the New York Telephone Company suggested that these latter observations were correct. Furthermore, information supplied by the supervisory personnel suggested that the same persons who were frequently absent constituted a disproportionate number of the individuals who were administrative problems for one reason or another. The present study was undertaken to investigate the distribution of absenteeism among a group of female employees and its relation to problems of administration and illness.

METHOD

For the purposes of this study a representative Division of the New York Telephone Company was selected in New York City. It comprises, in all, 19 central offices and one administrative division office. In this division there were approximately 1700 employees who had originally been hired as telephone operators. Nearly all of these women had been employed between the ages of 16 and 25. At the time of employment they were examined physically, and none had been accepted except those who were physically healthy or had rela-

tively minor defects. Most were telephone operators, but a small proportion had become clerks at some time in their careers. With regard
to working conditions, travel to and from work, income, and place of
domicile, the group could be considered relatively homogeneous. The
Sickness Benefit Plan under which these employees worked during
most of their career provided for payment from the eighth day of illness. For the period after 1940, all employees with more than two
years of service have been paid after the second day of absence. The
only types of absence which were excluded from the study were those
attributed to maternity leaves or administrative leaves of absence, and
excused short absences for such reasons as jury duty. The days lost,
therefore, included a small percentage of brief absences attributed to
personal or domestic causes. The results of this study were analyzed
statistically. In addition, the medical records of certain selected groups
of employees were carefully analyzed, and these employees were interviewed and examined in a manner which will be outlined.

RESULTS OF STATISTICAL STUDY

Complete records of attendance and complete medical
records were available on 1297 of the 1700 individuals. The average
lost time for this group of women in 1950 was 22.2 days. When the
group was analyzed in terms of the number of days lost by each during
the year and the results were graphed, it was found that they did not
group themselves around this average in a bell-shaped distribution
curve. Instead, it was found that the largest single group of employees
were those who had no absence. The distribution curve had a logarith-
mic shape with a long tail consisting of relatively few individuals with
many days of absence. Nine hundred and twelve individuals lay below
the average, and only 385 above the average. The 443 employees
(34.2 per cent) who had five days or less of absence in 1950 contributed a total of 856 days of absence (3.0 per cent). On the other
hand, the 418 employees (32.2 per cent) with 21 or more days of
absence during 1950 contributed 22,999 days (79.8 per cent) of
absence. Analysis of the group in terms of the number of times absent
gave a similar curve although the peak was somewhat less acute. In
terms of times absent it was evident that the 805 employees (62.1 per
cent) who were absent five times or less during the year contributed
1987 absences (31.0 per cent), whereas the 118 employees (9.1 per
cent) who were absent 11 times or more during the year contributed
1569 absences (24.4 per cent). In 1950, one-third of these women
accounted for four-fifths of the total days lost.

The lengths of service of the employees in this group range from
one year to 44 years. The initial year of service, therefore, covered a
range of years from 1906 to 1950, during which all sorts of business

conditions prevailed. When the employee group was analyzed in terms of number of days absent during the first year of service of each employee, the distribution of absence was more strikingly distorted than in the 1950 curve. In the first year of service the 850 employees with five days or less of absence contributed 1237 days of absence, whereas the 97 individuals with 21 days or more of absence contributed 3551 days of absence. That is to say, the 65.7 per cent of employees with lower absence contributed only 14.6 per cent of the absence during the first year, whereas the higher 7.5 per cent of the employees contributed 42 per cent. The distribution in terms of number of times absent during the first year of service was similar. Distribution curves for the number of times absent and the number of days absent in the second year of service produced further curves of the same type.

The question arose, did the same group of employees contribute a disproportionate amount of absence year after year? It had been suspected on the basis of medical records that some individuals had consistently high absence rates and other individuals had consistently low absence rates. The record of each of the 1297 employees was therefore analyzed in terms of the amount of absence each year throughout total service, and the total amount of absence. It was found that whereas the absence for each employee might vary in amount from year to year, the average absence for the employees throughout their totaled period of service was distributed in a manner similar to that for their first and second years. When employees were grouped according to the amount of absence which they had had in the first year of service, and this was plotted against the average number of days absent per year throughout the entire period of service, it was found that the points lay along a straight line. The employees with the least absence during the first year had the least average absence throughout their entire period of service, and so on, up to the employees with the highest absence during the first year, who had the highest average absence throughout their entire period of service. A predictability curve was also obtained when times absent during the first year was plotted against average times absent throughout the entire period of service. The predictability curve for average *days* absent was a straight line but that for average *times* absent was a curve tending to flatten out somewhat in the higher regions. It was felt that this flattening of the curve might be the result of the intervention of management; that is to say, among the group of individuals with 12 or more times absent during the first year, those who did not improve in subsequent years were separated from the payroll or resigned, and the remaining members of the group were those with improved attendance.

To determine if any correlation existed between the group of employees who are administrative problems and those who were attendance problems, arrangements were made to have these employees rated in terms of their performance in 1950. Employees were rated on attitude, ability to get along with others, and quality of work. The ratings were good, fair, and poor, in each category. These ratings were made by the chief operators of each of the 19 central offices. The chief operators had observed the employees under their supervision throughout the period of 1950; but they had not known most of them throughout their entire careers, because of the fact that employees are usually moved from one office to another in the Metropolitan Area of New York, the average stay in an individual office being several years. It was recognized that the rating of the chief operator might be influenced by her knowledge of the employee's attendance during the period in which the employee was under her observation. For this reason, the ratings as obtained were correlated not with absence during 1950, but with absence during the first year of service, however distant that may have been in the past. There was found to be a positive correlation between good attitude and good ability to get along with people in 1950, and low absence during the first year of service. There was some slight correlation in terms of quality of work. These findings suggested that attitude and ability to get along with others are affected by the same factors that affect absence. The poorer correlation of absence with quality of work may be a reflection of the intense administrative attention to work quality which has characterized this industry throughout the period studied. During this time supervisory personnel were much more prepared to tolerate poor attendance, poor attitude and poor ability to get along with others than they were to tolerate a poor quality of work. It is likely that those with a consistently poor work performance were rapidly dropped from the group.

MEDICAL STUDY OF SELECTED
GROUPS OF EMPLOYEES

In this group of 1297 employees there were 336 who had 20 or more years of service in 1950. It was decided to select from these 336, 20 who had had little absence throughout their service career, and 20 who had had a great deal of absence. These selections were made solely on the basis of attendance, without previous knowledge of the medical records of the employees. The groups were comparable in terms of both age and length of service. The average age of the women in the good attendance group was 48.8 years, and the average length of service was 28.8 years. The average age of the women in the poor attendance group was 46.1 years and the average length of service was 25.9 years. It had been intended that the 20 individuals with the most absence be compared with the 20 individuals with the least absence. However, one of the individuals assigned to the low absence group initially, was found after the study was partly completed to have somewhat more absence than had initially been indicated. She was not a high absence employee but an employee who did not fall into the lowest absence group. The weighting of the results by the presence of this employee tended to diminish rather than enhance the striking findings which were obtained and she was, therefore, allowed to remain a member of the group. As will be noted below, she contributed as much absence to her group as did the other 19 members of the good attendance group altogether.

Once the names of these employees had been obtained, their medical records were carefully scrutinized by staff physicians. These records contained notations covering almost every illness and disability from which each employee had suffered throughout her entire term of service. In connection with most of these illnesses there were visits to the Medical Department and descriptions of examinations made at that time. These were supplemented by notations of telephone reports from private physicians, certificates sent in by private physicians, and abstracts of hospital records. Because of the fact that the diagnostic statement of the private physician made in his initial certificate or telephone message might be incorrect for various reasons, careful evaluation of the signs, symptoms, and course of each illness was made in order to confirm or revise the stated diagnosis in accordance with the apparent facts as well as in accordance with the later knowledge provided by the advances in medical science. Medical diagnoses reported in these studies are, therefore, more accurate than they would have been had the raw data alone been utilized.

In addition to this scrutiny of the records, the 40 individuals were seen in the Medical Department, and were interviewed at length. A complete medical history was obtained. In addition, biographic data covering family history, cultural, social and economic background, and life history in detail were also obtained. The present life situation was investigated, and careful note was made of any evidences of disturbances of mood, thought, and behavior. These interviews, where possible, were supplemented by physical examinations and appropriate laboratory and diagnostic procedures.

It was found that the applicant examinations of these two groups of individuals provided no indication of the subsequent course of their health. The minor physical defects found in the various employees were distributed throughout the groups of good attendance and poor attendance employees.

Respiratory Disease

The employees with poor attendance greatly exceeded the employees with good attendance in all categories of subsequent illness. These categories of illness were grouped according to the major bodily organ systems. As had been expected, it was found that the respiratory illnesses were the largest group of disorders attributed to any single system. Minor respiratory infections were far more frequent in the poor attendance group than in the good attendance group, the ratio being about 12 to 1. In addition to this, it was evident that there was much more chronic respiratory disease and many more episodes of serious respiratory illness among the poor attendance group than among the good attendance group. In the poor attendance group there were found episodes of lobar pneumonia, bronchopneumonia, pleurisy with effusion, hemoptysis, bronchiectasis and asthma, whereas all of these more serious episodes had been absent in the members of the good attendance group. In addition to this, such disorders as chronic sinusitis, chronic post-nasal drip, chronic tonsillitis and chronic bronchitis were much more common in the group with poor attendance.

Gastrointestinal Disorders

Much the same pattern was found with regard to disorders of all of the other organ systems. In the gastro-intestinal system the episodes of such minor functional disorders as nausea, vomiting, hyperacidity, and constipation were much more frequent in those with poor attendance than those with good attendance. In addition, those with poor attendance included people with ulcerative colitis, cholecystitis, cholelithiasis, hiatus hernia (associated with severe symptoms), and peptic ulcer; whereas the good attendance group included only one individual who had duodenal ulcer and an episode of cardiospasm. All of the other members of the group were free of these serious manifestations, and had only a relatively small number of the minor functional disorders. It is interesting to note that the single individual with the duodenal ulcer and esophageal spasm was the one individual who was included in the good attendance group by mistake.

Gynecologic Disease

The most outstanding difference observed was that in the gynecologic disorders of the two groups of women. The women with a low absence rate had experienced phenomenally good health with regard to their genital systems. None had had any menstrual abnormality, and the only gynecologic disturbance found in the group was one instance of post-menopausal bleeding. There were serious menstrual irregularities in a large number of the women with a high absence rate, as well as other illnesses, such as uterine myomata, salpingitis, and spontaneous abortions. The so-called menopausal symptoms were entirely concentrated in this group, while the women with good attendance had all passed through menopause uneventfully.

Other Conditions

Among the disorders of skin, eye, ear, teeth, bones and joints, musculature, and the urinary system, and some miscellaneous conditions there was a similar concentration of illness in the group with poor attendance. This group had many more minor manifestations of illness in these systems, and nearly all of the major manifestations of illness.

In the cardiovascular system the results were somewhat less striking. There were five individuals with hypertension in the group with low absence and seven in the group with high absence. In the low-absence group all of the hypertension was asymptomatic, whereas in the high-absence group it was accompanied by many symptoms such as palpitation, extra systoles, tachycardia and headache. In this group also appeared an individual with two coronary occlusions and angina pectoris, as well as all of those individuals with disorders of the peripheral vessels, such as phlebitis and varicose veins. Obesity also was rather equally distributed between the two groups, but other metabolic disorders were much more frequent in the group with poor attendance.

There are relatively few occupational disorders associated with telephone operating, of which the only one seen in these two groups was a pressure sore of the ear caused by the pressure of the telephone ear-piece. There were five instances of this in three of the poor attendance women, and five instances in two of the good attendance women.

In both groups it was found that the disorders of feeling-state, thought and behavior which make up what is commonly called the "nervous and emotional" or "psychoneurotic" group of illnesses, were much more common than a simple recording of the diagnoses indicated by the private physicians would have shown. In past time it has been customary to disguise such disorders in terms of euphemisms, such as "functional endocrine," "fatigue state," "run-down condition," or simply as "grippe," or "virus." When the symptoms and manifestations of the various episodes of illness of these two groups of people were carefully evaluated, it was found that symptoms of tension, asthenia, anxiety, and mild depression were probably the most common of those encountered and the number of absences which could be attributed to such manifestations is as great as the number actually attributed to upper respiratory infections. In fact, in all of the group of employees in the poor attendance category these symptoms were almost constantly present throughout long periods of their employment. Because of their constant presence, symptoms of this nature colored all of the other absences. The excess of respiratory infections was somewhat exaggerated, and the total time lost was greatly exaggerated, by the simultaneous presence of disturbed feeling-states. A breakdown of the illness in terms of disorders of feeling-state, thought and behavior, revealed a remarkable prevalence of these manifestations. There were 492 instances of these disorders in the 20 poor attendance individuals. Manifestations of tension, asthenia, anxiety, and mild depression occurred in almost all of them, and more severe illnesses, such as paranoid schizophrenia, alcoholism, and phobic and compulsive states were also seen. There was a surprisingly high incidence of hysteric or conversion manifestations. Nine of these individuals exhibited 26 separate episodes of what could reasonably be termed hysteria.

In this category of illness, then, the findings were much the same as in all of the other categories of illness. There were only 23 instances of disturbances of feeling-state or behavior in the group with low absence as compared with 492 in the group with high absence. Again those manifestations which occurred in the low absence group were the minor manifestations such as anxiety, tension, insomnia, asthenia and mild depression, and these occurred on relatively few occasions; whereas similar manifestations were much more frequent in the group with poor attendance and the more severe disorders occurred solely in this group.

Accidents

The same pattern was apparent with regard to accidents. There were 133 accidents recorded in the poor attendance group and only 38 in those with good attendance. Nearly all of the accidents in the good attendance group were of a minor nature and led to no disability or lost time; whereas the major accidents such as fractured skulls, concussions, major burns, major lacerations, fractures of long bones, and severe contusions were all localized in the group with poor attendance. The group with poor attendance had lost a total of 2170 days because of accidents, whereas the group with good attendance had lost only 91 days.

Surgical Operations

In view of the larger incidence of illness in the poor attendance group it might be expected that the women in this group would have had more operations than those in the group with good attendance. This was found to be the case.

The total amount of absence attributed to the group with poor attendance was 24,185 days, whereas the total amount of absence attributed to the group with good attendance was 667 days. Of these 667 days, 333 days of absence were contributed by one woman with somewhat poorer attendance who was inadvertently included in the group.

Social Background

An effort was made to come to some understanding of why illness and absence so much predominated in one group as compared to the other. The results of these studies can be summarized here. It was found that the cultural and economic backgrounds of the two groups were similar. Both were made up of second-generation women of Italian or Irish background, and as such they are representative of the larger group of employees from which they were abstracted. In both groups it was found that there had been many instances of poverty and of the early death of one or both parents. It could not be determined from the information these women gave about their family histories that the parents of either group were more healthy, more long-lived, or more free of familial diseases than those of the other. Among the parents of the women who later became ill, there were somewhat more instances of such outstanding disorders of the personality as alcoholism, brutality and neglectfulness; but some instances of this were also seen in the parents of the group of well women. Likewise, there was no striking difference in the amount of childhood disease seen in the two groups. Bearing in mind the fact that probably some of the ill women tended to conceal earlier evidence of illness, nevertheless one could state that outstanding evidences of childhood illness also occurred in the group of women who were later well. The groups were similar also in terms of education. Nearly all had graduated from grammar school at about the age of 12 to 14 and had gone no further in their studies. Nearly all had gone to work at an early age and had held several jobs before becoming telephone operators at the age of 16 to 20.

The one outstanding difference in the histories of the two groups lay in the degree to which they had been exposed to what is broadly termed "life stress" throughout their period of employment. The well women had been content, comfortable and secure in their life situations. The ill women, however, had been made unhappy, insecure, and discontented by repeated frustrations, deprivations, unrewarded responsibility, and interpersonal conflicts throughout their adult lives.

Nearly all of the well women were women who had had no great desire to be married and who had been content with a career as single women and telephone operators. They were individuals who were able to make friends readily. They were "outward going" and capable of diffuse emotional attachments. In any group in which they found themselves they soon became happy and well liked. Among these women there were many instances of profound loyalty and deep attachment to parents, brothers and sisters, or husbands, but the loss of these individuals from their lives led to no prolonged disturbance of their mood or behavior. They were individuals with no unalterable goals in life. They had grown up without any settled idea of what they "should" or "should not" do in terms of a career and without any preconceived notions of what they wanted to do above all else. Some of them had been offered promotions from time to time in the past, but had refused these promotions simply because they felt more happy with the lack of responsibility and comfortable hours which they had attained in their present position. They rapidly adapted to being moved from one type of operating to another or from one office to another. Because of their capacity to make friends, their failure to complain, and their pliability with regard to assignments, they were well liked by their associates and by their supervisors.

The group of women who were ill were in great contrast to the group who had been well. This group of women had nearly all desired to be married and to have a family which was supported by a husband. They had gone to work as telephone operators with the idea that they would work for a few years, accumulate savings and a few worldly goods, and then be married and stop working. For one reason or another they had been frustrated in this goal. Some had been saddled with ill parents for whose care they were responsible. They had, therefore, felt unable or unwilling to be married, and had continued in a state of resentment and frustration thereafter. Others had married only to find that their marriages soon dissolved. In some instances this was the result of incompatibility and divorce, in some instances it was the result of desertion or lack of support by the husband, and in some instances it was the result of his early death. Some of these women were left with young children to support. Several, because of their religious beliefs felt precluded from obtaining a divorce or making another marriage. They had, therefore, returned to telephone operating as a necessary means of making a living. They had "struggled" through life, attempting to work and at the same time to raise a family or care for an ailing relative. Their moods were constantly those of frustration, resentment, depression, and anxiety which so characterized the so-called "nervous and emotional illnesses" present among them. They were not outward-going individuals, but tended to be defensive, suspicious, and somewhat hostile. They did not make friends easily, and drew little sustenance from the group among whom they worked. Nor were they readily deviated from their goals or their position in life. If moved from one office to another, or one job to another, they reacted to this with distaste and with complaints. As a group they were women of ambition. Once in the company, they had attempted to get ahead. They had accepted higher positions if these were proffered, and had resented it if they were not. They were, therefore, not well liked by those in supervision over them, and they reciprocated this dislike. As a group they were not happy with their jobs, and were, therefore, prepared to welcome any opportunity to be absent with a legitimate excuse. On the other hand, under the pressure of economic necessity, they were prepared to work. They tolerated their symptoms and their various illnesses in times of economic distress when there was some reason for them to fear that they might lose their jobs.

COMMENT

The results of these statistical studies confirm the earlier findings of Fulton, Johnson, and Gafafer which have been cited previously. It is evident that in any one work year about two-thirds of the absence in this group of employees was contributed by about one-third of the individuals. It becomes further evident from this analysis that the same employees contribute a disproportionate amount of the absence throughout their entire period of service, i.e., the group may be divided into employees with a consistently low absence rate and other employees with a consistently high absence rate. The two groups, of course, shade off into each other with no distinct point of separation. Furthermore, it is apparent that the group of employees with the consistently high absence rate includes a large proportion of the employees who are regarded by their supervisors as having a poor attitude and poor ability to get along with those around them.

The medical studies indicate that the women in the group with a high absence rate had far more illnesses of all types than those in the group with a low absence rate. Minor manifestations of illness of all types were seen in the women with a low absence rate, but these were many times more frequently seen in the women with a high absence rate. The severer manifestations of illness of all types were almost entirely confined to the women with a high absence rate. The women with a low absence rate had relatively infrequent accidents of a minor nature, rarely disabling. The women with a high absence rate had much more frequent minor accidents, and nearly all of the major accidents, which led to prolonged disability. There were only four surgical procedures in the women with good attendance, while there were 52 surgical procedures, many of them of a major nature, in the women with poor attendance. The two groups could, with great justification, be referred to as a "well group" and an "ill group," and it might also be said that the ill group was "accident prone."

Comparison of the medical records of the two groups of individuals confirms the fact that minor illnesses of all bodily systems are widespread throughout the general population, and occur in all individuals from time to time under appropriate circumstances of exposure to stress. This also holds true for the transitory disturbances of feeling-state, attitude, and behavior which are commonly termed tension, anxiety, asthenia or mild depression. The fact that the members of the high absence group tended to take more time off with these minor ailments because of their general attitude and feeling toward their work unquestionably entered into the high total number of days lost by the group with poor attendance. But no matter how much weight one gave to the effect of attitude on the length of individual illnesses of these employees, it was nevertheless evident that episodes of minor illness in all bodily systems were much more frequent in the people with poor attendance than in the members of the group who had good attendance. One would expect that the group of unhappy, tense and anxious women might have had more neurodermatitis, more complaints of minor abdominal pain, dysmenorrhea, and more visits to the Medical Department for minor bumps and bruises. Such manifestations might be regarded as a part of their pattern of behavior. However, it is also evident that these women had more herpes zoster, eczema, acne, otitis media, pyorrhea, nausea, vomiting, constipation, diarrhea, cystitis, menorrhagia, menstrual irregularity, osteoarthritis, asymptomatic goiters, and low back pain than did their co-workers in the good attendance group. Not only this, but also they had more frequent sprains, strains, bruises, minor lacerations and burns, than did the low absence group. Examinations in the Medical Department and descriptions of the lesions unequivocally bear this out.

A further striking fact is the concentration of serious illness almost entirely in the group with poor attendance. Such illnesses as lobar pneumonia, bronchial asthma, pleurisy with effusion, bronchiectasis, peptic ulcer, cholecystitis, cholelithiasis, ulcerative colitis, uterine fibromata, spontaneous abortion, severe uterine hemorrhages, pyelitis, coronary occlusion, angina pectoris, herniated nucleus pulposus, angiosarcoma, hyperthyroidism, tuberculous chorioretinitis, otitis media, epilepsy and severe dental caries, were all found almost entirely in the group with high absence. The only severe forms of bodily illness found in the group with good attendance were one peptic ulcer, one case of mild diabetes mellitus, and five instances of hypertension. It has been noted that the instance of peptic ulcer occurred in the one woman who was inadvertently included in the group. Likewise, the major manifestations of disturbed feeling-state, attitude and behavior were in the group with high absence, as well as all of the major bodily injuries. It was in this group that one found the alcoholic, the paranoid schizophrenic, the women with major symptoms of anxiety, tension, depression, asthenia, compulsions and phobias in whom a diagnosis of "psychoneurosis" had been made, as well as the two individuals who seemed clearly to fall into the category of conversion hysteria. It was also in this group that one found nearly all the episodes of fractured skull, fractures of long bones, major lacerations, contusions, abrasions and sprains, as well as nearly all the major surgical procedures.

Industrial absenteeism is not simply a reflection of physical disability. The amount of time which an individual spends away from work with each period of ailment is in part under his own conscious and volitional control. The fact that absence goes up when jobs are plentiful and goes down when jobs are scarce, the fact that it is high in offices with poor morale and low in offices with good morale, and the fact that it increases as sickness benefit programs are liberalized, are all indications of the actions of this factor. It is obvious that employees who are interested in their jobs and enjoy their work and their surroundings will tend to take as little time off because of illness as they reasonably can; whereas employees who are unhappy, dissatisfied, and do not like their jobs or their working conditions can be expected to exploit every reasonable opportunity which is given to them to be away from work with a legitimate excuse and the assurance of a steady income. Likewise, it could reasonably be expected that those who have fewer responsibilities and entanglements outside of their work would find less reason to be absent than those whose lives are primarily dedicated to the task at hand. In this sense it is, therefore, not surprising that this study confirms the fact that those employees in the group with good attendance were employees with "a good attitude" and that those employees with poor attendance were those with "a poor attitude." But it is also of great significance that those employees with "a good attitude" were those who were well, whereas those with "a poor attitude" were those who were ill.

The question of why some women are relatively well and happy all the time throughout their adult years whereas others are relatively unwell, unhappy and discontented, is not so easily answered. The family histories of the two groups of women were not notably different. It could not be discovered from the medical history that the group of well women had parents who were either more healthy or more long-lived than those of the ill group. Nor were the childhood experiences of these two groups entirely different. Most of the well women had had a good deal of security and happiness in childhood. The same was apparently true of some of the ill group; but some women in both the well and the ill group had been through notably difficult childhood experiences. It has been pointed out that the one obvious differentiating factor in the two groups lay in the fact that the women who were ill were dissatisfied, discontented, unhappy and resentful at their lot in life and that throughout their working years they were loaded with outside responsibilities, worries, and frustrations with which the well women were not burdened.

Searching for a physiologic explanation for these parallel phenomena of unhappiness, illness and inability to get along with others one may assume either that the ill group were people with innately less adaptability than those in the well group, or that something happened to the women in the ill group to render them subject to many bodily disturbances, and that this had not happened to the well group.

The latter appears to be the more likely explanation. During the course of the past 15 years an increasing body of medical evidence has indicated that many types of bodily disturbances may occur as a part of an individual's adaptive response to events and situations in his external environment. Physiologic and experimental studies have confirmed the great importance of such adaptations to life stress in producing dysfunctions of the gastro-intestinal tract, both upper[8] and lower,[9] in cardiovascular disorders,[10] in headache,[11] vasomotor rhinitis,[12] sinusitis,[13] changes in bronchial secretion and bronchial asthma,[14] in metabolic disorders such as obesity,[15] diabetes[16] and hyperthyroidism,[17] muscle tension,[18] and urticaria,[19] as well as others.[10] At the present time there is no unequivocal evidence to indicate that increased susceptibility to infection is a concomitant of chronic exposure to life stress, but present experiences with the effects of ACTH and the adrenal steroids on infection, as well as clinical impressions of long standing, would suggest that this may be true.

Likewise, the evidence that disorders of the eyes (except glaucoma), of the teeth, the urinary system, the joints, and the functions of the female genital tract may be seriously affected by adaptations to life stress, remains a clinical impression without much experimental evidence in support. However, one might reasonably expect that these systems would take part in bodily adaptations in the same manner in which other systems participate.

While these medical and physiologic data have been accumulating, parallel investigations in the realm of psychiatry during the past 50 years have produced increasing amounts of evidence that the disturbances of feeling-state, thought and behavior which are commonly known as the "psychoneuroses," or "psychoses," are also in large measure the result of the individual's attempt to adapt to various forms of life stress. Studies of the frequency of accidents among various groups of industrial employees have suggested that "accident proneness" is the result of disturbed adaptive reactions also.[20]

Therefore, it would appear that that group of individuals who are chronically exposed to life stress is the group in whom most of the illnesses will occur, and who will present the most difficult problems in interpersonal relations, and administration. As far as industry is concerned, it is apparent that certain steps may be taken to deal with these people for the mutual benefit of both employer and employee. The individual with a high illness and absence rate, with difficulty in interpersonal adjustments and in adaptation to office routine can be recognized soon after his employment. Early in his employment career a suitable assessment can be made not only of his physical condition, but also of the factors operating in his life to create stress for him. It can be determined whether the problems which he faces and the attitude with which he faces them are such as to make it likely that he will be a happy and productive employee, or whether perhaps he might better seek some other position in life. Likewise, various arrangements can be made with regard to his position, supervisors, location of work and type of work so that he will be able to attain his highest level of productivity. It is evident that such an early assessment of employees and arrangements to enable them to exploit their highest potentialities would be beneficial to all concerned. Such a course is especially desirable in industries in which the term of employment can be expected to be long, and where tenure of position and sickness benefits are provided for. Among employees who have been on the payroll for a long time and who have family and financial responsibilities of an important nature, it is obvious that every effort must be made to ameliorate the stresses to which the employee is exposed, insofar as these stresses pertain to employment and are within the reasonable potentialities of management. The alternative is obviously one of continued absence and poor performance to the detriment of the employer, and continued illness and ill health to the detriment of the employee.

CONCLUSIONS

1. A study was made of the absences of 1,297 telephone operators throughout their working careers. It was found that in any one year the distribution of absences in the group was such that the greater proportion was caused by a small proportion of the employees. This was true both in terms of total days absent and in terms of number of times absent.

2. It was found that the same employees fell into the high absence and low absence group throughout their entire period of employment. For the group, the relation between absence in the first year of service and the total absence throughout subsequent years of service showed a high positive correlation.

3. Of the employees in this group, 336 had had 20 or more years of service. From these 336, 20 of those with the greatest total amount of absence and 20 of those with the smallest total amount of absence were selected for intensive study.

4. Critical review of the medical records of these two groups indicated that the 20 women with high absence had had frequent minor illnesses pertaining to all bodily systems; and that they had had a large number of major illnesses pertaining to all bodily systems. They had had frequent and prolonged minor disturbances of feeling-state, thought and behavior, and a large number of major disturbances of this nature. They had had frequent minor injuries and a large number of major injuries causing lost time from work. They had had a large number of surgical operations, both major and minor. The women with a low absence rate, on the other hand, had had relatively few and scattered illnesses in all bodily systems, and few major bodily illnesses. They had had few and minor disturbances of feeling-state,

thought and behavior, and no major disturbances of this nature. They had had relatively few minor injuries leading to little lost time, and few major injuries. They had had few surgical operations.

5. The 20 women with a high absence rate were as a group discontented, unhappy, difficult to get along with, and difficult to supervise. The 20 women with a low absence rate were as a group contented, happy, easy to get along with, and easy to supervise. For the entire 1297 employees it was found that general attitude and ability to get along with others in 1950 had a positive correlation with attendance in the first year of service, however long ago that might have been.

6. It was found that the 20 women with a high absence rate had been exposed throughout their period of employment to life situations and experiences which were to them stressful; whereas the 20 women with a low absence rate throughout their period of employment had been exposed to relatively few experiences which they had interpreted as stressful.

7. In this group of telephone operators, absenteeism, bodily illness, psychologic disturbances, poor attitudes and administrative problems were concentrated in those members of the working population who were having difficulty in adapting to the situations and experiences to which they were chronically exposed throughout their period of employment.

1. Baetjer, A. M.: *Women in Industry*. Philadelphia, W. B. Saunders Co., 1948.

2. Fulton, W. J.: "Records—the 'Seeing Eye' of Industrial Medicine," *Indust. Med.*, 13:1, 1944.

3. Johnson, O. J.: "Public Health and Medical Relationship in Industrial Health." *Am. J. Pub. Health*, 32:1157, 1942.

4. Gafafer, W. M.: Absenteeism in *Manual of Industrial Hygiene*, U.S. Pub. Health Service. W. B. Saunders Co. Philadelphia, 1943.

5. Baetjer, A. M.: *op. cit.*, Page 131.

6. Newbold, E. M.: *Contribution to the Study of The Human Factor in the Causation of Accidents*. Great Britain Medical Research Council, Industrial Health Research Board Rep. 34, 1926.

7. Great Britain Medical Research Council: *The Personal Factor of Accidents*. Industrial Health Research Board Emergency Rep. 3, 1942.

8. Wolf, S., and Wolff, H. G.: *Human Gastric Function*. Oxford University Press, 2nd Ed., 1943.

9. Grace, W. J., Wolf, S., and Wolff, H. G.: *The Human Colon*. New York, Paul B. Hoeber Co., 1951.

10. *Life Stress and Bodily Disease*, Res. Pub. Assn. Res. Nerv. & Mental Diseases, Vol. 29, 1949, Part X.

11. Wolff, H. G.: *Headache and Other Head Pain*. Oxford University Press, 1949.

12. Holmes, T. H., Goodell, H., Wolf, S., and Wolff, H. G,: *The Nose*. Charles C Thomas, Springfield, Illinois, 1949.

13. *Idem*.

14. *Life Stress and Bodily Disease*, Page 566.

15. Bruch, Hilde: Psychological Aspects of Obesity. *Bull. New York Acad. Med.*, 24:73, 1948.

16. Hinkle, L. E., Jr., and Wolf, S.: The Importance of Life Stress in the Course and Management of Diabetes Mellitus. *J.A.M.A.*, 148:513, 1952.

17. Lidz, T., and Whitehorn, J. C.: *Life Stress and Bodily Disease*, Chapter 28, Page 445.

18. Holmes, T. H., and Wolff, H. G.: *Life Stress and Bodily Disease*, Page 750.

19. Graham, D. T.: *Life Stress and Bodily Disease*, Page 989.

20. Dunbar, Flanders: *Psychosomatic Diagnosis*. New York, Paul B. Hoeber, 1943.

Alcoholism in Industry*

HARRY LEVINSON, PH.D.

THE PROBLEM OF DRINKING

More than 68 million people in the United States drink alcoholic beverages.[1] Four and one-half million of them are alcoholics. More than two million of them, representing approximately 2 per cent of all workers, are employed in business and industry. Although the accuracy of these figures from the Yale Center of Alcohol Studies has been questioned,[2] they remain the most valid estimates available.

Some colleagues suspect that the Yale figures are too low. One study of 10 large industrial firms concluded that approximately 8 per cent of skilled, experienced workers between the ages of 35 and 45 showed outward signs of alcoholism.[6] From the same study it was estimated employee alcoholism reduced overall national productivity at least 2½ per cent. A study in the province of Ontario, Canada, reported that "six per cent of the personnel in ten typical companies (relatively small companies employing fewer than 200 workers) surveyed by the Alcoholism Research Foundation of Ontario were diagnosed as problem drinkers or alcoholics."[7] Further, "five and one-half per cent of all alcoholics uncovered by that foundation's survey of a typical Ontario county were found among the managers and owners of businesses and in the professional group . . . Sixty per cent of the alcoholics found were skilled, semi-skilled or white-collar workers in the upper income brackets. . . ."

Accepting the 2 per cent figure as being more representative than the 8 per cent extreme incidence on the one hand and the highly conservative estimate of half of one percent from a survey sponsored by Licensed Beverage Industries, Inc.,[16] on the other, then one out of every 50 employees is a problem drinker. The incidence of problem drinking, however, hardly begins to reflect its importance. The Yale figures[3] indicate further that the average problem drinker in industry is absent from his job 22 working days a year because of the effects of alcohol. He loses two days a year more for other illness than does the average of other employees, has twice as many accidents as the non-alcoholic, and loses 12 years of his life span when compared with the non-alcoholic. Contrary to the popular stereotype of the alcoholic as a vagrant, those men who visit outpatient clinics for alcoholism are a representative cross-section of the male population between 30 and 55 years of age.[4] Many problem drinkers are in responsible positions where mistakes, errors of judgment, and the public relations effects of their drinking are extremely costly. In addition, because of its insidious

* Reprinted in part by permission from a special issue of the *Menninger Quarterly*, 1957, Volume 11, pages 1–20. The author is Director, Division of Industrial Mental Health, Menninger Foundation, Topeka, Kansas.

development and because of the tendency to deny and conceal the problem, many men continue to function for a long time in inadequate and ineffective ways. In contrast to the Skid Row itinerant whose chronic alcoholism is all too apparent, the drinker in industry presents a problem precisely because his difficulty is so often concealed rather than blatantly demonstrated.

Taken altogether the cost of the problem in terms of absenteeism, inefficiency, and other forms of industrial handicap, apart from the personal cost to the man himself and his family, is indeed heavy.

THE PROBLEMS OF TREATMENT

Although there is considerable clinical understanding of the problem drinker,[8] problem drinking has been conspicuously and consistently resistant to medical and psychologic therapies. So overwhelming have been the failures by traditional psychiatric therapies that many psychiatrists do not treat alcoholics and those who do take only a highly select group of them.[9]

The reasons for these failures are many. One reason is that the symptom itself represents a flight from reality. The alcoholic while drunk has as little contact with the world around him as the most severely mentally ill patient. Characteristically he avoids or escapes treatment. So often it is much easier to obliterate troubles by drinking than to confront them, especially if confrontation seems to offer little chance for solution. Another reason is that the symptom often represents a last-ditch defense against complete psychic breakdown. For some it provides the only relief they know for the increasing tension which seems to threaten them with collapse. A third reason is that the physician traditionally has been unable to control the environmental conditions beyond the hospital or treatment center. While in recent years some progress has been made in this direction by the use of social workers in clinics and hospitals, few private physicians have social workers affiliated with them; the larger public institutions are so understaffed that adequate social work is all but impossible. After "drying out" or undergoing a course of treatment, the alcoholic returns to the same environment from which he came. The same pressures exist, and there is the same easy availability of solution to them. There are few, if any, external governing or motivating forces to take the place of the alcoholic's lack of motivation for treatment. Still another reason for the failures of physicians treating alcoholics is that, once the alcoholic has recovered from the acute stages of his illness, he is convinced he can remain sober by himself and no longer needs treatment. He often protests and resents a hospital staff which doubts his word and, unless committed, he usually leaves a hospital against medical advice.

To make a difficult therapeutic problem even worse, alcohol has been regarded as a moral and social problem rather than as a medical one. Alcoholism is not an illness itself any more than fever is an illness. It is a symptom of a severe underlying personality disorder, precipitated by many different problems and circumstances. Because it is a most troublesome symptom and a most obvious behavior deviation, and because the problems underlying it are usually unrecognized, many people regard alcoholism as an entity. For some it is a problem of will power. "He could stop if he wanted to." Others regard it as a question of morality, and for still others it is a question of responsibility. These conceptions have tended to create a general attitude of shame, rejection, futility, and even bland denial.

The difficulties in treatment and the false conceptions of the nature of alcoholism have resulted in the social rejection of the alcoholic and his problem. Although 41 states had by 1955 passed legislation supporting the development of clinics and hospitals for the treatment of alcoholism or creating commissions or other bodies to carry out programs of education and research,[10] facilities for treatment are painfully inadequate and most therapeutic efforts are stop-gap and emergency in nature.

In addition to the inadequacy of treatment and the lack of facilities for treatment, industry itself has been reluctant to face the problem. For many years firing the person who could not control his drinking was the easiest solution. Furthermore, by attributing the problem to the employee alone, industry could say, "It's his problem, not ours." The social stigma attached to drinking made it seem poor public relations for any company to recognize that within its organization were those who might be regarded as "drunks."

Few businesses had records which gave any idea of the extent of the problem within their own organizations. Most felt there were enough problems to deal with anyway. Then there were questions of cost and of interference with the personal lives of employees. A complex of many forces kept industry from attacking the problem.

NEW FORCES

Over the past 25 years four major developments have contributed to an accelerated attack on the problem. Alcoholics Anonymous,[11] a voluntary organization made up of recovered or "arrested" alcoholics, founded in 1935, has grown to an estimated 150,000 members in more than 5,000 local groups. The single requirement for membership is that the applicant be an alcoholic who desires help with his drinking problem. The members of the organization help each other. They will, on call, take an intoxicated alcoholic to a hospital or other facility and sit with a person who feels he is about to return to the bottle. They work for the development of treatment facilities, provide recreation centers for their membership, and undertake many other activities which, to the alcoholic, mean a new way of life and continuing support from other people. Alcoholics Anonymous makes possible an environmental control not previously available to the physician.

The second major event has been the development of the Yale Center of Alcohol Studies.[12] This has grown out of research in the Yale Laboratory of Applied Physiology (now the Laboratory of Applied Biodynamics) which began about 1930 to focus on the effects of alcohol. Ten years later, the recognition that the study of physiology was but one of many approaches to research in alcoholism and that a scientific clearing house for research in this field was needed, the separate unit called the Yale Center of Alcohol Studies was created. Its basic purpose is to establish physiologic, psychologic, and sociologic knowledge about alcoholism. It serves as a source of statistics on various aspects of the alcohol problem and has set up a model clinic known as the Yale Plan Clinic which gave rise in Connecticut to the first State Commission on Alcoholism. The Yale Center also issues publications, conducts educational programs for persons concerned with preventing alcoholism, and offers consultation services to governmental, voluntary, and business organizations concerned with the problem.

Third, in 1937, there was organized a Research Council on Problems of Alcohol[10] which for 12 years stimulated both research and public education, giving special impetus to a medical attack on alcoholism. Then, in 1949, this organization became the National Research Council Committee on Problems of Alcohol. Following this line of development various professional groups began to give some attention to alcoholism. The American Psychiatric Association, the American Medical Association, and the Industrial Medical Association all have committees on alcoholism.

A fourth major development was the creation of the National Committee on Alcoholism[14] (now the National Council on Alcoholism, Inc.), a voluntary citizens' movement to increase public understanding of alcoholism, organized in 1944 to distribute literature and provide information on alcoholism and facilities for treatment.

The development of these organizations has resulted in a rapid growth of public concern with alcoholism. In addition to the state agencies set up for public education and research, some 60 local community facilities have developed, mainly under the sponsorship of local committees on alcoholism.[13]

By making it possible to extend increased assistance to the alcoholic, and thereby to increase his chances of recovery, all these events have created a climate in which alcoholism is increasingly recognized as a health problem. With growing freedom, recovered alcoholics speak publicly about their experiences and the kind of help which has made it possible for them to become useful citizens again. At the same time increasing concern for the individual, the increasing investment of industry in ever more highly skilled and responsible personnel, and the continuing dearth of employees in many skilled fields combine to make industry more interested in and concerned with the conservation of human resources, including the person whose drinking has impaired his functioning.

1. Keller, M., and Efron, V.: The Prevalence of Alcoholism. *Q. J. Stud. Alc.*, *16:* 618–644, 1955.

2. Roberts, J. I., and Russo, E. A.: The Alcoholic in Industry—and his Rehabilitation. *Indus. Med. & Surg.*, 24: 269–272, 1955.

3. Jellinek, E. M.: What Shall We Do About Alcoholism? *Vital Speeches*, 13: 252–253, 1947.

4. Straus, R., and Bacon, S. D.: Alcoholism and Social Stability. A Study of Occupational Integration in 2,023 Male Clinic Patients. *Q. J. Stud. Alc.*, *12:* 231–260, 1951.

5. ———, Facts on Alcoholism in Industry. *Mgmt. Rev.*, *43:* 581, 1954.

6. ———, *Mgmt. Rev.*, 40: 70, 1951.

7. Robinson, Robert R.: Industry Can Cut Its Losses by Facing Up to Alcoholism. *Canad. Pers. & Indust. Relat. J.*, *2:* 12–21, 1955.

8. Menninger, Karl A.: *Man Against Himself.* New York, Harcourt, Brace and Company, 1938.

9. Hayman, Max: Current Attitudes to Alcoholism of Psychiatrists in Southern California. *Am. J. Psychiat.*, 112: 485–493, 1956.

10. Hirsch, Joseph: *State Programs on Alcoholism Research, Treatment and Rehabilitation.* New York, Licensed Beverage Industries, Inc., 1955.

11. ———, *Alcoholics Anonymous.* New York, Works Publishing Co., 1939.

12. ———, *The Yale Center of Alcohol Studies.* New Haven, Yale Center of Alcohol Studies, no date.

13. Straus, Robert, and Henderson, Ralph M.: Programs on Alcoholism in the United States, 1952, in *Alcoholism, 1941–1951: A Survey of Activities in Research, Education and Therapy.* Edited by the Staff of the Yale Center of Alcohol Studies. New Haven, Quarterly Journal of Studies on Alcoholism, 1952.

14. Mann, Marty: *Primer on Alcoholism.* New York, Rinehart & Co., 1950.

5. The Mothers and Their Children

RATES of maternal, infant, and child mortality have long been considered critical barometers of a society's health practices and status, and thus organized services to mothers and children are seen as basic to health protection and the growth of a healthy citizenry. Early and comprehensive pre- and post-natal care, the prevention, detection, and treatment of birth injuries and anomalies, nutrition and health promotion through proper child-rearing are among the foremost concerns of Public Health programs.

Much current biologic research focusses upon factors influencing growth and developmental patterns. Significant correlations between the mother's health status and fetal and infant growth are emerging constantly. In the area of socio-psychologic development, patterns of mother-child and child-environment interaction have been long known to be of critical importance, but in recent years they have been made the object of vigorous comparative researches.

In the papers that follow, both a broad view of maternal and child health status in the United States, and some significant biologic and behavioral studies are presented.

Deaths around Birth—The National Score*

MARTHA M. ELIOT, M.D.

DEATH IS ASSOCIATED with birth and being born in the United States more often than it is with any disease except heart disease, cancer, and cerebral hemorrhage. These deaths are among the most tragic, since they cut off life at its beginning or take a mother away from

* Reprinted, with omission of tables and figures, by permission from the June 21, 1958 issue of the *Journal of the American Medical Association,* Volume 167, pages 945–949. This paper was presented at the 57th Annual Meeting of the Association for the Aid of Crippled Children, New York, New York, April 30, 1956. The author, now retired, was formerly Chief of the Children's Bureau, Social Security Administration, U.S. Department of Health, Education, and Welfare, and more recently, Professor and Head of the Department of Maternal and Child Health, Harvard University School of Public Health, Boston, Massachusetts. Marian M. Crane, M.D., and Eleanor P. Hunt, Ph.D., of the Division of Research of the Children's Bureau, participated in the development of this report.

her family. In 1955, deaths in childbearing and being born numbered an estimated 165,376, of which 1,901 were maternal deaths, about 86,124 were deaths of infants before or during birth (if we take account of underreporting of such deaths), and 77,351 were deaths of liveborn infants in the neonatal period.[1]

Mortality, we know, is not the whole toll from sickness and misadventure in childbearing and being born. The aftermath for the mother may be chronic illness or repeated reproductive failure; for the infant, it may be irreparable damage, such as we see in children who suffer from cerebral palsy, epilepsy, mental retardation, and congenital malformations. In the United States today, mortality of the infant in the perinatal period, that is, in the period before, during, and soon after birth, is of vital concern to all who seek to conserve new life or who see in these fatalities a threat to continuing health in mothers and children.

Because there is much concern today with problems of maternal morbidity which result in premature delivery and with the causes of fetal and neonatal deaths, particularly those associated with congenital malformation, primary attention is given in this report to the whole perinatal period continuing to the end of the first month of postnatal life. The term perinatal mortality, as used here, embraces deaths of infants before or during birth (fetal death) in pregnancies of 20 weeks' duration or more and deaths of liveborn infants in the neonatal period (under 28 days), regardless of duration of the mother's pregnancy. This perinatal mortality rate is the number of such fetal and neonatal deaths per 1,000 births of live or stillborn infants. This rate is useful, since it helps us to view, as a whole, infant losses among mothers whose pregnancies are relatively advanced. Within this span, different intervals may be focused on separately, depending on the problem under study.

Perhaps at this point we should look back to see how far we have come in safeguarding mothers and babies during the maternity cycle and the first year of the infant's life. One of the reasons for the establishment of the Children's Bureau in 1912 was a nationwide concern about the deaths of infants and women during pregnancy and childbirth. At that time, the national score on infant and maternal mortality was not known. It was for this reason that one of the first activities of the young Children's Bureau was to work with the Bureau of the Census and the General Federation of Women's Clubs in establishing the birth registration area.

The first score was obtained in 1915. Although based on data from only a few States, it showed clearly that far too many mothers and babies were dying. For every 1,000 live births, six mothers died, and 100 infants, one out of 10, did not live to see their first birthday.

As we compare today's scores with those of 1915, we can feel considerable satisfaction in the accomplishments of the last four decades. Instead of six maternal deaths in 1,000 live births, now there are nearer five in 10,000. The infant mortality rate has dropped from 100 to 26 per 1,000. Seen in retrospect, the national score in 1955 looks extremely good.

Improved sanitation and standards of living, better nutrition, important discoveries in medicine, more and better hospital care and other health services—all these have contributed to this great saving of life. But, unfortunately, these benefits have not extended equally to all parts of the United States or to all groups of the population.

In many localities in the United States, progress in reducing infant and maternal mortality lags behind that for the country as a whole. For example, in isolated counties with no cities of 50,000 or more, the average annual infant mortality rate in the period 1951–1954 was 17 per cent higher than that in counties with such cities.

Most of the reduction in the national infant mortality score has been due to a decrease in deaths after the first month of life. These have dropped from about 56 per 1,000 live births in 1915 to just over seven in 1955. This saving of life has come about largely through the prevention and control of infectious and gastrointestinal disease.

But the death rate in the first month of life has dropped much more slowly. As we look at the principal causes of death in the neonatal period, we find that infectious and gastrointestinal disturbances are not important in the picture. The five main causes to which deaths in the first and later weeks of the neonatal period were attributed are prematurity, postnatal asphyxia and atelectasis, birth injuries, congenital malformations, and hemolytic disease of the newborn, which results chiefly from Rh incompatibility.

The mortality rates for these five causes were 5.2, 4.3, 2.9, 2.5, and 0.6 per 1,000 live births. The conditions responsible for these early infant deaths nearly all have their origin before or during birth and are, for the most part, associated with morbidity in the mother.

At least three out of five neonatal deaths are in infants whose mothers' pregnancies do not run to normal term. Although premature delivery is not usually thought of as evidence of maternal morbidity, surely some abnormality causes a mother to give birth before term. Premature delivery increases the risk of death in the newborn infant 20 times.[2]

The trend lines of the perinatal death rate and death rate for infants surviving the first month of life from 1942 to 1955, show that while the postneonatal mortality rate was cut in half, the perinatal mortality rate was reduced less than one-third. The perinatal death rate is now five times that of infants after the first month of life.

An indication of the national importance of present perinatal and maternal losses is seen in the fact that the frequency of such deaths is fourth among main causes at all ages in 1955 in the United States.

More and more evidence is accumulating that the same conditions that bring death to infants before, during, and soon after birth also may lead to chronic illness and handicap in many infants who survive. We do not know accurately how many children may suffer such results. But, from the limited information, a rough estimation is that probably 315,000 children have cerebral palsy,[3] 310,000 epilepsy, and 1,500,000 mental retardation. Something like 285,000 infants with congenital malformations are born each year (these estimations were made by the Children's Bureau to take into account underreporting).

More research is needed to discover how such chronic illness and handicap are related to the 350,000 premature deliveries that occur to mothers of liveborn infants each year, to other complications of pregnancy, labor, and delivery, or to the diseases and defects that each year take an estimated 163,475 infant lives in the perinatal period.

The greatest hazards to the baby occur just before birth and during his first three days of life. Since most of the babies who die soon after birth are born prematurely, our best chance to reduce deaths in these first few days lies in finding effective ways of insuring that the mother can carry her baby to term.

While fatal risks in the first three days of life have been cut little since 1942 (17 per cent), the neonatal death rate for infants surviving these days has been reduced 46 per cent since 1942. No doubt this reflects, at least in part, improvement in the care of newborn infants, especially in the care of premature infants.

In recent years, more than half of the states and territories made some special effort in behalf of premature infants through their maternal and child health programs. Twenty-one were either supporting special services for premature infants or otherwise contributing to development of good hospital care for these infants. While much has been and is being done to improve care of such immature infants, much more remains to be done.

Since 1942, the fetal death rate in the latter half of pregnancy has been reduced by nearly a third, from 25.0 to 16.8 per 1,000 births, live and still. Presumably, this is the result of better prenatal and obstetric care of mothers. Mothers have a better chance today of giving birth to a living child than they had a decade ago. Some infants who formerly would have died in utero or during labor are born alive. Many of them survive, though some are too feeble for independent existence and die within a few days.

In regard to the volume of perinatal loss recorded in 1955 in the United States, in relation to age at neonatal death and duration of pregnancy in which fetal death occurred, over half the neonatal deaths (52 per cent) were on the first day of life; 89 per cent occurred in the first week, 6 per cent in the second, 3 per cent in the third, and the remaining 2 per cent in the last week of the neonatal period. Of the 69,153 fetal deaths recorded in 1955 in pregnancies of 20 or more week, 32 per cent were in those reported as enduring 40 or more weeks.

RESEARCH

How can we attack the problem of carrying infants safely through the perinatal period? Research is one answer. Not only do we need research to discover how various handicapping conditions of childhood are related to maternal and perinatal illness and defect but we also need knowledge of the whole chain of events underlying these conditions.

Understanding the reproductive process calls for many different approaches. One approach, animal research, is producing important clues as to possible causes of congenital defects. We need many more such studies, together with studies showing the application of these findings to human beings.

Another approach lies in clinical and pathologic studies of untoward conditions during pregnancy and follow-up studies of surviving infants. For example, what are the causal factors in bleeding in early pregnancy, and how does this affect the fetus? Or, what are the significant events associated with premature labor? True, we know some of them, but, for the majority, we can only guess. In a study at Johns Hopkins University of premature deliveries, no explanation could be found in 60 per cent of the cases.[4]

The clinical and Public Health approaches to these problems can be combined in forward-looking studies of successive pregnancies from the beginning of each pregnancy through delivery with long-term and regular follow-up of the mother and her children. This is one way physicians can learn more about the immediate and long-run bearing of specific events in early pregnancy on the health of the mother and the development of her child. Studies of this sort are now being initiated in a number of clinics.

Obviously, research on reproduction calls for the knowledge and skills of many scientific disciplines: obstetrics, pediatrics, pathology, chemistry, physiology, embryology, genetics, biostatistics, Public Health administration, and others.

Many investigators believe that, although each of these specialties has its own approach to these studies, all specialists can work more fruitfully if their efforts are coordinated. This does not necessarily mean coordination through formal plans and agreements, but, the kind of coordination that occurs from exchange of ideas and from joint thinking about the problem when different approaches intersect or overlap.

Of some things we are certain. We know that good care for infants born prematurely saves many who would not survive otherwise. Services to provide such care should be available wherever infants are born.

We recognize the need for more extensive and more effective maternal and child health services, especially in rural areas and for the less fortunate socioeconomic groups. But just what is meant by more effective services? For one thing, a program that accepts prenatal care as one of its major functions is necessary. An analysis of the way Public Health nurses use their time shows that 40 per cent of it is devoted to maternal and child health, but, of this, only 10 per cent—4 per cent of the total time—is given to prenatal care.

More attention needs to be given to finding those expectant mothers who are less likely to seek care for themselves and who more often need intensive service. And we can give thought and study to how the nursing visit can be most meaningful.

Continuity in care throughout pregnancy and labor and the postpartum and interpregnancy periods is essential to the best maternity care. Commonly, continuity in medical care for the pregnant woman is provided by physicians in their private practice. The support and supervision thus given may be even greater if the plan of care provides also for visits to the family by a Public Health nurse. Often, however, when a mother seeks maternity care in a hospital or other clinic this continuity of medical care does not exist. She may be seen by more than one physician during a single pregnancy and be delivered by still another. Between pregnancies she may not be seen at all by either physician or nurse. Much attention needs to be given to this aspect of maternity care if premature delivery and perinatal mortality are to be reduced.

Studies of obstetric case histories usually reveal a certain proportion of women who have had repeated unsuccessful pregnancies. For a physician to dismiss such a woman after her postpartum examination may mean he is dismissing her at a time that she most needs study and treatment. By the time her next pregnancy is confirmed, it may be too late to do anything about helping her carry her baby to term.

In cases where a woman has had one or more unsuccessful pregnancies, careful diagnostic study of both husband and wife are indicated, with treatment as necessary, before another pregnancy occurs. The treatment may be psychologic, nutritional, or physical, with endocrine therapy when needed. Such study and treatment are best carried out by a team—physicians, nurses, social workers, nutritionists, and psychologists—each member contributing an important share.

An aspect of prenatal care too often neglected is the provision of hospital care when complications of pregnancy occur. Where good hospital care is available, a woman with toxemia or threatened abortion can often be carried through until the infant becomes mature enough to have a good chance for survival. Or, if toxemia in later pregnancy is too severe, the premature induction of labor may prevent a fetal death, possibly even a maternal death.

A few State health departments now make funds available for hospitalization of women with complications of pregnancy. These funds can be used more effectively in a program which has a carefully developed referral system and nursing follow-up.

For another thing, we need services directed especially to the socioeconomic groups that are most vulnerable. In Denver, a study of the women admitted to the hospital because of complications of pregnancy showed that a large proportion came from an area of low socioeconomic development in which the general health level was low. At the University of Aberdeen, Scotland, where nearly all of the women received the same maternity care, premature birth and perinatal death were found more often in infants of mothers from the lower socioeconomic groups than they were in those of upper social groups.[5]

In the United States, we have evidence that perinatal mortality is affected by the socioeconomic status of the mother. Perinatal losses are higher for the nonwhite population than for the white; the fetal death rate is 85 per cent higher among nonwhite mothers than among white, and the perinatal rate more than 67 per cent higher than for white. While some of these differences reflect the younger age and larger families of nonwhite mothers, undoubtedly they also represent differences in economic status and deficiencies in early and present environment. Similarly, in the careful study on incidence of congenital malformations reported from Babies Hospital and Sloan Hospital for Women in New York City, a significantly higher incidence was found among nonwhite as compared with white infants.[6]

SUMMARY

Today, the greatest loss of infant life occurs around the time of birth. Much of this fatality could be prevented if present knowledge were more widely and intensively applied. Medical, nursing, and hospital services should be more readily available ouside of cities. Too few good hospital services exist for premature infants. Maternity services should seek out and give special attention to the woman who has already had an unsuccessful pregnancy when, or even before, she becomes pregnant again. Early environment may affect a woman's ability to bear children successfully. Consequently, we must concern ourselves with the nutrition and health of all of the family if little girls growing up today are to bear healthy babies tomorrow.

1. *Vital Statistics of United States, 1955*, vol. 1, National Office of Vital Statistics, U.S. Department of Health, Education, and Welfare, U.S. Public Health Service, 1957. Baumgartner, L.; Wallace, H. M.; Landsberg, E.; and Pessin, V.: Inadequacy of Routine Reporting of Fetal Deaths: As Evidenced by Comparison of Such Reporting with Maternity Cases Paid for Under Emergency Maternity and Infant Care (EMIC) Program, *Am. J. Pub. Health* 39:1459–1552 (Dec.) 1949.

2. *Selected Studies: Weight at Birth and Its Effect on Survival of Newborn in United States, Early 1950*,

vol. 39, no. 1, National Office of Vital Statistics, U.S. Department of Health, Education, and Welfare, U.S. Public Health Service, July 23, 1954.

3. Altman, I.: On Prevalence of Cerebral Palsy, *Cerebral Palsy Rev.* 16:4, 25 (July–Aug.) 1955.

4. Eastman, N.J.: Prematurity from Viewpoint of Obstetrician, *Am. Pract.* 1:343–352 (March) 1947.

5. Baird, D.: Preventive Medicine in Obstetrics, *New England J. Med.* 246:561–568 (April 10) 1952.

6. McIntosh, R., and others: Incidence of Congenital Malformations: Study of 5,964 Pregnancies, *Pediatrics* 14:505–521 (Nov.) 1954.

Epidemiologic Investigations of Some Prenatal Factors in the Production of Neuropsychiatric Disorder*

BENJAMIN PASAMANICK, M.D.

IN THE NATURALISTIC TYPE of epidemiologic investigation, an attempt is made to isolate the independent variable in the experimental population by selecting a control population similar in all conceivable aspects except for the variable under scrutiny, and then determine how the populations differ in the dependent variables. This is in contrast to the experimental type of study in which both experimental and control samples are drawn from the same population and the independent variable is intentionally altered. The latter type of study is invariably prospective, and it is much more likely to offer definitive conclusions. Unfortunately, the naturalistic study is frequently the only type of method available for research upon human populations, particularly in the chronic disorders. However, it is possible to strengthen the evidence for a chain of causality by forging one link

* Reprinted by permission from *Comparative Epidemiology of the Mental Disorders*, edited by Paul H. Hoch, M.D., and Joseph Zubin, Ph.D., (The Proceedings of the Forty-Ninth Annual Meeting of the American Psychopathological Association, held in New York City, February 1959), published by Grune & Stratton, Inc., 1961, Chapter 14, pp. 260–275. The author is Professor of Psychiatry, Ohio State University College of Medicine, and Director of Research, Columbus Psychiatric Institute and Hospital, Columbus, Ohio.

to another, and interweaving additional factors to the point where the total mass of evidence is so weighty and strong that no other conclusion seems possible under the circumstances.

Offered for your consideration is a chain of studies, still incomplete, but which, even at this stage, would seem to warrant serious consideration as evidence of a potent precursor of neuropsychiatric disorder. The hypothesis basic to the series of studies to be described stems from a number of propositions which may be summarized as follows: Inasmuch as prematurity and complications of pregnancy are associated with fetal and neonatal death, usually on the basis of injury to the brain, there must remain a fraction so injured who do not die. Depending upon the degree and location of trauma they do go on to develop a series of disorders extending from cerebral palsy, epilepsy, and mental deficiency through all types of behavioral and learning disabilities which are a result of lesser degrees of damage sufficient to disorganize behavioral development and lower thresholds to stress. Further, these abnormalities of pregnancy are associated with certain life experiences, usually socioeconomically determined, with the consequence that they themselves and their resulting neuropsychiatric disorders find greater aggregation in the lower strata of our society.

Because of space limitations, methodologic considerations and detailed discussions of findings are impossible, so discussion will be limited to a description of our studies, as they presented themselves chronologically.

We first became interested in the influence of prenatal factors during the course of a longitudinal study of Negro child development in New Haven.[1] In a cohort of Negro infants born during one of the middle war years, it was found that adaptive behavioral development was proceeding at white rates according to the Gesell developmental techniques. Not only was this finding contrary to previous published studies, but, in addition, no explanation of this disparate finding could be found in environmental associations such as education or geographic origin of the parents, number of siblings, quality of housing, or skin color. It was not until the growth curves were examined that a hypothesis for the fact that these infants followed the white norms presented itself. Also contrary to previous findings, it was noted that from birth the subjects were progressing according to the best published white rates in both weight and height. On the basis of this, it was hypothesized that the mothers of these infants had received an apparently adequate prenatal diet because of war-time rationing and employment which bettered economic status. This hypothesis was supported by further examinations of these children which continued into the eighth year of life. The only significant associations that could be found were those with growth, that is, physical status at birth and after.[2] At 7 years of age, this group of Negro children had a mean intellectual functioning equal to that of the mean white scores as measured on the Stanford-Binet and Arthur Performance tests.[3]

It should be added parenthetically that in two areas of behavioral development, language and gross motor behavior, significant differences from white norms were noted. The lowered language scores at 2 years were shown to be due to impaired verbal responsiveness, possibly a result of inhibition caused by a white examiner, while verbal comprehension remained unimpaired.[4] During the course of another study, to be described later, we found that the seeming acceleration in gross motor behavior which had also been described by other investigators was not present. It was discovered that apparently both white and Negro infants at the midcentury have comparable motor behavior, significantly accelerated over the norms established a decade or two ago and possibly owing to differing child rearing methods. However, no definitive explanation is available at this time.

Following upon this investigation, we embarked upon a series of retrospective studies seemingly with a much different hypothesis in mind, except for the fact that prenatal variables were involved. However, the results of these studies indicate that maternal diet may be a common factor.

In this particular series of studies of seven neuropsychiatric disorders—cerebral palsy, epilepsy, mental deficiency, behavior disorders, reading disabilities, tics, and speech disorders—the prenatal experience of children presenting them was examined. A large population of children diagnosed as having the particular clinical entity under scrutiny was selected from the case files of hospital out-patient clinics, institutions, and public schools. The clinical data from the case histories were abstracted and coded for internal comparison studies. The birth certificate register maintained by the Bureau of Vital Statistics was then searched to locate children born in Baltimore. A series of control infants with whom the cases could be compared was also selected. In all but one of the studies, the control infant was the next infant of the same race, sex, and socioeconomic status in the birth certificate register to have survived the newborn period, who was born in the same hospital to a mother of the same age. In the behavior disorder study, the control was the next child, alphabetically, of the same sex in the same school class, automatically controlling for race, since this study was done in Baltimore prior to integration. In the process of obtaining the necessary data on these children, pertinent information was derived from the birth certificates regarding their parents and socioeconomic status variables. For those children born in hospitals, the hospital records were abstracted and data were gathered on such items as number of previous pregnancies, abortions, stillbirths, premature and neonatal deaths, length of labor, complications of delivery, birthweight, and neonatal course.

In retrospective studies of this type, direct comparisons of current behavior between cases and controls are not made. Frequently, as in these studies, no actual examination of patients is done, but information that has been recorded in the past is examined. By this method, associations between prior conditions and current clinical entities can be demonstrated. Differences between cases and controls are usually demonstrated on the basis of significant differences in the incidence of various prior conditions or abnormalities under consideration, and not in absolute terms of presence or absence of abnormality. Those cases selected as controls from the birth certificate files were not known to have any of the clinical neuropsychiatric entities under investigation. However, they might well have had some disease. If this were so, any difference in the histories between the cases and the controls would be more significant in the face of the possibility that the control patient group was contaminated by clinical cases. Furthermore, abnormalities of the prenatal and paranatal periods will undoubtedly be found in the mothers of the control patients as well as in the mothers of the cases. The point has been raised repeatedly that studies of this nature are inherently flawed by the poor quality and almost universal under-reporting of complications or abnormalities. Hospital records are undoubtedly imperfect. It must be recognized, however, that this fact presents a bias against the hypothesis being tested, since if the hypothesis has any validity, and the rate of under-reporting or omission of data is the same in test and control groups, the true differences would be much greater than were actually found. There is obviously no reason to believe that having or not having a neuropsychiatric disorder later in life would have led to selection for the recording of abnormalities of pregnancy. Thus it should be apparent that, while associations might be obscured or missed in this type of investigation, when they are found they are much more likely to be true relationships.

FINDINGS

Only the major findings in these studies and their implications will be presented and discussed.

Thus far, five clinical entities in children have been found to be significantly associated with complications of pregnancy and prematurity. These are cerebral palsy,[5] epilepsy,[6] mental deficiency,[7] behavior disorders,[8] and reading disabilities.[9] A sixth condition, tics,[10] was found to be significantly associated with complications of pregnancy but not of prematurity. The seventh entity, that of childhood speech disorder,[11] when dissociated from cerebral palsy or mental deficiency, was not found to be associated to any significant degree with abnormalities of pregnancy or with prematurity, although differences in the predicted direction as far as pregnancy abnormality was concerned were found.

Two general observations should be made. First, the incidence of abnormalities of pregnancy is much higher in the nonwhites than in the whites. This was true whether the patient was a control or a case. Second, the differences between the cases and the controls tend to be greater in the more severe clinical conditions, e.g., cerebral palsy, and to decrease as the handicap becomes milder in nature. It is also interesting to note that no difference was found between the cases and controls in the incidence of prolonged and difficult labor and of operative procedures at the time of delivery, such as mid or high forceps, Caesarian section, breech extraction, or internal version and extraction, the types of situation that have previously been hypothesized as responsible for birth trauma. Rather, the associations occurred with the prolonged and probably anoxia-producing complications of pregnancy such as the toxemias and bleeding.

As in most epidemiologic studies, there were a number of by-products which permitted us to examine other possible etiologic factors and to seek for the internal consistency so necessary to help support the major tests of the hypothesis.

In the investigation of epilepsy, we found that, although differences between cases and controls were in the expected direction among Negroes, they were not statistically significant. This was probably at least partially attributable to the fact that the rate of abnormality of pregnancy among Negro mothers and their offspring, both in cases and controls, was so high that a much larger number of cases than were available would have been necessary to obtain statistical significance. In addition to direct evidence from morbidity statistics that postnatal insult following such conditions as lead intoxication, head injury, and infection is probably more common among Negroes than among whites, there is indirect evidence also for this in the findings of this study.[12] The younger a patient at the onset of convulsive seizures, the more likely is the condition to be due to brain damage sustained early in the development of the individual. In the white patients, there was a positive association between prenatal-paranatal complications and the onset of seizures in the first year of life. In the Negro epileptics, however, this relationship between age and onset of seizures and abnormalities of pregnancy was not observed.

Since we had data available on the occurrence of epilepsy in the families of our cases, we thought it might be fruitful to see what light might be cast on the genetic hypothesis. It is reasonable to assume that if prenatal and paranatal factors play a significant role in the causation of epilepsy, the cases in which these factors were absent should have more epileptic parents than those cases in which these factors were present. This was not found to be true, and makes it necessary to re-examine the genetic hypothesis in epilepsy. May not the familial aggregation of epilepsy be a reflection of the occurrence of familial aggregation of the prenatal and paranatal factors under discussion in this report? Prematurity, stillbirth, and neonatal deaths have been so described, and the socio-economic factors with which these and other abnormalities are associated is, of course, usually a life-long experience to which these mothers are subjected.

Similar to the situation in epilepsy, it was found in the study of mental deficiency that, although there was significantly more prematurity among the retarded Negro children, there was no significant difference between cases and controls as far as complications of pregnancy were concerned. When the relationship of these abnormal maternal and fetal factors was studied according to the degree of mental deficiency, however, a most revealing association was discovered.[13] In those Negro children with I.Q.'s under 50, almost every child had been exposed to one or more abnormalities of pregnancy. In those above I.Q. 50, no important difference existed between cases and controls. This is in contrast to the white cases where differences existed at all levels of deficiency. The most likely explanation for these results is probably the widespread socio-cultural retardation in the Negro children. The organically retarded Negro group with I.Q.'s in the upper ranges from 50 to 80 must have been diluted by including in it children who had no real brain disease but who merely reflected their cultural heritage. We also found that the very young mothers and the older women had a significantly higher risk of producing mentally defective children. Increasing birth order also increased the risk of developing mental deficiency.

Among the behavior disorders investigated, the highest association with the complications of the prenatal and paranatal periods was found in those children called hyperactive, confused, and disorganized in both racial groups.[14] These accounted for 40 per cent of the referrals to the Baltimore Division of Special Services of the Department of Education, to which 4 per cent of the school population is referred. When this diagnostic category of hyperactivity, confusion, and disorganization was removed from the white cases, there were no longer any significant differences between the cases and controls: In the Negroes, however, differences were still present for the remainder of the cases, even after this diagnostic category was removed. It may be that in the nonwhites cerebral injury is so pervasive that it infiltrates all of the types of behavior disorder.

SOCIO-ECONOMIC FACTORS

It was possible to examine a number of socio-economic and familial variables in a sample of the behavior disorder group, and compare them to controls from the same geographic area. Items previously incriminated by other writers, such as family composition, parental age and education, employment, and housing were not found to be different among the cases and controls.[15]

The reading disorder investigation was confined to white children, since the Negro children in the school system, with reading disorders, would have been heavily contaminated with socio-cultural causation.[16] As a test of internal consistency, we looked at association with degree of reading disability. It was found that the greater the disability, the more abnormalities of pregnancy in the background.

In the study of speech disorders, during which no significant association was found with complications of pregnancy, we encountered a finding which helped confirm previous impressions. Contrary to our expectation, there was no greater incidence of speech disorders among males, which was in marked contrast to the other neuropsychiatric disorders studied. This sex ratio may be one further lead to the etiology of brain injury as a precursor of these disorders. We also found a significantly higher proportion of multiple pregnancies among the speech disorder cases as well as an increased risk in the higher birth orders, both explainable on psychologic grounds.

It has been known for some time that the neuropsychiatric disorders thus far discussed are much more common among the lower socio-economic strata of our population, including Negroes and other minority groups with similar socio-economic disadvantages.[17] In addition, it was suspected that there is evidence of important socio-economic distinctions in terms of the complications associated with the neuropsychiatric disorders. Of particular interest to us was prematurity and the complications of the prenatal and the paranatal periods.

By studying the distribution of prematurity in Baltimore according to socio-economic status as defined by census tract, a significant negative correlation with socio-economic status in the white groups was demonstrated.[18] The incidence was 5 per cent in the highest economic tenth compared to 7.6 per cent in the lowest. In the non-whites, it was 11.4 per cent. Similarly, because of the inordinately high rates of complications of pregnancy and delivery noted in the Negro control population as compared to the whites—of the order of 2 to 1—it was felt that an examination of the relationship of the socio-economic status to these complications in the white population might give some possible leads to etiology. Since census tract data are rather crude, only the lower and upper economic fifth were compared in order to be as certain as possible about socio-economic differences. The findings were striking.[19] The incidence of complications of the prenatal and paranatal periods in the white upper economic fifth was 5 per cent and in the white lower fifth 14.6 per cent. In the nonwhites, it was 50.6 per cent. This is a ratio of 1 to 3 to 10.

These high rates of prematurity and complications of pregnancy among Negroes over even the lowest white socio-economic group are so marked that some workers in this field maintain that they must be attributable to some innate racial characteristic. Since Negro socio-economic status is lower than that in the lowest white groups, it seems much more parsimonious, scientifically, to eliminate the postulated racial factor, and to hypothesize that prematurity and pregnancy complication rates increase exponentially below certain socio-economic thresholds.

PROSPECTIVE STUDIES

Thus far, except for the longitudinal study of Negro child development, we have been discussing a series of retrospective investigations of associations. These are subject to the possibility that the dependent variable studies might have helped produce the independent variable through some other means than the one hypothesized. A somewhat better test of the hypothesis is possible through the prospective investigation in which the dependent variable of the retrospective studies becomes the independent variable and the independent, in turn, the dependent variable examined repeatedly through time. Some seven years ago we entered upon such a study, in which the independent variable was prematurity and during which a socio-economically stratified sample of 500 prematurely born children, delivered in one year in Baltimore, and their full-termed matched controls were followed from birth. Again, as previously, a detailed description of the study design and analysis has already been published and need not be described here.[20] Some of the pertinent findings of the Gesell Developmental Examination at 40 weeks of age, however, are germane to our present discussion. When adjustments were made for differences between the whites and nonwhites in the distribution of the birth weights, no significant differences were found between the races in the incidence of neurologic and intellectual defect.[21] Intellectual potential as in our New Haven study was essentially the same. However, as was predicted by our hypothesis, the incidence of abnormality increased as the birth weight decreased. The frequency of serious neurologic abnormality was significantly higher in the prematures as compared to the controls, and there was a high negative correlation of intellectual potential with degree of prematurity. Of the infants with birth weights under 1500 gm., 44 per cent at 40 weeks of age had an abnormal condition of sufficient magnitude to cause serious concern about the prognosis for future development. The comparable incidence for the rest of the premature group was 8.6 per cent, and for the full-term infants, 2.6 per cent.

In addition, significantly more of the prematures exhibited the syndrome of "minimal damage." This syndrome describes a group of children who in infancy show distinct and definite deviations in neurologic patterning, but in whom clinical experience indicated complete compensation for the neurologic abnormalities would occur with maturation. These children, found among both prematures (16.3 per cent) and controls (10 per cent), are the ones who would, according to the hypothesis, exhibit at a later date the integrational defects seen in behavior and learning disorders. We have recently had occasion to do an item analysis of the 46 individual neurologic patterns investigated in our study of prematures, which has given us a clinical picture of what may be a fairly specific entity and which is now being tested by further studies.[22]

At 40 weeks of age, the general developmental quotient was 105.4 and 104.5 for the white and nonwhite controls, respectively. It is noteworthy that the distribution of the general developmental quotients was not affected by differences in the education of the parents, by economic status, or by race. When the first 300 of the approximately 1,000 children involved in the Baltimore Study were re-examined, at approximately 3 years of age, distinct racial differences were observed. The mean developmental quotient for the white controls rose significantly to 111.2 while it fell to 98.9 for the nonwhites. This indicated the need for a special analysis of the data to see whether this change could be explained.

One method of evaluating this change with age between the two racial groups was to compare the distribution of the intellectual potential of the infant population with the distribution of intelligence tests as found in school-age children.[23] The distribution of general developmental quotients representative of the infant population of Baltimore was evolved by adjusting for differences in birth weight, race and economic status in the infant sample. The resultant distribution showed that approximately 90 per cent of the infant population had developmental quotients between 90 and 120. When the distribution thus derived was compared with that found on the Stanford-Binet testing in the literature, there was evidence of a widening band in the older age group. Two points about this widening are important. First, relatively little increase occurred at the upper range of the intelligence quotient scale in contrast to marked increase in the percentage of older children who had I.Q.'s less than 85. In addition, in the infant group, there was a sharp, abrupt rise at a level of 80 or 85, while in the older group this curve was relatively smooth and the increase starts at a lower level in the 50 to 55 I.Q. range. The increase in the percentage of school-age children with intelligence quotients below 85 occurred largely in the group between 50 and 70, who are frequently considered retarded on a genetic basis, but increases also occurred in the group with I.Q.'s between 70 and 85, those ordinarily felt to be part of the normal human variation but who occupy their position in the curve on the basis of inferior hereditary endowment.

Another method of evaluating the increase of number of children with I.Q.'s below 80 was by means of an analysis of the individual infants in the Baltimore group who had developmental quotients below 80. Almost all of these infants were organically impaired either neurologically or physically. They also had a history of a significantly higher proportion of the chronic complications of pregnancy and a markedly higher percentage of birth weights less than 1500 gm. compared to the remainder of the infants. In contrast, as already stated, older children are called in a high percentage of cases "familial morons" because of the absence of any objective neurologic findings as well as the result of the fact that other members of the family are also considered intellectually dull because of their inferior socioeconomic status. These findings tend to confirm those of our retrospective study of mental defectives, and our impression that measures of intelligence used in later life are greatly influenced by learning and affected by life experiences, which tend to limit opportunities for acquiring the kinds of information that the tests seek to evaluate. They even raise the question as to whether the distribution of intelligence really follows the normal curve that has been found for biologic characteristics. While the evidence is obviously far from complete, it tends to support the view that the range of normal human intellectual potential is much narrower than has been thought. Except for a few hereditary clinical deficiencies and for exogenous injury to neural integration, behavioral variation does not seem to be the result of genetically determined structural origin. We believe that it is now possible to entertain a new *tabula rasa* theory which hypothecates that at conception individuals are much alike in intellectual endowment except for a few rare hereditary neurologic defects. It appears to be life experience and the socio-cultural milieu influencing biologic and physiologic function which, in the absence of organic brain damage, makes human beings significantly different behaviorally from each other.

SEASONAL VARIATIONS

I would like now to turn to a fourth group of studies which apparently add to the chain of evidence, and at the same time strengthen the links already available. This last group revolves largely about the effect of summer heat on conception and the fetus. It has been known for some time that there existed a greater risk of developing mental deficiency in children born in the winter months. A number of hypotheses were advanced by way of explanation. However, with the feeling that whatever damage was incurred in most cases of mental deficiency occurred during the third fetal month, since molecular differentiation was at its height during this period, we examined the month of birth of all the children admitted to the Columbus State School from 1913 to 1949. We also found a significant peak in the births of mental defectives in the first three months of the year corresponding to a summer occurrence of the third month of pregnancy.[24] We hypothesized that this was associated with summer heat which, either by reducing maternal protein intake or by direct stress effect through the hypothalamico-pituitary-adrenal cortical axis, produced fetal damage. If this were the case, hotter summers should produce more mental defectives than would cooler summers. This was precisely what was discovered. Indeed, cooler summers were not associated with an increased risk of mental defect at all.

In our previous studies, we had found that complications of pregnancy were associated with mental deficiency, that season of birth apparently was associated with the same condition, that maternal diet also seemed to play a role in infant development, and in turn was associated with socio-economic status. There existed the possibility, then, that complications of pregnancy also varied seasonally. By examining a systematic sample of New York City birth certificates, we found that there was indeed a statistically significant higher rate of complications of pregnancy in the mothers who delivered in the winter months. Interestingly enough, they were precisely the same complications we had previously found to be associated with brain damage, that is, toxemias and bleeding.[25] The other complications on the whole did not even approach significance.

Because of the relationship of low socio-economic status to both mental deficiency and complications of pregnancy, there existed the possibility that we were dealing primarily with an increased rate of lower socio-economic births in the same winter months. We were able to test this by examining the variation in birth rates for a five-year period in Baltimore, using census tract of residence as the criterion of socio-economic status, and were able to rule this out.[26] As a matter of fact, the lower socio-economic strata, both white and Negro, had fewer deliveries in the winter months. There was marked variation in the seasonal birth rates by socio-economic status, with a large dip coinciding with summer conceptions for the lower socio-economic strata, and little or no variation throughout the year for the upper economic group. A variety of socio-economically determined factors may be operating to create these disparities, including the ability of the higher status groups to significantly modify the effects of climate. These may operate to a much stronger degree on the lower groups either by way of disinclination to coitus, heat amenorrhea, maternal dietary deficiency, or direct effect on the viability of sperm or fetus.

Having found this apparent association of birth rates with season of conception, it was thought that there might well exist a geographic difference as well, because of differences in summer climate. We therefore examined all the 1955 births in this country by month and our expectations were completely fulfilled.[27] The southern States show a marked decline in births during the spring months. The midwestern and northeastern States show only a slight trough in spring births. The northwestern States of Washington and Oregon exhibit no spring trough at all, and are indeed even slightly higher in spring births than expected. The data also indicate, but not at all conclusively, that male births are fewer just prior to and during the descending curve of the spring depression. You may recall that it has been demonstrated that males are apparently much more at risk of being brain injured pre-natally than females. We have also found that the peak neonatal death rate occurs in the spring, again coinciding with a summer conception.

Through the National Office of Vital Statistics, we were able to secure the seasonal distribution by birth weight for all the children born in the United States in one year. It was thought that if maternal diet would show any effect upon birth weight, it should appear in the children born during the summer, since it has been demonstrated repeatedly that dietary intake, particularly protein, decreases during summer weather and that the weight of the fetus is largely accumu-lated during the last trimester of pregnancy. Again, the predicted association was found. Children born in the summer time are signifi-cantly lighter in weight.[28] In another study in Baltimore, we had found previously that twin births are less frequent in the lower socio-economic white segments of the population.[29] If this could be due to the greater risks of abortion in multiple pregnancy, it was thought that this might also appear as a seasonal variation. Using the same Baltimore data, we did find the lowest rate of twinning in the first quarter of the year, and confined to the lower socio-economic strata. The peak rates of twinning occurred in the spring quarter, coinciding with summer conception, with the possibility that this might be due to the teratogenic effect of heat stress upon the embryo. I would like to remind you that multiple births are associated not only with a significantly higher incidence of prematurity, but also with a signifi-cantly higher infant mortality, and that twinning was much more common among our cases of neuropsychiatric disorder.

We are continuing our investigations of seasonal variation in mul-tiple births since the numbers in our Baltimore study are compara-tively small and require the confirmation of larger numbers. These, as well as other studies, are in progress. We are now analyzing data on the seasonal variation in the births of schizophrenics, since it had been previously demonstrated that they too have a peak rise in the winter months. Should association with higher summer temperature be found, it may well indicate that the lowered threshold to stress following brain injury may serve as an additional organic precursor to breakdown in the individual who, as Kallmann has shown, is already genetically predisposed.

It might be well to mention that we have embarked upon other investigations of the same variables. We are in the second year of a study similar to the premature study in design in which we are following prospectively a large group of infants born to mothers with toxemia, bleeding, and influenza during pregnancy. Another series of investigations deals experimentally in animals with the possible effects of a large number of variables upon the behavior of the resulting offspring. These will include all types of stresses, immunologic, physical (such as radiation and temperature), endocrinologic, and others, as well as deprivations of dietary constituents, oxygen, and so on.

On rereading this somewhat discursive discussion, I found it impossible to summarize adequately what has been essentially a series of summarizing abstracts, tied together by the thin thread of time and the common theme of prenatal experience. However, I would submit that the epidemiologic evidence offered for your consideration is sufficiently strong to indicate that there exists a continuum of reproductive insult, at least partially socio-economically determined, resulting in a continuum of reproductive casualty extending from death through varying degrees of neuropsychiatric disability. I would also submit that this evidence, which supports studies with similar findings and conclusions, is strong enough to warrant the institution of preventive programs in the prenatal period and perferably before conception. Hopefully, these would be established on a controlled experimental basis so that the hypotheses offered this afternoon could be tested definitively.

1. Pasamanick, B.: A comparative study of the behavioral development of Negro infants. *J.Genet.Psychol.* 59: 3–44, 1946.

2. Knobloch, H., and Pasamanick, B.: Further observations of the behavioral development of Negro infants. *J.Genet.Psychol.* 83:137–157, 1953.

3. Nash, E. H., Knobloch, H., and Pasamanich, B.: Unpublished data.

4. Pasamanick, B., and Knobloch, H.: Language development in Negro children and some implications for the testing of intelligence. *J.Abnorm. & Social Psychol.* 50:401–402, 1955.

5. Lilienfeld, A. M., and Pasamanick, B.: The association of prenatal and paranatal factors with the development of cerebral palsy and epilepsy. *Am.J.Obset.&Gynec.* 70:93–101, 1955.

6. ————: Association of maternal and fetal factors with the development of epilepsy, I: Abnormalities in the prenatal and paranatal periods. *J.A.M.A.* 159:155–160, 1955.

7. Pasamanick, B., and Lilienfeld, A. M.: Association of maternal and fetal factors with the development of mental deficiency, I: Abnormalities in the prenatal and paranatal periods. *J.A.M.A.* 159:155–160, 1955.

8. ————, Rogers, M. E., and Lilienfeld, A. M.: Pregnancy experience and the development of childhood behavior disorder. *Am.J.Psychiat.* 112:613–618, 1956.

9. Kawi, A., and Pasamanick, B.: The association of factors of pregnancy with development of reading disorders in childhood. *J.A.M.A.* 166: 1420–1423, 1958.

10. Pasamanick, B., and Kawi, A.: A study of the association of prenatal

and paranatal factors with the development of tics in children: A preliminary investigation. *J.Pediat.* 48:596–601, 1956.

11. ———, Constantinou, F. K., and Lilienfeld, A. M.: Pregnancy experience and the development of childhood speech disorders: An epidemiologic study of the association with maternal and fetal factors. *A.M. A.Am.J.Dis.Child.* 91:113–118, 1956.

12. ———, and Lilienfeld, A. M.: Maternal and fetal factors in the development of epilepsy, II: Relationship to some clinical factors of epilepsy. *Neurology* 5:77–83, 1955.

13. Lilienfeld, A. M., and Pasamanick, B.: The association of maternal and fetal factors with the development of mental deficiency, II: Relationship to maternal age, birth order, previous reproductive loss and degree of mental deficiency. *Am.J.Ment.Deficiency* 60:557–569, 1956.

14. Rogers, M. E., Lilienfeld, A. M., and Pasamanick, B.: *Prenatal and Paranatal Factors in the Development of Childhood Behavior Disorders.* Copenhagen, Denmark, E. Munksgaard, 1955.

15. Pasamanick, B.: The epidemiology of behavior disorders of childhood. In *Neurology and Psychiatry in Childhood* (Research Publications of the Association for Nervous and Mental Disease). Baltimore, Williams and Wilkins, 1956, chap. 16.

16. Kawi, A., and Pasamanick, B.: The Association of Factors of Pregnancy with the Development of Reading Disorders in Childhood (Monograph of the Society for Research in Child Development, 1959; and Pasamanick, B., and Knobloch, H., The contribution of some organic factors to school retardation in Negro Children. *J.Negro Educ.* 27:4–9, 1958.

17. Pasamanick, B., Knobloch, H.: Some early organic precursors of racial behavioral differences, *J.Nat. M.A.* 49:372–375, 1957.

18. Rider, R. V., Taback, M., and Knobloch, H.: Associations between premature birth and socioeconomic status. *Am.J.Pub.Health* 45:1022–1028, 1955.

19. Pasamanick, B., Knobloch, H., and Lilienfeld, A. M.: Socioeconomic status and some precursors of neuropsychiatric disorders. *Am.J.Orthopsychiat.* 26:594–601, 1956.

20. Knobloch, H., and Pasamanick, B.: A Development Questionnaire for Infants 40 Weeks of Age: An Evaluation (Monograph 61 of Society for Research in Child Development). Yellow Springs, Ohio, Antioch Press, 1956.

21. ———, Rider, R. V., Harper, P. A., and Pasamanick, B.: The neuropsychiatric sequelae of prematurity: A longitudinal study. *J.A.M.A.* 161:581–585, 1956.

22. ———, and Pasamanick, B.: The Syndrome of Minimal Damage. *J.A.M.A.* 170:1384–1387, 1959.

23. ———: Intellectual potential in an infant population. In Epidemiology of Mental Disorder (Symposium of the American Association for the Advancement of Science). Washington, D.C. (In press)

24. ———: Seasonal variation in the births of the mentally deficient. *Am.J.Pub.Health* 48:1201–1208, 1958.

25. Pasamanick, B., and Knobloch, H.: Seasonal variation in complications of pregnancy. *J.Obstet.& Gynec.* 12:110–112, 1958.

26. ———, Dinitz, S., and Knobloch, H.: Socio-economic and seasonal variation in birth rates. *Millbank Memorial Fund Quarterly* 38:248–254, 1960.

27. ———: Geographic and seasonal variation in birth rates. *Pub. Health Rep.* 74:285–288, 1959.

28. ———: Variation in Birth Weight by Season. (In manuscript)

29. Lilienfeld, A., and Pasamanick, B.: A study of variations in the frequency of twin births by race and socio-economic status. *J. Human Genet.* 7:401–402, 1955.

6.   Youth and the Community

GOALS of Public Health include not merely the elimination of disease but the maximizing of human functioning, social satisfactions, and feelings of usefulness of all the population. Paul Goodman, a poet, social critic, and psychotherapist, searchingly analyzes the factors underlying much "problem behavior" of young people today. Dr. Deschin's study demonstrates the value of using social science approaches in seeking new answers to traditional but persistent Public Health problems.

Growing Up Absurd—Jobs*

PAUL GOODMAN, PH.D.

I

IT'S HARD to grow up when there isn't enough man's work. There is "nearly full employment" (with highly significant exceptions), but there get to be fewer jobs that are necessary or unquestionably useful; that require energy and draw on some of one's best capacities; and that can be done keeping one's honor and dignity. In explaining the widespread troubles of adolescents and young men, this simple objective factor is not much mentioned. Let us here insist on it.

By "man's work" I mean a simple idea, so simple that it is clearer to ingenuous boys than to most adults. To produce necessary food and shelter is man's work. During most of economic history most men have done this drudging work, secure that it was justified and worthy of a man to do it, though often feeling that the social conditions under which they did it were *not* worthy of a man, thinking, "It's better to die than to live so hard"—but they worked on. When the environment is forbidding, as in the Swiss Alps or the Aran Islands, we regard such work with poetic awe. In emergencies it is heroic, as when the bakers of Paris maintained the supply of bread during the French Revolution, or the milkman did not miss a day's delivery when the bombs recently tore up London.

* © Copyright 1960 by Paul Goodman. Reprinted from *Growing Up Absurd—Problems of Youth in The Organized System*, by Paul Goodman, Chapter 1, pp. 17–35, by permission of Random House, Inc. The author is associated with the Institute for Gestalt Therapy in New York, N. Y., and Cleveland, Ohio, and is a writer of fiction and social commentary.

At present there is little such subsistence work. In *Communitas* my brother and I guess that one-tenth of our economy is devoted to it; it is more likely one-twentieth. Production of food is actively discouraged. Farmers are not wanted and the young men go elsewhere. (The farm population is now less than 15 per cent of the total population.) Building, on the contrary, is immensely needed. New York City needs 65,000 new units a year, and is getting, net, 16,000. One would think that ambitious boys would flock to this work. But here we find that building, too, is discouraged. In a great city, for the last 20 years hundreds of thousands have been ill housed, yet we do not see science, industry, and labor enthusiastically enlisted in finding the quick solution to a definite problem. The promoters are interested in long-term investments, the real estate men in speculation, the city planners in votes and graft. The building craftsmen cannily see to it that their own numbers remain few, their methods antiquated, and their rewards high. None of these people is much interested in providing shelter, and nobody is at all interested in providing new manly jobs.

Once we turn away from the absolutely necessary subsistence jobs, however, we find that an enormous proportion of our production is not even unquestionably useful. Everybody knows and also feels this, and there has recently been a flood of books about our surfeit of honey, our insolent chariots, the follies of exurban ranch houses, our hucksters, and our synthetic demand. Many acute things are said about this useless production and advertising, but not much about the workmen producing it and their frame of mind; and nothing at all, so far as I have noticed, about the plight of a young fellow looking for a manly occupation. The eloquent critics of the American way of life have themselves been so seduced by it that they think only in terms of selling commodities and point out that the goods are valueless; but they fail to see that people are being wasted and their skills insulted. (To give an analogy, in the many gleeful onslaughts on the Popular Culture that have appeared in recent years, there has been little thought of the plight of the honest artist cut off from his audience and sometimes, in public arts such as theater and architecture, from his medium.)

What is strange about it? American society has tried so hard and so ably to defend the practice and theory of production for profit and not primarily for use that now it has succeeded in making its jobs and products profitable and useless.

II

Consider a likely useful job. A youth who is alert and willing but not "verbally intelligent"—perhaps he has quit high school at the 11th grade (the median), as soon as he legally could—chooses for auto mechanic. That's a good job, familiar to him, he often watched them as a kid. It's careful and dirty at the same time. In a small garage it's sociable; one can talk to the customers (girls). You please people in trouble by fixing their cars, and a man is proud to see rolling out on its own the car that limped in behind the tow truck. The pay is as good as the next fellow's, who is respected.

So our young man takes this first-rate job. But what when he then learns that the cars have a built-in obsolescence, that the manufacturers do not want them to be repaired or repairable? They have lobbied a law that requires them to provide spare parts for only five years (it used to be 10). Repairing the new cars is often a matter of cosmetics, not mechanics; and the repairs are pointlessly expensive—a tail fin might cost $150. The insurance rates therefore double and treble on old and new cars both. Gone are the days of keeping the jalopies in good shape, the artist-work of a proud mechanic. But everybody is paying for foolishness, for in fact the new models are only trivially superior; the whole thing is a sell.

It is hard for the young man now to maintain his feelings of justification, sociability, serviceability. It is not surprising if he quickly becomes cynical and time-serving, interested in a fast buck. And so, on the notorious *Reader's Digest* test, the investigators (coming in with a disconnected coil wire) found that 63 per cent of mechanics charged for repairs they didn't make, and lucky if they didn't also take out the new fuel pump and replace it with a used one (65 per cent of radio repair shops, but *only* 49 per cent of watch repairmen "lied, overcharged, or gave false diagnoses").

There is an hypothesis that an important predisposition to juvenile delinquency is the combination of low verbal intelligence with high manual intelligence, delinquency giving a way of self-expression where other avenues are blocked by lack of schooling. A lad so endowed might well apply himself to the useful trade of mechanic.

III

Most manual jobs do not lend themselves so readily to knowing the facts and fraudulently taking advantage oneself. In factory jobs the workman is likely to be ignorant of what goes on, since he performs a small operation on a big machine that he does not understand. Even so, there is evidence that he has the same disbelief in the enterprise as a whole, with a resulting attitude of profound indifference.

Semiskilled factory operatives are the largest category of workmen. (I am leafing through the U.S. Department of Labor's *Occupational Outlook Handbook*, 1957.) Big companies have tried the devices of applied anthropology to enhance the loyalty of these men to the firm, but apparently the effort is hopeless, for it is found that a thumping majority of the men don't care about the job or the firm; they couldn't care less, and you can't make them care more. But this is *not* because of wages, hours, or working conditions, or management. On the contrary, tests that show the men's indifference to the company show also their (unaware) admiration for the way the company has designed and manages the plant; it is their very model of style, efficiency, and correct behavior. (Robert Dubin, for the U. S. Public Health Service.) Maybe if the men understood more, they would admire less. The union and the grievance committee take care of wages, hours, and conditions; these are the things the workmen themselves fought for and won. (Something was missing in that victory, and we have inherited the failure as well as the success.) The conclusion must be that workmen are indifferent to the job because of its intrinsic nature: it does not enlist worth-while capacities, it is not "interesting," it is not his, he is not "in" on it; the product is not really useful. And indeed, research directly on the subject, by Frederick Herzberg on Motivation to Work, shows that it is defects in the intrinsic aspects of the job that make workmen "unhappy." A survey of the literature (in Herzberg's *Job Attitudes*) shows that Interest is second in importance only to Security, whereas Wages, Conditions, Socializing, Hours, Ease, and Benefits are far less important. But foremen, significantly enough, think that the most important thing to the workman is his wages. (The investigators do not seem to inquire about the usefulness of the job— as if a primary purpose of *working* at a job were not that it is good *for* something! My guess is that a large factor in "Security" is the resigned reaction to not being able to take into account whether the work of one's hands is useful for anything; for in a normal life situation, if what we do is useful, we feel secure about being needed. The other largest factor in "Security" is, I think, the sense of being needed for one's unique contribution, and this is measured in these tests by the primary importance the workers assign to being "in" on things and to "work done being appreciated." (Table prepared by Labor Relations Institute of New York.)

Limited as they are, what a remarkable insight such studies give us, that men want to do valuable work and work that is somehow theirs! But they are thwarted.

Is not this the "waste of our human resources"?

The case is that by the "sole-prerogative" clause in union contracts the employer has the sole right to determine what is to be produced, how it is to be produced, what plants are to be built and where, what kinds of machinery are to be installed, when workers are to be hired and laid off, and how production operations are to be rationalized. (Frank Marquart.) There is *none* of this that is inevitable in running a machine economy; but *if* these are the circumstances, it is not surprising that the factory operatives' actual code has absolutely nothing to do with useful service or increasing production, but is notoriously devoted to "interpersonal relations"; (1) don't turn out too much work; (2) don't turn out too little work; (3) don't squeal on a fellow worker; (4) don't act like a big-shot. This is how to belong.

IV

Let us go on to the Occupational Outlook of those who are verbally bright. Among this group, simply because they cannot help asking more general questions—e.g., about utility—the problem of finding man's work is harder, and their disillusion is more poignant.

> *He explained to her why it was hard to find a satisfactory job of work to do. He had liked working with the power drill, testing the rocky envelope of the shore, but then the employers asked him to take a great oath of loyalty.*
> *"What!" cried Rosalind. "Do you have scruples about telling a convenient fib?"*
> *"No, I don't. But I felt uneasy about the sanity of the director asking me to swear to opinions on such complicated questions when my job was digging with a power drill. I can't work with a man who might suddenly have a wild fit."*
> *. . . "Why don't you get a job driving one of the big trucks along here?"*
> *"I don't like what's in the boxes," said Horatio sadly. "It could just as well drop in the river—and I'd make mistakes and drop it there."*
> *"Is it bad stuff?"*
> *"No, just useless. It takes the heart out of me to work at something useless and I begin to make mistakes. I don't mind putting profits in somebody's pocket—but the job also has to be useful for something."*
> *. . . "Why don't you go to the woods and be a lumberjack?"*
> *"No! they chop down the trees just to print off the New York Times!"*
>
> (*The Empire City*, III, i, 3.)

The more intelligent worker's "indifference" is likely to appear more nakedly as profound resignation, and his cynicism may sharpen to outright racketeering.

"Teaching," says the *Handbook*, "is the largest of the professions." So suppose our now verbally bright young man chooses for teacher, in the high school system or, by exception, in the elementary schools if he understands that the elementary grades are the vitally important ones and require the most ability to teach well (and of course they have less prestige). Teaching is necessary and useful work; it is real and creative, for it directly confronts an important subject matter, the children themselves; it is obviously self-justifying; and it is ennobled by the arts and sciences. Those who practice teaching do not for the most part succumb to cynicism or indifference—the children are too immediate and real for the teachers to become callous—but, most of the school systems being what they are, can teachers fail to come to suffer first despair and then deep resignation? Resignation occurs psychologically as follows: frustrated in essential action, they nevertheless cannot quit in anger, because the task is necessary; so the anger turns inward and is felt as resignation. (Naturally, the resigned teacher may then put on a happy face and keep busy.)

For the job is carried on under impossible conditions of overcrowding and saving public money. *Not* that there is not enough social wealth, but first things are not put first. Also, the school system has spurious aims. It soon becomes clear that the underlying aims are to relieve the home and keep the kids quiet; or, suddenly, the aim is to produce physicists. Timid supervisors, bigoted clerics, and ignorant school boards forbid real teaching. The emotional release and sexual expression of the children are taboo. A commercially debauched popular culture makes learning disesteemed. The academic curriculum is mangled by the demands of reactionaries, liberals, and demented warriors. Progressive methods are emasculated. Attention to each case is out of the question, and all the children—the bright, the average, and the dull—are systematically retarded one way or another, while the teacher's hands are tied. Naturally the pay is low—for the work is hard, useful, and of public concern, all three of which qualities tend to bring lower pay. It is alleged that the low pay is why there is a shortage of teachers and why the best do not choose the profession. My guess is that the best avoid it because of the certainty of miseducating. Nor are the best *wanted* by the system, for they are not safe. Bertrand Russell was rejected by New York's City College and would not have been accepted in a New York grade school.

V

Next, what happens to the verbally bright who have no zeal for a serviceable profession and who have no particular scientific or artistic bent? For the most part they make up the tribes of salesmanship, entertainment, business management, promotion, and advertising. Here of course there is no question of utility or honor to begin with, so an ingenuous boy will not look here for a manly career. Nevertheless, though we can pass by the sufferings of these well-paid callings, much publicized by their own writers, they are important to our theme because of the model they present to the growing boy.

Consider the men and women in TV advertisements, demonstrating the product and singing the jingle. They are clowns and mannequins, in grimace, speech, and action. And again, what I want to call attention to in this advertising is not the economic problem of synthetic demand, and not the cultural problem of Popular Culture, but the human problem that these are human beings worked as clowns; that the writers and designers of it are human beings thinking like idiots; and the broadcasters and underwriters know and abet what goes on—

> *Juicily glubbily*
> Blubber *is dubbily*
> *delicious and nutritious*
> *—eat it, Kitty, it's good.*

Alternately, they are liars, confidence men, smooth talkers, obsequious, insolent, etc., etc.

The popular-cultural content of the advertisements is somewhat neutralized by *Mad* magazine, the bible of the 12-year-olds who can read. But far more influential and hard to counteract is the *fact* that the workmen and the patrons of this enterprise are human beings. (Highly approved, too.) They are not good models for a boy looking for a manly job that is useful and necessary, requiring human energy and capacity, and that can be done with honor and dignity. They are a good sign that not many such jobs will be available.

The popular estimation is rather different. Consider the following: "As one possible aid, I suggested to the Senate subcommittee that they alert celebrities and leaders in the fields of sports, movies, theater and television to the help they can offer by getting close to these [delinquent] kids. By giving them positive 'heroes' they know and can talk to, instead of the misguided image of trouble-making buddies, they could aid greatly in guiding these normal aspirations for fame and status into wholesome progressive channels." (Jackie Robinson, who was formerly on the Connecticut Parole Board.) Or again: when a mass cross-section of Oklahoma high school juniors and seniors was asked which living person they would like to be, the boys named Pat Boone, Ricky Nelson, and President Eisenhower; the girls chose Debbie Reynolds, Elizabeth Taylor, and Natalie Wood.

The rigged Quiz shows, which created a scandal in 1959, were a remarkably pure distillate of our American cookery. We start with the brute facts that (a) in our abundant expanding economy it is necessary to give money away to increase spending, production, and profits; and (b) that this money must not be used for useful public goods in taxes, but must be plowed back as "business expenses," even though there is a shameful shortage of schools, housing, etc. Yet when the TV people at first tried simply to give the money away for nothing (for having heard of George Washington), there was a great Calvinistic outcry that this was demoralizing (we may gamble on the horses only to improve the breed). So they hit on the notion of a real contest with prizes. But then, of course, they could not resist making the show itself profitable, and competitive in the (also rigged) ratings with other shows, so the experts in the entertainment-commodity manufactured phony contests. And to cap the climax of fraudulence, the hero of the phony contests proceeded to persuade himself, so he says, that his behavior was educational!

The behavior of the networks was correspondingly typical. These business organizations claim the loyalty of their employees, but at the first breath of trouble they were ruthless and disloyal to their employees. (Even McCarthy was loyal to his gang.) They want to maximize profits and yet be absolutely safe from any risk. Consider their claim that they knew nothing about the fraud. But if they watched the shows that they were broadcasting, they could not *possibly*, as professionals, not have known the facts, for there were obvious type-casting, acting, plot, etc. If they are not professionals, they are incompetent. But if they don't watch what they broadcast, then they are utterly irresponsible, and on what grounds do they have the franchises to the channels? We may offer them the choice: that they are liars or incompetent or irresponsible.

The later direction of the investigation seems to me more important, the inquiry into the bribed disk-jockeying; for this deals directly with our crucial economic problem of synthesized demand, made taste, debauching the public, and preventing the emergence and formation of natural taste. In such circumstances there cannot possibly be an American culture; we are doomed to nausea and barbarism. And *then* these baboons have the effrontery to declare that they give the people what the people demand, and that they are not responsible for the level of the movies, the music, the plays, the books!

Finally, in leafing through the *Occupational Outlook Handbook*, we notice that the armed forces employ a large number. Here our young man can become involved in a world-wide demented enterprise, with personnel and activities corresponding.

VI

Thus, on the simple criteria of unquestioned utility, employing human capacities, and honor, there are not enough worthy jobs in our economy for average boys and adolescents to grow up toward. There are of course thousands of jobs that are worthy and self-justifying, and thousands that can be made so by stubborn integrity, especially if one can work as an independent. Extraordinary intelligence or special talent, also, can often carve out a place for itself—conversely, their usual corruption and waste are all the more sickening. But by and large our economic society is *not* geared for the cultivation of its young or the attainment of important goals that they can work toward.

This is evident from the usual kind of vocational guidance, which consists of measuring the boy and finding some place in the economy where he can be fitted; chopping him down to make him fit; or neglecting him if they can't find his slot. Personnel directors do not much try to scrutinize the economy in order to find some activity that is a real opportunity for the boy, and then to create an opportunity if they can't find one. To do this would be an horrendous task; I am not sure it could be done if we wanted to do it. But the question is whether anything less makes sense if we mean to speak seriously about the troubles of the young men.

Surely by now, however, many readers are objecting that this entire argument is pointless because people in *fact* don't think of their jobs in this way at all. *Nobody* asks if a job is useful or honorable (within the limits of business ethics). A man gets a job that pays well, or well enough, that has prestige, and good conditions, or at least tolerable conditions. I agree with these objections as to the fact. (I hope we are wrong.) But *the question is what it means to grow up into such a fact as: "During my productive years I will spend eight hours a day doing what is no good."*

VII

Yet, economically and vocationally, a large population of the young people are in a plight more drastic than anything so far mentioned. In our society as it is, there are not enough worthy jobs. But if our society, being as it is, were run more efficiently and soberly, for a majority there would soon not be any jobs at all. There is at present nearly full employment and there may be for some years, yet a vast number of young people are rationally unemployable, useless. This paradox is essential to explain their present temper.

Our society, which is not geared to the cultivation of its young, *is* geared to a profitable expanding production, a so-called high standard of living of mediocre value, and the maintenance of nearly full employment. Politically, the chief of these is full employment. In a crisis, when profitable production is temporarily curtailed, government spending increases and jobs are manufactured. In "normalcy"—a condition of slow boom—the easy credit, installment buying, and artificially induced demand for useless goods create jobs for all and good profits for some.

Now, back in the Thirties, when the New Deal attempted by hook or crook to put people back to work and give them money to revive the shattered economy, there was an outcry of moral indignation from the conservatives that many of the jobs were "boondoggling," useless made-work. It was insisted, and rightly, that such work was demoralizing to the workers themselves. It is a question of a word, but a candid critic might certainly say that many of the jobs in our present "normal" production are useless made-work. The tail fins and built-in obsolescence might be called boondoggling. The $64,000 Question and the busy hum of Madison Avenue might certainly be called boondoggling. Certain tax-dodge Foundations are boondoggling. What of business lunches and expense accounts? fringe benefits? the comic categories of occupations in the building trades? the extra stagehands and musicians of the theater crafts? These jolly devices to put money back to work no doubt have a demoralizing effect on somebody or other (certainly on me, they make me green with envy), but where is the moral indignation from Top Management?

Suppose we would cut out the boondoggling and gear our society to a more sensible abundance, with efficient production of quality goods, distribution in a natural market, counterinflation and sober credit. At once the work week would be cut to, say, 20 hours instead of 40. (Important People have already mentioned the figure 30.) Or alternately, half the labor force would be unemployed. Suppose too— and how can we not suppose it?—that the automatic machines are used generally, rather than just to get rid of badly organized unskilled labor. The unemployment will be still more drastic.

(To give the most striking example: in steel, the annual increase in productivity is 4 per cent, the plants work at 50 per cent of capacity, and the companies can break even and stop producing at *less than 30 per cent* of capacity. These are the conditions that forced the steel strike, as desperate self-protection. (Estes Kefauver, quoting Gardiner Means and Fred Gardner.)

Everybody knows this, nobody wants to talk about it much, for we don't know how to cope with it. The effect is that we are living a kind of lie. Long ago, labor leaders used to fight for the shorter work week, but now they don't, because they're pretty sure they don't want it. Indeed, when hours are reduced, the tendency is to get a second, part-time, job and raise the standard of living, *because* the job is meaningless and one must have something; but the standard of living is pretty meaningless, too. Nor is this strange atmosphere a new thing. For at least a generation the maximum sensible use of our productivity could have thrown a vast population out of work, or relieved everybody of a lot of useless work, depending on how you take it. (Consider with how little cutback of useful civilian production the economy produced the war goods and maintained an Army, economically unemployed.) The plain truth is that at present many of us are useless, not needed, rationally unemployable. It is in this paradoxical atmosphere that young persons grow up. It looks busy and expansive, but it is rationally at a stalemate.

VIII

These considerations apply to all ages and classes; but it is of course among poor youth (and the aged) that they show up first and worst. They are the most unemployable. For a long time our society has not been geared to the cultivation of the young. In our country 42 per cent have graduated from high school (predicted census, 1960); less than 8 per cent have graduated from college. The high school trend for at least the near future is not much different: there will be a high proportion of drop-outs before the 12th grade; but *markedly more* of the rest will go on to college; that is, the stratification will harden. Now the schooling in neither the high schools nor the colleges is much good—if it were better more kids would stick to it; yet at present, if we made a list we should find that a large proportion of the dwindling number of unquestionably useful or self-justifying jobs, in the humane professions and the arts and sciences, require education; and in the future, there is no doubt that the more educated will have the jobs, in running an efficient, highly technical economy and an administrative society placing a premium on verbal skills.

(Between 1947 and 1957, professional and technical workers increased 61 per cent, clerical workers 23 per cent, but factory operatives only 4½ per cent and laborers 4 per cent.—Census.)

For the uneducated there will be no jobs at all. This is humanly most unfortunate, for presumably those who have learned something in schools, and have the knack of surviving the boredom of those schools, could also make something of idleness; whereas the uneducated are useless at leisure too. It takes application, a fine sense of value, and a powerful community-spirit for a people to have serious leisure, and this has not been the genius of the Americans.

From this point of view we can sympathetically understand the pathos of our American school policy, which otherwise seems so inexplicable; at great expense compelling kids to go to school who do not want to and who will not profit by it. There are of course unpedagogic motives, like relieving the home, controlling delinquency, and keeping kids from competing for jobs. But there is also this desperately earnest pedagogic motive, of preparing the kids to take *some* part in a democratic society that does not need them. Otherwise, what will become of them, if they don't know anything?

Compulsory public education spread universally during the 19th century to provide the reading, writing, and arithmetic necessary to build a modern industrial economy. With the overmaturity of the economy, the teachers are struggling to preserve the elementary system when the economy no longer requires it and is stingy about paying for it. The demand is for scientists and technicians, the 15 per cent of the "academically talented." "For a vast majority [in the high schools]," says Dr. Conant in *The Child, the Parent, and the State,* "the vocational courses are the vital core of the program. They represent something related directly to the ambitions of the boys and girls." But somehow, far more than half of these quit. How is that?

IX

Let us sum up again. The majority of young people are faced with the following alternative: Either society is a benevolently frivolous racket in which they'll manage to boondoggle, though less profitably than the more privileged; or society is serious (and they hope still benevolent enough to support them), but they are useless and hopelessly out. Such thoughts do not encourage productive life. Naturally young people are more sanguine and look for man's work, but few find it. Some settle for a "good job;" most settle for a lousy job; a few, but an increasing number, don't settle.

I often ask, "What do you want to work at? If you have the chance. When you get out of school, college, the service, etc."

Some answer right off and tell their definite plans and projects, highly approved by Papa. I'm pleased for them, but it's a bit boring, because they are such squares.

Quite a few will, with prompting, come out with astounding stereotyped, conceited fantasies, such as becoming a movie actor when they are "discovered"—"like Marlon Brando, but in my own way."

Rarely somebody will, maybe defiantly and defensively, maybe diffidently but proudly, make you know that he knows well what he is going to do; it is something great; and he is indeed already doing it, which is the real test.

The usual answer, perhaps the normal answer, is "I don't know," meaning, "I'm looking; I haven't found the right thing; it's discouraging but not hopeless."

But the terrible answer is, "Nothing." The young man doesn't want to do anything.

—I remember talking to half a dozen young fellows at Van Wagner's Beach outside of Hamilton, Ontario; and all of them had this one thing to say: "Nothing." They didn't believe that what to work at was the kind of thing one *wanted*. They rather expected that two or three of them would work for the electric company in town, but they couldn't care less. I turned away from the conversation abruptly because of the uncontrollable burning tears in my eyes and constriction in my chest. Not feeling sorry for them, but tears of frank dismay for the waste of our humanity (they were nice kids). And it is out of that incident that many years later I am writing this book.

Teenagers and Venereal Disease*

CELIA S. DESCHIN, PH.D.

RECENT INCREASES in venereal disease among adolescents in the United States—a rise of 130 per cent in reported cases from 1956 to 1960—make it imperative to clarify our own as well as the young people's attitudes toward sex; to replace ignorance wtih knowledge, and community apathy with appropriate action; and to take a critical look at the laissez-faire attitude of some Public Health authorities toward physicians who do not report the venereal disease patients they treat in private practice. The history of medicine makes it clear that attitudes toward disease have constituted significant factors either in facilitating or impeding control. Therapy alone—even when effective —has not proved sufficient to control disease unless supplemented by education, and by appropriate changes in social institutions and in human behavior.[1]

With this in mind, the American Social Health Association in co-operation with the New York City Department of Health undertook a study of the attitudes of teenaged venereal disease patients for the Public Health Service, U.S. Department of Health, Education, and Welfare. Begun in September 1958, the study was completed in March 1961. It involved interviews with 600 teenagers attending the social hygiene clinics of New York City, and visits to the homes of 100 of them.

Although the study was designed to include the patients of private physicians as well as of clinics, too few of the former were referred to the study to make any comparisons possible. This was a reflection of physicians' traditional reluctance to report their patients—a major factor in hampering efforts toward eradication of the disease, and in preventing precise calculation of how many teenaged patients there may be in the nonclinic population.

Some preliminary field work indicated that venereal disease patients, including teenagers, were treated as if the disease existed apart from a human being. To be sure, the patients were urged to return should they become reinfected. However, a clinic policy of moral neutrality can be misinterpreted by the young patient as a quasi-acceptance of the sexual activity through which he has become infected.

At the time the study was initiated, little was known about the teenaged venereal disease patients in New York City. As director of the study, I was warned by both social hygiene clinic personnel and

* Reprinted with some minor additions, by permission, from *Children* (July-August 1962), Vol. 9, pp. 144–148, U. S. Department of Health, Education, and Welfare, Social Security Administration, Children's Bureau. The author is Associate Professor, School of Social Work, Adelphi College, Garden City, Long Island, New York.

social workers in community agencies dealing with problems of youth that such teenagers were "delinquents" from demoralized families with little potential for rehabilitation, and that they would certainly not talk to adults about their sexual behavior or related aspects of their lives. It was suggested that young interviewers be engaged, and some form of payment be provided to the interviewees.

Not entirely convinced, I did some exploratory interviewing in one of the city's social hygiene clinics in a district health center where the physician in charge did not share these stereotyped views. From the beginning, the response of the teenagers was friendly, interested, and cooperative, despite some initial resentment at having to prolong a visit to the clinic that sometimes took up to three hours, because of the un-avoidable delays common to busy, walk-in clinics. Similar cooperation was subsequently met by the study interviewers—all of them adults who were trained and experienced social workers. In order to obtain 600 voluntary interviews, we had to approach 610 teenagers. Only three of the 10 refused outright to be interviewed; five were persuaded by persons close to them not to participate in the study; and two with-drew. Word soon got around that the study was a "Junior Kinsey," and that the interviewers were "OK." No one was paid, and the teen-agers were told that any results could not come soon enough to be of direct benefit to them. Where problems were revealed with which they or their families needed help, referrals were made through the charge nurse to appropriate agencies. The young people seemed eager to make a contribution to the study.

THE INTERVIEWS

In each interview, the objectives of the study were out-lined briefly and simply, and the importance of accuracy was stressed. The young people were given an opportunity to withdraw at any point if reluctance or serious inconsistencies were noted. The interview schedule, which was evolved during the exploratory interviewing, took from an hour to an hour and a half to complete. The teenagers were asked to provide data concerning their socioeconomic and cultural backgrounds; family status; education; religious affiliation and church attendance; leisure-time activities; employment; sexual activities, knowledge, and attitudes; feelings of guilt or religious conflict con-cerning their behavior; self-evaluation; and socially deviant behavior, sexual included, to their identifications with adults, their goals and self-images.

Parents accompanying teenagers to the clinics were interviewed as were parents in their homes.

The social workers involved in the interviewing were given training in research. The confidentiality of the information obtained in the clinic interviews was protected by having the home visits made by a social worker who did not do any clinic interviewing. In view of the limited knowledge available concerning the teenaged venereal disease patients, and the unpredictability of the flow of patients in the clinics, we decided to interview all who came to the clinics during the period the primary data were being collected—February through August 1959. This means, of course, that the findings cannot be generalized until validated or invalidated by follow-up studies in New York with nonclinic patients and by comparable studies elsewhere.

Essentially exploratory, the study had as its major objective that of determining factors contributory to the increase in venereal disease among adolescents, and was designed to answer questions pertinent to the epidemiologic aspects of control, including the following:

> *What kinds of teenagers are involved in venereal disease? From what kinds of families and social backgrounds do they come?*

From the above flowed a variety of specific questions. One was:

> *Are there significant differences in their social behavior depending upon their social background as a whole; or depending upon age, ethnic group, religion, family stability, education, employment, self-image, aspirations, and adult identifications?*

A question of a general nature, included to bring out some of the extrafamilial influences that conceivably might be having an influence on both teenagers and their parents, was:

> *Are there trends in 20th-century American life that tend to exert pressure on the adolescent toward premarital sexual experimentation?*

In the final report of the study,[2] this question is answered in the affirmative on the basis of a comprehensive analysis of the kinds of stimuli and social sanctions which induce young people to experiment sexually in the absence of comparable stimuli toward experimentation in nonsexual activities.

METHOD

The data from the teenagers were obtained in depth interviews by trained, experienced social workers in the clinics, using an interview schedule containing both pre-coded and open-ended questions. Interviews with parents were largely unstructured, and were designed to provide information as to the characteristics of the home and neighborhood; the relationship of parents to children; parents' knowledge and attitude regarding sex and venereal disease characteristics of the parents; clues to the marital relationship; identifying data concerning family setting, parents' employment, source of income, religious affiliation and attendance and use of leisure time on the part of the family as a whole. The latter identifying data were used as a measure of the reliability of comparable data obtained from teenager. Parents were told that visits to the home were in connection with a study of adolescent behavior. This caused no problem and many volunteered knowledge of their adolescent's venereal exposure or infection as a problem of concern, along with other types of disturbing or antisocial behavior.

FINDINGS AND IMPLICATIONS

Who were the teenagers and from what kinds of families did they come? To what extent did identification of both fit the prevailing stereotypes?

While it is not possible here to describe findings that cover four chapters in the published report,[2] some significant findings and implications can be highlighted.

While all the teenagers interviewed had had sexual relations, only 63 per cent were found by the clinic to have had one or more venereal infections. Of these, 70 per cent were boys; 30 per cent, girls. Among the infected group, numbering 379 teenagers, 159 reported one previous infection; 55 reported two or more.

Promiscuity, defined as casual, frequent, and depersonalized sexual relations, was a predominantly male phenomenon in the study universe. It was determined on the basis of number of sexual partners, length of time the teenager had been engaging in sexual activities, and personalization of the partner. The 600 teenagers—aged 12 through 19—were more evenly divided between boys and girls, 352 and 248, respectively, than the differences in promiscuity reflect. Only two girls were in the most promiscuous group as against 60 boys, while five times as high a proportion of the girls, than of the boys, were in the least promiscuous group. While society's greater acceptance of promiscuity among males may have occasioned some exaggeration on the part of the boys, and some underreporting on the part of the girls, there is little reason to believe that this appreciably affects these comparisons.

Homosexuality was also much more prevalent among boys, with only nine girls so involved out of a total of 115 teenagers who reported homosexual activity.

Tabulations to check the reliability of responses, checks for consistency, and the information obtained in the home visits confirmed the interviewers' impressions that the teenagers provided essentially accurate data—subjective as well as objective. Additional confirmation of interpretation of the differences in promiscuity between the sexes is to be found in correlations showing that promiscuity among the males was not significantly related to socially deviant behavior, while it was so related among the females. It should come as no surprise that promiscuity correlated significantly with venereal disease, especially among the boys.

STEREOTYPES

Although nonwhites accounted for 71 per cent of the universe, Puerto Rican teenagers, 16 per cent, and other whites, 13 per cent, promiscuity was found in all three groups with no essential difference. Contrary to a prevailing stereotype, the white teenagers were the new residents in the city. A majority of the nonwhite, and most of the Puerto Rican patients, were either long-term or lifetime residents of the city. In some instances physicians in the clinics failed to inform white teenagers about the research interview, and these were not, therefore, included in the study.

A majority of the young people interviewed came from low-income, minority group families. However, only one-sixth were dependent, in part or in whole, on public assistance. More than one-sixth of them came from families of lower middle-class status, and 28 per cent from families with middle-class aspirations. Their social class status was confirmed by the home visits and by indices of parental control. For example, over two-thirds of the teenagers reported that their parents were interested in knowing where they went, expected them to be home at a certain time, and set standards for their behavior, even if unable to insure that these were carried out at all times.

The stereotype of demoralized families with little potential for rehabilitation does not stand up under the study's findings. Most of the parents who were interviewed expressed concern over the behavior which had resulted in their child's illness, though often they did not seem to know about other socially deviant aspects of his or her behavior. The social worker who interviewed parents in their homes encountered requests for help and many evidences of a desire to improve their situations. For example, there were many indications of attempts to transform slum apartments into attractive, livable homes.

VISITS TO THE HOME

The 100 home visits could not be made on a random basis since visits had to be initiated while the interviewing was still in progress. Permission for a home visit was the last question in the interview. The visits were found to be representative for sex and religious affiliation. Among the significant findings were confirmation of the essential reliability of the data obtained from the teenagers, insight into the problems parents had—both of a general nature and specifically in relation to the adolescent about whose behavior they were already concerned, awareness of their own ignorance of sex and their inability to provide wholesome education concerning sex and venereal disease, as well as their inability to help their children aspire to and achieve more meaningful goals.

More than three-fourths of the teenagers interviewed—79 per cent —were over 16 years of age; 62 per cent were 18 years old. In religion, 62 per cent were Protestant; 32 per cent were Catholic; 2 per cent were Jewish; the remainder were either unaffiliated, or belonged to miscellaneous religious groups. Almost half the young people reported that their parents attended religious services, while slightly more than 25 per cent of the teenagers themselves did so.

The educational and cultural levels of most of these young people can only be characterized as impoverished. While 537 had entered high school, only 72 had graduated, and an additional 18 went on to college. Few reported any use of New York City's neighborhood libraries and the cultural opportunities available in the schools and in community centers.

The major school problems reported were lack of interest in subjects, reading difficulties, failure to achieve promotion, and lack of interest on the part of the teachers. As one teenage girl put it: "My teacher would sometimes say, "I get paid whether you learn or not. I don't have to teach you!" This girl, like many of the other teenagers, had been involved in truancy before becoming involved in sexual activities. Repeated truancy was reported by 80 per cent.

Of the 439 teenagers not in school when interviewed, only 176 had had any work experience, part- or full-time.

The teenagers revealed their concerns over lack of a meaningful role in answers to questions designed to get at their self-image. When asked what they did in their spare time, 509 replied: "Nothing!" This is not in contradiction to their having indicated that they spent some time in recreational and other types of activities—including sexual; it is a frank—if somewhat devastating self-appraisal. Having nothing to do—in the sense of having few meaningful and socially useful responsibilities—means, essentially, to be nothing. To what extent this lack of role and the resultant *anomie* may be related to promiscuity can only be raised as a question for further investigation.

SOCIAL CONTROLS AND BEHAVIOR

Despite the availability of technics for mechanically processing research data, relating social controls to behavior is still a major problem for the social sciences. The status of today's knowledge of human behavior and its interaction with environment calls for caution in interpreting statistical associations, especially in an exploratory study. Because of this and the subjective nature of interview data, probability levels were set high in the tests for statistical significance, and reservations were made in the interpretation of correlations.

Many indices of social control generally regarded as having an influence on behavior reflected significant relationships to promiscuous and socially deviant behavior, with variations according to sex and ethnic group. Among these indices were: psychologic atmosphere of the home (rated as favorable if the teenager spent considerable time there, took his friends there, and did things with his family); teenagers' religious attendance; whether the teenager lived with his family; and whether the teenager was still in school. School status reflected the most statistically significant influence.

Attempts at classifying the teenagers as living in a "favorable" or "unfavorable" environment were unsuccessful, since most of them lived in evironments having both favorable and unfavorable aspects.

Educational level correlated significantly with what was rated as a "very good" knowledge of the facts about venereal disease. However, only 10 per cent of the young people had this kind of knowledge—not surprising in the light of the generally low level of educational attainment.

Despite their involvement in sexual activities, these young people exhibited little understanding of the meaning of sex. Peers constituted the source of sex knowledge for 64 per cent of these young people, while parents were the source for 21 per cent; other adults, for 15 per cent. Relatively fewer of the teenagers who obtained their sex knowledge from parents or adults with whom they had a positive identification were promiscuous.

Ignorance is transmitted with the same ease as knowledge. At one point, the cost of the transmission of ignorance has to be weighed against the cost of improved education for parents and professional persons, as well as for teenagers.

While many of the teenagers had been involved in "delinquent" behavior, the group as a whole could not be characterized as delinquent. More than half the young people reported they had driven cars without a license and had done some stealing; 27 per cent had been involved in street fighting; 38 per cent had come to the attention of the police; but only 7 per cent had been taken to court.

The interviewers were impressed with the frankness with which the teenagers revealed illegal actions and other aspects of their behavior that did not present them in a favorable light. They were also impressed with the frequent expressions of guilt and religious conflict.

SOME CONTRASTS

The difficulties in establishing a typology for differentiating these teenagers, their general ignorance about sex and venereal disease, and the wide range of their behavior, both social and sexual,

suggest the need not only for more education but also for greater individualization of these teenagers. Consider the contrasts in the following young people who were among those interviewed in the social
hygiene clinics:

A shy, withdrawn, guilt-laden honor student of 18, who lives with
his grandmother, had his only sexual experience with a prostitute to
test his "virility."

An 18-year-old drug addict, who lives with both parents, has had at
least 25 sex partners toward whom he feels no personal attachment.
He feels sorry only for having been "caught."

A highly intelligent high-school girl, who lives with both parents,
had infrequent sexual relations with her steady boy friend, but caught
syphilis from him after he had impulsively had relations with a
"pickup," following a lover's quarrel.

A recent arrival in New York, where she has no family ties, has
gradually drifted into prostitution.

A 17-year-old girl from a closely knit family, who was goaded by
her girl friends into having sexual relations with her fiance, found
herself both pregnant and infected, and is in an anguish of guilt and
fear for the future.

A 15-year-old boy from a broken home and a special school for
problem children became infected from engaging in homosexual
activity for money. He says he has no goals, does not care about anyone, and has no idea what he wants out of life.

One need all these young people had had in common was for
better education about sex and venereal disease. On the surface, this
should present little or no problem. The issue is, however, beclouded
by emotionally charged, conflicting, and controversial attitudes toward
sex in society at large, as well as among the teenagers who have contracted the disease. Constructive sex education requires a point of
view and sanctions for codes of behavior to which society expects its
youth to adhere. Such education should not only help to prevent the
behavior which results in infection, but should facilitate cooperation
from the young patient in the contact interview and prevent repeated
infection. It can only succeed, however, if ways can be found to involve such youth in opportunities for more education generally, the
cultural life of the community, and, above all, in meaningful work
and social responsibility.

The findings suggest that if more effective control of the venereal
disease is at stake, the cultural sanction for sexual experimentation on
the part of boys as well as girls will require critical reevaluation.
Similarly, the findings that more indices of social control are reflected
in acceptable social than sexual behavior suggest the importance of
critical examination of the trends in the culture that tend to exert a
pressure on the adolescent to experiment sexually. This suggests the

need to make available to the teenagers in the study universe opportunities to experiment in other aspects of their lives important in the socialization process, if the objectives of more effective control and a beginning in prevention of the venereal diseases are to become a reality.

This has to go back to the behavior (socialization of the sexual drive) and not merely to symptoms—venereal disease and illegitimacy. Ways must be found to help parents, teachers, and professionals in the health and welfare fields to overcome their apathy in the matter of bringing adolescents into the main stream of community life, by insuring adequate education and preparation for maturity, and by setting standards for behavior, including in this social as well as sexual behavior.

Whether these implications are soundly based will, in the near future, be a matter of objective report. As a result of the study, an adolescent clinic has been initiated in the health center in which the exploratory interviewing took place. A social worker has been assigned to provide counseling and make referrals to rehabilitation agencies, and plans are underway for the provision of psychiatric services, a youth employment counselor, and courses in family life education. Moreover, even before the study was completed, changes in attitude were discernible among those responsible for operating the social hygiene clinics.

It is good to see these beginnings in a period during which it has become fashionable to emphasize man's potential for evil, and to assume that control of the sex drive during adolescence is not only not essential to mature development, but impossible to achieve. Teenagers like those in the study have been held responsible for conduct traceable to the failure on the part of adults to facilitate and sanction controls. Twentieth-century psychologic theories that have been exploited to support sexual license, almost to the debasement of human values and personal relations, need to be reexamined if followup studies and the experimental clinics confirm the findings of this study.

In 1947, Dr. Stokes warned that even a perfect cure would not eradicate the venereal diseases since "their onset is often obscure, often invisible and nonincapacitating," and that "conduct not treatment is the key to control."[3] It is hoped that this study may stimulate more attention to the social aspects of venereal disease without which efforts at control are undermined. Stokes' warning and Scheele's statement more than a decade ago that "what is needed is increased research on the part of those in psychiatry and the social sciences to determine the factors underlying the spread of venereal infection and the social deviations related to their spread,"[4] are even more pertinent today.

1. Deschin, Celia S.: *The relation of socioeconomic and cultural factors to an understanding of illness*, Ph.D. dissertation. Center for Human Relations and Community Studies, New York University, 1958.

2. Deschin, Celia S.: *Teenagers and venereal disease; a sociological study*. American Social Health Association, New York: March 1961. Reprinted by the U. S. Department of Health, Education, and Welfare, Public Health Service, Communicable Disease Center, Venereal Disease Branch, Atlanta, Ga.

3. Stokes, John H.: The course in health and human relations: its origin and its purposes. *Educational Outlook*, January, 1947.

4. Scheele, L. A.: We are moving forward. *Journal of Social Hygiene*, March, 1949.

7. The Mentally Ill in Social Perspective

ONE of the dramatic changes of recent social history is the vast interest in mental illness, and the growth of a more optimistic outlook on its treatment, rehabilitation, and prevention. Underlying this change has been an accumulating body of research which has provided tools for the management of some forms of mental disorder, and which gives promise of unlocking the mysteries of others.

Dr. Gruenberg's paper considers how Public Health methods may be applied in the prevention and control of mental illness. As the mentally ill recover, their rehabilitation and re-entry into the population necessitate a full gamut of coordinated community health and welfare services. These will be reviewed in later Sections that deal with social and community psychiatry, as an important discipline in the Public Health framework.

Application of Control Methods to Mental Illness*

ERNEST M. GRUENBERG, M.D.

WHAT CAN BE DONE to control mental disorders among the people of a community?

The answer to this question emerges from an estimate of our knowledge regarding the etiology and epidemiology of various mental disorders. The unhappy situation regarding our ignorance about the schizophrenias outlined by Hoch[1] should not discourage us unduly. Public health has scored victories in the past on the basis of simple empiric procedures, identifying a key link in the natural history of a disease or an observation regarding the association of a disease with a particular modifiable feature of the environment. We cannot do all that we would like to do, but we should, at least, make certain that we are doing what we know how to do to reduce the burden of mental disorders.

* Reprinted by permission from the August 1957 issue of the *American Journal of Public Health*, Vol. 47, pp. 944–952. Copyright by the American Public Health Association, Inc., 1790 Broadway, New York 19, N. Y. This paper was presented before the Mental Health Section of the American Public Health Association at the Eighty-fourth Annual Meeting in Atlantic City, New Jersey, November 13, 1956. The author is Professor of Psychiatry, College of Physicians and Surgeons, Columbia University, New York, New York.

The Public Health approach to mental disorders is the same as the Public Health approach to any other group of illnesses: first, prevent what we know how to prevent; second, terminate or mitigate illnesses that we know how to terminate or mitigate; third, reduce the disabilities suffered as a result of illness where we know how.

Although concern with mental health in a health department may be new, we should not assume that only new programs will affect the mental health of our communities. If our concern for mental health is new, we have probably been unaware of effects old programs have had on mental disorders. A review of our knowledge reveals that some well established Public Health programs have probably been yielding mental health dividends which we do not take into account when estimating their value. The absence of morbidity data as an index of program effectiveness keeps us from placing emphasis on activities in accordance with their mental health values.

In addition, some new programs, whether in health departments or in other community agencies, can be expected to have an effect. Community mental hygiene clinics, general hospital psychiatric units, mental health consultants to health departments, parent education programs, and other activities are frequently advocated as "answers" to the mental health problem which many recognize as one of the nation's leading Public Health problems. While each of these services has a value,[2] none of them alone, nor even all together, will produce a reduction in the size of the mental health problem in a community unless it devotes itself to activities that will actually improve the mental health of the people. An orientation regarding the activities which will produce this kind of effect is needed in order to allocate resources in the light of present knowledge.

PRIMARY PREVENTION
The Public Health Agencies

MATERNAL AND CHILD HEALTH SERVICES. Are we fully using present knowledge in attempting to reduce the number of children born with lifelong handicaps of brain functioning?

We have no clear evidence to this effect. Health departments measure the effectiveness of their maternal and child health programs with yardsticks not designed to rate success or failure in terms of chronic illness. If such scales were developed, would we feel so sure of the effectiveness of present programs? Declining maternal and infant death rates show that these programs have been "successful," but there is evidence that these savings in life have often been bought at the cost of increases in the numbers of blind, palsied, epileptic, and mentally deficient children. Death rates, which have served so long as the sole measure of the improvement of a community's health, are insufficient measures of today's Public Health programs.

These are costly and tragic penalties to pay, particularly when a great deal could be done to avoid these preventable mental illnesses. Thus a maternal and child health program should include preventive treatment for syphilis when it is present—(How many infants were born with congenital syphilis? How many were truly not preventable?); for protection against the consequences of Rh factor incompatibility—(How many cases of unanticipated erythroblastosis occurred?); for protection against rubella during pregnancy; and for the development of optimal nutrition in pregnant women. There is excellent evidence that these preventive measures will reduce the incidence of children born with damaged brains, damage which will show up in cerebral palsy, epilepsy, mental deficiency, and behavior disturbances.

Surely a nutrition program for mothers-to-be which concerns itself exclusively—or even mainly—with obesity indicated that the sponsoring health department is ill-informed on the relationship of maternal nutrition to the incidence of toxemia and between toxemias and mental deficiency, behavior disorders, and epilepsy,[3] apart from the actual nutritional status of the young women of its community.

No one would wish to see death rates rise again, but can we tell what we are doing, and whether we are doing enough, without better data on the morbidity we prevent? Evidence regarding the frequency with which children develop lifelong mental handicaps because of inadequacies of these programs should be cited here, but our mechanisms for recording these forms of morbidity are too weak to provide reliable data on this question. The only way to know how many preventable cases of illness are occurring is to record them, report them, and count them, for our ability to develop control programs often depends upon the availability of knowledge regarding our failures to apply effective measures. Death certificates and even maternal death conferences, great as their value might be for other purposes, are of no value here. We need morbidity data and we will have to develop such data. The national health survey[4] will provide a welcome start in this direction, but it is obviously only a start. Health departments that think there is no need to strengthen their maternal and child health services so as to prevent a larger proportion of the cases of fetal infection with syphilis and rubella, of injury due to Rh incompatibility, or of fetal malnutrition are remaining blind to the issues. If they take account of preventable cases of mental deficiency, cerebral palsy, epilepsy, and behavior disorders they will probably find that their programs need great intensification if they are to prevent these forms of mental illness.

CONTROL OF ENVIRONMENTAL HAZARDS. Iodine deficiency,[5] poisoning,[6] brain injuries,[7] and drug intoxication[8] cause mental disorders which are preventable. Their control is usually assigned to the division of environmental sanitation of our health departments. Are these divisions apprised of these hazards so that they can prevent these mental disorders? Are they fully aware of the consequences of the failure to put their knowledge and resources to work? It is hard to see how they could be, since there exists so little information on the incidence of mental disorders which could be reduced by intensifying the division's action in this area. Those with experience in transforming knowledge into community programs for the betterment of health will think of many ways of strengthening old and creating new programs so as to control preventable cases of mental disorder arising from inadequate community health protection.

The hazards to fetal brain development created by ionizing radiation and food additives also need evaluation. Evidence on the consequences of failure to act is needed in order to create the concern and energy which will lead to action.

NUTRITION. Poor nutrition during pregnancy is not the only kind of nutritional deficiency related to mental disorder. Delirium tremens and some confusional psychoses, particularly of the elderly, are other examples. Pellagra, now a rarity in our country, is another example. Nevertheless, there are States whose mental health consultants continue to ignore the small stream of pellagra psychoses which come to their mental hospitals. A mental health consultant who does not call attention to such an opportunity to prevent mental disorders is using a questionable concept of priorities. While all health workers have a responsibility for contributing to the prevention of mental disorders, the mental health consultant should be especially alert to the action the health department could take, but is not now taking, to preclude these disorders.

Alcoholism is a serious social and health problem. Sometimes great efforts are made to rehabilitate alcoholics or to prevent alcoholism. Despite the urgency of the problem, the sincerity of the workers in the field, and the credibility of some of their theories, it must be admitted that the campaign against alcoholism is an uphill fight with little assurance that the expended efforts will prove effective. However, were some of this energy devoted to maintaining the nutritional state of alcoholics, it would appear that delirium tremens could be prevented (9). This devastating syndrome, which causes such severe disability, is so readily preventable that it might be profitable to focus upon this objective, even if the underlying alcoholism cannot be controlled.

Mental Hospitals have long been reporting that many elderly psychotic persons are admitted in a poor nutritional state. They also report that many confusional states disappear following a regimen of a good diet with supplements (10). Getting good nutriments to elderly people should be a challenge to the nutrition workers in our Public Health agencies, since it is obviously much more than a health education problem. How can one overcome such problems as financing the older person's food budget, or his limited energy and capacity for shopping? How to supply him with dentures comfortable enough to chew the needed yet costly proteins? Food preparation and sometimes chewing itself taxes his energy. There is often loneliness at meal times, and since eating is a social activity, many people do not have an adequate appetite for food in the absence of the social stimulation to eat. A program for improving the nutrition of the elderly requires the combined efforts of many community agencies besides the health agencies. Even in the United States, a community can expect to improve the mental health of its members by improving their nutrition, bettering its control of infectious diseases, and strengthening its environmental sanitation. Yet we have the highest per capita consumption of proteins, vitamins, and calories in the world.

These are the main activities of health departments with conventional programs that can reduce the incidence of mental disorders. These are programs which exist and which we know how to operate. Yet they all present the same problem. Because their relationship to mental health is ignored, because their value in controlling preventable mental disorders is not appraised, the result has been to undervalue the results of these activities. Attention to mental health responsibilities should lead to a strengthening of these activities. It will inevitably lead to the development of better data on mental disorder so that eventually program planners will be able to assess a program, not merely in terms of deferred deaths or public popularity, but in terms of the amount of mental disorder prevented.

WELFARE DEPARTMENTS AND SOCIAL AGENCIES

"There is no substitute for family life" (11). Although this is one of the best established facts about personality development, it seems to be more fashionable today to pay attention to the possible consequences of unhealthy family situations. The result is that many children have no family life. (For example, New York City is said to have a roster of 1,322 children awaiting long-term placement for whom no homes are available, as reported in *News*, January, 1957, published by the Citizens Committee for Children of New York City, Inc.) We are not preventing mental disorders if we let adoptable young children remain in nonfamily settings. Whether placement failures are due to administrative difficulties in locating homes, or the inability to persuade families to take in homeless children, or because of thoughtless legal or policy barriers, such failures should be considered missed opportunities to prevent mental disease.

Deprivation symptoms can follow maternal illness or death, parental desertion or imprisonment. Opportunities for prevention occur when children lose their continual family associations because of broken homes. Can we say that our resources for maintaining family life for young children are in proportion to our resources for placing children in foster homes or institutions? Do we hospitalize young children, and their mothers, rather than bring medical, nursing, and housekeeping assistance to them in their homes? It would seem worth while for all Public Health, welfare and mental health departments to look into this question in their own communities. Little information is available regarding the present state of affairs because current practices have not been examined thoroughly in the light of this knowledge. Conversations with various authorities in the child-rearing field leads one to believe that there is no consensus of experts regarding the causes of preventable failures to assure young children with a continuous family life experience. The only point which every expert makes is that he knows the causes and what should be done. Unfortunately, what each expert knows is entirely different from what the other experts know. Under these conditions there is need to develop the epidemiology of familyless early childhood (12), if such a term may be coined. Of course, it is important to keep in mind that, so far as we know, damage to personality development is as likely to follow too many family lives as none at all; that is, repeated placements in unstable foster homes need to be avoided as assiduously as the lack of placement.

SECONDARY PREVENTION
Early Diagnosis and Effective Treatment

The disease experience of a population may be reduced by lessening its incidence, by shortening its duration, or by preventing its progress. Secondary prevention by definitive treatment of identified cases has played an important role in improving the people's health with respect to diabetes, epilepsy, tuberculosis, syphilis, and malaria. Which mental disorders today are subject to ready diagnosis and effective treatment, so that the progress of illness may be halted or its duration shortened? It would have been convenient for the purposes of this article to have been able to cite a recent authoritative review of the question. None has been found, however. The following not too authoritative list is given, not as a definite answer to the question, but as a prod to others, indicating what the author believes to be a minimum list from available evidence. Treatment known to limit the duration or retard the progress of illness is available today for depressive states of a certain type and intensity regardless of the diagnosis, and for general paralysis, pellagra, toxic deliria, conversion hysteria, cretinism, and phenylpyruvic acid oligophrenia.

In order to provide for early diagnosis and treatment of these conditions it is necessary to conduct case-finding and arrange for definitive treatment. Yet no local mental health program is known to have done this. Agencies are not now organized to recognize and treat these conditions on a priority basis, for priorities in the use of diagnostic and treatment services are not in practice based on a list of disorders subject to secondary prevention. There is much public health experience to draw upon in organizing secondary prevention programs. Thus, providing readily available treatment is a first step. Getting the people in need of treatment to the treatment is a second. Other tested public health devices are campaigns to educate and alert physicians, public health nurses, pastors, and others likely to be sought as first resources when illness strikes. Could not such a secondary prevention program be applied to mental health? The answer appears to be negative unless those who operate treatment services can be induced to set up definitive treatment programs for the illnesses most subject to secondary prevention. Recently, a highly dramatic suggestion was made that ferric chloride be sprinkled on the diapers of newborn infants before they leave the hospital as a simple mass screening device for identifying the rare cases of congenital disorders of phenylpyruvic acid metabolism (13). (The originator was not certain that the disorder is manifested that early, and proposed the procedure only to oppose it on the grounds that this would increase the incidence of phenylpyruvic acid disorders in the next generation!)

While some disorders can neither be prevented nor arrested by treatment, recurrent patterns of illness can be disrupted by treatment between episodes of illness. For example, there is considerable evidence (from some trials of uncertain conclusiveness) that electric shock treatments given monthly to remitted schizophrenics delay remissions (14). This promising approach to secondary prevention deserves further trial.

TERTIARY PREVENTION
Reduction of Disability

Illnesses than can neither be prevented nor shortened in duration can sometimes be made less disabling through various means. The fact that we cannot prevent schizophrenia, for example, nor shorten its course, should not blind us to the fact that we have a number of powerful technics for reducing the disability of schizophrenes. At present, mental health has three types of tools for lessening the amount of disability experienced by a population. First, there are many social measures which can be taken, such as the formation of patient clubs, the rearrangement of hospital organization in the direction of therapeutic communities, the education of the public to tolerate the disabilities of chronically disabled patients, and the creation of various forms of social protection for disabled patients (committees to care for property and prevent exploitation of work and of sex, sheltered workshops, supervised residences, etc.) Second, there are educational and psychotherapeutic methods for reducing disability: teaching disabled persons to use undamaged latent skills, teaching them to avoid hazards arising from their disabilities, and teaching them to make use of the social resources mentioned above. Third, there are pharmacologic methods for reducing disabilities due to impulsiveness, insomnia, anxiety, restlessness, or inertia.

DEATH. The final disablement is, of course, death. While mortality rates have long been regarded as indexes to the health progress of a community, mental health programs rarely have used these rates in self-appraisal. Nonetheless, we know that some mental disorders can lead to death and at times psychiatric treatment is determined by estimates regarding the danger to life created by an illness. Thus, our certification laws lean heavily on the concept of the patient's "danger to himself or others"—the danger referred to being largely the danger of suicide or murder. Public anxiety regarding the dangers arising from mental illness has played a large role in creating and maintaining the present policy of overinstitutionalization, so that progress in the reduction of disability of the mentally ill will require systematic alleviation of this anxiety. To do so, it will be necessary to educate people to understand that violence in the community is not primarily a product of mental disorder, and that few mental disorders will increase the likelihood of violence. It must also be made clear that present knowledge does not make it easy for psychiatrists to predict who will commit violence against his own or another's person, and that professionals cannot undertake to provide perfect community protection from physical violence.

However, as our knowledge increases regarding the prognosis of certain illnesses and our therapeutic armamentarium develops, we shall become more capable of identifying these persons and more effective in our treatment and rehabilitation of them. Since many suicides are associated with depressive states amenable to early treatment, it should be expected that a mental health program should reduce the incidence of suicide, although it is not entirely preventable with present knowledge (15). So far as is known, only a small proportion of homicides are attributable to definable mental disorders amenable to early diagnosis and treatment. It is to be hoped that our knowledge will increase sufficiently to make homicide a declining phenomenon, an anachronistic form of human behavior.

HOSPITALIZATION. Hospitalization is to be regarded here as a severe form of disability. While it is true that some treatments are best obtained in hospitals (and hence there are instances of persons overcoming a chronic disability through a short term in hospital), mental hospitals have had so many uses other than therapeutic that it must be pointed out that few of the patient days spent in mental hospitals are spent there in order to obtain diagnosis and treatment. The situation is rapidly changing today, but in many communities a great number of persons in mental hospitals do not need to be there for treatment or protection, or for the protection of the community. This is not because of the failure of any particular group or profession, but is the consequence of a social heritage of misconceptions about the nature of mental illness and about the proper organization and use of mental hospitals. If we wish to emancipate ourselves from this heritage we will need a concerted effort by mental hospital staffs, health and welfare departments, the media of mass communication, and by those who are responsible for transmitting social inheritance to the next generation—the schoolteachers.

There is reason to believe that some communities have experienced a rapid decline in mental hospitalization over the past two decades without there having been introduced some new definitive treatment to account for this change. These drops in the prevalence of institutionalization are apparently due to a few outstanding personalities who have taken seriously the generally forgotten teachings of Pinel regarding the mental functioning of psychotics. One such individual is Rees, who has been putting Pinel's ideas into action at the Warlingham Park Hospital in Croyden, England. Key to this concept of mental illness, which apparently underlies the shift in rates, is the belief that the capacity for taking social responsibility atrophies, like muscle, with disuse (16). Dr. Rees makes systematic efforts during all stages of patient care to identify areas of life in which they may continue to exercise responsibility, and invents technics to permit them to do so. The result is that social behavior does not decay so rapidly and that a much larger proportion of patients proceed in a shorter time to regain the capacity to lead independent responsible lives than patients treated in the usual mental hospital manner. This conceptual change in treatment can be looked upon as paralleling the change that occurred in physical medicine following the introduction of the concept of early ambulation; without adequate understanding of the processes involved, it has some of the same inherent dangers.

Of course, this principle cannot be applied by a mental hospital receiving persons from a fearful community which believes that the function of the hospital is to keep ill persons out of sight and mind. The hospital cannot change its basic practices unless the community's officials and its leading citizens produce a concomitant change in community attitudes. In addition, the relationships between hospital and community will need to change since both patients and professionals will become much more closely intertwined with the people of the community.

The new tranquilizing drugs have appeared at the same time as the social changes have been brought to the attention of the professional world. They will undoubtedly increase our ability to help mentally ill persons live in the community. The drugs have been embraced at a much greater speed than the changes in social organization and practice referred to above; both the social changes and tranquilizers appear to reduce the duration of hospital stay and to reduce the amount of disturbed behavior. Little is known about the independent effect of these tranquilizers for there has been little exploration by staffs working in community-oriented mental hospitals. However, from what is known, it is clear that they are a valuable new tool for reducing disability, particularly from schizophrenia.

MAINTENANCE OF SOCIAL ROLES. The above remarks assume that being hospitalized is a severe form of social disability, since persons in hospitals are prevented from participating as active, responsible members of the community. A less severe form of social disability is represented by persons who cannot take part in two major types of social enterprise—attendance at schools and at work.

The child who is excluded from school because of a mental disorder is more disabled than a child with the same disorder who manages to stay in school. As was previously noted, there exist three methods for reducing the number of children excluded from school because of mental disorders. Thus we find that modification of schools as social institutions, to make them more adaptable to the various emotional needs of children, has long been going on under the slogan of "the child-centered school." Whatever else this movement does, it does make it possible for a larger proportion of children whose mental functioning is reduced in flexibility or toughness to find a place in the school and a way of living with it. Again, various measures have been devised for helping children to adapt to school life early in their student careers. Such devices as kindergarten, play-school, counseling about anxieties during the first week of school, and permitting mothers to stay with their children during the first weeks of school are social procedures which make for an inclusion of a greater number of children in the school. The development of new methods of teaching the physically, mentally, or emotionally handicapped child decreases the number of children with unprevented chronic disorders who are excluded from school. Educational and psychotherapeutic methods are also used to reduce childhood school disabilities; here the program needs to be directed toward teacher, mother, and child.

Adult disability from work because of the presence of unprevented or interminable mental disorder can also be reduced by social, educational, psychotherapeutic and pharmacologic methods. There are many known technics for accomplishing these objectives, but what is needed is a systematic review of available technics for reducing the proportion of persons with mental disorders who are disabled from holding social roles either at school or at work. Since it is not fashionable for the clinical specialists to define their function in such limited and specific terms there is no current authoritative statement of what technics have been established for reaching these goals. Obviously, however, if a community mental health program seeks to reduce the amount of disability produced by mental disorders and exclusion from school and work situations is regarded as a form of serious disability, then such a statement is needed.

Disability for other social roles can also be reduced by present technics. Inability to carry family responsibilities of child rearing, contributing financially to the upkeep of a home, doing housework, etc., could be specified, and many of our present educational and psychotherapeutic methods, many of our procedures for improving participation in social organizations, and some of our pharmacologic technics could be used to reduce the number of mentally disordered persons who are disabled in these ways. In order to do this, one must differentiate between the disorders one is seeking to terminate, and disorders one does not know how to terminate, and concentrate available resources on achieving the greatest possible reduction in morbidity and in disability in the population for whom a mental health program is designed.

CONCLUSION

It should be emphasized that while most clinic staffs would agree with these statements, they would not regard them as an adequate set of goals in light of the clinic's relationship to its case load. What one considers worthwhile goals, depends, of course, on one's point of view. I have tried to point out that from the Public Health approach it is worthwhile to give first priority to preventing what is preventable, and second and third priority to reducing disability from disorders which have not been prevented, terminated, or arrested.

These are the things that can be done to control mental disorders in a community. It is clear that most are not being done so well or so intensively as they should be done. Other steps can be taken with mental disorders: we can undertake detailed psychologic and psycho-dynamic studies, biochemical analyses, autopsies, epidemiologic studies, and other research to get new knowledge to strengthen our skills in controlling mental disorders; we can remove dangerous persons from freedom to do harm; and we can tell the public how good or how bad are mental hospitals. But only by preventing the truly preventable disorders, terminating the terminable disorders, and reducing disability experienced from mental disorders will we control mental disorders among the people of a community.

1. Hoch, Paul H.: The Etiology and Epidemiology of Schizophrenia. *American Journal of Public Health,* September, 1957, 47, No. 9, pp. 1071–1076.

2. *Elements of a Community Mental Health Program.* New York, Milbank Mem. Fund, 1956.

3. Thompkins, W. T., Wiehl, D. G.: Toxemia and Maternal Nutrition. *Promotion of Maternal and Newborn Health.* Proceedings of the 1954 Annual Conference. New York, Milbank Mem. Fund, 1955, pp. 62–79.

Pasamanick, B., Lilienfeld, A. M.: Pregnancy Experience and the Development of Behavior Disorders in Children. *American Journal of Psychiatry,* February, 1956, 112, pp. 613–618.

Lemkau, Paul V.: Factors in the Evaluation of Mental Retardation—Epidemiological Aspects, in *The Evaluation and Treatment of the Mentally Retarded Child in Clinics.* New York, National Association for Retarded Children Inc., 1956, pp. 16–34.

4. The National Health Survey Act. *Public Health Reports,* January, 1957, 72, pp. 1–4.

5. Mayer-Gross, W., Stater, Eliot, Roth, Martin: *Clinical Psychiatry.* London, Cassel, 1955, p. 80.

6. *Ibid.,* Chap. VIII.

7. *Ibid.,* pp. 398 ff.

8. *Ibid.,* pp. 347 ff.

9. *Ibid.,* pp. 338 ff.

10. Noyes, Arthur P.: *Modern Clinical Psychiatry,* ed. 4. Philadelphia, W. B. Saunders Co., 1953, p. 278.

11. Bender, Lauretta: There Is No Substitute for Family Life. *Child Study* 23:74 (Spring) 1946.

12. Mental Health Research Unit Technical Report. Albany, New York State Department of Mental Hygiene, 1957, p. 21.

13. Cawte, J. E.: A Note on the Future of Phenylketonuria. *Journal of Mental Science,* October, 1956, 102, pp. 805–811.

14. Stevenson, G. H.: Prophylactic Electroshock—A Five-Year Study. *American Journal of Psychiatry,* April, 1951, 107, pp. 743–746.

Cameron, Ewen: The Changing Role of the General Hospital Psychiatric Unit, in *Programs for Community Mental Health.* New York, Milbank Memorial Fund, 1957.

15. Parnell, R. W., Skottowe, Ian: Towards Preventing Suicide. *Lancet,* 1957, 272, pp. 206–208.

16. Rees, T. P.: Personal Communication to the author.

8. The Mentally Retarded

Mental Retardation*

LUTHER W. STRINGHAM

MENTAL RETARDATION is a condition, characterized by the faulty development of intelligence, which impairs an individual's ability to learn and to adapt to the demands of society.

The failure of intelligence to develop normally may be due to diseases or conditions—occurring before or at the time of birth, or in infancy or childhood—that damage the brain. It may also be due to factors determined by heredity that affect the development of the brain. It is sometimes accentuated by home or social conditions which fail to provide the child with adequate stimulation or opportunities for learning.

DEGREES OF RETARDATION

The degree of retardation varies greatly among individuals. It can be so severe that the afflicted person must have protective care throughout his life. In others the retardation is so mild that many tasks can be learned and a measure of independence in everyday life can be achieved. In a substantial number of cases the affected persons can adjust in a limited way to the demands of society, and in many instances can, wth help, become productive members of the labor force.

There is no fully satisfactory way of characterizing the degrees of retardation. They range, according to one classification, from profound to mild, and are related to intelligence quotient (I.Q.), developmental characteristics, potential for education and training, and social and vocational adequacy as shown in the following table:

* Reprinted by permission from the June 1962 issue of *Health, Education, and Welfare Indicators*, pp. V–XV. This article was prepared with assistance from members of the Secretary's Committee on Mental Retardation and the staff of the President's Panel on Mental Retardation. The author is the Director, Office of Program Analysis, Office of the Assistant Secretary (for Legislation) and Chairman of the Department's Committee on Mental Retardation.

Developmental Characteristics of the Mentally Retarded

Degrees of Mental Retardation	Pre-School Age 0-5 Maturation and Development	School Age 6-20 Training and Education	Adult 21 and over Social and Vocational Capabilities
Profound (I.Q. below 20)	Gross retardation; minimal capacity for functioning in sensorimotor areas; needs nursing care.	Some motor development present; cannot profit from training in self-help; needs total care.	Some motor and speech development; totally incapable of self-maintenance; needs complete care and supervision.
Severe (I.Q. 20-35)	Poor motor development; speech is minimal; generally unable to profit from training in self-help; little or no communication skills.	Can talk or learn to communicate; can be trained in elemental health habits; cannot learn functional academic skills; profits from systematic habit training.	Can contribute partially to self-support under complete supervision; can develop self-protection skills to a minimal useful level in controlled environment.
Moderate (I.Q. 36-52)	Can talk or learn to communicate; poor social awareness; fair motor development; may profit from self-help; can be managed with moderate supervision.	Can learn functional academic skills to approximately 4th grade level by late teens if given special education.	Capable of self-maintenance in unskilled or semi-skilled occupations; needs supervision and guidance when under mild social or economic stress.
Mild (I.Q. 53-68)	Can develop social and communication skills; minimal retardation in sensorimotor areas; rarely distinguished from normal until later age.	Can learn academic skills to approximately 6th grade level by late teens. Cannot learn general high school subjects. Needs special education particularly at secondary school age levels.	Capable of social and vocational adequacy with proper education and training. Frequently needs supervision and guidance under serious social or economic stress.

Another classification, used in relation to educational programs, makes use of a three-way division as follows:

Level	Intelligence Quotient
Below 25	I. Custodial
About 25–50	II. Trainable
About 50–75	III. Educable

Other classifications group the retarded in somewhat different ways and make use of other terminology. Nevertheless, all of them recognize gradations of mental retardation, although the exact boundary lines vary. Regardless of the particular classification used, however, it should be understood that seldom, if ever, is I.Q. the only determining factor in mental retardation. Other factors that affect intellectual competency are emotional control and social adaptability.

THE CAUSES OF MENTAL RETARDATION

Based on present knowledge the causal factors in mental retardation may be divided into two broad categories: (1) mental retardation caused by incompletely understood psychologic, environmental, or genetic factors without any evident damage of the brain; and (2) mental retardation caused by a number of specifically identified conditions or diseases. The causal and contributing factors included in each of these categories are as follows:

1. Mental Retardation Caused by Incompletely Understood Psychologic, Environmental, or Genetic Factors without Any Evident Damage of the Brain

This group contains 75 to 85 per cent of those diagnosed as retarded. It consists of individuals who show no demonstrable gross abnormality of the brain and who are persons with relatively mild degrees of retardation. In general, the prevalence of this type of retardation is greater within the less favored socioeconomic groups within our culture.

A variety of factors may be operating within this large category. It is believed that some members of this group are products of complex mechanisms of heredity, reflecting the fact that human beings show genetic variability in any characteristic, including measured intelligence. Environmental factors such as the psychologic circumstances of life, social interaction patterns, and the richness of the environment with respect to intellectual stimulation play an important definitive or contributory role within this group. Finally, a variety of unfavorable health factors—including maternal health and prenatal care, nutrition, the conditions of birth, and other illnesses or injuries which may produce minimal and undemonstrable brain damage— probably contribute to a lower level of performance in many cases.

The total effect, thus, is a complex one, involving the action or the interaction of genetic factors, psychologic experiences, and environmental influences. At the present time, it is impossible to assign clear weights to each of these general causative factors. It is known that all of them operate more strongly in the underprivileged groups than among those more favorably situated in society. The prospects for prevention and amelioration should not be discouraging since many of the environmental and psychologic variables are subject to control, opening up the possibility of preventing some of the retardation, especially of milder degree, based upon this class of causation. Some of these conditions are preventable if treatment can be instituted early enough in the child's life. Most of the remainder can be ameliorated through a combination of resources, medicine, social work, education, and rehabilitation.

It should be clearly stated that these same factors also affect retarded individuals whose difficulty stems from the more specific etiologies enumerated in category 2 below.

2. Mental Retardation Caused by Specifically Identified Conditions or Diseases in which There Is Demonstrable Brain Damage

In approximately 15 to 25 per cent of diagnosed cases of mental retardation, a specific disease entity can be held responsible. The impact of such diseases can be most readily demonstrated in those instances where there has been gross brain damage and where the degree of retardation is severe. As mentioned above, it is uncertain to what extent these "organic" factors may operate to produce minor impairment among the less severely retarded groups. Such "organic" factors fall within seven general classes:

a. DISEASES DUE TO INFECTIONS IN THE MOTHER DURING PREGNANCY OR IN THE INFANT AFTER BIRTH. German measles, occurring during the first three months of pregnancy, is known to result in mental retardation as well as other abnormalities. Other infections occurring during pregnancy have also been implicated. A number of the infectious diseases of infancy and childhood may cause brain injury resulting in retardation.

b. BRAIN DAMAGE RESULTING FROM TOXIC AGENTS WHICH ARE INGESTED BY THE MOTHER DURING PREGNANCY OR BY THE CHILD AFTER

BIRTH. Jaundice of the newborn due to Rh blood factor incompatibility and carbon monoxide or lead poisoning are examples.

c. DISEASE DUE TO TRAUMA OR PHYSICAL AGENT. Brain injury occurring as a result of difficult delivery and asphyxiation due to delay in the onset of breathing at the time of birth are common causes. They occur with particular frequency in premature babies. Brain injury in childhood, especially from automobile accidents, is an added factor.

d. DISEASES DUE TO DISORDERS OF METABOLISM, GROWTH OR NUTRITION. A number of disorders of metabolism, some of which are determined by heredity, produce mental retardation. Some of the most important of these disorders are phenylketonuria and galactosemia in which there are abnormalities of amino acid chemistry in the body.

e. ABNORMAL GROWTHS WITHIN THE BRAIN. A number of rare conditions, some determined by heredity, are characterized by tumor-like and other abnormal growths within the brain and produce mental retardation.

f. DISEASES DUE TO UNKNOWN PRENATAL FACTORS. Recent discoveries prove that mongolism results from abnormal grouping of chromosomes probably at the time of formation of the ovum in the mother. Other congenital malformations have a similar basis. For some, however, an undetermined prenatal mechanism must be responsible.

g. DISEASES DUE TO UNCERTAIN CAUSES BUT WITH EVIDENT DAMAGE OF THE BRAIN. A sizable group of mentally retarded children have evident damage to the brain which is presumed to be linked to the mental retardation. The causes of the pathologic changes of the brain in this sizable group remain unknown.

Data on patients in institutions show a higher prevalence of pathologic conditions among the more severely retarded. Retarded children have other defects more often than the average child. They are often smaller than average, and have poorer muscular coordination. They have a greater than ordinary percentage of defects, such as hearing and vision, and have probably greater difficulty in perceiving what the sense organs bring to their minds. Thus, many of them are multihandicapped in a degree.

SCOPE OF THE PROBLEM

As stated above, mental retardation is defined as impairment of ability to learn and to adapt to the demands of society. These demands are not the same in every culture. In fact, even within our own community they vary with the age of the individual. We expect little, in terms of intellectual pursuits, from the preschool child. During the school age, the individual is evaluated critically in terms of social and academic accomplishment. In later life, the intellectual basis of social inadequacy again may be less evident. Numerous surveys directed toward determining the frequency and magnitude of the problem of mental retardation have shown that the number of individuals reported as retarded is highest during the school age. Less than one-fifth as many children in the age group 0–4 were reported by these surveys as mentally retarded as were reported in the age group 10–14. Similarly, only one-fourth as many persons in the age group 20 and over were identified as mentally retarded as compared with the number identified in the age group 10–14.

This varying prevalence by age is to some extent determined by differential survival rates and other demographic factors. However, the high prevalence at ages 10 to 14 is due primarily to the increased recognition of intellectual handicap of children within the school systems. The low number of infants from 0 to 1 year old identified as retarded is in part at least due to the fact that their intellectual deficiency is not yet apparent. Only gross impairment is evident in early childhood. Of striking significance is the fact that half of the individuals considered retarded during adolescence are no longer so considered in adulthood.

In view of these considerations, only the most crude estimates of the overall magnitude of the problem can be established. One such estimate may be derived through the use of intelligence quotients, and obtained from the samples upon which our intelligence tests have been standardized. The numbers of mentally retarded persons by this criterion can be calculated roughly on the basis of this experience with intelligence testing. On most tests standardized nationally, experience has shown that virtually all persons with I.Q.s below about 70 have significant difficulties in adapting adequately to their environment. About 3 percent of the population score below this level.

Based on this figure of 3 percent, it is estimated that, of the 4.2 million children born each year, 126,000 are, or will be, classed as mentally retarded.

Of the 126,000, some 4,200 (0.1 percent of all births) will be retarded so profoundly or severely that they will be unable to care even for their own creature needs. About 12,600 (0.3 percent of all births) will suffer from "moderate" retardation—they will remain below the 7-year intellectual level. The remaining 110,000 (2.6 percent of births) are those with mild retardation and represent those who can, with special training and assistance, acquire limited job skills and achieve almost complete independence in community living.

Applying these same percentages to the total population it is estimated that there are approximately 5.4 million mentally retarded persons in the population. Of this number:

60,000 to 90,000 are persons, mostly children and adolescents, so profoundly or severely retarded that they cannot survive unless constantly cared for and sheltered.

300,000 to 350,000 are moderately retarded children, adolescents, and adults who can assist in their own care and can even undertake semi-productive endeavors in a protected environment. They can understand the meaning of danger. However, they have limited capacity to learn, and their shortcomings become evident when they are called upon to understand the meaning of symbols as used in the written language. These people can learn many tasks when patiently and properly taught.

Some 5,000,000 are mildly retarded children, adolescents, and adults who are able to perform more adequately, adjust in a limited way to the demands of society, and play a more positive role as workers.

ECONOMIC COSTS OF MENTAL RETARDATION

There are no reliable estimates of the total cost to the Nation, both direct and indirect, of mental retardation. The direct costs to families and to communities include those for institutional and home care and for special services. Indirect costs include the losses that result from the absence of earning capacity and inability to contribute to the production of goods and services.

Only 4 per cent of the mentally retarded are confined to institutions. Yet, their care costs relatives and communities some $300 million annually. Additional amounts are required for the construction of facilities for custodial and educational purposes. The cost of institutional care, facilities construction, and special care in the family home totals more than $1 billion per year.

THE DEVELOPMENT OF NATIONAL CONCERN

Mental retardation thus is a serious problem affecting many aspects of our society. The host of problems presented by these people—to themselves, to their families, and to their communities—include biologic, psychologic, educational, vocational, and social areas of concern. Mental retardation must be approached through the whole life cycle, from consideration of genetics and conception through pregnancy, delivery, childhood, adolescence, adulthood, and old age.

Since 1950, interest in the problem of mental retardation has grown rapidly. During the past decade increased activities have been stimulated by a few foundations, by the demands of parents, by interested lay and professional groups, and by members of legislative bodies who have been convinced of the urgent need for programs in this field.

Today, private efforts and public programs at all levels of government—local, State, and Federal—take eight basic forms:

1. DIAGNOSTIC AND CLINICAL SERVICES. There are over 90 clinics specializing in services to the retarded. Well over half were established within the past five years. These services need still greater expansion. The 20,000 children aided in 1960 represent only a small fraction of those who need the service.

2. CARE IN RESIDENTIAL INSTITUTIONS. Today there are over 200,000 mentally retarded patients in such institutions, approximately 10 percent more than there were five years ago. But the average waiting list continues to grow, and the quality of the service often suffers from limited budgets and salary levels. Increases in both facilities and manpower are necessary.

3. SPECIAL EDUCATION. The number of mentally retarded enrolled in special education classes has been doubled over the past decade. In spite of this record, we are not yet meeting our existing requirements, and more such facilities must be provided. Less than 25 percent of our retarded children have access to special education. Moreover, the classes need teachers specially trained to meet the specialized needs of the retarded. To meet minimum standards, at least 75,000 such teachers are required. Today there are fewer than 20,000, and many of these have not fully met professional standards.

4. PARENT COUNSELING. Counseling of parents is now being provided by private physicians, clinic staffs, social workers, nurses, psychologists, and school personnel. Although this service is still in an experimental stage of development, it offers bright prospects for helping parents to meet their social and emotional problems.

5. SOCIAL SERVICES. Social services provided mentally retarded children and adults include case work, group work, and day care. These services are an integral part of clinical, rehabilitation, and other mental retardation programs. Social workers are also active in community organizations and in working with parents groups.

6. VOCATIONAL REHABILITATION. In the past five years the number of mentally retarded rehabilitated through State vocational agencies has more than tripled—going from 1,094 in 1957 to 3,562 in 1961. In terms of the number who could benefit from rehabilitation services, this number is small. However, new knowledge and new techniques

are needed, for over 25 percent of those coming out of the special classes still cannot be placed.

7. PREPARATION OF PROFESSIONAL PERSONNEL. The Federal government is now promoting the training of leadership personnel in education, rehabilitation workers, research personnel, and medical and welfare specialists. In addition, programs are being provided that will increase the competence of the health professions in providing services for retarded persons. Nevertheless, shortages of qualified personnel remain one of the major bottlenecks in providing services to retarded persons and their families.

8. RESEARCH. Support for research in the causes and amelioration of mental retardation has been greatly increased, especially during the last five years. Progress has been made in identifying specific conditions and diseases and in establishing basic problems of behavior and learning, but major research breakthroughs must be achieved before there will be adequate understanding of the pathologic, genetic, psychologic, environmental, and other aspects of mental retardation.

PROGRAMS OF THE FEDERAL GOVERNMENT

Primary responsibility within the Federal government for activities relating to mental retardation is located in the Department of Health, Education, and Welfare. Within the Department these programs are administered by four operating agencies—the Public Health Service, Office of Education, Social Security Administration, and Vocational Rehabilitation Administration—and may be grouped under four main categories: (1) research and studies; (2) professional preparation; (3) services; and (4) construction of a limited number of facilities that qualify for assistance under the hospital and medical facilities construction (Hill-Burton) program.

Research activities include (1) the intramural and extramural support programs of the National Institute of Mental Health, the National Institute of Neurological Diseases and Blindness, and the Center for Research in Child Health of the Public Health Service; (2) the Office of Education programs of studies, surveys, and cooperative research; (3) special project grants under the maternal and child health program of the Children's Bureau, Social Security Administration; and (4) the research and demonstration projects of the Vocational Rehabilitation Administration.

Professional preparation is supported through (1) Vocational Rehabilitation Administration grants to educational institutions for training of personnel for all phases of rehabilitation; (2) teaching and training grants of the National Institutes of Health; (3) intramural training programs of the Public Health Service; and (4) Office of Education training grants to colleges and universities and State educational agencies for leadership positions in the education of the mentally retarded.

Services include consultation and technical assistance in their respective areas of competence by (1) the Children's Bureau, under the maternal and child health and the child welfare services programs; (2) Vocational Rehabilitation Administration to State rehabilitation agencies; (3) the National Institute of Mental Health through its regional office staffs; and (4) the Office of Education to State and local school systems, educational personnel and voluntary groups. In addition, financial assistance to States is provided under the Federal-State programs of public assistance, and benefit payments for the disabled are made under the Federal program of old-age, survivors, and disability insurance.

In the 1963 fiscal year, the Department of Health, Education, and Welfare anticipates expenditures in excess of $28 million from general funds for research, training, and services in the field of mental retardation. This total represents an increase of $4.3 million over the estimated level of funds available for this purpose for fiscal year 1962 and more than doubles the $12.4 million spent by the Department five years ago. In addition, it is estimated that over $63 million will be paid from the old-age, survivors, and disability insurance trust funds to persons with diagnosed mental deficiency—primarily adults who have had disabilities from childhood.

MENTAL RETARDATION AND THE FUTURE

The acceleration of effort—private and public—already has produced some encouraging results. Progress has been made in identifying specific disorders and their treatment, in training personnel, in providing additional facilities, and in improving services generally. Special education classes have multiplied. More rehabilitations have been completed, and parents get better counseling.

Even though such progress is gratifying, mental retardation will continue to be a problem of national concern. Unless there are major advances in methods of prevention, there will be as many as one million more mentally retarded persons by 1970.

Improved and more extensive prenatal, obstetric and pediatric care have brought about marked increases in the infant survival rate in the Nation over the past 20 years. Such efforts, along with increasing the chances of survival of all infants, have also increased the survival rates of infants who are premature or who have congenital handicaps or malformations. Since mental retardation is one of the major conditions associated with such handicaps in infants, improved care has to an extent also increased the number of the retarded for whom special services will be needed.

Disease control, new drugs, and higher standards of living have steadily increased the life span of most Americans. While the mentally retarded as a group fall below the average life expectancy, the number of years the average retarded individual lives has been increasing proportionately with the overall average. This increase in life span adds materially to the number of mentally retarded persons, particularly in the upper age levels. With the increased availability of health services, the life span of mentally retarded persons may continue to increase and move closer to the average life expectancy of the general population.

The increased survival rates of retarded infants will probably bring with it an increase in the number of retarded persons who have associated physical handicaps. Current reports from clinical programs dealing with retarded children under six years of age indicate that even now in this group, 75 per cent have associated physical disabilities. Likewise, because the older individuals are now living longer, we can expect many of them to present the physical problems of the aged in the general population.

Because of changing social and economic conditions, some of the problems of mentally retarded persons will become more acute in the future:

1. *Families are growing larger* and in fewer instances will a retarded child be an only child.

2. *More mothers of young children are in the labor force.* Many times the factors that induce mothers to work are even more forceful for the mother who has a retarded child. Substitute care for the retarded child, however, is more difficult to obtain. Frequently, too, the retarded child is less able to understand the need for a parent substitute, which makes planning more difficult to carry out.

3. *More children are going to school longer.* The general level of education is rising in the Nation. As this trend continues, the mentally retarded whose disability shows itself in this area will be more marked. As educational standards and achievements continue to rise, a greater number of individuals who cannot keep up or achieve these levels will be discovered and will demand attention.

4. *Machines replace unskilled labor.* In the past, the majority of the mentally retarded children completing special classes for the educable in urban areas were able to find jobs on their own. There is some question whether this will continue to be so in the next 10 years without additional special help. Increased industrial specialization, automation and the intensified tempo of industrial production, pose new problems. Elevated educational standards in rural areas also are adding to the problem. Farming, which years ago provided a field of

employment for many of the retarded, has become so highly specialized that persons who would have been employed in the past have a difficult time finding employment at all now.

THE PRESIDENT'S PANEL ON MENTAL RETARDATION

Thus the problem of mental retardation presents a major challenge to society: to find causes, to seek prevention, and to provide the best possible assurance for lives of maximum usefulness. Manifestly, the needs remain great for more knowledge, more personnel, more facilities, and more services.

In October, 1961, President Kennedy appointed a panel of physicians, scientists, educators, lawyers, psychologists, social scientists and other leaders to review present programs and needs, to ascertain gaps, and to prescribe a program of action. The President has asked the Panel to formulate a national plan to combat mental retardation and to report to him on or before December 31, 1962. The Panel's recommendations will provide the guidelines for future efforts and further progress in the years to come.

9. The Migrants

GEOGRAPHIC mobility among workers is characteristic of America's
labor force in the '60s, the space scientist and unskilled worker alike.
Particularly for unskilled and itinerant laborers, migrations produce
or intensify multiple health problems. Shafer and his colleagues review the health needs of an important group—agricultural workers
who follow the crops and pose a serious challenge to Public Health.

Health Needs of Seasonal Farmworkers and their Families*

JAMES K. SHAFER, M.D., DONALD HARTING, M.D.,

AND HELEN L. JOHNSTON

THE PAST 10 or even 20 years have brought few improvements in the
lives of migrant farmworkers and their families. A Public Health
Service report of 20 years ago and a 1960 report from California
describe the same lack of health care for nearly a million U.S. citizens.
In 1940, the situation was summarized in these words. "The effect of
transients on community health is to increase the hazard of ill health
to residents and to raise the incidence of most of the communicable

* Reprinted by permission, with the omission of one illustration, from the
June, 1961 issue of *Public Health Reports*, Vol. 76, pp. 469–474. This
paper is based on a speech by Dr. Shafer at the Conference on Families
Who Move With The Crops, San Jose, California, October 23–24, 1960.
The authors are, respectively, Health Adviser, Office of Emergency Plan-
ning, Executive Offices of the President, Washington, D.C., formerly
Chief, Division of Community Health Practice, Public Health Service,
U.S. Department of Health, Education, and Welfare, Washington, D.C.;
Director, Center for Research in Child Health, National Institutes of
Health, Bethesda, Maryland, formerly Assistant Chief, Division of Com-
munity Health Practice, Public Health Service, U.S. Department of
Health, Education, and Welfare, Washington, D.C.; Deputy Chief,
Migrant Health Section, Division of Community Health Services, Bureau
of State Services, Public Health Service, U.S. Department of Health,
Education, and Welfare, Washington, D.C., formerly Public Health
Adviser, Public Health Administration Branch, Division of Community
Health Practice.

diseases. This results chiefly from the fact that transients are not given equal consideration in community programs of sanitation, preventive medicine, and isolation of infectious cases of communicable disease."[1]

Eleven years later a Colorado physician remarked: "We know that communicable diseases are present among the migrants. The fatalistic acceptance of the situation, plus their poverty, makes the problem of medical care a critical one."[2] And a Florida observer commented: "Many of the older ones just accept sickness as part of life, just as they do being out of work or living in a shack."[3] The California reports in 1960 summed it up as "the almost complete nonavailability of medical care and the inadequacy of preventive services available to this group of workers."[4]

Another California study indicated that about one out of five adults among itinerant farm laborers included in a recent study by the State vocational rehabilitation service had some kind of disability.[5] Half of these disabled adults suffered seriously reduced earning capacity. The report concludes: "Due to their standard of living, they are . . . apt to have serious unresolved health problems and major disability."

HOUSING

In many areas, the usual living and working conditions of seasonal farmworker families contribute to disease and disability. Some families live in large, well-built, well-maintained, and well-managed farm labor camps with good toilets, adequate water supply, and regular garbage and trash collection. Others live in rows of makeshift units where there is little regard for human health, safety, or decency. Ditchwater is used for drinking and washing, filthy privies for human waste, and the camp and its surroundings for dumping garbage. Heating and cooking equipment improvised from discarded oil drums or other makeshift materials constitute both a fire and an accident hazard.

In the unincorporated communities and fringe areas of towns where some of these families own or rent their own housing, conditions are often as bad as in the worst camps.

Young children brought to local clinics show the results in severe burns, diarrhea, impetigo, and respiratory infections. There is no effective way to quarantine the results of poor housing within the particular area where the housing exists. When families move, the consequences of a bad situation may go with them, and filthborne diseases may be spread to others even though all presently live in a good camp.

As they travel for long distances, the families need overnight shelter and places to use as rest stops. In many parts of the country, this need is completely overlooked. No stops may be made for journeys of several hundreds of miles because the driver is told to move on wherever he attempts to park his bus or truck. As a result, the families must use the side of the road between towns for infrequent rest stops.

FIELD SANITATION

Large-scale agriculture of the type that employs migrant farmworkers is a notable exception to the rule requiring the mainte-nance of sanitation standards at work locations. In other businesses and industry, we do not tolerate a complete lack of toilets, drinking water, or handwashing facilities where people are employed all day. This is still the widely accepted practice in commercial agriculture.

Testimony offered early in 1960 at the Cobey Committee hearings in California indicates that although slight risk to the health of con-sumers results from the lack of field facilities, a sound field sanitation program would have definite psychologic benefits to consumers and sociological benefits to the workers. It seems likely to be only a matter of time until consumers will insist upon good sanitation practices being followed in fields and orchards. Their esthetic sense, if nothing more, will be offended beyond the point of tolerance as they become increas-ingly aware of the conditions under which some of their food is picked.

The workers themselves also object to the lack of field sanitation facilities. One picker told a representative of the California Council of Churches: "There were no restrooms in the fields where we worked last season. We went down the row far away where there was nobody working and nobody could see us. The women do not like to work in the fields because of this."

Both the housing and the field sanitation situations introduce con-flict into migrant health programs. On the one hand, we health workers may try diligently to care for patients with diarrhea when they come to our attention, but we are treating only a symptom if we neglect the poor sanitary conditions which are the underlying cause. From time to time we also try to teach the workers how to maintain their own health. But what good is it to teach a worker about safe water if his only supply is obviously unsafe? And of how much value is education about good personal health practices if the only toilet is between rows of field crops or a filthy privy?

OCCUPATIONAL HEALTH

Control of occupational hazards is notably lacking in com-mercial agriculture. In still another respect, this type of enterprise has a strange immunity. Children under 15, working or not, are seldom seen in a large factory. Yet children under 15, some of them workers, suffer each year from disabling accidents in industrial agriculture. Sometimes the mangled hands or arms suffered by young children who get caught in harvesting machinery have alerted a community to the larger migrant health problem.[6,7]

Occupational risks arise not only from machines, ladders, and other farm equipment but also from agricultural poisons. Sometimes crops are sprayed while workers are in the fields, or without regard for the proximity of workers' housing. Pickers sent into the fields too soon after spraying may also suffer from poisoning. Cases of parathion poisoning affecting 70 crop workers were reported in the *Journal of the American Medical Association*.[8] Last summer a 2½-year-old boy died in a labor camp in Illinois, apparently because he drank from a jar that still contained a little of the milky liquid used to spray cabbages.

Transportation to and from the labor camp or nearby town to the worksite, as well as long-distance transportation, is still another hazard of agricultural work. Such transportation may be by rattletrap bus or other makeshift vehicle.

On the east coast, discarded school buses, some of them decked in bright new coats of paint, are replacing many of the trucks that were used to haul workers to and from the fields as well as from State to State. Some crewleaders are making an honest effort to meet the recent regulations of the Interstate Commerce Commission.[9] In many places, however, there is no regulation to govern short hauls of farmworkers.

HEALTH SERVICES

In a study of a group of Spanish-speaking migrants, sponsored by Texas, Michigan, and the Public Health Service, few if any had previously had contact with a Public Health agency.[10]

Our experience in Texas and Michigan showed that there can be no assurance that a service started in one location will be completed in another, even when a migrant follows instructions. One family, for example, had their first immunizations without charge in a local health department clinic in Texas. The mother went to the local health department in the north, as she had been instructed, but was referred to a private physician since the health department did not give inoculations. The physician charged a fee for each of the children for the second injections. The mother did not return for the third. This is hardly surprising in view of the typically uncertain income of such families and their lack of conviction of the value of such preventive services as vaccination.

Followup may be difficult even when a community makes an effort.

The results of chest X-rays, for example, often become available after migrant families have moved to a new location. Local health workers in the new area may find that the information forwarded to them about the time the family will arrive or the place where they will work is incomplete or inaccurate. Even if the sick person is found, it may be hard to persuade him to go to a hospital. He may have a strong compulsion to work while work is available so that his family will have something to live on for the rest of the year. Moreover, his fear of disease may be far less than his fear of an "Anglo" hospital where rules bar him from seeing his family and friends.

Fear and lack of understanding or acceptance of our health ways are factors that must be considered in trying to adapt the usual community health services to the special circumstances of seasonal farmworkers and their families. These reasons, rather than neglect, may explain why few of these families have had immunizations and why cases of illness they bring to a physician or clinic may be far advanced. In the Texas-Michigan project the use of folk remedies for treatment of a young infant delayed the family's taking her to a hospital for about a week. The baby died on the same day she was finally taken to a hospital.

Some conventional health methods make little sense when looked at from the migrant family's point of view. Special clinics, for example, held at different times and places for different purposes are time consuming, costly if a family must arrange and pay for transportation, and result in loss of income if time must be taken from work, since a migrant paid on a piece rate or hourly basis earns only while he works.

Our earlier example of the mother whose children needed to complete their immunization series is another case in point. The conditions under which the first injections were obtained were quite different from those in another location. Generally we expect the migrant to make all the adjustments as he seeks needed health care in one work area after another.

CURRENT MIGRANT HEALTH ACTIVITIES

The West Side clinics in Fresno County, Calif., have circumvented some of these problems by the excellent cooperative relationships maintained over the years among the medical society, county hospital, health department, local growers, welfare department, and other groups. The clinics have been possible because of the grant from the Rosenberg Foundation that helped get them started and the continuing interest and wholehearted support of many local citizens.

At first, it wasn't easy to encourage the families in Fresno County to take advantage of clinic services. There were more staff than patients at a few of the early clinic sessions, and the first patient at an early maternity clinic was a man. The clinic staffs gradually learned, through experience, that papa and his needs had to be considered, as well as mama and the children, if Spanish-speaking migrant families were to use the health services offered. Furthermore, clinics had to be scheduled in the evening so that people wouldn't lose time from work.

Now the Fresno County clinics are proud that mothers come for prenatal care before the sixth month of pregnancy. Before the clinics started, some mothers would have gone without medical care even at the time of delivery. The clinics have also turned out to be a good device for tuberculosis and venereal disease casefinding, in part because the relationship between the families and the physicians and nurses encourages visits to the clinic for care when symptoms first appear rather than after an emergency develops. The frequent friendly contact of the county health department's nurses with families in the labor camps is still another important factor in the Fresno County operation and may be one of the keys to the success of the West Side clinics.

There are few demonstrations such as that in Fresno County elsewhere in the Nation. Health services for migrant families are usually sporadic, unplanned, and unorganized within as well as between communities.

If the million-plus migrants, including domestic workers and their families and foreign workers, were all settled in one place, they would be surrounded by an organized network of services to protect and maintain health. Instead, the people are scattered and groups of varying size and composition travel to widely separated counties of the same State or different States to work each year. Each new community that becomes their temporary home has its own unique network of services, adapted to the needs and convenience of its own permanent residents. Usually built into this network are restrictions that limit the services available to outsiders.

LOCAL AND STATE ACTION

To improve the health of migrants, many different types of action might be taken. The improvement of housing seems a good place for most communities and States to start, since this would automatically relieve some other problems. A start on several fronts could logically be made.

1. Educate the community, including growers and migrant families, as to the basic requirements for providing and maintaining safe, healthful housing. This would be a first step toward developing understanding and relationships that would support good housing and crowd out bad. At present the grower who provides good housing receives no sure reward, and the one who neglects his workers' housing suffers no

sure penalty. Even where housing codes set standards, inspections may be infrequent and cursory.

2. Determine the elements of motivation, planning, and management that make it financially possible, and perhaps profitable, for some employers to provide good housing in the same area where others provide rudimentary shelter.

3. Develop simple construction plans and mass-production techniques, if they do not exist, to reduce the cost of acceptable housing.

4. Develop methods of financing housing adapted to (a) the migrant himself if a permanent farm-labor-supply pool is needed in a particular area; (b) growers and their associations; or (c) the community, if a public authority of some type would be the appropriate agency to provide, maintain, and manage housing.

Another greatly needed step is for large-scale agriculture to accept more of the responsibilities long ago assumed by large-scale industry. California has taken a step in this direction by its extension of workmen's compensation coverage to agricultural employment. In field sanitation, control of work hazards, and other matters pertinent to the health and well-being of workers and families, growers generally have a long way to go.

Agriculture differs from other industry in some important respects. Nevertheless, this difference does not justify a do-nothing policy.

In the provision of health services, a California physician warns that a "major roadblock to solving the health problems of seasonal farmworkers is the ease with which we can, if we let ourselves, pass the problem on to someone else, and not tackle it as it must be tackled—as a community health problem."[11] Certainly, the community where a person lives at a particular time is the place where he can best receive the health care he needs. Moreover, the community where a migrant makes an economic contribution owes him some assurance of service on a par with that received by other local citizens while he works in the area.

NATIONAL RESPONSIBILITY

Although emphasizing local and State responsibility is appropriate, the periodic shifting of workers and families from one community to another implies the added need for national leadership and assumption of responsibility. The separate action of single communities and States is likely to result in the duplication of some services to migrant families and gaps in others. Interstate planning and exchange, across the continent if necessary, can be facilitated by active national leadership and participation.

Recent Public Health Service efforts devoted solely to migrant workers have consisted of limited consultation and technical assistance, chiefly what three people in the Division of Community Health Practice could do on a part-time basis. Other programs have included migrant health within their scope, but this has not been their major focus. Some of us feel that our past effort has been grossly inadequate in view of the fact that the migrant health situation represents an indefensible gap in the application of knowledge we have long ago applied to the general population.

We in the Public Health Service also feel quite strongly that waiting for the problem to disappear is no way to deal with it. The Service report of 20 years ago and the California report of 1960 bear out this contention. The problem recurs with the same regularity as the crop seasons. Mechanization and other changes in farming and employment practices have radically changed some local situations. They have not affected the national situation materially in recent years. The fluctuations in local and State situations seem to us, however, to add to the necessity for national leadership in order to keep what is done adjusted to current needs.

Some have felt that the number of persons in the farm migrant population as compared, for example, with those affected by chronic diseases and automobile accidents make their health needs negligible for consideration at the national level. We do not share this view. Instead we look at the situation as evidence of about a half-century lag in the application of existing knowledge to a sizable population, one as large as the 1960 census shows for any one of more than a dozen States.

Moreover, the size of the migrant population is not an accurate measure of the extent of the problem. Each time a person moves with his family he must have adequate shelter, safe drinking water, and safe methods of disposal of human and other waste at his new location. Each new community must also be ready to provide him with health services according to his need while he is in the local area. For these reasons, we feel that a more accurate measure of the national problem can be obtained by multiplying the population by at least the number of times the people move each season. Using two as a multiplication factor would be conservative.

In 1960 the president of the American Public Health Association submitted a proposal to the Senate Subcommittee on Migratory Labor.[12] The Public Health Service has endorsed the principles outlined in the association statement. We agree that there is urgent need for health aid for migrants, including preventive health measures, arrangements for medical care, training for health leadership within the migrant group, and further study to determine cultural blocks and other difficulties that restrict provision and acceptance of health care.

The health needs of seasonal farmworker families are as broad as those of other families. Accordingly, the health aid available to them should encompass the range of preventive and curative services offered by communities to their permanent residents. The experience of many years has demonstrated, however, that without adaptation the usual community services often fail to reach seasonal farmworker families. To be effective in meeting their health needs, services must be geographically accessible, geared to the families' living and working situation, culturally acceptable, and planned in a way that relates the services of one area to those for the same families elsewhere.

Family health services alone, of course, are not the answer. With these must go services to safeguard living and working conditions in order to prevent needless illness and disability. With the further addition of a strong health education focus to both types of activities, the worker and his family will be helped most effectively. They will then be on the road to assuming responsibility for their own health needs in an effective way.

1. Blankenship, C. F., and Safer, F.: *A study of medical problems associated with transients.* Pub. Health Bull. No. 258. Washington, D.C., U.S. Government Printing Office, 1940, 132 pp.

2. Thomas, H. E., and Taylor, F.: *Migrant farm labor in Colorado.* New York, National Child Labor Committee, 1951, 116 pp.

3. Koos, E. L.: *They follow the sun.* Jacksonville, Fla., State Board of Health, 1957, 55 pp.

4. *Background information for the western interstate conference on migratory labor.* Berkeley, Calif., State Department of Public Health, 1960.

5. *Itinerant farm labor project.* Sacramento, Calif., State Department of Education, Vocational Rehabilitation Service, 1960, 10 pp. (Mimeographed.)

6. Work Injuries in California Agriculture. San Francisco, Calif., State Department of Industrial Relations, 1957, 25 pp.

7. Bishop, S.: Health problems of migrant children. *Am. Child.* 39:6, 12, January, 1957.

8. Quimby, E., and Lemmon, A. B.: Parathion residues as a cause of poisoning in crop workers. *J.A.M.A.* 166:741–746, Feb. 15, 1958.

9. *An act to provide for the regulation of the interstate transportation of migrant farm workers.* P.L. 939, ch. 905, 84th Cong. Washington, D.C., U.S. Government Printing Office, 1956.

10. Atwater, J. B.. et al.: *Texas-Michigan migrant health project.* Washington, D.C., Public Health Service, 1961. (To be published.)

11. Jessup, R. B.: Health of migrants. *California Health* 17:177–184, Apr. 15, 1960.

12. Letter by Malcolm Merrill, M.D., President APHA, to Hon. Harrison Williams, chairman, Senate Subcommittee on Migratory Labor, April 15, 1960. *In Hearings before Subcommittee of the Committee on Appropriations,* U.S. Senate, 86th Cong., 2d sess., H.R. 11390, p. 992.

10. The Travelers

Satisfaction and Stress in Working Overseas*

THE PSYCHOLOGIC rewards for the person who decides to take an overseas assignment are many. At first sight, the work may represent mainly an opportunity for personal advancement, escape, or variety. But no matter what the immediate motivation, the chance to live and work outside one's own country over a period of time often satisfies a deep human need to have personal experience of the world beyond one's horizon.

There is of course the satisfaction of the particular work accomplished. Then there are additional satisfactions for the man with specific interest in foreign affairs, cultural studies, political science, economics, or language studies. There is a reward for the person interested in world-wide cooperation in specific areas of business or science. There can be special pleasure for those who love to teach or to be taught. There are others who derive their satisfaction from patriotic motivations, as well as those who particularly seek rewards in the form of honor, status, or prestige. Some derive much-needed financial security in the form of higher salaries and pensions, as well as others who go abroad at considerable personal self-sacrifice for a specific humanitarian reason. The motivations are many and varied; the rewards may be great or small, depending upon the individual himself and upon circumstances he cannot foresee or control.

In general it may be said, however, since the majority of persons (except those in governmental or military service) go abroad of their own free choice to live and work, that the rewards of working overseas are obvious and real to those who choose to go. Nevertheless, even for them, there are psychologic stresses, which are not either apparent or anticipated.

ENVIRONMENTAL CHANGES AND "CULTURE SHOCK"

When an individual moves from his home to *any* new and unfamiliar place, it involves certain basic changes in his habits, relationships and sources of satisfaction, and produces a different pattern

* Reprinted in part, by permission, from *Working Abroad: A Discussion of Psychological Attitudes and Adaptations in New Situations*, formulated by the Committee on International Relations of the Group for the Advancement of Psychiatry, Inc., Report Number 41, published by the Group, New York, New York, December 1958, pages 491–495.

of stresses from the ones to which he had become accustomed. When the change is the still larger one of moving to a different country and culture, the adaptation required assumes even greater significance. Inherent in such a move, of course, is the opportunity to leave behind, if only temporarily, one set of relationships and life-patterns, and to enrich one's life by establishing new ones, with new satisfactions. Nevertheless, even the well-integrated person sent overseas is likely, especially at first, to have a sense of geographic dislocation or isolation, a feeling of "being out of things;" he often finds an intensified need for communication with home, a sense of frustration over the inevitable slowness of establishing the feeling, of "belonging" locally, and a feeling of boredom brought about by the monotony and limitations of social life.

"The overseas employee and his family are required to adjust to the foreign situation with its frequently more difficult climate, poor sanitation, lack of formal entertainment, inadequate housing, circumscribed social activity; they are expected to work effectively with people who have a different temperament, language, religion, culture . . . different ways of doing things, different values . . . different concepts of time, etc. The most difficult jobs are those which require the employee to work extensively or exclusively with the indigenous people with minimal supervision or support."[1]

Primarily, the success or failure of the adjustment to the overseas situation depends upon the individual's personality, temperament, and capacity for adaptation. (This is not meant to exclude group and social factors which will be considered later.) Generally it has been found to hold true that if a man has been able to live and function happily and effectively at home, he is likely to be successful in his transition to overseas life. When there are unsettled psychologic or emotional difficulties, these are usually transferred to the new situation. Occasionally, the new environment may be favorable for the individual and his particular emotional difficulty, but far more frequently the difficulty becomes aggravated. This likelihood emphasizes the importance and value of careful screening with special reference to the nature of his work and the country to which he will be sent.

Surveys show that those who have worked well and happily abroad generally have the following qualities: flexibility, personal stability, social maturity, and "social inventiveness." They either have fewer prejudices or a greater awareness of them, and the ability to tolerate the objects of their prejudice.

An important psychologic factor relating to emotional stress abroad is the degree of reality in the individual's expectations. Some persons' anticipations are unrealistic, even grandiose. For instance, some people with adolescent phantasies take overseas jobs hoping to "save the world." They have irrational concepts of "self," of others, and of the amount of time required for changes in attitudes and habits. For the person whose expectations of himself or of his job are excessive, the frustrations may be so great that he will find it hard to concentrate on the work to be done, or to see his role in it in proper perspective.

If an individual is unable to relate his new expreiences to his old ones, to see the foreign situation in terms of his own country's past development, to see the needs of another country through its own eyes, or to reach desired objectives through new or still-to-be-discovered methods, he may become disappointed, frustrated, and discouraged. Such feelings are then often expressed in the form of bitter criticism and hostility toward the foreign country, and are not recognized as the result of his excessive optimism, or his lack of realistic understanding of the problems, or of himself.

THE ROLE OF THE FAMILY

Marital situations may also cause either special psychologic distress or satisfaction overseas. Ordinarily the man who goes abroad with his family finds that he is thrown into a more intense relationship with them than he had at home. For some Americans, this greater proximity results in greater intimacy and understanding than had been the case at home. For others, basic difficulties within a family relationship become accentuated in the closer living, with fewer opportunities for diverse activities or substitute outlets.

Many men who go overseas find a continuity in their work, which makes a bond between their life at home and the life abroad; some even feel a greater sense of usefulness overseas than at home. Certainly many men find their new job extremely challenging and their time fully occupied. But some wives, particularly those who may have given up jobs or careers in order to accompany the family, experience a greater change of living habits than their husbands. Most wives find housekeeping radically different abroad with entirely new problems to cope with, e.g., having either much more or much less free time than they had at home, or completely new relationships with servants. Problems of schooling, shopping, transportation, can defeat even the most devoted and resourceful wife. And there are such matters as face-saving and "squeeze"—i.e., being obliged to pay higher prices due to lack of knowledge of local language and resources, and being dependent on certain local persons—which she must be prepared to meet. Often when she calls on her husband for help, he may not know what to do any more than she does, and he may take refuge in his own work and his more pressing problems.

For these reasons, agencies which send employees abroad tend nowadays to consider the prospective applicant *and* his family as a *unit,* and try to determine not only the man's but the *wife's* and the *family's* readiness for life and work overseas. In the words of one

Foreign Service officer, "The adjustment and training for overseas for wives is as important as the adjustment and training of the men. I have seen men overseas, doing well at their jobs, become unhappy and dissatisfied because their wives became dissatisfied."

Still another source of psychologic reward or distress for the individual may arise from the living arrangements and customs of the group with whom the American employee is to associate. While technical assistance and voluntary agency personnel often live separately because of the nature of their work, the majority of Americans working abroad tend to live within American groups. When, for example, the employing organization provides organized housing, many Americans overseas derive considerable security from being able to live in circumstances of physical comfort and safety, not too different from those at home, in a small community of fellow-Americans to which they can "really belong." Often, however, such "colonies" or "compounds" interfere with any real contact with the native population, and may involve social ostracism of individuals who have the interest or desire to make such contact. The U.S. citizen who derives sufficient satisfaction from his work, his family relationships, and the limited community, may feel content. On the other hand, the individual who was inclined to go abroad in the first place because of his interest in or curiosity about other cultures, or out of a sense of adventure, may find himself seriously limited and frustrated.

In considering the psychologic rewards and stresses for anyone going overseas to work, one should not make the mistake of emphasizing only rewards and stresses as the determining factors in the ultimate state of mental health for any individual. They are probably only of somewhat greater significance overseas than at home. In the overseas situation, the primary factors in an individual's mental health are his already existent *personality*, his degree of satisfaction or adaptation in his family, his work, his social contacts, his *recreational* situation, and the particular dynamic balance among them.

1. "Observations of Some Aspects of Performance and Adjustment of MSA and TCA American Personnel in Asia," by Dr. Mottram Torre, 1953, unpublished.

PART THREE

The Settings: Arenas of Health Service

1. Health Administration in Federal Government   275
2. Health Administration in Other Jurisdictions   308
3. The Hospital and Regionalization   332
4. The School: A Primary Setting   346
5. The Armed Services   360
6. The Voluntary Health Agency   374
7. Cooperation among Agencies   390

PUBLIC HEALTH has developed a complex planning and administrative machinery to carry out its goals of disease prevention and health promotion. This machinery, in Reichert's words,[1] "enables Public Health to study all aspects of health and disease in any population group or in the physical and social environment; to maintain a flow of information about changing health needs and resources; to render service or to give protection anywhere in the human life cycle through its own services or through arrangements with other social institutions; to focus its intervention on individuals, groups, communities or their environments; to deploy its manpower in response to shifting priorities and changing techniques."

This complex machinery, the functional roles and relationships of Public Health agencies and cooperating community groups constitute the main subject-matter of this Section. The statutory foundations of Government agencies, and the programs and functions they have evolved are reviewed by leading officials. All the varied interrelationships of financing, standard-setting, demonstration, and program development cannot be fully set forth in brief papers, but the many-faceted programs and issues are outlined here.

The ultimate test and product of Federal and State activities are to be found on the local level—city, county, and regional. Dr. James' comprehensive account of a large city's multiple activities describes the application of most of the instrumentalities of investigation and action in the Public Health armory. Obviously, smaller cities cannot do all or many of these things; but the paper illustrates how Public Health resources can be marshalled and deployed against the needs of an urban complex.

The role of a major resource in community health service—the Hospital—is considered, along with regional hospital planning, which has become an important method for the more adequate and equitable distribution of services.

The importance of the School Health Service for the detection and prevention of disease in a natural setting is discussed, and illustrated. The contributions to health knowledge of Armed Service programs of research and care are reviewed by Dr. Francis. Aspects of voluntary agency collaboration in Public Health care are considered by Drs. Katz and Hamlin. Of major significance to Public Health are the expanding programs of medical care for the needy, collaboratively organized by public departments of health and welfare, which are described in the concluding papers in this Section.

1. Reichert, Kurt: "Application of Public Health Concepts and Methods to the Field of Social Work," *1963 Proceedings, Annual Program Meeting*. January 1963 (Council on Social Work Education).

1. Health Administration in Federal Government

Role of the Public Health Service in Medical Care in the United States—Trends in Medical Care*

GOVERNMENTAL MEDICAL CARE ACTIVITIES

A trend to be considered in our review of medical care activities is the increasing number and complexity of governmental activities in this field. In recent decades there has been a growth in direct governmental health and medical services, in governmental financial support of private medical services, in public aid for the construction of facilities, and in public regulation of medical care personnel and facilities. All levels of government—Federal, State, and local—have participated in these programs, with the problem of coordinating the various activities becoming increasingly great.

Public hospitals have long included municipal and county general hospitals, and specialized institutions for tuberculosis patients and the mentally ill. Federal hospitals for many years have served such special beneficiary groups as military personnel, veterans, merchant seamen, and American Indians. In recent years the use of these public hospitals has increased at almost the same rate as the population. For example, in 1950, there were 4,991,000 admissions to Federal, State, and local governmental hospitals, at a rate of 33 per 1000 population; in 1959 this figure was 6,106,000, at a rate of 35 per 1000 population. In the intervening years the average daily census increased from 942,000 to 973,000, the rate per 1000 population changing from 6.3 to 5.5.[1,2]

Public health nursing, a traditional part of the local Public Health department's activities, has assumed growing importance with the development of organized home care programs for the chronically ill and aged. Health department nurses, in cooperation with nurses employed by voluntary visiting nurse associations, can be expected to

* Reprinted, in part, with omission of one table, by permission from *Medical Care in The United States—The Role of the Public Health Service*. Report to the Surgeon General from the National Advisory Health Council, March 1961, published by the U.S. Department of Health, Education, and Welfare, Public Health Service, pp. 17–22.

provide an increasing amount of bedside care, as well as carrying on their traditional preventive health functions.

Public health and medical programs for mothers and children, crippled children, persons in need of vocational rehabilitation, and those with tuberculosis or other infectious diseases have a fairly long history. Of more recent origin have been the community-oriented programs for the promotion of mental health and for the detection of diabetes and other chronic disease. Other governmental programs have provided financial aid for construction of hospitals and related medical facilities.

In recent years, a growing variety of governmental programs has emerged to help in financing private medical services. Examples of Federal support are the "home-town care" programs of the Veterans Administration and the Medicare program of the Department of Defense, each of which pays for care of Federal beneficiaries through private medical resources. Many State and local welfare authorities make payments for private medical care of public assistance recipients, with partial matching from Federal funds. These payments are scheduled to be expanded under newly established Federal grants for medical aid to the aged. The recently adopted program of health insurance for Federal employees is financed jointly by employee and Government funds.

In relation to total health and medical care expenditures, governmental expenditures grew more rapidly in the early 1930's than they have since that time. In recent years their rise has just about paralleled that of private expenditures in this field. In a few areas, such as local Public Health services, governmental expenditures have actually lagged behind the growth of the population.

Although the medical profession still carries the largest responsibility for maintaining adequate standards of medical practice by individual doctors and in medical care institutions, there has been growing recognition of the need for public participation in promoting adequate standards. State licensing of health personnel, already highly developed for doctors, dentists, and nurses, is being extended gradually to cover such allied health groups as physical and occupational therapists, medical laboratory technicians, optometrists, pharmacists, practical nurses, and others, The Food and Drug Administration requires that pharmaceutic products meet increasingly high standards of safety and purity.

The demand for public regulation of health insurance plans can be expected to grow further as the number and size of such plans increase. At present, in most States, the regulation of health insurance plans is centered in State insurance commissioners who are concerned primarily with the financial soundness of the plans. However, public opinion is increasingly demanding that greater emphasis in the regulation process be placed on the kinds of benefits provided and that greater recognition be given to the interrelationship of financial mechanisms and the quality and quantity of care provided.

Among the governmental programs relating to medical care, those of the Public Health Service, which range from the multimillion dollar hospital survey and construction grant program to small experimental studies in the use of particular types of health manpower, are now described and analyzed.

CURRENT PUBLIC HEALTH SERVICE
ACTIVITIES IN MEDICAL CARE

The Public Health Service plays a significant role in many medical care activities, both in the direct provision of personal health services to certain Federal beneficiaries and in the evaluation or support of medical care resources available to the population generally. Important among its activities bearing on medical care resources for the people of the Nation are those relating to health status measurement, personnel, facilities, expenditures and financing, organization of services, and related aspects of medical services. Examples of activities in these fields are considered in the following discussion.

Analysis of Health Status and Use of Services

Several Public Health Service programs provide information on the health status of the Nation, the use of medical care services, and their relationships to socio-economic factors. Within the National Center for Health Statistics, the National Health Survey Program[3] and the National Office of Vital Statistics[4] compile and analyze data on the volume of medical care. In various parts of the Service, studies have been conducted dealing with the medical care needs of the aged,[5] of migrant workers,[6] and residents of rural counties.[7]

Indices such as those developed by the National Health Survey give a better understanding of the use of medical services and facilities, in relation to such factors as age, economic status, and insurance coverage.[8] Studies have been conducted of the factors that motivate people toward seeking health examinations.[9]

Personnel

The recruitment and training of health services manpower are among the highest priority problems in the field of medical care. The Public Health Service has given these problems considerable attention in recent years.

In addition to the activities of the Surgeon General's Consultant Group on Medical Education,[10] the Service has made numerous studies of supply, need, and education for other health professions including the preparation of manpower source books on physicians, dentists, nurses, social workers, and other personnel.[11] Traineeships and fellowships are provided in such areas as professional nursing, mental health work, and hospital and medical care administration.[12]

Among present studies are those relating to the training and utilization of dental assistants and practical nurses. A manual has been prepared to aid hospitals in making the best use of nursing personnel.[13]

Facilities

Over the past decade significant Federal support has been given to hospital planning and construction, under the Public Health Service's Hospital and Medical Facilities Construction (Hill-Burton) Program. The program has included assistance for the construction of general, tuberculosis, mental, and chronic disease hospitals. Recently, increased aid has been channeled to nursing homes, diagnostic and treatment centers, rehabilitation facilities, Public Health centers, and other facilities offering care outside hospitals.[14]

Currently the Service is conducting studies of Progressive Patient Care,[15] a program designed to furnish better care through organization of hospital services around the medical and nursing needs of the patient. Illustrative of the extramural research activities sponsored by the Public Health Service are the current studies of the regionalization of health care services, and a study of the hospital as a community health center.

Prominent among present Public Health Service activities relating to facilities are studies of nursing homes and related facilities with particular reference to such matters as the characteristics of the patients, the standards of facility construction, the quality of care provided, the methods of organizing and financing the homes, and licensing procedures.[16]

Expenditures and Financing

Apart from the necessary financial analysis that accompanies the administration of grant programs, Public Health Service studies of the details of medical care expenditures and financing have been piecemeal. Recently, however, there has been some compilation and analysis of consumer expenditures for medical care,[17] of services in prepaid dental care plans,[18] and of medical care costs in relation to public health.[19]

Organization of Services

The Public Health Service has demonstrated its concern with the organization of medical care services at the community level through its studies and promotion of organized home care programs,[20] homemaker services,[21] patient-referral systems, regionalization of health services,[22] and studies of group practice.[23]

Standards of Quality

The Service's attention to standards of quality has been focused mainly on nursing personnel and facility standards. In the latter area, the hospital and medical facilities construction program has given impetus to State licensure of hospitals and related medical facilities.

Personal Health Practices

Much of the health education activity in which the Public Health Service participates is aimed toward the improvement of personal health practices. In the area of restorative services, booklets have been developed to show patients how to further their own physical rehabilitation and reduce the disability from stroke[24] or arthritis.[25] Activities to stimulate State and local programs for diabetes and glaucoma screening and for cervical and breast cancer examination have as one of their objectives the encouragement of such preventive health practices as periodic health appraisal by a physician.

Expenditures for Medical Care Research

The Public Health Service is currently spending about $2.5 million to support research on the administration of hospital and medical care services. Voluntary agency and foundation spending in this area is probably somewhat less. This means that altogether perhaps $4–5 million, or 2/100 of 1 per cent of all health expenditures, is being invested in attempts to understand how a $25 billion industry functions and how to improve its operations.

Conclusion

These few examples of activities in which the Public Health Service is currently addressing itself to the problems of medical care suggest that in most of the areas of interest—personnel, facilities, organization, finance, standards—the Service can demonstrate some creditable program activity. In relation to the need for leadership, however, the present activities tend to be fragmentary, uneven, and lacking in focus. Some of the programs whose titles appear comprehensive (e.g., "Public Health traineeship program," "chronic disease demonstrations"), are found when scrutinized to be minute in relation to the magnitude of the problems with which they deal. Medical care administration is a complex process which includes the planning, organizing, financing, coordinating, and evaluation of all resources and services that a medical care program comprises. Few of these elements have received adequate attention and little attention has been paid to the totality of medical care administration.

1. Hospitals. V. 25, No. 6, Part 2. *Administrators Guide Issue,* June, 1951. Table 3.

2. Hospitals. V. 34, No. 15, Part 2. *Administrators Guide Issue.* August 1, 1960. Table 2C.

3. U.S. National Health Survey. *Health Statistics,* Series A-D. Washington, D.C., 1958 to present.

4. U.S. National Office of Vital Statistics. *Vital Statistics of the United States,* 2 Vols. Washington, D.C. Published annually.

5. Confrey, Eugene A., and Goldstein, Marcus S. "The Health Status of Aging People." *In Handbook of Social Gerontology.* Edited by Clark Tibbetts. University of Chicago Press, 1960. pp. 165–207.

6. Robinson, Norma J. "The Public Health Program for Mexican Migrant Workers." *Public Health Reports,* V. 73:851–860 (September 1958).

7. Harting, Donald, et al. "Public Health Needs and Practices in a Great Plains County." *American Journal of Public Health,* V. 49:1591–1595 (December 1959).

8. U.S. National Health Survey. Health Statistics from the National Health Survey: Interim Report on Health Insurance, United States: July–December 1959. *Public Health Service Publication* No. 584–B26. Washington, D.C., December 1960.

9. Borsky, Paul N., and Sagen, Oswald K. "Motivations Toward Health Examinations." *American Journal of Public Health,* V. 49:514–527 (April 1959).

10. Surgeon General's Consultant Group on Medical Education. Physicians for a Growing America. *Public Health Service Publication* No. 709. Washington, D.C., 1959.

11. U.S. Public Health Service. Health Manpower Source Book, Sections 1–10. *Public Health Service Publication* No. 263 (Sections 1–10). Washington, D.C., 1952–1960.

12. U.S. Public Health Service. Professional Nurse Traineeships. Parts I and II. *Public Health Service Publication* Nos. 675 and 676. Washington, D.C., 1959; ——. The Training Program of the National Institute of Mental Health, 1946–57. Washington, D.C., 1958.

13. U.S. Public Health Service. How to Study Nursing Activities in a Patient Unit. *Public Health Service Publication* No. 370. Washington, D.C., 1954.

14. U.S. Public Health Service. Ten Years of the Hill-Burton Hospital and Medical Facilities Program, 1946–56. *Public Health Service Publication* No. 616. Washington, D.C., 1958.

15. Haldeman, Jack C. "Progressive Patient Care: A Challenge to Hospitals and Health Agencies." *Public Health Reports,* V. 74:405–408 (May 1959).

16. Solon, Jerry, et al. Nursing Homes, Their Patients and Their Care. *Public Health Service Publication* No. 503. Washington, D.C., 1957; and U.S. Public Health Service. National Conference on Nursing Homes and Homes for the Aged, Feb. 25–28, 1958. *Public Health Service Publication* No. 625. Washington, D.C., 1958.

17. Mushkin, Selma. "Characteristics of Large Medical Expenses." *Public Health Reports,* V. 72:697–702 (August 1957).

18. Pelton, Walter J., and Rowan, John C. Digest of Prepaid Dental Care Plans, 1958. *Public Health Serv-*

ice Publication No. 585. Washington, D.C., 1958.

19. Unpublished Study of the World Health Organization.

20. A Study of Selected Home Care Programs: A Joint Project of the Public Health Service and the Commission on Chronic Illness. *Public Health Service Publication* No. 447. Washington, D.C., December 1955.

21. Homemaker Services in the United States: A Report of the 1959 Conference. *Public Health Service Publication* No. 746. Washington, D.C., 1960.

22. Mountin, J. W., Pennell, E. H.,

and Hoge, V. M. Health Service Areas: Requirements for General Hospitals and Health Centers. *Public Health Bulletin* No. 292. Washington, D.C., 1945.

23. Pomrinse, S. David, and Goldstein, Marcus S. "Group Practice in the United States." *Group Practice*, V. 9, No. 11 (November 1960).

24. U.S. Public Health Service. Strike Back at Stroke. *Public Health Service Publication* No. 596. Washington, D.C., 1958.

25. U.S. Public Health Service. Strike Back at Arthritis. *Public Health Service Publication* No. 747. Washington, D.C., 1960.

Federal Legislation Relating to Food*

GOVERNMENTAL protection for the consumer dates back to at least 300 B.C. when an Indian law prohibited the adulteration of grain, scents, and medicines. English laws of 1215 and 1597 provided for the seizure of certain harmful foods before they could reach the consumer.

In the United States the first laws passed by Congress for consumer protection dealt primarily with imports. An act passed in 1890 prevented the importation of adulterated food. The early legislation regulating foods and drugs produced in this country was enacted by individual States. At the turn of the century, however, an increasing proportion of foods and drugs was being shipped between States. The States were limited in their power to regulate foods from other areas and producers found it increasingly difficult to comply with the labeling provisions and other requirements which varied among States. Further, the consumer wanted protection from unscrupulous practices, while enjoying the wholesome products provided by reputable food producers. It became apparent that federal legislation was needed.

The first major legislation regulating food in this country was the Federal Food and Drugs Act (sometimes called the Pure Food Law) passed in 1906. The purpose of pure food legislation has been summed

* Reprinted, with omission of one illustration, by permission from *Food Additives—What They Are/How They Are Used,* published by the Manufacturing Chemists' Association, Inc., Washington, D.C., 1961, pages 37–44.

up by George P. Larrick, Commissioner of Food and Drugs, Department of Health, Education, and Welfare, writing in the 1959 Yearbook of Agriculture:

"Federal food laws for more than half a century have been dedicated to safety, wholesomeness, and the type of labeling that will permit citizens to make intelligent selections in their purchases. Telling people what to eat is attempted by education rather than regulation. Their choices affect the whole food industry, for in the long run the practices of manufacturers reflect consumers' wishes."

Two agencies in the government share responsibilities for insuring a safe and wholesome food supply. The Food and Drug Administration, which is a unit of the Department of Health, Education, and Welfare, is responsible for the enforcement of the Federal Food, Drug, and Cosmetic Act. The Department of Agriculture administers the Federal Meat Inspection and Poultry Products Inspection Acts and certain other laws relating to agriculture. A third governmental agency, the Federal Trade Commission, among other duties, has jurisdiction over false and misleading advertisements to the public regarding food.

THE EVOLUTION OF THE CURRENT FEDERAL FOOD, DRUG, AND COSMETIC ACT

This act, which regulates the purity of food, is an outgrowth of the Federal Food and Drugs Act of 1906. The 1906 law underwent a complete revision in 1938, and since then has had several major amendments.

THE FEDERAL FOOD AND DRUGS ACT, AS ORIGINALLY ENACTED IN 1906, made illegal the adulteration of food and drugs entering into interstate commerce. (Food and drugs produced locally for local consumption continued to be regulated by the individual states.) Adulteration of a food was defined to include the addition of poisonous and deleterious substances to foods, the extraction of valuable constituents, the concealment of inferiority, substitution of other articles or the mixture of substances which would adversely affect quality or strength.

The law contained some labeling restrictions. At that time the law was administered by the Secretary of Agriculture.

The law was recognized as good for its time. However, as conditions changed and advances were made in medical science and food technology, it became obvious that the law needed modernizing. A new bill was introduced in Congress in 1933; and after years of legislative hearings and many revisions, the Federal Food, Drug, and Cosmetic Act of 1938 was adopted.

THE FEDERAL FOOD, DRUG, AND COSMETIC ACT OF 1938 retained the provisions of the original act and added new provisions to meet the requirements of consumer protection under then current conditions. The 1938 Act, which is still the basic Federal legislation in this field, applies to exports and imports, and to commerce between the States and within the District of Columbia and the territories. While the law is a long and highly technical document, these points relating to food are pertinent to consumers.

Food is defined as "Articles used as food or drink for man or other animals, chewing gum, and articles used for components of any such article." While water is a drink and therefore a "food" under the act, public drinking water is usually the concern of the U.S. Public Health Service and State and local health departments.

The adulteration of food is prohibited. Food containing an added poisonous or deleterious substance is deemed to be unsafe unless the added substance is required or cannot be avoided by good manufacturing practice and a safe level of use has been established. Adulteration is also defined to include all kinds of cheating such as: the addition of a substance to increase bulk or weight, or to reduce strength or quality, or to make an article appear of greater value; the removal of a constituent which would ordinarily be expected to be present; the partial or complete substitution of one product for another; or concealing an inferior or damaged product.

Truthful labeling is made mandatory. The label must tell what is in the package, list the weight or volume of the contents, and must not be false or misleading in any way. Sometimes labels have been termed "misleading" when they fail to tell certain facts that the consumer has a right to expect. The label must give the name and place of business of the manufacturer, packer, or distributor. Required statements must be prominently placed on the label so as to be easily read.

Definitions and standards for foods are authorized whenever, in the judgment of the Secretary of Health, Education, and Welfare, such action will "promote honesty and fair dealing in the interest of consumers."

Standards of identity establish what a given product is—that is, what the consumer had a right to expect when he or she asks for the food by its common name. For example, the standard of identity for fruit preserves and jellies requires not less than 45 parts of fruit or fruit juice to each 55 parts of sugar. If less than that proportion of fruit or fruit juice is used, the product must be labeled "imitation." The standard of identity for any food contains a listing of both required and optional ingredients.

Standards of quality for a number of canned fruits and vegetables have been established. These minimum standards and specifications are for such factors as tenderness, color, and freedom from defects. If the food does not meet the standards, it must be labeled "Below Standard in Quality," followed by a statement such as "excessively broken" or another term to describe why the product fails to meet the standard.

Standards of fill of container tell the packer how full the container must be to avoid deception of the consumer. These standards are especially important for products that may shake down or settle after filling. Standards of fill have been established for such foods as shellfish, and some canned fruits and vegetables.

Some Foods for Which Definitions and Standards Have Been Published

Chocolate and cocoa products
Wheat and corn flour and related products
Macaroni and noodle products
Bakery products
Milk and cream
Cheese and cheese products
Dressings for food—mayonnaise, French dressing, salad dressing
Canned fruit and canned fruit juices
Fruit butters, jellies, preserves and related products
Shellfish
Canned tuna fish
Eggs and egg products
Oleomargarine, margarine
Canned vegetables and vegetable products

THREE MAJOR AMENDMENTS TO THE 1938 LAW

(1) THE MILLER PESTICIDE AMENDMENT to the Food, Drug, and Cosmetic Act of 1938 was passed in 1954. This Amendment establishes a procedure for the setting of safe amounts (generally referred to as tolerances) for residues of pesticides which may remain on fresh fruits, vegetables, and other raw agricultural commodities when shipped interstate. Under this Amendment, the Department of Agriculture certifies that the pesticide proposed by the manufacturer for use in killing insects, disease organisms, weeds, or other crop pests is useful for the purpose claimed. The Food and Drug Administration sets the tolerances for the quantities that may remain in or on the food. These tolerances are based on an evaluation of scientific evi-

dence (including results of animal tests) submitted by the pesticide manufacturer.

(2) THE 1958 FOOD ADDITIVES AMENDMENT to the Food, Drug, and Cosmetic Act had a two-fold purpose: (1) to protect the Public Health by requiring proof of safety before a substance may be added to a food, and (2) to advance food technology and improve the food supply by permitting the use in foods of substances which are safe at the levels of intended use.

The food and chemical industries as well as many consumer groups testified before congressional committees in support of the principle that safety testing should be required by law. Reputable manufacturers and users of food additives had always made thorough tests for safety and, prior to the 1958 legislation, had often consulted with Food and Drug officials during their investigations. There was, however, no provision in the law that made this pretesting or consultation mandatory, except in the case of certified colors. The use of an unsafe additive constituted adulteration, but to stop such use (after the food containing the additive was already being sold to the public), Food and Drug officials were required to demonstrate that such substances might be harmful or deleterious in some quantity.

Food additives which are subject to the Amendment are "any substance the intended use of which results or may reasonably be expected to result directly or indirectly in its becoming a component or otherwise affecting the characteristics of any food . . ." excluding those generally recognized by qualified experts as safe (GRAS in the Washington jargon) under the conditions of their intended use.

Under the Food Additives Amendment of 1958, before an additive may be used, the proponent of the additive must establish the safety of the proposed use of the additive, and must obtain from the Food and Drug Administration a regulation permitting that use. He must also satisfy the Administration that the additive will perform the function claimed for it and, if a limit is necessary, that the amount to be used is not greater than is reasonably required to achieve the intended effect. The regulation, when issued, may, if appropriate, place a tolerance (or quantity limitation on the amount which the food may contain) and must specify any other conditions of use that may be necessary to protect the Public Health.

The Amendment forbids issuance of any regulations permitting the use of any substance in any amount whatever which "is found to induce cancer in man or animals." This clause has caused a great deal of controversy. Many scientists feel the clause does not permit the exercise of scientific judgment and bars the use of substances for which safe tolerances or levels of use could be determined.

The definition further excludes color additives and substances used as pesticides on raw agricultural products (pesticides are covered by the provisions of the Pesticide Amendment of 1954), pesticide chemicals to the extent that they are intended for use or are used in the production, storage, or transportation of any raw agricultural commodity, and any substances used in accordance with any sanction or approval granted prior to the enactment of the Food Additives Amendment, pursuant to the Act itself or the Poultry Products Inspection Act, or the Meat Inspection Act.

Obviously, the definition of a food additive, as contained in the Amendment, is somewhat complicated and highly technical. The definition used in the publications of the Food Protection Committee of the National Academy of Sciences is perhaps more meaningful so far as the general public is concerned. The Committee defines a food additive as "a substance or mixture of substances, other than a basic foodstuff, which is present in a food as a result of any aspect of production, processing, storage, or packaging. The term does not include chance contaminants."

(3) THE COLOR ADDITIVE AMENDMENTS OF 1960 were enacted for several reasons. Prior to this legislation, coal-tar colors were controlled by a special provision of the Pure Food Law while all other colors added to food were covered under the Food Additives Amendment. All colors are now covered under the Color Additive Amendments.

Until this Color Additive Bill became effective, coal-tar colors could not be used unless the FDA listed them as "harmless and suitable for use." The provision provided further that each batch of the color must be certified for harmlessness by the FDA. No provision was made for tolerances for safe amounts. As a result, some colors which were completely safe in actual use were removed from the approved list because massive doses were shown to be harmful to experimental animals.

Under the Color Additive Amendments, a color additive is a substance which, when added to a food, drug or cosmetic, or to the human body, is capable of imparting color thereto. However, substances which are used solely for purposes other than color are not included in the definition of color additives under this amendment.

The Color Additive Amendments, like the Food Additive Amendment, permit industry to apply for tolerances for any colors if scientific evidence shows that the colors will be safe under normal conditions of use. Also like the Food Additives Amendment, no color may be approved in any amount whatsoever if it is found to induce cancer in man or animals.

The Color Additive Amendments provide that whenever a question arises as to whether a color additive may induce cancer, a scientific advisory committee will be established at the initiative of the FDA or at the request of any person who may be adversely affected by the FDA's decision. The advisory committee is to be composed of experts selected by the National Academy of Sciences. The committee is authorized to examine and report upon any matter arising in connection with the question of whether the additive will induce cancer, if such matter requires the exercise of scientific judgment.

OTHER LAWS AFFECTING FOOD ENTERING INTO INTERSTATE COMMERCE

THE FEDERAL MEAT INSPECTION ACT, passed in 1906, makes it illegal to ship meat and meat food products in interstate or foreign commerce unless they have been inspected and bear the stamp of approval of the Federal meat inspector. This act also requires the inspection of all cattle, sheep, swine, and goats before entering the slaughtering house. The slaughtering house itself is also subject to inspection. The inspection applies to all parts of carcasses intended for human consumption, and to processed and manufactured meat and meat food products such as smoked ham and bacon, and to cooked meats of all kinds, such as sausage and canned products. Meat may be inspected any time during processing or manufacturing.

Any product that fails to pass inspection must be destroyed or reprocessed to satisfy inspection standards. If products are found to be unsuitable for human food, they are marked "Inspected and Condemned" by the inspector.

Specific uses of additives which had been approved under the Meat Inspection Act prior to the Food Additives Amendment are exempted from further approvals by the Food and Drug Administration under the Amendment. Before a new food additive can be used in a meat or a meat food product, its safety must be established to the satisfaction of the Meat Inspection Division as well as the Food and Drug Administration. Research required and supporting data are the same type as outlined previously. The law is administered by the Agricultural Research Service of the Department of Agriculture.

THE IMPORTED MEAT ACT, a section of the Tariff Act of 1930, provides that all imported meats shall be inspected under the same standards as domestic meats.

THE POULTRY PRODUCTS INSPECTION ACT, which became effective in 1959, applies not only to poultry and poultry products produced for interstate and foreign commerce, but also to those used in major consuming areas whether they move across State lines or not. The Secretary of Agriculture may designate such consuming areas.

The Act provides that such poultry and poultry products must be inspected and stamped indicating that they are approved for wholesomeness. Adulteration is prohibited. A product is not deemed adulterated if it contains a substance unavoidably present under good manufacturing practice, or that is permitted by other provisions of the Federal law which sets tolerances for such a substance.

OTHER ACTS define certain foods. For example, butter was defined in a 1923 act. Non-fat dry milk was defined in a 1956 amendment to a 1944 act. Filled milk was defined in a 1923 act, and is unlawful. The term "filled milk" means any milk, cream, or skimmed milk (in any form) which has been blended with any fat or oil other than milk fat so that the resulting product is an imitation or semblance of milk, cream, or skimmed milk. The definition exempts certain proprietary compounds not readily mistaken for milk, used customarily by physicians and stated groups such as hospitals and child welfare associations.

STATE AND LOCAL LAWS   In general, foods and drugs are transported across State lines are not subject to Federal laws and regulations. The States have their own pure food laws to prevent the adulteration and misbranding of foods. These vary greatly from State to State depending on local needs and conditions. Some are patterned very closely after the Federal laws, and in many States the enforcing agency is given the power to accept or adopt the Federal definitions and regulations not only for foods and drugs, but also for pesticides and other dangerous materials that might find their way into foods. Many of the States are at present in the process of adopting food additive laws closely following the provisions of the Federal amendments. Cities and counties also may have laws and ordinances to prevent the adulteration and misbranding of foods.

Medical Research: Past Support, Future Directions*

DALE R. LINDSAY AND ERNEST M. ALLEN

THE HEALTH status of the nation is a complex matter, involving many factors. Cancer, tuberculosis, heart disease, pneumonia and influenza, arthritis, blindness, deafness, mental illnesses, diabetes—these are only a few of the hundreds of diseases and disabilities that have long afflicted mankind and that still persist as greater or lesser health problems in this and other countries.

New diseases have appeared in the world from time to time, and the industrial age has brought with it environmental health problems not dreamed of by earlier generations. Left to themselves these influences, together with the greater opportunities for the spread of contagion in a crowded urban society, would have brought our national health level to a new low, beneath that of the preponderantly rural society of a century ago. Yet, as we are all aware, such have been the advances in the broad attack upon these influences that there has been a steady improvement in the health status of the nation.

The picture has not been one of uniform improvement on all fronts, as may be seen in the death rates of 291 and 127 deaths per 100,000 for our two major killers, heart disease and cancer. We find encouragement, on the other hand, in figures for tuberculosis, influenza-pneumonia, and gastro-intestinal inflammatory disease. Still other diseases have declined to so low a level of importance in the total health picture that they must be looked for only among the fine details. Typhoid fever, malaria, and smallpox, once scourges, have been tamed. The hookworm problem is steadily diminishing in importance in areas where hookworm was once so prevalent. Pellagra is almost a thing of the past.

HEALTH PARAMETERS

We may feel the need for an over-all measurement that expresses or reflects the nation's present health status and permits us to evaluate past and future change. One that is informative is the age-adjusted death rate in our population for deaths from all causes. It

---

* Reprinted by permission, with the omission of six tables, from the December 22, 1961 issue of *Science*, Vol. 134, pp. 2017–2024. Copyright 1962 by the American Association for the Advancement of Science. The authors are, respectively, Deputy to the General Director (for Research Administration) and Executive Secretary, Committee on Research, Massachusetts General Hospital, Boston, Massachusetts, formerly Chief, Division of Research Grants, National Institutes of Health, Public Service, U.S. Department of Health, Education, and Welfare, Bethesda, Maryland; and Grants Policy Officer, Public Health Service, U.S. Department of Health, Education, and Welfare, Washington, D.C.; formerly Associate Director for Research Grants, National Institutes of Health, Bethesda, Maryland.

stands now at only 44 per cent of the death rate at the beginning of the century and has gone down appreciably even in the past several years.

Another over-all measurement, a different health parameter of the population, is the average life span, known technically as the "life expectancy at birth." It stands at the highest figure in our history, is among the highest in the world, and has risen noticeably in even so short a period as the past 8 or 9 years.

Further information, of a different sort, dealing with the prevalence of *all* illnesses, not just those that have a fatal outcome, might be had from figures on the average number of days per person per year lost from work or other normal activity because of illness—the average days of "incapacity." No information from which to compute this additional parameter is available for the past decade, but we may anticipate that such data for coming years will be available in the future.[1]

The death rate, average life span, and average days of incapacity are not, of course, the only informative parameters of the health of a population that one might desire. The summary data that are available and that are given here, however, do reflect the generally favorable trend observed in the past half century and more. They also bring to sharp focus a challenge: It is necessary that the trend, where favorable, be continued or even accelerated, and that every effort be made to reverse the present trend in the incidence and outcome of diseases, such as heart disease and cancer, which have not yet responded favorably.

To accept such a challenge, it is necessary to understand the factors responsible for the improvement in health that has taken place. One factor is surely the higher economic level of our society: A rising per capita income has made possible a larger investment in health measures, both by the individual and by philanthropic agencies and the state. We shall not attempt to evaluate the magnitude of the contribution of this factor. It may be large, and in the short view it may be even larger than that of the other major factor, research. In short, most or much of the improvement could conceivably be a "catching up," a putting to good use the research findings of the past.

Certain it is, however, that for the improvement to continue, research and ever more research will be necessary. Without it the upward progress in health would necessarily level off to a plateau.

The National Institutes of Health has played a significant part in the support of medical research for only a decade and a half, but its role seems destined to be of even greater significance in the decade to come. In view of the growing importance of NIH on the biomedical research scene, it seems fitting to present a brief account of the growth of research support provided through NIH in the past, of what has been achieved, and of what seems to lie ahead.

HISTORICAL BACKGROUND

At the beginning of the century the part played by the federal government in the drama of medical research was small indeed. Philanthropic granting agencies and universities, with some participation by industry, together with private individuals, constituted the main sources of research support. The federal government's participation traces back only to 1887, when a one-room laboratory, a "laboratory of hygiene" devoted to bacteriologic studies on returned seamen (studies of cholera, tuberculosis, typhoid fever, diptheria, and so on), was established in the Staten Island Marine Hospital. In 1891 this laboratory was moved to Washington, and in 1905, with a greatly expanded research mission—that of investigating "infectious and contagious diseases and *matters pertaining to the public health*"—it moved into its new laboratory building at 25th and E Streets, adjoining the Naval Hospital. It had come to be known officially, in the meantime, as the "Hygienic Laboratory." The research areas into which it extended its activities further increased in number thereafter; cancer was included in 1922, and mental hygiene in 1930. In the latter year the laboratory, with its several divisions, was rechristened the National Institute of Health—a name which was changed in 1948 to the present National Institutes of Health.

It was not until 1938 that the federal medical research effort expanded beyond the confines of government-operated laboratories. The expansion was through grants-in-aid to universities and other private research institutions under the newly inaugurated "research grants program." In that fiscal year the effective appropriation was $91,000. In the next several years, ending with 1945, appropriations for research grants remained at or below this level, but in 1946 an "*expanded* research grants program" came into being, with $780,000 in funds. The next year (1947) the program experienced an increase that was spectacular for the time, to $3.4 million, and now, 14 years later (fiscal year 1961), it stands at $287 million. The "intramural" research effort, within the confines of the National Institutes of Health, grew in the same period from $2.3 million in fiscal year 1946 to $98.4 million in 1961.

It is important to note that, in the same period, *non*federal support of medical and related biologic research also underwent a substantial increase (for example, from $60,000,000 in fiscal year 1947 to $333,-000,000 in 1960). Clearly, the great expansion of federal support has by no means acted to dry up nonfederal funds; it is reasonable to believe, on the contrary, that the increased harvest of research accomplishments brought about by the federal outlay has actually stimulated support of medical research through voluntary channels. Certainly both federal and nonfederal support have risen, each at an unprecedented rate, in the last 15 years, and particularly in the last decade.

RESEARCH ACHIEVEMENTS

What has been achieved with this unprecedented outlay of federal and private funds? In the first place, to name an intangible but important achievement, there has been a great expansion and intensification of public interest in medical and related biologic research. New research findings, if they have news value, are likely to be reported to the general public by the science writers for our newspapers and other periodicals. The average citizen is, accordingly, better informed on health matters than ever before, more "research-minded," more aware of the hopes that research can offer, more insistent that we "get on" with the task of research toward beneficent ends. With this growth in alertness to the promise and importance of medical research has come a willingness to contribute to its support—a willingness to have a greater share of the tax dollar invested in medical research and a willingness to make additional contribution to this urgently necessary activity through nonfederal channels. This aroused interest and willingness to contribute must be regarded as a major achievement of the greatly expanded research effort that has come about, under federal leadership, in the last decade and a half, and particularly in the past 10 years.

BASIC RESEARCH. A second result of the developing research-mindedness of the American public is the greater public understanding of the essential part played by basic research in our effort to conquer disease. Basic research may be likened to the submerged part of an iceberg: It does not call attention to itself, but it provides indispensable support for all applied research directed toward the control or conquest of disease.

NIH-supported research. Although both federal and nonfederal funds for medical research are fundamentally from the same source, differing only in route, it may seem important to attempt to give "credit" to the National Institutes of Health (as to other federal agencies) for the research accomplishments resulting from its grants to universities and other research centers and from the research conducted within this great medical center itself. It is easy enough to enumerate some of the more important discoveries in the medical and related biologic sciences that have been made in the past decade or so, and to list specifically some that have been made in the course of work supported by research grants from the NIH. This is done elsewhere in this article. It is important, however, first to understand federal support as it has influenced the total body of medical research, regardless of the source of support.

Research expenditures by the National Institutes of Health in fiscal year 1950 represented approximately 18 percent of the total national outlay for medical research. For fiscal year 1960, the percentage stands at an estimated 40 per cent, or double the earlier figure. An average of the two, expressed roughly as "one out of three," may be taken as representing the entire 10-year period. One out of every three dollars spent for medical research in the decade was spent via the NIH. Certainly during the latter part of the decade, it may be presumed, one out of every three research findings—big or little, basic or applied—came to light during work financed through NIH support.

But the other two out of three research findings were not isolated—quarantined as it were—from scientific contact with the one. On the contrary, each of these, and indeed every research finding, owes something to other findings that have preceded it. A recent quick count of the number of bibliographic references appended to each of five papers in ten representative journals in the medical sciences reveals that one scientific paper refers, on the average, to between 25 and 30 previously published papers. These papers have contributed either to the investigator's conception of the problem he has attacked, or to his method of attack, or to his interpretation of his findings, or to all three. His work, like the capstone of a pyramid, rests upon the work of others. He has seen findings reported in recent issues of journals, heard them reported at scientific meetings, and even learned about new findings in private conversation with fellow scientists in the same general field of interest.

In short, this "one recent research finding, out of every three," that may conservatively be attributed directly to NIH support has itself undoubtedly been an essential step leading toward the other two, or to *some* other two in the total body of advances in medical research. To disentangle the research achievements clearly creditable to NIH support from the achievements to which NIH support has contributed indirectly by making them possible as "a next step," is quite an artificial separation. To use a phrase from Scripture, "the little leaven leaveneth the whole lump" and cannot thereafter be extracted from it. It must be said that in recent years NIH-supported research has been an important factor, has played an inextricable part, in the general advance in knowledge and practice toward the control of disease, in every area in the total field of medicine and related biology.

The picture would be distorted if the presumably even greater influence *on* NIH-supported research arising from research supported by other agencies—60 per cent of the national total, as estimated for 1960—were not also pointed out.

NUMBER OF PROJECTS SUPPORTED. The influence of NIH-supported work has surely permeated the whole body of modern research in the medical and related biological sciences, but is it possible to sharpen the focus a bit? Can one be more specific about what the nation has got for the tax money channeled through the NIH? How many research projects have been supported? How many papers have been published? What of importance has been discovered?

The number of separate research "projects" given NIH support in each of the years in the past decade may be seen in Table 1, column 6. The average "dollar size" of a project (col. 2) can also be computed for each year, by dividing the total amount of funds granted by the number of projects. It is recognized, of course, that there is a wide spread in the annual dollar size of individual projects supported by the NIH. Some cost less than $1000 for 1 year; others cost more than 100 times as much. They also vary correspondingly in personnel and equipment, ranging from a single investigator with his microscope to half a dozen interdisciplinary teams, each working with complicated and costly facilities, in half a dozen scattered research centers.

The number of NIH-supported research projects can be appreciated better when it is viewed as a component of the estimated total number of medical and related biologic research projects in the nation (Table 1, col. 3). These estimates have been computed by dividing the estimated total medical research expenditure[2] for the nation by the "average dollar size" of an NIH-supported research project— that is, the average dollar outlay per year per project (col. 2). The estimates in columns 4 to 6 have been similarly computed. Underlying these computations is, of course, the assumption that the average dollar size of a project, in NIH experience, can be used as an estimate of the average for medical research in general (see Table 1, footnote *).

The NIH supported 10,700 projects in universities and other research institutions in 1960, out of a national total estimated at 38,500 projects.

NUMBER OF PAPERS.   On publication of a paper from NIH-supported research, the author is asked to (and usually does) supply a reprint for the NIH files. These files are, unfortunately, incomplete prior to 1957; the count for 1957 shows 5,230 papers, and that of 1960, a total of 11,000.

A backward extrapolation of these figures is speculative but suggests that the number of papers from NIH-supported research for the year 1950 was in the neighborhood of 2000. The total for the 11 years ending with 1960 is conservatively estimated to be 50,000 or more.

Each paper reports from one to several research findings in its field.

There is reason to believe that the findings from NIH-supported research are of somewhat greater than average scientific importance, for, although the judgment of the mature and experienced investigator

Table 1.

Average size of projects (in dollars) and number of medical and related biologic research projects for fiscal years 1950 through 1960.

Fiscal year	Average* size of project ($)	ACTIVE MEDICAL RESEARCH PROJECTS (NO.)			
		Throughout the nation†	All nonfederal†	Federal (including NIH)†	NIH extramural research‡
1950	9,649	15,300	9,100	6,200	1,400
1951	10,601	15,400	8,500	6,900	1,500
1952	10,658	16,200	8,800	7,400	1,700
1953	10,261	19,800	10,400	9,400	2,000
1954	11,203	20,100	10,500	9,600	2,600
1955	11,379	21,100	10,700	10,400	3,000
1956	12,470	22,900	12,000	10,900	3,100
1957	14,209	28,000	14,900	13,100	5,700
1958	15,300	32,100	17,300	14,800	6,500
1959	16,584	35,400	17,900	17,500	8,500
1960	18,584	38,500	18,000	20,500	10,700

* "Average" means the average for all projects supported by NIH research grants. These averages were used as estimates of the national average in calculating entries in columns 4 to 6. For the separate institutes, averages for fiscal year 1960 were as follows: Arthritis and Metabolic Diseases, $16,200; Neurological Diseases and Blindness, $21,700; Cancer, $21,100; Dental Research, $13,500; Allergy and Infectious Diseases, $15,000; General Medical Sciences, $18,200; Heart, $19,300; Mental Health, $21,600. The NIH averages in column 2 may possibly be somewhat higher than averages for the nation.
† Estimates, calculated by dividing the figures for total reported research outlay (not shown) by the amounts in column 2. Discrepancies are due to rounding of figures.
‡ NIH research grants program.

of scientific standing is, and should continue to be, sufficient certification of the importance—indeed, the necessity—of any research he proposes, every project supported by an NIH research grant has, nevertheless, been in a sense doubly certified as to its scientific importance and necessity.[3] Each project awarded an NIH grant has been endorsed by a "jury" of from 10 to 20 distinguished scientists who have studied the proposal, and has been given further consideration by an advisory council of equally distinguished members and recommended by them to the surgeon general of the Public Health Service for grant-in-aid support.

It is reasonable to believe that research undertakings that have been so competently scrutinized and screened constitute, as a body, an aggregate research effort of superior worth and promise. Even if the results from NIH-supported research were not identifiable as such in the vast output of the nation's research laboratories and only the total forward march of research achievement could be perceived, it could still be said with assurance that most of the work coming out of the laboratories receiving NIH support (together with research supported by other agencies using similarly effective screening mechanisms) must be in or near the forefront of the procession.

Listed below are a few research findings from the thousands of significant advances in medicine and related biology that have been made in the past decade in the course of research supported by the NIH.[4] It should be pointed out again that such findings are but capstones of "pyramids" of findings by many workers, supported by many agencies. These peak findings will, of course, be built in turn into the lower levels of other such pyramids, to be capped by further achievements.

SOME RESEARCH FINDINGS

Prednisone, a synthetic relative of the steroid cortisone, was found to be as effective as cortisone or hydrocortisone, or more so, for treating rheumatoid arthritis, and to cause less edema or none at all.

The folic acid antagonist methotrexate has been found to have pronounced beneficial effects in cases of choriocarcinoma, a variety of cancer.

With the albino hamster as the experimental animal, it has been shown that dental caries can be both infectious and transmissible. The organism is a streptococcus. A different study has shown that fluoride (1 part per million) in drinking water has a dramatic preventive action in children.

The hemadsorption viruses, members of the parainfluenza group, were isolated and shown to cause many of the acute respiratory infections in children, from afebrile infections to such conditions as croup and pneumonia.

It has been shown that giving codliver oil to pregnant rats reduces the incidence and severity of congenital anomalies caused by deficiency of vitamin E in their diet. A change in the balance of the remaining vitamins in the diet apparently compensates to some extent for deficiency of the single vitamin.

The adrenocorticotrophic hormone (ACTH), a protein hormone containing 23 amino acids, was synthesized from the natural amino acids. This is the largest protein molecule yet synthesized.

Convincing evidence that the onset of acute multiple sclerosis, in a case of the disease in man, resulted from injection of rabies vaccine (containing elements of nervous tissue) has strengthened the view that multiple sclerosis, as it ordinarily occurs, is an autoallergic disease representing an immunologic response to some unknown chemical constituent of the patient's own nervous tissue.

Raising the brain's concentration of gamma-aminobutyric acid (GABA), a normal constituent of the brain, has been found to give protection against convulsive seizures.

Scientists studying epilepsy were handicapped by their inability to reproduce it in any laboratory animal until it was found that, after a simple surgical operation in which alumina cream is applied to a small area of the brain surface, the experimental animal for some months becomes an "epileptic," having typical epileptic attacks.

A viral agent associated with mouse leukemia has been found to acquire such potency in serial passage in tissue culture that it can produce *multiple* primary tumors in mice and sarcomas in hamsters and rats. This discovery strengthens the view that viruses may be at least one of the causes of cancer in man.

Chloroquine and pyrimethamine were shown to be suppressive, and primaquine was shown to be curative, of malaria. These drugs have now been adopted for use in the U.S. military forces.

It has been shown that the placenta will, if necessary, deplete levels of vitamins B_{12}, B_6, C, and iron in the mother's blood in maintaining these nutrients at more nearly normal levels in the fetal blood stream.

It has been shown that forced oral (or intravenous) administration of large quantities of a solution of one teaspoon of table salt and one-half teaspoon of baking soda in a quart of water can serve in cases of burn shock as an emergency substitute for plasma. In another study it has been shown that, of individuals treated with balanced salt solution and individuals treated with whole blood, more of the former survive.

A living virus, the "tobacco mosaic virus," has been taken apart, into its skeleton of ribonucleic acid and the latter's protein envelope, and reconstituted. The ribonucleic acid is the primary source of the infectious activity of the virus. These findings will lead to a better understanding of the pathogenicity of viruses.

Two specific tests, each based on the bentonite flocculation procedure, now permit diagnosis, in a few minutes, of rheumatoid arthritis and lupus erythematosus.

Mapping of the gene locations in the chromosomes of the red bread mold *Neurospora* is continuing and will contribute information that will ultimately be useful in the effort to unravel the mystery of the action of deoxyribonucleic acid and ribonucleic acid as code-determinants of the hereditary structure and function of all organisms.

It has been found that galactosemia is due to the absence of the enzyme P-Gal transferase—a genetic defect. A quick test on the blood permits diagnosis and prompt institution of a galactose-free diet.

A culture medium of chemically defined composition has been developed that has made it possible to maintain cultures of cells from a variety of tissues (such as normal skin, bone, kidney, connective tissue, and cancers) indefinitely.

It has been shown that production of the fetal type of hemoglobin is favored by oxygen and glucose deficiencies.

A new drug, phenazocine, first conceived on the "drawing board" and then synthesized, has been found to be many times more potent than morphine in relieving pain.

An erythropoietic factor is formed by goats exposed to a stimulated altitude of 22,000 feet and is secreted in the milk. Injected into rats, it raises the blood hemoglobin and the reticulocyte count.

A new pathway for sugar metabolism, the "hexosemonophosphate shunt," has been discovered. It bypasses the citric acid cycle and contains several previously unknown sugars.

Evidence has been obtained that liver changes similar to those in carbon tetrachloride poisoning can be brought about by central stimulation of the sympathetic nervous system.

Two independent investigators have won Nobel prizes for nucleic acid synthesis—the one for discovering an enzyme that synthesizes desoxyribonucleic acid, the other for discovering an enzyme that synthesizes ribonucleic acid. These two nucleic acids code-control bodily structure and function, apparently throughout all animal and plant life.

A molded plastic replica of a normal mitral valve of the heart has been constructed and used successfully to replace a diseased valve in man.

This list could be greatly extended.

RESEARCH ACHIEVEMENTS SUMMARIZED. We might summarize research achievements through NIH support as follows.

1) In 1950 the number of published papers from NIH-supported research projects appears to have been in the neighborhood of 2000 or 2500 (reliable figures are not available); in 1960 the number is reliably estimated at 11,000. The total number of such papers from (and including) 1950 through 1960 is conservatively estimated at 50,000.

2) In 1950 the number of active research projects receiving NIH support through its program of research grants to medical schools and other institutions conducting medical research amounted to 1400, out of a national total of medical research projects estimated at 15,000; in 1960 the number had grown to 10,700, out of a national total estimated at over 38,000.

There is every reason to believe that this NIH-supported research (and research supported by other granting agencies with similarly effective screening mechanisms) has, on the average, been of superior scientific merit and importance.

3) The number of research findings reported in papers published in the period 1950–60 that give credit to NIH for support cannot be estimated. At a minimum it would be expected to equal the number of research papers published in the period (estimated at 50,000) and might well be two or three times that number.

4) NIH-supported research has made an inextricable contribution to the total progress of medical science and its achievements in the last 10 or 15 years. The past 10 years' research supported by this and other granting agencies active in the medical and health research field has, without much doubt, played a part in the fall in death rate and the rise in life expectancy that have occurred even in the same decade. It is reasonable to expect that continued or expanded biomedical research in the next decade will have an increasingly important impact on the health of the nation.

FUTURE RESEARCH OPPORTUNITIES

Let us now look beyond the periphery of present biomedical knowledge and mention a few of the areas where it appears that intensive exploration would be rewarding.

It should be understood that no attempt at complete coverage of research opportunities will be made here, and no attempt to shape the pattern of the discussion into conformity with any pre-existing formulation, such as the balanced pattern of program interests of the several institutes of the NIH. An attempt will be made, however, to convey the restrained enthusiasm of many of the group of competent scientists who have left their laboratories in order to render a broader service to medical science through their office in the Division of Research Grants of NIH.[5]

Instrumentation. The objectives of instrumentation and automation research have been succinctly stated as follows: "to measure (and record) more things, more accurately, and automatically."

It has long been said in science that the ability to measure some important quantity with greater precision by one more decimal place opens up a new era of advance in the scientific field. To be conservative, one might amend the saying to read "two more decimal places" —measurements 100 times more precise. The core of truth in the saying is that the progress of biologic science is ultimately dependent upon development of ever more sensitive instruments and methods for making ever more precise measurement of an ever wider variety of things, and that an explosion of new research follows a new and important development in instrumentation. A modern example is the burst of research progress in cell biology that has resulted from invention of the electron microscope and development of the technics of immuno- and microchemistry, the electron microscope making visible cell structures a thousand times more minute than those visible without it, and microchemical methods making possible more and more progress in the chemical analysis of these minute structures.

Instrumentation (including science technology in general) has been given first place in this survey of important and promising avenues of research effort because it stands at the doorway to progress in science.

Further advances in the sensitivity of instrument types now in use, development of new types of instruments, and further adaptation for biologic use of instruments used in other areas may be expected in the next decade, and, with each development, an explosion of new research in the corresponding scientific area. Great advances are to be expected in the coming decade in the adaptation of computers to medical and related biologic research. The use of electronic computers for analyzing the complexities of interrelated biologic data is in its infancy.

Efforts will surely be intensified to develop improved methods for storing and retrieving scientific data, and for analyzing and interpreting them. The further use of computers in the analysis of data from x-ray crystallography of proteins and nucleic acids may be cited as an example.

Quantification and evaluation of the information-input capacity of the various senses may be achieved. Progress may be expected in the development of computer analogs or models for the simpler brain functions. More instrumentation will undoubtedly be developed for continuous measurement and recording of some of the many variables undergoing simultaneous change in the body in response to stress or other change in conditions, or to disease or therapeutic measures, both for purposes of research and for diagnosis and observation in medical practice. The use of computers in the further development of mathematical biology and for further progress toward ultimate automatic translation of foreign scientific literature may be expected.

PROSTHESIS. Related to instrumentation and associated techniques is the area of prosthesis—a term referring here, in the broadest sense, to artificial substitutes for, or aids to, body parts and functions. Further investigation directed toward the following objectives may be expected: developing artificial heart valves; improving extracorporeal blood oxygenating and circulating units; perfecting techniques for maintaining some part of the body (for example, a cancerous extremity) under a separate circulation with a high concentration of some remedial agent; devising a means of aiding or replacing failing kidney function; improving dental filling and bonding materials; devising a substitute (possibly tactile) for lost vision or for a lost sense of equilibrium.

TISSUE AND ORGAN TRANSPLANTS. Research may be expected to continue on the problem of the rejection of skin grafts and organ transplants (for example, kidney), which now occurs except in cases where the recipient and the donor of the transplant have near-to-identical genetic backgrounds. Blood and bone-marrow transfusions regardless of serological type may be an associated development, if and when the general problem of immunological rejection of foreign tissue is ever solved. The same process of rejection is, of course, altogether beneficent when the body combats the "foreign tissue" of an invading pathogenic organism.

Tissue culture of bone marrow for purposes of transfusion may be brought nearer in the next decade. "Tooth banks" and tooth transplants are a hoped-for possibility.

Associated with the objective of successfully making tissue and organ transplants is that of regenerating lost tissues. A breakthrough toward controlled and useful regeneration of lost tissues in mammalian forms is hardly to be expected in the next decade, but as a long-term goal it will surely be kept in view, as research is continued on suitable lower species.

HUMAN ECOLOGY AND ENVIRONMENTAL HEALTH. A vast terrain remains to be explored in the general research area of man and his environment, both animate and inanimate—the mutual balance of environmental factors, beneficent and harmful, as they affect health and disease, longevity, performance levels, and even evolution. Important in this field are also the health interactions between human populations and interactions of these with other populations of animal and plant life.

One of the most important problems in environmental health is protection against unwanted radiation effects. Research has been pressed in the past several years and will surely be intensified in the coming decade.

The problem of making desired food additives safe and of determining a safe tolerance level for adventitious additives (chiefly residues left in food from insecticidal crop sprays) has become increasingly more acute in recent years, as agricultural chemicals and various substances required in food processing and packaging have multiplied. A vast amount of research will be needed to make sure the public is protected. The continued search for better biologic tests that are equivalent to lifetime exposure for man is a prime necessity in such efforts.

Closely related to the foregoing problems are the problems of pollution of air and water by substances harmful to health. "Smog" is only one among many such harmful agents. Of prime interest is the pollution of urban air from products of the motor age. Identification of such products and knowledge of their long-term biologic effects, with development of suitable control measures, are objectives of pressing importance. The possibility that some of these products of incomplete combustion may be implicated in the steadily growing incidence of malignancy of the lower respiratory tract gives such research added importance. Progress can be hastened through accelerated research in instrumentation; the need for such acceleration indeed pervades all research areas.

The atom bomb is a potential environmental hazard that warrants more health-related research than appears to be in prospect.

CANCER. The search for the cause or causes of human cancer and for means of prevention and better means of therapy has been pressed in recent years to an extent that almost entitles this to be called a crash program. Crucial knowledge is slowly but surely being accumulated.

Demonstration of the virus etiology of a variety of cancers (including leukemia) in certain laboratory animals has renewed our hope for an early breakthrough toward control of this dread disease and has already led to more intensified research in this direction. There is also growing, if not indeed conclusive, evidence that carcinogenic substances can reach the body through the inspired air—evidence that relates the cancer problem to the general problem of environmental health. Research in this direction is being pushed and will surely be increased in the coming decade.

HOST-PARASITE RELATIONS. The area of research on host-parasite relations encompasses all the relationships between man (and other animal and plant hosts) and the beneficent, neutral, and harmful plant and animal parasites that infest and infect, including viruses, bacteria, protozoa, and other parasitic organisms. An extension of the parasite concept can, of course, bring the invasive cells of cancer into the same category. Research will continue on a broad front on the pathogenic parasitic organisms, on their nutritional requirements and metabolic processes, and on the evolution of pathogenic forms and the development of pathogenicity in forms that were previously inactive (in the carrier state) or harmless or even beneficent (for example, the colon bacillus). The interaction between host and parasite, in particular the effects of the parasite upon the host and the mechanism of these effects, will continue to engage the attention and effort of research workers, as will the continued development of control measures, including antibiotics and other chemotherapy. The development of parasite resistance to such therapy in the course of an infection—a heartbreaking event—and the perpetuation of such resistant strains thereafter to endanger the lives of others are twin problems that will call for intensified further research. The restraint upon one parasitic population that results from the presence of another also deserves more study.

This research area is obviously one of extraordinarily broad scope, including as it does all the infectious diseases. A vast amount of work has already been done, during nearly a century of research, but the area remains at or near the top of any list where priority is determined by pressing need or promising opportunity.

TISSUE IMMUNE REACTIONS. Closely related to the great research area just discussed is that of the reaction of the body to substances foreign to it—a reaction of either defense or neutralization or acceptance. The preponderance of research in the past has properly been directed toward strengthening the mechanisms for defense, for here lies the greatest need; but when the defense is against a skin graft or a transplanted kidney donated to an individual in dire need, the same beneficent mechanism can act blindly as a liability. The next decade should see an intensification of work in both directions—toward strengthening the body's defense mechanisms on the one hand and toward holding them in check on the other.

Inseparable from the objective of strengthening the body's natural defenses is that of adding new defense factors, chemically tailored to general or specific needs. Research toward this end holds continued promise of future rewards.

ANTIMETABOLITES, ANTIBIOTICS, OTHER CHEMOTHERAPEUTIC AGENTS. Although they have been referred to incidentally in the previous discussion, antimetabolites, antibiotics, and other chemotherapeutic agents deserve special mention. Antimetabolites are among the most promising of the agents being tested for anticancer action, and they also offer continued promise in the attack on invading disease organisms. The last several years have seen the testing of all manner of chemical compounds, many thousands of them, for possible anticancer activity. The next decade will see a continuation of such testing and of research toward the development of new antimetabolites and antibiotics and of other compounds for effective chemotherapy.

HEART, CIRCULATION, AND BLOOD. We may expect further advances yearly in heart surgery and prosthesis, in techniques of localized perfusion, in diagnosis and relief of vascular insufficiencies of various body areas, in the control of clotting, in understanding and controlling the processes in hematopoiesis, and in our knowledge and control of the basic causes of atherosclerosis.

Reproduction. The well-being of the new individual will continue to be the dominant practical objective in research on reproduction, where progress will be dependent upon a clearer understanding of the processes involved and the factors that influence them. Reduction in fetal wastage and deformity (biochemical as well as anatomic will remain an important immediate objective. Overpopulation and associated hunger in some world areas will continue to stimulate interest in developing more effective measures of birth and population control.

The Brain. The outlook for brain research in the next decade is one of continuing investigation with the oscillograph, the electroencephalograph, and other instruments; of localized short-term and long-term brain stimulation and the placing of minute brain lesions, precisely localized; of continued exploration of the biochemistry and the pharmacology of limited areas and of brain secretion of hormones; of deeper delving into the biophysics and biochemistry of excitation in studies on single neurons (and other types of cells); and of continued efforts to extend the limited analogies between brain activity and the function of computers (as a class) in information storage, organization, and retrieval. Both in the field of neurology and in that of mental health, advancement toward the control of disease will be promoted by such research.

BEHAVIORAL SCIENCE, MENTAL HEALTH. During the next 10 years we may expect to see more research in which attempts are made to relate mental phenomena to the underlying biochemistry, biophysics, and endocrinology of the brain; more study of the behavioral patterns in the lower animals; and further study of the factors affecting and determining the course of development of the child, enabling him to assume the responsibilities of the adult as a member of society.

Cross-cultural and other studies are needed to determine the influence on mental health of such factors as patterns of thought and behavior, systems of personal and social values, the structure of the family and other social groups, patterns of interaction in the family and community, levels of aspiration in relation to the attendant environmental and economic potentials, and hygienic practices of populations. Such research will promote control of mental disease and control of the development of such patterns of deviance from social norms as alcoholism, accident-proneness, and juvenile delinquency. Research in some of these areas is practically in its infancy.

AGING. Research directed toward discovery of the fundamental processes in aging will be pursued further by investigators experienced in the field of cell biology. It may be hoped that the biochemical, biophysical, and structural differences between the aged and the youthful cell, and the effects of these differences, will begin to be understood. As for the diseases so prevalent among the aged—heart and vascular and collagen disease (including excessive fibrosis)—and the "natural process" of progressive shrinkage of the various functional cell populations of the body with advancing age, no dramatic "breakthrough" is in sight; but as the coming decade advances, the slow accumulation and piecing together of bits of knowledge gained through basic research will surely bring us nearer to an answer to the problems of aging.

CELL AND MOLECULAR BIOLOGY. Reference has been made to improvements in instrumentation that have permitted examination of finer structural detail and chemical analysis of more minute portions of material than was previously possible. The electron microscope and the developments in microchemistry and in x-ray crystallography, together with technical developments in other areas (for example, immunochemistry), have opened up for study the single cell and its constituent structures. Researches on cell morphology, physiology, biochemistry, biophysics, pharmacology, pathology, radiobiology, and genetics are in progress and will undoubtedly be greatly extended in the coming years.

More detailed study of disease processes may be expected, with further exploration of the precise architectural structure of molecules in disease states as contrasted with their structure in the state of health. Although the importance of the precise architecture of molecules in biologic processes has long been appreciated, particularly in the fields of enzymology and immunology, molecular biology as a research field is still in its infancy. It will undoubtedly grow in stature in the next decade, as its newly conceived sibling, submolecular biology, just begins to stir.

NUCLEIC ACIDS. If the research areas in the whole of medicine and related biology were represented as mountain peaks in a vast terrain yet to be fully explored, the Mount Everest in that little-explored country would surely be "Mount DNA." Deoxyribonucleic acid (DNA) and ribonucleic acid (RNA) are the two nucleic acids that are found, singly or together, in the cellular units of all living organisms so far examined, from viruses, bacteria, and other plant forms through all animal forms up to and including man. The most challenging research in the future will be that directed toward the biosynthesis and function of these nucleic acids; for out of such studies will come the revolutionary answers to long-standing questions regarding the phenomena of genetic reproduction (replication) of cell structure and function and the biosynthesis of the proteins, the most important structural components of living systems. Possibly, too, from such studies will come the answers to questions regarding the fundamental nature of cell differentiation, the development in each individual of such different cell populations as those of nerve and liver from an original single cell—the fertilized ovum. New technics in the study of the nucleic acids have been developed in the past 10 years, and it is certain that research on these compounds will be vigorously carried on for many years to come. This research is so basic that dividends can flow from it in almost any direction. One could well be in the direction of cancer control.

GENETICS. Closely related to, even inseparable from, research on DNA and RNA is research on the gene population (the "genotype") in the original single cell from which a cell progeny is derived, whether this be a clone community of bacteria in a flask or a cell aggregate making up one human being. What genes are present in the parent cell, what factors determined their presence together, and what bodily attributes (including hereditary disease or susceptibility to disease) each gene or gene group controls—these are some of the challenging questions in genetics. New techniques for visualizing the entire complement of chromosomes in a single cell and identifying each by its peculiar characteristics now make possible a surge of new work on hereditary disease and susceptibility to disease. Control of the complement of genes with which each individual starts his existence is a visionary objective, even though probably unattainable as a goal.

The genetics of new pathogenic strains of organisms; of the first malignant cell to appear in an individual who develops cancer; of the development of resistance to chemotherapy in a viral, bacterial, or cancer cell population—these fields, too, present challenging problems on which more research is urgently needed.

Much of the promise of achievement yet to come from medical and related biological research rests upon the further development of interdisciplinary team work, now well under way. A more extensive development of great research centers for categorial and general research in the coming decade is a strong possibility.

BASIC AND APPLIED RESEARCH. The amount of applied research carried on from year to year in the coming decade should be in homeostatic equilibrium with the amount of (pre-existing) basic research, for each is dependent upon the other.

Applied research has as its objective some achievement that can be put to "practical" use in some way other than as a step toward further research. Basic research contributes new variables to science, quantitates them, identifies (and quantitates) new causal relationships between variables, and points out new spatial and temporal groupings of variables and new sequences in their changes in value.

The motivation and justification and the basis of evaluation are the same for applied research in general and for any one project in applied research: They are, respectively, the practical objective and the extent to which it is attained. For basic research, the motivation is scientific curiosity—an almost monastic dedication to the pursuit of learning. The justification (in the eyes of the onlooker, including the one who supplies the funds) is that the stream of applied research dries up unless it is fed by basic research. The merit of any one achievement in basic research is measured by the extent to which it clarifies pre-existing knowledge, contributes toward establishing a new generalization, or simply leads to new research.

The interdependence of applied and basic research has been pointed out. No matter what the practical objective of any applied research is, "spade work" (equated here with basic research), unless it has already been done, is found to be necessary. An enormous amount of basic research may yet have to be carried out before death rates from heart disease and cancer can be substantially improved. Thus, the need for applied research stimulates support of basic research, and the findings of basic research ultimately open the doors to more applied research. There is no reason to believe that this symbiosis will be in any way disturbed in the coming decade.

1. The data are being collected by the U.S. National Health Survey, which was begun back in 1957.

2. This figure is not shown in Table 7 but can be obtained by multiplying entries in column 2 by those in column 3.

3. This can also be said, of course, of work supported by other agencies that have a similarly effective review mechanism.

4. "Research supported by the NIH" includes both grant-supported and intramural research.

5. Grateful acknowledgment is made here for the contribution of these scientists.

2. Health Administration In Other Jurisdictions

Effective Community Health Services*

GEORGE JAMES, M.D.

THE CHALLENGE OF CHANGE

The rapid expansion of knowledge and the public's growing sophistication make one fact clear to those in the health and social service fields. As professional workers, we must concentrate on services for the individual which meet his particular needs. We were not hired to plan and execute programs, develop agencies, stimulate coordination among agencies, improve teaching programs, or develop new tools, except as these activities may be useful in serving people. The effect, immediate or ultimate, on each citizen is the measure of our effort, and the only measure by which we will eventually be judged.

In this light one can discuss Public Health or social work with a minimum of slavish adherence to traditions, charters, laws, and agencies. One can give maximum attention to epidemiologic questions: what are the needs of our population, the resources available to satisfy these needs, and the modifying influences on community attitudes. We must develop effective services for the citizen while we continue to improve present resources and community attitudes.

This emphasis upon service to the individual, against the backdrop of his particular family and community environment, assures a tailor-made approach to local health services. It means that no two communities will need or should have identical health programs. It means that no person in the community need have exactly the same services as another. It means that with the rapid changes in the social, economic, and scientific life of our time no single community can keep exactly the same pattern of health services for two consecutive years. Hence, all who practice Public Health are students. All of us are floating on seas of change, driven by variable main currents, tossed in swirling eddies. All our programs on behalf of health are adaptations. True, many of them have been devised and pretested in stable labora-

* Reprinted, by permission, from *Public Health Concepts in Social Work Education*—Proceedings of Seminar held at Princeton University, Princeton, New Jersey, March 4–9, 1962. Published by the Council on Social Work Education in cooperation with the Public Health Service, Department of Health, Education, and Welfare, pp. 39–68. The author is Commissioner of Health, The City of New York, New York.

tories. But until they are tried in one's own community, upon each person in need, their real value in any particular area cannot be accurately assessed.

I am reminded of a personal experience in a southern State which was attempting to build up its child health services. Each local health officer was urged to obtain more funds for child health clinics and immunization programs. In one county roads were so poor that neither families nor clinic teams could reach any central service point during the rainy season of each year. Strange as it seemed to some of our Public Health colleagues, we made no request for special funds for child health services; instead, we urged increased expenditures for local highways. In terms of real and meaningful health resources, better roads were more useful in that area at that time than more doctors, nurses, social workers, vaccines, clinic quarters, health education, or anything else.

An important principle governs the development of local services, including health services: for the foreseeable future, the needs of our citizens will remain insatiable. Under our present value systems, there are not sufficient resources to satisfy all human needs for housing, health, welfare, highways, education, museums, recreation, and those other community services we have come to believe essential. That human needs are insatiable means that communities must develop priorities for service. These will depend greatly upon human values, upon the specific crises and enthusiasms that develop, and on new scientific discoveries. Since each factor which will modify and affect priority is itself greatly subject to change, it is evident that a community's priorities for the various services will also change. Current program emphases on air pollution, radiologic health, and case-finding in diabetes and glaucoma were generally unknown two decades ago, although from a strictly scientific viewpoint the needs existed to approximately the same degree as now.

One cannot predict today exactly what will be tomorrow's major health priorities. It is essential that each community be so organized as to maintain constant contact with and understanding of the factors influencing change in community and health priorities. This organizational structure need not follow any fixed pattern. One has only to look around the nation to see many patterns and to realize that dogmatism in the organization of health services has no place in our current plan of action. The test of any organization must be its effectiveness in meeting the needs and priorities for each community.

DISEASES THAT KILL

Any discussion of local Public Health services must therefore start with the needs of the local population. We use the normal epidemiologic principle of stressing those conditions which do or can affect the most citizens. First come the major causes of death.

Heart Disease

The leading cause of death, by far, in all areas of this nation is "diseases of the heart." They kill at least 40 per cent of those who die each year. Although the group includes rheumatic heart disease and syphilitic heart disease, both now increasingly well controlled, the greatest killer is disease of the coronary arteries. Long-term prospective studies seem to indicate that coronary heart disease occurs more often in obese individuals who have high blood pressure, a high serum cholesterol level, and a generally sedentary occupation. The serum cholesterol level seems to be related to the amount of dietary saturated fatty acid, a food element commonly supplied by animal fats. Several important scientific groups have recommended that these individuals reduce obesity, eat food lower in saturated fat, and increase their routine exercise. It is true that our civilization devalues exercise as a daily component of life; transportation is the rule, and walking almost a lost art. Commenting on our present retreat from exercise in a recent television broadcast entitled "The Fat American," Dean Mayer noted a high school near Boston which has made half its athletic field into a parking lot for the students!

While we are not yet prepared to make firm recommendations for the prevention of heart disease in adults, it looks as if some of the ideas arising from recent research on exercise and diet must be tested in demonstration programs, for eventual practical use. In the meantime, a huge number of patients with heart disease require medical care and present a host of major social problems to the community.

Cancer

The number two cause of death in this country is cancer. Cancer is responsible for about one in every seven deaths. No discussion of this health problem can be meaningful unless we categorize our remarks according to cancer sites. Man has made his greatest progress in controlling cancer of the cervix. It is believed that fully two-thirds of those now dying from this disease could be saved if early detection programs were developed. Each physician can check for cancer of the cervix as part of a routine examination program, or we can use mass methods by taking Papanicolaou smears on all women admitted to general hospitals and outpatient departments. It has been estimated that a single case of fatal cervical cancer costs the City of New York $10,000 from the time of discovery to the time of death. In our experience half the patients with cervical cancer would not have been detected without the smear, and of these more than two-thirds can be saved at the time of diagnosis. In New York City, therefore, the screening of 75,000 women at each of the two hospitals where we now have active programs is expected to save as much as $2,750,000 per year— $2,750,000 saved every year by a program estimated to cost less than a tenth of that.

The story of cancer of the lung is a dismal one because our biologic knowledge offers us highly effective technics which our social sophistication cannot accept. By itself cancer of the lung is about number eight among the causes of death. In New York City it kills 1,600 persons per year, more than twice the number of those who lose their lives in automobile accidents. Among men it is a leading cause of deaths from cancer. The most serious epidemic disease in our civilization, it sharply increases year by year among both men and women. Fourteen retrospective and three large prospective studies during the last 15 years have indicated an association between this disease and the habit of cigarette smoking. Although other factors such as air pollution may be significant, epidemiologists believe at least three-quarters of all deaths from cancer of the lung could be prevented if the cigarette-smoking habit were stopped. Despite these facts, no community to my knowledge has been successful in decreasing the number of cigarette smokers. On the contrary, cigarette sales continue to increase year by year in complete disregard of the risks involved. Faced with this gloomy picture, health departments have decided to concentrate on the youthful smoker, hoping to prevent the habit in those beginning to experiment with it.

Other cancers present other problems. Cancer of the stomach is decreasing as a cause of death; no one really knows why. Studies are attempting to ascertain the reason for this decrease in the hope that the downward trend might be accelerated if we knew the factors responsible.

Cancer of the breast still has not responded as well as expected to health education aimed at early case-finding. Although there are some small indications of progress in the saving of life, these at best are minor; there is much more we must learn about this condition if we are to bring it under control.

Cancer of the gastrointestinal tract is diagnosed in its early stages more often now than formerly. Health educators have stressed the significance of bleeding from the gastrointestinal tract and the importance of proctologic examination, which can detect small cancers and precancerous polyps of the rectum.

Leukemia, still a mystery, is invariably a fatal condition. The association of an increased incidence of leukemia with undue exposure to x-rays underscores the need to protect operators of x-ray machines from overexposure and to avoid the use of intensive radiation in certain therapeutic procedures for the very young.

Stroke

The third large category in the causes of death is stroke. This condition is responsible for about 7½ per cent of all deaths. Although there are obvious epidemiologic differences between this disease and coronary heart disease, it is generally believed that many of the same factors obtain in both. High blood pressure seems to play a definite role, and elevated serum cholesterol may be of some significance. At present there are no clear-cut recommendations for prevention of stroke, even for use in a demonstration program. Moreover, the stroke patient who recovers presents an enormous community problem in rehabilitation. Most of the local health departments have begun programs in this field.

Respiratory Infections

In New York City the fourth leading cause of death is the influenza-pneumonia group, which is responsible for about 4 per cent of the deaths each year. Many occur among the old, and chronically ill, who lack the stamina to withstand an acute respiratory infection which settles in their lungs. It is known that old people readily lose their immunity to influenza; if this immunity can be maintained by booster doses of influenza vaccines, however, they may be in a better position to withstand an attack of disease. Development of the sulfa and antibiotic drugs has improved the patient's chances against pneumonia, even those of the aged. In general, health departments maintain services for the influenza immunization of old people and other high-risk groups such as pregnant women. Moreover, the care of persons ill with such respiratory infections comes under the general heading of medical care services.

Diseases of Early Infancy

The fifth leading cause of death is a general category called "certain diseases of early infancy." Most are not now amenable to either treatment of prevention. On the other hand, as obstetric and early infant care improve we can expect further progress in this field. Proportionately, there are four times as many nonwhites in this group as there are whites. This certainly seems to indicate that the lower socio-economic status of non-white parents is a major influence in many of the deaths among their offspring. Although these diseases are fifth among the causes of death for all persons in New York City, they are sixth for whites and third for non-whites. Local health services providing early prenatal care for the mother, the best hospital delivery care, and prompt and adequate child health clinic services for the infant are essential.

Accidents

Sixth among the leading causes of death are accidents. Health departments have done a great deal to prevent death from poisons by poison information centers. Day or night, anyone in the world can call the center in New York City and find out exactly what chemicals are involved in any material. A large library contains information on a whole host of household substances never meant to be ingested, so that a physician can be told what hazardous chemical is involved and what treatments might be effective if a child should swallow one of them. Improperly operating gas appliances also caused some deaths from carbon monoxide poisoning in New York City until health education, combined with inspection and regulation of appliances, relegated this problem to minor status.

Even after these hazards have been checked, the largest group of accidental deaths remains: automobile accidents and most home accidents from falls and fires. Although obvious measures can prevent each such occurrence, it is extremely difficult to develop effective programs of prevention in the community. Recently the relationship between alcoholism and auto accidents has become increasingly certain. What is not certain, however, is whether stringent punishment or any other so-called deterrent to drunken driving is effective. Using the experience of our Scandinavian friends as an example, we first must deplore social drinking before driving and incorporate this attitude in our values system. Although falls in the home can be minimized by meticulous attention to slippery rugs, lack of hand-holds in bathrooms, and faulty appliances, health department efforts in these fields are still halting, tentative, and experimental, and they have not yet been shown to be effective.

Cirrhosis of the Liver

The number seven cause of death is generally believed to be associated with alcoholism. It is estimated that there are over 300,000 alcoholics in New York City, a truly staggering proportion of our 7,700,000 inhabitants. Many communities have devoted much effort to the prevention and control of alcoholism. Although several studies show dramatic improvement in individual patients, no one claims that any major impact has been made upon the total community problem. At least we have come to recognize that alcoholism is a complex problem, and have attempted to provide medical care and mental health care for the alcoholic.

Diabetes Mellitus

The eighth leading cause of death is increasing in importance despite the availability of insulin as a therapeutic agent for over 40 years. Although concrete proof is lacking, most medical scientists believe insulin and diet, by which the patient keeps his diabetes under control, effectively inhibit serious complications. These complications, which relate to atherosclerosis of coronary, renal, cerebral, and peripheral blood vessels, are responsible for most loss of life from diabetes. Most health departments, believing adequate control is essential to avoid complications, have begun diabetes detection programs. These are aimed at finding the disease in its earliest stage, when it can cause abnormally high blood sugar without necessarily producing symptoms. If the diabetic then receives good medical attention and cooperates by regulating his diet and taking prescribed medications, it is hoped that we can add immeasurably to his survival and continued self-sufficiency.

In addition, health departments are now becoming interested in another group: those who have a small distortion of blood sugar without presenting enough evidence to warrant a diagnosis of diabetes. These potential diabetics or "prediabetics" are now being studied to see whether special treatment might prevent their developing diabetes altogether. Screening would thus be a way of locating the individual at risk of developing diabetes so that measures could be taken to keep him free of the disease.

Certain additional groups are particularly prone to diabetes: individuals with a family history of the disease, the obese, and women whose infants weigh more than ten pounds at birth. Epidemiologic efforts are aimed at locating these individuals and seeing that they receive annual tests for diabetes. So far, although many communities have these programs, none has been able to demonstrate a major decrease in deaths chargeable to diabetes through these efforts.

Generalized Arteriosclerosis

Pathologic changes in blood vessels, probably similar to those in coronary arteries, is the ninth cause of death. We know little about the causes of atherosclerosis in other than the coronary arteries; there may well be influences other than diet, lack of exercise, and high blood pressure. Moreover, many deaths charged to this condition might have been charged to heart disease if the patients had been more thoroughly studied.

Congenital Malformation

At present our effort to prevent the tenth leading cause of death lies in instituting the best rehabilitative and medical care. Research now under way should help us understand the genetic mechanisms in these conditions. Much has already been discovered, and some day we may be able to prevent congenital malformations. With gamma globulin, health officials can now prevent German measles in pregnancy and thus prevent malformations in many fetuses.

Other Causes of Death

Tuberculosis, eleventh cause of death in New York City, dropped in 1959 for the first time from the list of the top 10. Although tuberculosis decreases year by year as a cause of death, there is still a large reservoir of undetected cases in most urban centers in this country. No longer a major disease of young women, its primary target is now older men of the low socio-economic class, whose rehabilitation is often complicated by the need for total social rehabilitation. Alcoholism, poverty, homelessness, physical defects, and other chronic diseases make social rehabilitation difficult.

Cases are found in mass surveys or in routine x-raying of patients admitted to the general services of hospitals or outpatient departments. It is standard epidemiologic procedure to x-ray families and contacts of known cases. The tuberculin test is used to measure the prevalence of the infection among various age groups, and to find cases among the young. It is now recommended that young children with positive tuberculin reactions receive isoniazid treatment as a preventive measure.

In New York and other large centers, tuberculosis must be continuously sought among nonwhites, Puerto Ricans, and inmates of homes for the aged, nursing homes, correctional institutions, and shelters for homeless men. Whereas the prevalence of tuberculosis in mass surveys is now well below one per thousand in New York City, the rate has been as high as 16 per thousand among those admitted to a welfare shelter for homeless men.

Suicides, number 12 among causes of death, and homicides, number 18, represent groups in the community who are suffering from various social and emotional diseases. To prevent these deaths the health department must act in close association with many other community agencies. An interesting development in suicide control has been undertaken in several areas, where 24-hour counseling and guidance are available to the individual who feels he needs support. At present much more epidemiologic knowledge is needed about suicides. It has been suggested that persons who attempt suicide and fail are particularly in need of mental health services.

To prevent most of the other causes of death—ulcer, number 13; hypertension, number 14; other diseases of circulatory system, 15; chronic nephritis, 16; hernia and intestinal obstruction, 17; benign and unspecified neoplasms, 19; and hyperplasia of the prostate, 20—the major resource is good medical care. This means prompt diagnosis of the condition, effective treatment, and follow-up care.

PRIORITIES FOR PREVENTION

In summary, we can make a few general comments about the 20 leading causes of death as Public Health problems. Public Health can do a great deal to prevent two of the 20. Although some mysteries still exist, we can save a significant number of those suffering from the influenza-pneumonia illnesses. With influenza vaccine and prompt, adequate treatment of pneumonia we prevent many deaths. State and federal laboratories can isolate new forms of influenza virus which appear in the community and promptly prepare vaccines for widespread use. We still have undiscovered cases of tuberculosis and our present methods of control could be applied more thoroughly.

We are essentially powerless, however, against 18 of the 20 leading causes of death unless we can discover new and potent weapons. Although the biologic facts may be known—as for the prevention of deaths from lung cancer—we have so far been unable to apply them in any community to any measurable degree. Insulin for the diabetic, and diet low in saturated fat for the heart patient may some day offer promise, but research and demonstration are needed now to indicate that this is really so.

Cancer of the cervix and certain conditions of early infancy are amenable to control, and effective measures should be taken by local health officers. The exact nature of the programs will depend upon many factors, but in nearly every community an effective start can be made.

Nevertheless, it is not yet possible to prevent most of the major causes of death in our present civilization. Our priorities must be:

1. Research to discover new resources which might be effective.
2. Demonstrations of promising new approaches to see if they are truly effective and acceptable to the population, and to ascertain their impact upon other programs.
3. Medical care to ameliorate the condition, postpone its degenerative aspects, and rehabilitate the patient to the highest possible degree of self-sufficiency.

DISEASES THAT DISABLE

In addition to the major causes of death as determinants of the health program, there are a number of major non-fatal causes of disability. Leading the field are the mental diseases, which are responsible for half the patients in hospital beds in this nation. Most communities have mental health clinics; their over-all effectiveness is as yet largely unproved. Nevertheless, we must continue to offer mental health services in order to learn more about the mental illness and in the hope that our services will be somewhat effective.

Non-fatal stroke is another condition of importance; since World War II an enormous amount of attention has been devoted to the rehabilitation of stroke victims. Glaucoma, number one cause of blindness in this country, is detectable in its early stages; if treated early, most patients can be helped and blindness prevented. Arthritis, a rather mysterious condition, is being attacked by research in both laboratory and epidemiologic studies; present rehabilitation efforts show some good results.

A number of infectious diseases, such as the common cold, hepatitis, and measles, are major causes of temporary disability. The search continues for a greater understanding of these conditions and for effective vaccines. We may be on the threshold of effective vaccines for hepatitis and measles and for some, but by no means all, of the common respiratory diseases.

Dental caries is another significant condition which results in disability. We know how to prevent two-thirds of the dental caries by fluoridating public water supplies. Although nearly one-fifth of the U.S. population is now consuming fluoridated water, many large urban centers have not seen fit to adopt fluoridation. It has been estimated that one engineer responsible for the fluoridation of the public water supply in New York City could prevent more cavities in children's teeth than the city's 8,000 dentists could fill, even if they worked at the problem full time.

ACCENT ON REHABILITATION

Rehabilitation has meant much to Public Health in this decade. Ingenious new technics have made rehabilitation services more effective; the concept of rehabilitation itself has led to a major shift in Public Health philosophy. Whereas in the past we emphasized prevention and cure as major parts of a Public Health program, today we begin our rehabilitation programs with a frank admission of our inability to prevent and cure. We emphasize that despite his disease the patient can be brought to a greater degree of self-sufficiency if we apply special varieties of medical care. Hence, we can have two individuals with the same degree of arthritis, the same degree of farsighted vision, the same degree of high blood pressure, and yet one may be confined to bed and the other be a relatively active and productive citizen. We cannot find the difference between them by minutely assessing physical condition organ by organ, but by studying the total adaptation each has been able to make between his physical and mental status on one side and life's challenges on the other. Patients must be helped to adapt and thereby increase their level of activities of daily living.

The concept of rehabilitation has led us to accentuate the positives, not the negatives, in mental and physical health. Instead of stressing what is wrong with the patient, we stress what is right. It is not important in daily living that he can bend his knee only a little; the important thing is that he can bend it enough to walk and go up and down stairs. It is not important that he has lost 40 per cent of his vision; what is significant is that he can read effectively with strong spectacles. In New York City it is usually not enough that a disabled man be able to hobble around a little on crutches; until he can walk fast enough to cross a New York City street in 45 seconds, before the traffic light changes, he cannot ordinarily move about in our community. In a less hectic place, the demands upon him would be far less and he could be more self-sufficient. The concept of rehabilitation is geared to the individual in the particular situation in which he finds himself or in which we place him. Rehabilitation, more than anything else in Public Health, has made us concentrate upon the individual and forced us to plan each man's program in terms of his locus, abilities, goals, and potentialities.

There is a huge cost factor in rehabilitation. With an adult we are often working against time—time which seems to degenerate our patient faster than we can rehabilitate him. Rehabilitation has a practical goal—to return the patient to the activities of daily living—and we must be equally practical in deciding how much rehabilitation care we can afford to invest in each patient. In New York City we are studying the dimensions of the problem through a community-wide program in one section with a 200,000 population.

I predict that rehabilitation services will take on increasing importance as the years go by. No matter what happens to our list of the 20 leading causes of death, there will always be patients needing rehabilitation. With each we must weigh the cost of improvement against the ultimate social and economic value of the improvement.

FIVE CRITERIA OF GOOD MEDICAL CARE

No matter how we look at the health problems affecting large numbers of our people, the importance of good medical care is paramount. We recognize five criteria of a good medical care program.

The first is *comprehensiveness*. A program is comprehensive when it makes available to each patient all the technics and services he requires for adequate medical care—doctors, hospitals, vaccines, drugs, speech therapists, physiotherapists, or dentists.

The second principle is *continuity of care*. Each patient should be cared for by a single physician or team of physicians through his entire medical care program. If this is impossible, the next best thing is to send his new physician or team an up-to-date, complete, and accurate medical and social record showing exactly what has already been done for him. This is not done routinely, as it should be; in many parts of the country it is actually easier to repeat complicated x-ray and laboratory procedures on a new patient than to obtain his record from another institution. Moreover, many of our major social welfare programs are geared to destroy continuity of care by forcing patients to change physicians and institutions when the patients are shifted from one type of assistance to another.

The third criterion is that medical care should be *family-centered*. Instead of fragmenting the family among many different clinics and physicians, there is much to be gained by centering the care of the entire family in one medical group. Not only is disease often a family phenomenon, but certainly its effective treatment and rehabilitation should make use of any community strength which may exist. His family is still a major source of community strength for any individual. Removing him from his family, ignoring other family problems as we plan his care, often leads to defeat for health workers. For example, recently we had proof that a child is far more likely to smoke when both parents smoke; any attempt at educating him in school to avoid the habit seems doomed to failure if he returns home to see parental smoking.

The fourth criterion of a good medical care program is that it should emphasize *preventive services*. Many hospital patients could be offered such preventive services as diabetes, glaucoma, cancer, and tuberculosis detection if such programs were available. Many go routinely to specialty clinics such as those limited to ear, nose, and throat, but may have other significant medical conditions, such as cervical cancer or tuberculosis, of which the specialty clinic is unaware. Every patient receiving care from any medical group is a candidate for comprehensive care, including the full range of preventive services.

The last criterion is that all medical care should be of the *highest quality*. Surgery should be performed only by competent surgeons, hospitals should meet full accreditation standards, and all the benefits of the teaching hospital should be available to the community. Although 90 per cent of medical care takes place away from the hospital bed, most of our high-quality physicians spend the greater portion of their time working with patients in teaching-hospital beds. The bene-

fits of this high-quality care must be extended to outpatient departments, home care programs, home visiting, nursing homes, and homes
for the aged.

In general, then, medical care must be oriented to the patient, not
to the treatment facility. As Dr. Breslow says, "The right patient must
be in the right bed at the right time and must be receiving the right
treatment." This should be true for all, rich or poor. Many of our
poorest, most fragmented medical programs are all that are available
to the well-to-do. The practice of fragmenting programs by organizing
them around the agency which pays for them is highly reprehensible.
In most cases this results in episodic medicine, in purchasing a given
piece of medical care of a certain category permissible under federal,
State, or local legislation.

A study now under way in New York City highlights many aspects
of this problem of fragmented medical care. For example, it has demonstrated that 80 per cent of those on our welfare rolls go off the rolls
in any given year; sooner or later, most of them return to welfare. But
during the time they are not receiving public assistance, their medical
care is handled in an entirely different way by different groups of
physicians. Recently we found that one man with six children, each of
whom was going to a different outpatient clinic, was spending his entire day sitting in clinic waiting rooms. When his children were
brought together in a family-centered program, the man went back to
work and the entire family was removed from the welfare rolls.

TYPES OF SERVICE
Outpatient Care

The outpatient department is an important element in the
scheme of medical care activities. Fragmentation of services by specialty, an outgrowth of the past, must give way to an integrated,
family-centered approach. Outpatient care must become part of a continuum with hospital and home care. Visits to emergency rooms in
New York City's municipal hospitals have increased 74 per cent in
the last six years; visits to outpatient clinics have increased only 26 per
cent. Patients have learned that the wait in emergency rooms is
shorter, that they will be cared for any time, day or night. Emergency
rooms give the most fragmentary kind of episodic services, of course.
To correct this problem in New York City, we are trying to establish
branch clinics of overcrowded institutions either in other hospitals or
in health department facilities; here, physicians of the home hospital
operate the clinic in cooperation with the agency owning the structure.
This brings clinic care closer to the patient's home and high-quality

medicine to a wider area of the community, maintains continuity of care, avoids overcrowding.

New York City is also expanding its day clinics for mentally ill patients. We have found that these patients, who might otherwise have to be hospitalized, can be treated effectively during the day and returned home for evenings and weekends. The program is family-centered. Often the psychiatrists find that the patient under treatment at the day clinic for hallucinations and delusions is not the only mentally ill person in the family, but simply the one with overt symptoms. Sometimes a strong-willed and seemingly well-integrated person is really the sickest member of the family and the major cause of the patient's disease. The day hospital program gives the psychiatrist an opportunity to work with the whole family, often with startling results.

Home-care services are an important addition to the armamentarium of medical care. At first it was believed that a strong home was essential for the maintenance of home-care services. But we have found that a single person can be given home care when the community will add homemaker or housekeeper services. The total cost is much less than the cost of hospitalization, and the patient can be helped more readily toward self-sufficiency. The New York City Department of Health, in cooperation with other community agencies, is undertaking a number of programs in housing projects that will offer tenants improved health maintenance and home-care services. It has been surprising to us how many of these people had never received adequate medical care for the many conditions with which we find them suffering.

Nursing homes are another important part of the medical care program. It is essential that a nursing home be affiliated with a medical center so that the highest quality of medical care can be offered to the patients in the home. With rehabilitation the goal, the nursing home is part of the complex of medical care along with the hospital, the clinic, and the home-care program. A patient can be moved between nursing home and hospital to assure the best care at each stage of his illness, convalescence, or relapse.

General Maintenance of Health

So far I have discussed the major causes of death and disability and the ways that health departments seek to prevent or ameliorate disease and otherwise care for the sick. Most health departments also provide a number of *general maintenance services*. One relates to the control of communicable diseases. Many of these diseases, once major scourges, are now largely controlled. The health department must maintain this control and keep the diseases from increasing in significance again. Smallpox reappeared in 1947; this year it appeared in India and Pakistan, whence it spread to England, Germany, and Switzerland. All port cities have been urged to step up their routine vaccination programs of hospital employees because most smallpox in western Europe and the United States in recent years was transmitted by undiagnosed cases in hospitals. There is also an extensive program of surveillance of those who have been in infected areas to see whether any develop smallpox after arrival in this country. Control of diphtheria and whooping cough must be maintained by ensuring that immunizations are up to date.

We are concerned about certain groups in the community who do not take advantage of the widespread polio immunization services available to them. Our efforts in these fields must continue and all promising leads must be explored. For example, we have given Public Health nurses syringes of polio vaccine so that when they visit a home they may immunize children on the spot. In most cases we find no resistance, just lethargy about taking advantage of the immunization procedure, which is widely available in clinics throughout the city.

Typhoid, cholera, plague, and rabies have essentially been wiped out as major threats to our population, but we must keep on the alert to prevent their recurrence. A few cases of typhoid continue to appear, spread by carriers in our community. Dog bites are frequent and rabies always a fear; with the recent discovery of rabies in bats in various parts of the country, this disease has taken on added significance. We now realize that there is an ever-present reservoir of rabies infection in our midst.

Another general maintenance service is the control of nutritional diseases. Although most major diseases born of malnutrition have been conquered, there are still groups in the population who are not receiving optimal amounts of common nutrients. Pregnant women must pay careful attention to their diet. The aged, because of low income, general lethargy, or cultural diet patterns, often do not maintain an adequate diet; lack of teeth and particular disorders of the gastrointestinal tract in this age group also add to the problem.

Prenatal Services

The provision of adequate services for pregnant women is a program of the highest importance in every community. Even in New York, replete with facilities, about one-fifth of the pregnant women have no prenatal care at all or receive care late in pregnancy. A recent study gave us the reasons: ignorance, a false sense of security because they had already had children, difficulty in getting away from the family when there are small children at home, and inadequate attention in clinics often not geared to their particular needs. Efforts are now being made to have prenatal clinics in the evening or to invite patients to bring their preschool children to daytime child health clinics. The Department of Health has developed a number of prenatal clinics in cooperation with hospitals to give more family-centered care. Most health departments have dropped isolated prenatal services in the belief that a woman should be cared for in the clinic of the hospital which will deliver her baby. This good arrangement is bettered when the hospital operates a branch clinic in the health department, thereby bringing services closer to the home.

Services to Mothers and Babies

The importance of continuous follow-up of infants and preschool children in child health conferences is well-known. All need immunizations and many require treatment because of physical defects. In addition, behavior problems evidenced during the preschool period can prove serious in later life if help is not given to the family. In New York City we study the attitudes of the mother toward the child, and, in the child health clinic, attempt first to discover what troubles her and take steps to be of assistance. On the other hand, if she has no particular difficulties and her child is well, the clinic team does not spend as much time with her. This is another indication of our attempt to gear the service to the patient. A problem that disturbs us in child health clinic care is the large number of "drop-outs"— children who come for a while and then stop coming. This is being studied to discover why it occurs and to take steps to correct it.

Services to the Child in School

The health of the school-age child requires the full use of all community resources. In some areas this health program comes under the auspices of the health department, in others under the department of education. In either case no one department can do the task alone; in fact, many community agencies must take part. The school is a convenient place where children can be studied and followed with a minimum of administrative difficulty. Those with chronic rheumatic heart disease can be supervised to see that they take their daily penicillin tablet. At school we have an opportunity to study a defect and the effect of corrective measures. School is also an excellent place to observe early manifestations of diseases which if untreated, would become significant in later life. Among these is obesity, since it has been shown that the obese child is apt to become the obese adult. Dietary habits can be established in these children which will have great importance in their later years. It has been shown that many children establish the habit of smoking between the ages of 11 and 14; it may be possible to prevent this habit in many by working with children in this age group and with their parents. Habits of physical exercise should be inculcated in this group if we want them to maintain an exercise program when they are adults. The emphasis upon inter-school athletics should not distract us from encouraging each child to develop his own physical exercise program on a permanent basis.

Nor should we lose sight of the enormous educational importance of demonstration during the school years. A hasty, ill-conceived, poorly done physical examination of a high school student merely leads that student to believe little can be expected from a physical examination later on in life. It is important that we show the school-age child only the highest quality of health services, including counseling and mental health services.

Services for Adults

General maintenance services for adults are receiving greater attention now than ever before. In our early industrial hygiene programs we attempted to assure the continued health of the worker. Soon we discovered that many of the major conditions affecting the American worker were directly traceable to the home. For example, industry made great strides in preventing factory accidents but not in reducing worker absenteeism caused by accidents at home. Instead of providing clinic service only in illness, we now try to attract adults to clinics for general health maintenance. Some areas provide clinic services for the aged, since they suffer from a large number of physical and mental defects. In several New York City housing projects, health services are offered to aged tenants in an attempt to maintain them in their homes in maximum health, and to prevent disease from advancing to the point where hospitalization is the only hope. Although it is too early to report tangible results, we know that these health maintenance programs are extremely popular and that many patients are receiving necessary medical care for the first time in years.

Most health departments provide laboratory services: performing actual tests, training local laboratory scientists, developing new tests, inspecting and consulting with local laboratories. Again, in keeping with the desire of modern Public Health workers to be coordinators, it is not necessary for the health department to perform each service itself if it can help to raise the quality and ability of others and thereby ensure the adequacy of essential laboratory services.

Housekeeping Services

These health services maintain the cleanliness of the community as a means of preventing disease and providing an esthetic and attractive environment. In insisting on sanitary food and milk, health departments not only prevent the spread of diseases such as typhoid, paratyphoid and dysentery, but also provide a wholesome, palatable product. It is important that the taste and odor of a water supply be inoffensive, even if they are not significant in preventing disease.

In our major cities, pollution of harbor waters has recently received greater attention. Unless pollution can be reduced and controlled, the recreational use of waters for bathing may be seriously impaired. General environmental sanitation—adequate housing, rat control, sufficient heat in apartments—is also a program that citizens have come to demand. It is obvious that the urban apartment-dweller cannot handle these problems by himself.

Other housekeeping services relate to environmental problems of increasing importance—radiation and air pollution. Although there has been much in the papers recently about radioactive fallout, by far the greatest source of unnecessary human exposure to radiation comes from the improper use of x-ray machines. A recent survey in New York City found 90 per cent of these to be defective, either in construction or operation. Most health departments are undertaking major programs of radiation control to prevent unnecessary dosages of radiation. When properly used, x-rays, a potent device for the detection and treatment of disease, need give us no concern. On the other hand, it is unnecessary to spray portions of the population with scatter radiation which serves no useful purpose in medicine and can cause ultimate genetic damage to the human race.

Although the health implications of air pollution are not entirely known except in major disasters such as occurred at Donora and London, the citizen demands a clean atmosphere for the enjoyment of life and property. Studies are under way to elucidate the importance of air pollution in chronic pulmonary disease and lung cancer. That air pollution plays some role in the development of these diseases seems fairly certain, but the exact relationship and the relative importance of air pollution requires much further study.

Finally, the health department provides certain services largely because they are socially desirable. Certification of births and deaths is one such service. The collection and tabulation of vital statistics enable us to analyze various facets of the Public Health situation and to derive new approaches to old problems. For example, several years ago we began to look to the birth certificate for information on congenital defects in newborn infants, and this has been helpful in planning rehabilitation programs for these children.

AVENUES TO PUBLIC HEALTH

What approaches are used by health departments in offering service to people? One is *direct service* by physicians, nurses, dentists, and social workers to prevent and treat disease. Another is *service on behalf of people.* For example, sanitation inspections of restaurants and public water supplies and the introduction of fluoride into a water supply system are services which aid people, often without their being aware of them.

A third approach is *health education* to stimulate greater use of health services. Health education is often aimed at special groups, sub-cultures in a community. For example, one study in New York City discovered that people from Czechoslovakia were twice as willing to accept medical care when symptoms of illness occurred as were those from Ireland. Such a cultural difference in the acceptance of medical care is extremely important, if we wish to emphasize early diagnosis and prompt treatment for chronic disease.

Health education has its limitations, and it is important that health departments realize this. Recently social scientists studied whether health education technics were useful in persuading patients to get chest x-rays during a mass survey in the Bronx. Repeated studies of this population failed to reveal that health education technics were effective. Of far greater effectiveness were (a) a loud-speaker at the site of the x-ray unit blaring forth Calypso music, (b) good weather, and (c) location of the x-ray bus where large numbers of people congregated, such as shopping centers. Another example of health education which failed was Edinburgh's extensive effort to point out the danger of lung cancer. Despite an amazing amount of community cooperation, no change occurred in the smoking habits of Scotsmen.

One of the approaches used by local health departments is *coordination.* Because of its broad mandate, the health department is often in the best position to take leadership among many agencies and bring them together on behalf of a given health program. The Queensbridge Housing Project program, organized by a district health officer, has five city agencies and several voluntary agencies working together for 1,000 aged persons who live in the project. The Department of Health has not determined the roles of these agencies, but has brought them together to concentrate on the specific problem; and in working together each group defines its own role. There are other examples in our area where the Department of Health has taken the first step in working with voluntary and municipal hospitals to develop joint programs for continuous, comprehensive, and, we hope, eventually family-centered care for groups in the population.

A health department can play a major role in *research and demonstration* for health. Research is essential if we are to provide new services to fill gaps. Although much research is undertaken by medical schools and other institutions, many major problems in chronic disease lend themselves to the epidemiologic approach. Health officers have the opportunity to study large numbers of presumably well people and to observe them when they develop the earliest signs and symptoms of disease. These prospective studies might give us much information about the development of disease, enabling us to take steps to control it.

Research is also needed if we are to streamline existing services. We can no longer continue to pour men and material into traditional programs when these resources are desperately needed for new programs. For example, a few injections of penicillin cure venereal disease better than a year and a half of arsenic and bismuth, and free a large amount of manpower for new services. Likewise, development of the three-in-one vaccine cuts the number of clinic visits for infants and preschool children, and frees clinic time and personnel for other activities.

If we are to bring more services to people who are not taking advantage of those now available, we may have to *redesign the package.* If all the polio vaccine in the world were on top of Mount Everest, few cooperative persons would come for vaccination—Tensing and Hillary and the four who followed later. For many, perhaps, the health services now available are really on Mount Everest. Let us bring them down. Let us find out how to locate and package our services to make them immediately available to all our people. Perhaps some do not take advantage of them because of ignorance, cultural blocks, inconvenience. Giving polio vaccinations in homes is a different way of packaging services. Bringing medical care into a housing project for the aged is another. The usefulness of any package depends upon the total problem, the local value system, and the particular group we are trying to serve. We must become involved with the specific problems, and keep an open mind about alternate solutions, if we are to achieve success.

Another approach is *evaluation.* Whenever we undertake a health program, we arrange for feedback of the results so that we can make indicated modifications. Periodically we become dissatisfied with a program and try a new approach, as we did in the control of cancer of the cervix in New York City.[1] We began in 1947 with a cancer detection clinic in a teaching center. Most of the patients were Jewish women, the group with the lowest incidence of cancer of the cervix in our city. Nonwhites and Puerto Ricans, whom we wanted to attract, did not come to the clinic. Result: we found few cancers of the cervix. We then opened a cancer detection clinic in East Harlem, heart of the Negro and Puerto Rican area, and still had a clientele composed mostly of Jewish women; only a quarter of the patients were in the high-prevalence risk groups. Noting that our social hygiene clinics served many in the high-risk groups, we began taking Papanicolaou smears along with gonorrhea smears and cultures. Although we found a high yield of cancer of the cervix, we still reached only a fraction of the New York City women who were developing the disease. We therefore extended the detection service to all women admitted as outpatients or inpatients to two large municipal hospitals in the area of highest prevalence. This resulted in the detection of an appreciable number of cancers of the cervix. Eventually we shall expand the program to the remainder of the city.

The information fed back to us from each clinic spurred the Department of Health to change its approach and modify its program. Once we thought we would have to blanket the city with cancer detection clinics; now we know this would be an inefficient way of finding cancer. Instead, routine screening of general hospital admissions in areas of high prevalence is now the method of choice.

ORGANIZATION OF PUBLIC HEALTH SERVICES

More than 20 years ago Haven Emerson studied the pattern of local health services in this country and recommended the creation of a finite number of county and district health departments. His blueprint, based largely on recommendations from state health departments concerned about jurisdictional limits and home rule, was then used as a basis for the creation of new local health departments. To some degree his recommendations were accepted, but frequently they were ignored.

Local health departments expanded after World War II, but now seem to have reached a plateau. A study of Kit Carson County, Colorado,[2] shows that many citizens are receiving adequate services without an organized local health department. Elsewhere, communities with organized health departments are known to receive inadequate services. Our emphasis therefore has shifted from organization to service. The National Advisory Committee on Local Health Departments, formed in 1940 to implement Dr. Emerson's report, now recommends that we work toward the goal of adequate community health services, not toward the creation of a fixed organizational structure.

It is obvious that much is done to improve the nation's health by other than official health agencies. Nearly every governmental program has some health component. The police are concerned about safety, alcoholism, juvenile delinquency, narcotic addiction, and the enforcement of some Health Code provisions for cleanliness. Fire departments are interested in safe construction. Education departments are interested in school health, health education, and vocational rehabilitation. Welfare departments are often responsible for medical care of welfare recipients. Labor departments are interested in industrial hygiene. Departments of parks are interested in recreation and exercise, departments of markets in the cleanliness and wholesomeness of food, mental health departments in a significant part of the total health picture.

Voluntary agencies also carry on many effective health programs. Some have specific health goals: control of cancer, heart disease, muscular dystrophy, venereal diseases, tuberculosis, polio and birth defects. For others, the health goal is not paramount, though important. For example, Lions Clubs are concerned about the problem of blindness; Boy Scouts, Girl Scouts, and Camp Fire Girls stress health and safety; and Kiwanis Clubs and the Junior and Senior Chambers of Commerce frequently sponsor specific health projects of significance nationally or in particular areas.

There is no automatic, sure way of ascertaining which agency, public or voluntary, is best able to accept responsibility for a particular health program. Organizational patterns differ widely from locality to locality, and a given health program may be sponsored here by one agency, there by another. Nor is there a rule which says this category of personnel must be governmental or voluntary. Even sectarian personnel—chaplains, for example—are found on government payrolls in State and municipal hospitals.

Today we see the emergence of new patterns in health programing. New Jersey's Hunterdon County is showing how a large county hospital can detect chronic disease and raise the level of medical care for an entire county, with results far superior to those obtained in most communities with organized local health departments. Northern California's small counties buy their health services from the State health department. Labor's health centers are delivering adequate health services to union members, and certain industries have developed health programs of note.

To reiterate, it is not important that a particular local health structure meet a given organizational criterion. It *is* important that the health service received by our people be of excellent quality. That is the true measure of success. Is the service adequate, effective, efficient, comprehensive, family-centered? These questions must be answered as we evaluate a health program and seek to improve it.

CONCLUSION

How does one steer a course through this maze of organizations, policies, goals, disciplines, technics? In the interest of efficiency, we must argue for some coordination of effort. Although research may require many different approaches and thrive on competition, service programs generally are injured by competition because it inhibits free communication and concentration upon all aspects of the changing problem. Competition and lack of coordination fragment services for individuals who were never created to be served in a fragmented fashion and whose needs are not fragmented. Fortunately, affiliations are developing between health centers and hospitals, child health clinics and hospitals, school health programs and hospitals. The child whose defects are detected in a school health program can now be treated in the hospital by the same physician who serves the school.

Our welfare recipients would benefit from a similar liaison between the health and medical care programs in the community. One cannot buy medical care for welfare recipients as one buys a pound of spinach; spinach is generally as good in one store as in another. We will never have comprehensive, continuous, preventive, high-quality, family-centered health care so long as we think of it as so much spinach.

In New York City the director of welfare medical care is an employee of the Department of Health on full-time loan to the Department of Welfare. He calls upon the full resources of the Department of Health and of other city and voluntary agencies which can be useful in developing a program that works. In addition to the welfare medical director, the Department of Health has assigned several other employees to other agencies. One physician is developing a home care program in a city hospital. Another is developing a program of research and demonstration in community medical care for a voluntary hospital. We have a separate Department of Mental Health, although the Department of Health operates many programs with mental health implications. To handle these properly, we have requested the Commissioner of Mental Health to assign a psychiatrist with Public Health experience to the Department of Health. In developing these mental health programs, he will look to the Department of Health for administrative supervision, to the Commissioner of Mental Health for technical guidance.

I end this paper as I began—by emphasizing the individual's need as the proper point of reference and evaluation. I have mentioned the Queensbridge Housing Project, where five municipal and five voluntary agencies cooperate in bringing health services to 1,000 needy aged tenants. Once a month representatives of these agencies meet to hear the medical staff discuss problem cases. Recently I heard three cases, each offering the array of difficult problems peculiar to the economically depressed aged and neglected person. Each agency representative remarked at least once when a particularly difficult problem arose, "We can't do anything about this particular problem. Our agency doesn't cover this sort of thing." Before the discussion was over, however, each was suggesting how his agency could be of help after all. Something upsets our cherished notions when we leave our desks and face a person in need.

The road to success in community programs is not paved with agency policies, principles, manuals, and regulations. These are necessary, of course. But when there is human need, when resources are at hand, precedents, traditions, rules must bend before the appeals for help. The impact of a small discrete demonstration on the agency's overall program is not immediately drastic. There is time to modify, slowly and methodically. In this way the new service can develop within the agency without disturbing the integrity of normal, routine programs.

If we believe we can solve health problems by evolution rather than revolution, then let us arrange ourselves so that we can respond to these pressures for service. Let us cooperate with all others who can help. Let us learn to work together as we learn how best to serve people in need.

Cooperation and coordination are not merely desirable principles, signs of an advanced civilization. If we could be successful working alone, then by all means let's stop this infernal round of committees, conferences, communications, and interagency discussions. But we cannot. The problems of medical care, rehabilitation, health maintenance, and health inspection are too complex to be solved by any single agency. Man's present health problems cannot be solved by fragmented approaches. "Unite and conquer" is the slogan of this age of ecology. The insatiable social and health needs of our many different populations demand this of us. The least we can do is meet each other halfway, flexible of mind, dissatisfied with current methods, continuously aware of the problem itself. A real willingness to work with all useful individuals and agencies will come. It *must* come if we are to succeed in local Public Health service during this present era.

1. George James, "Program Planning and Evaluation in a Modern City Health Department," *American Journal of Public Health*, 51:1828–40, December 1961.

2. Donald Harting and Others, "Public Health Needs in a Great Plains Country," *American Journal of Public Health*, 49:1591–95, December 1959.

3. The Hospital and Regionalization

Hospital Regionalization in Perspective*

MILTON I. ROEMER, M.D., AND ROBERT C. MORRIS

REGIONALIZATION of hospital services has become a popular theme in the United States. Since 1947, State master plans for hospital construction under the Federal Hill-Burton Act have been based on this concept. Regional and metropolitan hospital councils are set up in 11 States. Insurance commissioners, faced with rising Blue Cross premiums, have called for regional coordination of hospitals to reduce costs.[1] A series of conferences has been held across the Nation on planning hospital systems, in which regional organization is the key problem. Seasoned hospital leaders call for more research in the field.[2]

But the meaning of "hospital regionalization" is not always clear. To some it is simply an approach to making decisions on where hospital buildings are needed and how many beds should be provided at each location. To others it means a systematic scheme for cooperation among hospitals in their day-to-day operations. To a European, it usually implies unified management of a network of hospitals in a geographic region. And there are other defined points in the range of possible meanings.

In fact, hospital regionalization has had different meanings historically, and it has different meanings today in different parts of the world or different places in the United States. Perhaps the only common note in all the interpretations is an element of coordination, in planning construction or in actual operations or both, among a group of hospitals in a geographic region. Ways of expressing this coordination vary greatly. The intention is always to give the hospital program a rational structure in order to improve the quality of service or reduce the costs or both. But whether this goal has actually been achieved by regionalization efforts or how it might be best achieved are questions to which we do not have answers.

If we take a closer look at the hospital regionalization movement,

* Reprinted by permission from the October, 1959, issue of *Public Health Reports*, Volume 74, pages 916–922. The authors are Professor of Medical Care Administration, School of Public Health, and Professor of Preventive Medicine and Public Health, School of Medicine, University of California, Los Angeles, formerly Director of Research, Sloan Institute of Hospital Administration, Graduate School of Business and Public Administration, Cornell University, Ithaca, New York; and Research Associate on the staff of the Sloan Institute of Hospital Administration.

we may gain perspective in designing research to answer these questions.

HISTORICAL BACKGROUND

It is customary in the United States to trace the origin of the hospital regionalization idea to the program of the Bingham Associates Fund operating in Maine since 1936.[3] Here was an effort to bring first-class modern scientific medicine to residents of the rural areas and small towns of Maine. The emphasis was on improved resources for medical diagnosis. The base center is in Boston, where patients with difficult cases are sent. Then there are two regional or district hospitals in the principal cities of Maine and 38 cooperating small community hospitals around them. More recently western Massachusetts has been added to the program. In this area four larger hospitals, lying close together, jointly serve as a regional center for 10 smaller community hospitals. Laboratory specimens and X-ray films are sent from the community hospitals to the regional centers for examination, and consultants go outward from the centers to advise the rural doctors. Physicians are encouraged to come to the centers for postgraduate education. Consultation is also offered in nursing, dietetics, medical record-keeping, and other aspects of hospital administration.

This program, with its two-way flow of patients and services, now the hallmark of the regionalization concept, was built with outside philanthropic support. Certainly the quality of services in the smaller hospitals has been improved, but we have little, if any, idea of the relative costs, and whether the same end might be served in other less expensive or more effective ways.

The basic idea of hospital regionalization, however, is much older than the Bingham program. In Denmark, around 1912, the decision was made to avoid further building of rural hospitals and to bring patients with complicated illnesses from rural areas to the central hospitals. A network of institutions was developed, centering in Copenhagen and branching out to the whole country.[4]

In 1920, there appeared an English study on improving hospital services which described the basic scheme embodied in the British National Health Service 28 years later. The Dawson report called for establishment of a network of hospitals within which all services could be integrated. It defined primary and secondary health centers and recommended that the smaller units, staffed mainly by general practitioners, be supervised by the larger ones, staffed mainly by specialists. The report even sketched prototype centers, showing buildings and layouts and listing services to be performed.[5]

Military medical establishments have long been organized on a regional scheme, with base hospitals, division or theater-of-operation hospitals, and field stations. Highly systematized, of course, these hospitals demonstrate the feasibility of actual administration of many institutions by a central authority.

Colonial governments have likewise operated hospital systems through central authority. In Asia and Africa, there are capital and district hospitals, with small health centers or mobile clinics at the periphery. Countries liberated from crown domination, such as India or Indonesia, have usually retained and developed these regional hospital networks.

With one or two exceptions, Catholic sisterhoods do not operate regional hospital networks, but have long exercised central authority over certain aspects of their hospitals which may be located in scores of far-flung communities. Funds are pooled which may be channeled to provide construction and equipment wherever it is most needed, and uniform administrative policies are usually enforced.

These are expressions of the hospital regionalization concept originating many years ago. In fact, if we think of regionalization as a range of activities, we must go back even farther. For any step of a hospital from isolation and self-sufficiency toward interdependence with other agencies or organizations is fundamentally a move in the direction of regionalization.

Thus we can visualize a hospital in colonial America, such as the Pennsylvania Hospital in 1751, as an institution quite alone. The staff may not have grown their own food for hospital use, but surely they made most of their own bandages and supplies. There was, moreover, little to be purchased from the commercial market. There were ideas brought from Europe, but their implementation was entirely up to the small staff working in this solitary structure.

As other hospitals were established, as industry grew, as medicine developed, the hospital obviously became less isolated. Equipment and supplies were produced by industrial companies. Educational institutions trained skilled personnel needed to staff the hospital. A Public Health laboratory did tests on hospital patients. A State agency was given legal authority to approve certain aspects of hospital construction or operation. Money to support services for certain beneficiaries was derived from diverse public and voluntary agencies. Associations of hospitals were formed for educational and promotional purposes.

In different countries, this process of dynamic inter-relationship among hospitals has evolved in different ways and to varying degrees. In general, the process has gone farther in countries where governments at all levels, national, provincial, or local, have become largely responsible for the ownership and operation of hospitals. This is, indeed, the predominant pattern in Europe, Latin America, Asia, and in fact the entire world outside the United States and Canada.[6]

Even in the United States, however, the regionalization process has been clear and gaining momentum. Much of it has been on a casual, spontaneous basis. Patients are transferred from one hospital to another. Equipment is sometimes lent. A radiologist based in one hospital interprets films sent by another. A blood bank in one hospital sends a pint of blood to another.

Other expressions of the process toward integration and coordination of hospitals have been more formal and systematic. The Bingham program has been mentioned, and it is historically important not only for the specific mechanisms it pioneered, but also for the attention it focused on the need for improved medical care in rural areas.

As America has become industrialized and urbanized, the rural areas have, in a sense, been left behind. The same is true all over the world. A special consciousness of the problems of rural medical care emerged in the 1930's. The first conference on rural medicine was held at Cooperstown, N.Y., in 1938. The Bingham program in Maine got started. The Commonwealth Fund launched its program of building rural hospitals and supporting medical education for rural youth. Improved Public Health organization in rural counties was promoted. The U.S. Department of Agriculture started its medical care program for low-income farmers.[7]

It was during World War II that the regionalization idea matured as an approach to improved hospital service for rural people. Public understanding grew and plans were made for a federally subsidized construction program. In 1945 the Commonwealth Fund promoted the Council of Rochester Regional Hospitals.[8] Immediately after the war, in 1946, the National Hospital Survey and Construction Act was passed, providing not only funds to subsidize hospital construction, but requiring a master plan to be drawn up by each State establishing priorities for different localities. Virtually everywhere the rural areas received top priorities because their relative bed shortages were greatest.[9]

Under the impetus of the Hill-Burton Act, planning groups studied bed needs in all the States. A formula calling for 4.5 and 5.5 general hospital beds per 1,000 population in a State made planning for construction purposes relatively easy. Planning for coordinated hospital operation, however, was not so easy. Attractive charts portrayed networks of regional, district, and community hospitals in each State, implying the classic two-way flow of patients and services. In practice, the State hospital construction agencies were seldom in a position to bring life to the charts in day-to-day hospital operation.

COORDINATED OPERATIONS

Nevertheless, the introduction of rationalism into construction planning stimulated voluntary groups to do something about coordinating hospital operations.

National attention was focused on the regionalization experiment around Rochester. Elsewhere in New York State regional hospital councils were organized, not simply to process applications for construction funds but to promote interhospital cooperation.[10]

State hospital associations became organized or revitalized. They conducted educational and informational programs for their members. Training institutes were held for hospital trustees and administrators as well as for nurses, dietitians, medical record librarians, laboratory technicians, and business office personnel. Uniformity was introduced into accounting practices so that hospitals could deal effectively with third-party payers, such as governmental welfare agencies or Blue Cross hospital insurance plans.

The hospitalization insurance movement did a great deal to bring autonomous hospital administrations together. Through boards of directors of regional Blue Cross plans, hospital advisory committees, and other mechanisms, administrators discussed common problems of hospital operation. Many of these problems are expressed ultimately in per diem costs which the prepayment plan is expected to meet. To sell Blue Cross insurance policies, premiums must be kept as low as possible, and yet premiums are based on hospital operating costs. While costs have indeed been rising, in line with the continued improvement in the content and quality of hospital service, the Blue Cross program in recent years has exerted moderate pressure toward economy and efficiency in hospital operation.

It is true that some observers doubt if paying agencies are doing enough to induce economic operation of hospitals. It is even claimed that prepayment has led to extravagance. The challenge of the State insurance commissioners has been mentioned. Representatives of organized workers, who make up a large proportion of the Blue Cross membership, have been skeptical of the efficiency of hospital administration. In any case, public pressure created by a vast extension of prepayment for hospital care is doing much to bring hospitals together to explore common problems of effective administration.

One expression of this is the organization of joint purchasing arrangements. While the development is still modest, in some large cities hospitals have agreed on standard specifications for linens, laundry supplies, antiseptics, certain drugs, and the like, and have achieved lower prices through mass purchasing. The Hospital Bureau of Standards and Supplies, Inc., is a national organization devoted to this purpose. A nonprofit organization, it purchases many commodities for its hundreds of members, does product testing, and issues informational bulletins. Similar group purchasing activities are conducted by the hospital councils in Rochester, N.Y., and Pittsburgh, Pa., by the Federation of Jewish Philanthropies of New York City, and by others. The purchases made in this way, however, usually constitute only a small percentage of the total made by the cooperating hospitals.[11]

Another measure of cooperation is the pooling of resources for educating nurses. Certain types of didactic instruction are given to the student nurses of one hospital in the training school of another. Students from many general hospital schools of nursing may receive practical training in mental disease, pediatrics, or obstetrics in "affiliated" hospitals specializing in these fields. In Saskatchewan, Canada, in Massachusetts, and elsewhere, centralized lectures for students from many nursing schools have been given in universities.

Medical schools have taken the initiative in a number of places to promote postgraduate education of physicians through the local hospitals in a region. Programs around the medical schools at Buffalo, Richmond, New Orleans, and Berkeley have been outstanding. Rotation of interns and medical residents from a university hospital among several surrounding community hospitals is a growing practice which helps elevate the quality of service in the smaller institution, while it gives the young physician insight and experience in a simple grassroots setting.[12]

Regional and metropolitan hospital councils with full-time staffs in the United States have increased from the first one at Rochester, N.Y., in 1945, to 23 in 1958.[13] Their functions vary greatly, but they all represent a pooling of interests by several institutions to achieve improvement in hospital service. The majority of the councils have been organized in large metropolitan cities, where a dozen or more hospitals are found. Their scope of activity changes from year to year, but there has been a clear tendency to progress from an original primary concern with construction planning to the wider problems of the content of hospital service.

Even so, hospital council activities are still oriented more to administrative problems than to elements of direct patient care.[14] Programs depend on council members and their needs of the moment. While the Syracuse council, for example, regularly summarizes vital statistics for hospitals of the region, it also does many one-time jobs, such as preparing a booklet to recruit young people for work in the hospital field. The Buffalo council supplies a clearinghouse for employment. The Philadelphia council does much to encourage uniform accounting procedures. The Pittsburgh council is now deeply involved with reorganizing activity to comply with the Pennsylvania Insurance Commissioner's ruling of 1958.[1] The Chicago council is making arrangements with the telephone company and the many local fire and police departments for coordinated hospital action in the event of disaster. The Swift Current council in Saskatchewan provides consultant services in X-ray technology, pharmacy, dietetics, and accounting to its member hospitals.[15]

Thus, hospital councils are in a stage of vigorous growth. Aside from their basic services, they are laying the groundwork for greater cooperation among sovereign hospitals in the future.

Evolution of interhospital cooperation to the point of unified management of several institutions has occurred only in a handful of places in the United States. Federal hospital systems for veterans, Indians, merchant marine, and similar groups under the Veterans Administration, Public Health Service, and other agencies, are, of course, highly rational. These programs, however, started out on a centrally organized basis under uniform rules and regulations. They do not include community hospitals open to all persons.

The closest thing to regional management of a network of community hospitals is seen in the Miners Memorial Hospital Association of the United Mine Workers of America. Supported by the welfare and retirement fund of this union of coal miners, the association operates 10 hospitals in the Appalachian Mountain States. There are regional and peripheral hospitals in the system. Authority is centralized with a branching-out of delegated responsibilities. Functions involving direct patient care are, of course, locally based, while supportive activities, such as accounting and payroll, specialized plant maintenance, purchasing, and staff hiring are done regionally for the entire group. Financial functions are centralized to an even further degree; they are performed with electronic equipment at the United Mine Workers headquarters in Washington, D.C.[16]

In the Adirondack section of New York, there is a group of three small hospitals, set up by the Noble Foundation, under single management. Some church missions operate a network of small hospitals in the southwestern United States. In western Pennsylvania, the hospital division of Grenoble Hotels, Inc., is a private organization engaged in the business management of 11 general hospitals under voluntary auspices. Five independent hospitals in Newark, N.J., have just consolidated their administration as the United Hospital Association.

The Commonwealth of Puerto Rico, with the support of the Rockefeller Foundation and the Public Health Service, is developing a regional hospital system under central direction. A large regional center, three district hospitals, and about 14 small community hospitals are in the network. Not only is the management of all these hospitals unified, but even medical services throughout the region are supplied or directed by a staff of qualified specialists located at the regional center.[17]

DISCUSSION

This, then, is a brief review of where we stand in the United States in the broad range of hospital regionalization activities. A great deal is going on and established ideas of hospital services are obviously in ferment. Yet the surface of the possibilities of regionalized hospital services through teamwork in natural trading regions has hardly been scratched.

The chief determinants of the degree of inter-hospital cooperation are philosophic and technical. The philosophic or ideologic determinants are found, of course, in our whole system of free enterprise in health service. They include the existence of two types of sovereignty: the autonomy of the boards of directors of voluntary hospitals and the independence of the practicing physicians who staff the hospitals.

We have seen how small bits of these sovereignties have been yielded through increased cooperative activities among hospitals. Professional independence also has been modified by the widening group discipline within the medical staff organization in hospitals. Appointment of full-time chiefs of clinical services, centralized medical audit procedures, diligent tissue committees, and limitations of privileges have all helped to introduce a collective conscience into the practice of medicine in hospitals.

These two levels of sovereignty are central features of American health service, and they will doubtless be part of our life for a long time. Yet we are finding that cooperation and teamwork among hospitals does not reduce the dignity of the individual patient, doctor, board member, or administrator.

It is, however, the second determinant of any interhospital cooperation, the technical aspects, that will ultimately be most decisive. How much is really to be gained in effective hospital service by more highly organized relationships among institutions in a region? How much can the quality of care be improved by joint action and how much can costs be reduced?

To answer these large questions, they must be broken into many smaller parts. There are perhaps 15 to 20 principal activities involved in hospital service: nursing care, laboratory service, dietetics, business management, and plant maintenance, to name only a few. Under each of these are dozens or even hundreds of subdivisions. The activities in a laboratory service, for example, include the establishment and maintenance of equipment, the supervision and judgment exercised by a pathologist or laboratory director, the training of technicians of many types, the procedures for doing hundreds of tests, the review of technical performance to assure accuracy, the issuance of reports, and the like. Certain laboratory examinations, moreover, are highly complex and can be done only in technical centers, while others are simple and can be done in the most modest setup.

If the advantages of regional cooperation are to be evaluated, each of these many units of hospital service must be considered objectively. Measurements must be made in which cost is one dimension and patient need another. Under the latter, one must consider the frequency of need for a specific service and the importance of time. A corollary of time is distance and the feasibility of transportation.

These questions are familiar in other contexts, especially in the organization of industry. They are the bread-and-butter problems of students of production and industrial engineering. Are there secrets in American technology which have not been applied to the production and distribution of health services?

There is need to take a closer look at the organization of hospital services in geographic regions from the viewpoint of technical effectiveness. One must not overlook the patient, for his welfare must always remain in the center of the picture. One must likewise not lose sight of ideologic realities in American culture. But research focused on the technical aspects of hospital regionalization is urgently needed to evaluate properly the advantages to be gained through cooperative efforts.

If clear-cut technical advantages to specific forms of teamwork among hospitals can be shown, half the battle will be won. To the extent that gains are demonstrable, the American mind usually finds ways of application. If more highly developed expressions of hospital regionalization can be shown to yield better hospital services at the same or lower costs than prevail in the United States today, we are bound to find ways of implementing these approaches which will be philosophically acceptable and consistent with our social values.

1. Smith, F. B.: *Adjudication pursuant to hearing on the filing of the Associated Hospital Service of Philadelphia*. Harrisburg, April 1958.

2. Bugbee, G., and Pattulo, A.: A foundation views hospital problems. Report of the Hospital Advisory Committee of the W. K. Kellogg Foundation. *Hospitals* 32:39–43, Apr. 1, 1958.

3. Smillie, W. G., and Curran, J. A.: *The unmet needs in medical care of rural people*, State of Maine, 1956. Bethel, Maine, Bingham Associates Fund, 1957, pp. 1–7.

4. *Social Denmark. A survey of the Danish social legislation*. (Translated into English by W. E. Calvert, 1947.) Copenhagen, Socialt Tidsskrift, 1945.

5. Consultative Council on Medical and Allied Service, Great Britain: *Interim report on the future provision of medical and allied services*. Parliament Command Paper 693. London, His Majesty's Stationery Office, 1920.

6. Roemer, M. I.: *Medical care in relation to public health*. Geneva, World Health Organization, December 1956, pp. 89–97.

7. Mott, F. D., and Roemer, M. I.: *Rural health and medical care*. New York, McGraw-Hill Book Co., 1948, 608 pp.

8. Rosenfeld, L. S., and Makover, H. B.: *The Rochester Regional Hospital Council*. Cambridge, Mass., Commonwealth Fund, 1956.

9. Abbe, L. M., and Baney, A. M.: *The Nation's health facilities*. Ten years of the Hill-Burton hospital and medical facilities program, 1946–1956. PHS Pub. No. 616. Washington, D.C., U.S. Government Printing Office, 1958, 181 pages.

10. Bourke, J. J., and Wagner, H.: Regional council: Valuable aids in statewide planning. *Hospitals* 24: 65–68, March 1950.

11. What are the facts about group purchasing? (Symposium.) *Mod. Hosp.* 88:63–72, April 1957.

12. Rosenfeld, L. S., Kramer, N., and Wadman, R.: *Preliminary report on survey of regional organization of health services*. Presented before the medical care section, American Public Health Association, Cleveland, Ohio, October 1952.

13. American Hospital Association: *Roster of hospital association officers.* Chicago, October 1958.

14. Morris, R. C.: *Toward the full potential of hospital regionalization.* Ithaca, N.Y., Cornell University, Graduate School of Business and Public Administration, Sloan Institute of Hospital Administration, June 1959. (Mimeographed.)

15. Rickard, P., and Roemer, M. I.: Canada's first regional hospital council. *Hospitals* 31:45–49, Sept. 16, 1957.

16. Miners Memorial Hospital Association: [A series of three articles.] United Mine Workers' hospitals—part 1. Hospital chain [parts 2 and 3]. *Architectural Forum* 99:132, August; 99:150, September; 99:132, November 1953.

17. Ferrer, R. A.: *Annual report for fiscal year 1957–58 of the Project for the Regionalization of Health and Welfare Services of the Bayamon Area.* San Juan, P.R., Department of Health, Regional Office for Coordination and Research, August 29, 1958.

The Hospital and Its Patients*

RICHARD M. TITMUSS, D.SC.

FOR A NUMBER of reasons, and I shall mention only one or two, these advances of science into the hospital have made it harder to treat the patient as a person. One reason is that more science has meant more division of labor and, inevitably, of course, more professional fragmentation as specialisms have developed and new groups of workers have banded themselves together as professional groups. An increase in the division of labor means that more people with different functions and skills to perform are brought into contact with the patient. Each separate function to be performed, for out-patient as well as in-patient, involves the sick person in a personal contact with more people—more 'experts' (for that is how they often appear to the patient). All this happens at a time when the patient, sick perhaps in mind as well as in body, with fears and anxieties about himself and his family, with more questions and uncertainties in a mind disturbed by illness, is less able to cope with the strain of entering into new personal contacts with many strange individuals endowed with all the authority and mystery which surround the hospital and its gift of survival. As most of us know, to feel ill is to feel unadventurous, to want to retreat from life, to have one's fears removed and one's needs met without effort. Physical illness can play queer tricks with our

---

* Reprinted, in part, by permission, from *The Welfare State*, published by George Allen & Unwin Limited, 1958, Chapter 7, "The Hospital and Its Patients," pp. 124–125. The author is Professor and Head of the Department of Social Science and Administration, The London School of Economics and Political Science, London, England.

thought and our behavior. This does not mean, as some all too easily suppose, that we are neurotics. In being querulous and ungrateful, demanding and apathetic in turn, we are in fact behaving as ill people. The demands that people make on society are greater when they are ill than when they are well. Yet the advent of science has made it more difficult, in social and psychologic terms, for the hospital as part of society to meet these demands. More science means more division of labor and more experts—more of the mysteries of blood counts, X-rays, test-meals, investigations, case history taking and so forth. These, in turn, mean more departmentalism and, all too often, more departmental thinking. As A. N. Whitehead warned us, the fixed person for the fixed duties in a fixed situation is a social menace. He is particularly a menace to the sick person who is more in need, rather than less, for explanation and understanding. But the departmentalism which stems from a division of labor—from a dividing up of services rendered to a patient—is given more to silence than to communication. Silence from those in authority, from doctor, sister, nurse, administrator, clerk, technician and so on often means a want of imagination: silence consents to fear among those who have great need for explanation and reassurance.

What is it that patients complain of more than anything else in relation to the hospital—'No one told me anything'—'Nobody asked me'—'I don't know'. How often one comes across people who have been discharged from hospital, bewildered, still anxious and afraid; disillusioned because the medical magic has not apparently or not yet yielded results, ignorant of what the investigations have shown, what the doctors think, what the treatment has been or is to be, and what the outlook is in terms of life and health.

Hospitals and the Tragedy of Unused Medical Knowledge*

LEONA BAUMGARTNER, M.D.

SIGNS OF HOSPITAL FERMENT

There are many signs of ferment inside hospitals which need to be watched, copied, modified, and evaluated.

1. The Concept of Progressive Patient Care

The conventional system of putting a patient in a hospital bed and offering him the same service whether he is on a critical list or simply in to get some tests, costs too much in dollars, staff time and unhappiness for the patient who is well able to move around and get his own meals. The new approach of progressive patient care must be expanded and accelerated.

2. More Imaginative Exploration of Methods of Handling Hospital Routines of All Kinds, Despite the Protestations of Administrators

American industry has been more ingenious in devising housing, servicing and feeding arrangements in motels and airplanes than we have been in trying anything from disposable sheets to frozen meals in hospitals. These prosaic matters are not so far removed from conventional medicine as they may seem.

The whole field of the collection, storage, retrieval, and use of medical information might be revolutionized by developments in the field of information control. This might solve the problems of the patient's going from the clinic to a bed in the same hospital, without his outpatient record's ever getting into the hands of the in-patient physician. Also, it might help solve the shortage of stenographers or the proverbial illegibility of physicians' notes.

3. Further Explorations of the Application of Electronics to the Physiologic Monitoring of Patients

How can we apply the lessons of space technology to hospital care? If the vital signs of an astronaut 100 miles or more in space can be electronically monitored from a remote ground station,

---

* Excerpted in part, by permission, from the August 16, 1961 issue of *Hospitals*, Vol. 35, pp. 67–70, 158–159. This paper was delivered at the 150th Anniversary Convocation of the Massachusetts General Hospital, Boston, Massachusetts, February 1, 1961. The author is Assistant Administrator, Agency for International Development (AID), U.S. Department of State, Washington, D.C., formerly Health Commissioner, New York City Department of Health, New York, New York.

isn't there something useful to be learned about monitoring patients in beds only a few feet away from a nursing station?

4. Ambulatory Care of All Kinds Needs All Our Ingenuity

Too long have outpatient departments been the step children of the hospital, a basement operation, literally and figuratively. We have sent them the least skilled people, the least satisfactory equipment, the leftovers of available resources, the least of our imagination, and almost none of our enthusiasm.

The depressing waiting rooms and offices, the lack of privacy, and the hours of waiting on hard benches have been an outward reflection of our own lack of interest.

Increased Expenses of American Hospitals*

COST OF OPERATING American hospitals increased nearly $1 billion in 1961, according to statistics in the 1962 Guide Issue of *Hospitals*, Journal of the American Hospital Association. The cost was $9,387,-242,000, compared with $8,420,986,000 in 1960. Hospital admissions rose also in 1961, to 25,474,370, nearly a half million more than in the preceding year.

The average cost per patient-day increased in all categories of hospitals. In non-Federal short-term general hospitals, which admit 91.7 per cent of all patients, the average cost climbed $2.75, from $32.23 in 1960 to $34.98 in 1961. This average included voluntary hospitals, $36.04; proprietary, $33.29; and State and local governmental, $32.27. In long-term non-Federal hospitals, the average cost in psychiatric institutions was $5.53; in tuberculosis hospitals, $14.72; and in general long-term hospitals, $14.49. Federal hospital average was $23.34.

Payroll, $6.2 billion in 1961 and $5.6 billion in 1960, accounted for nearly two-thirds of the costs. The increase reflects additional hospital employees, 1.6 million in 1960 compared with 1.7 million in

---

* Reprinted by permission from the January 1963 issue of *Public Health Reports*, Vol. 78, p. 26. The statistics appeared initially in the 1962 Guide Issue of *Hospitals*, Journal of the American Hospital Association.

1961, as well as higher salaries for the more highly skilled personnel needed to give today's specialized care. Expanding research, continued education of health personnel, higher prices for equipment, and the continually growing number of outpatients (whose visits are not counted in admissions) also boosted hospital expenses.

4. The School: A Primary Setting

School Health Programs*

TODAY, HEALTH PROGRAMS for school-age children are community ventures. They utilize the health and the educational facilities of the community as a whole in a partnership consisting of school personnel, school and private physicians, parents, dentists, nurses, Public Health workers, and other paramedical personnel.

It is obvious that such comprehensive community programs, which utilize the talents and knowledge of so many professions, cannot be based solely on the school. Nevertheless, because the opportunities for guidance and health supervision offered by the school are so great, health programs for the school-age child remain centered, fundamentally, in the public and parochial schools.

According to the Report of the Committee on School Health of the American Academy of Pediatrics, published in October 1959:

> The major purpose of a school health program is to maintain and improve the health of the school-age child. The program should include adequate supervision of the physical, mental, emotional and social aspects of school life. It also includes planning the course content and instruction in nutrition and health education, including accident prevention, recreation and physical education. School buildings and grounds should be safe and healthful.
>
> The child's need for health care, either physical, developmental, emotional or social, should be discovered as promptly as possible. If it has not been recognized at home, such need should be brought to the attention of the parents. If parents are unable to arrange for care or are irresponsible, arrangements should be made through the local or county medical society or an appropriate community health service.

Some health authorities believe that proper school health programs will prevent not only acute illness but also chronic conditions, and help pupils avoid crippling ailments which in later life might require constant medical care and even permanent residence in medical institutions.

THE BEGINNING

The close relationship between the school and the well-being of children became more clearly recognized during the last century as the role of Public Health assumed greater importance. In

* Reproduced, with omission of two illustrations and one table, from Pfizer *Spectrum*, Vol. 7, No. 10, © copyright 1959, Chas. Pfizer & Co., Inc.

1872, the Board of Education of Elmira, N.Y., appointed a "sanitary superintendent" to check "an alarming prevalence of small-pox." Two decades later, Boston sent fifty physicians, aptly titled "medical visitors," into its schools "to examine all children thought by their teachers to be ailing." New York City appointed a public school medical officer about 1892 and in 1897 set up an inspection service of 134 physicians. Five years later, the city added a corps of school nurses to help in the control of communicable diseases.

Early in the 20th century, mass immunization, improved sanitation, and innumerable other advances in medicine and Public Health had brought communicable disease under control. As a result, there was a shift in emphasis in school health programs from protection against and control of disease to discovery and correction of childhood defects. In the last decade this concept of "the health of the school-age child, not school health" received additional impetus through the organization of the School Health Service as a section of the Public Health Service.

By the middle of the 20th century, health programs in schools were no longer considered an innovation or even an elective activity. By 1950, all cities of over 100,000, and 90 per cent of other large cities, had some type of school health service ranging from nominal inspection by teachers and nurses to comprehensive programs under either the Board of Education or the Health Department, or both (e.g., New York, Los Angeles, Philadelphia, and Denver).

BASIC CONCEPTS

When school medical services were started in this country, the principal objective was to control contagious and nuisance diseases through frequent medical inspection of the schools and the pupils. As the tides of contagion were stemmed, emphasis shifted to examinations for hearing and vision defects, and soon school physicians began to probe for other physical defects.

Although physical examinations were, and still are, of tremendous importance for detection of symptoms of illness, today the emphasis is often educational—to teach children and their parents the principles of basic hygiene and the importance of periodic consultations with a family physician. Indeed, Arthur J. Lesser, Director of the Division of Health Services of the United States Children's Bureau, has said of this half century of development that "for many schools, health educathis is considered the principal reason for having school health services." The same opinion is generally held by Public Health and public education leaders today.

Robert W. Culbert, Director of the Bureau of School Health, New York City Department of Health, stresses the need to inquire into the nature and extent of adverse health conditions exhibited by school children following major events such as economic depression, war, shifts in population, changes in social attitudes, and major advances in medical science. He notes that the approach to school health has changed:

> The emphasis was changed from the finding and correcting of physical defects to the health appraisal of children as individuals in the solution of over-all general health problems. The important entity was not the physical defect, but the living child who needed attention. To us, this has been a more satisfactory approach to solving school health problems.

Harold Jacobziner, Assistant Commissioner of the New York City Department of Health, has said, "In the search for defects, the child was almost lost in the shuffle. A large number of annual examinations were done and the service was defect-centered." In Jacobziner's view, noting the partial results achieved by a partial approach, the present stress must be placed on the child "as an individual and on his total personality needs." The current school health program, at least in ideal, is now regarded as a crucial element in public or community health. He says:

> "the child's health and development of his total personality are not isolated incidents but are significantly dependent on the health of the family and of the community . . . school health services must become family-centered and family-oriented. . . . The ultimate objective of the school health services is to maintain, protect, and promote the optimal health—physical, mental, emotional and social—of the school-age child."

MODERN FUNCTIONS

What then should be the functions of the school health program? The Joint Committee on Health Problems in Education of the National Education Association and the American Medical Association lists these functions:

1. To appraise the health status of pupils and school personnel.
2. To counsel pupils, parents, and others concerning findings.
3. To encourage the correction of remediable defects.
4. To assist in the identification and education of handicapped children.
5. To help prevent and control disease.
6. To provide emergency service for injury or sudden sickness.

These functions should be adapted to meet the needs of the individual community and should follow the patterns of medical services available to the child and his family.

The conflict between the need to expand health facilities and the democratic ideal of family responsibility for the rearing of children has emphasized the need for a definition of proper and reasonable functions of a school health program. The United States Department of Health, Education and Welfare, in a discussion of this problem in a pamphlet, "Better Health for School-Age Children" (U.S. Children's Bureau, 1951) has stated its basic philosophy:

Experience has clearly shown that success comes more often when health programs for children are carried out in the American tradition of cooperation between public and private groups and are adapted to local needs and resources. All such programs should supplement the health care which parents provide their children, since all of us recognize that the responsibilities of parents for such care come first.

PROGRAMS IN LARGE CITIES

To furnish part of the background for this special school health issue, *Spectrum* explored how one city (New York) has attempted to solve the problem of coordinating school and community services in its school health program. New York was chosen, not because it is representative of U.S. cities and not because its program can be considered a typical one, but because in its unique size and complexity New York City presents, for all practical purposes, a microcosm of the United States.

At present, New York has a large, comprehensive system of health services available to about 1,250,000 children. It is estimated that during 1959, in the elementary and junior high schools alone, a total of 742,000 pupils are registered in public schools and 308,000 in parochial schools.

Services to schools are provided under joint administration of the Department of Health, which provides medical, nursing and special health services; the Board of Education, which is responsible for "health day" routines, initial vision and hearing screening, health instruction and guidance, physical activities, and continuing health surveillance, through the cooperation of health counselors, principals and teachers; and the respective parochial systems.

Essentially, the New York City program of health services is designed to discover the child in need of health guidance and to direct him to proper care. It includes:

Periodic, complete health examinations conducted by family or school physicians for: newly admitted pupils; upper grade pupils (6th grade); pre-high school entrants (8th or 9th grade); and high school seniors (pre-graduation).
Case-finding through teacher observation and teacher-nurse con-

ferences whereby pupils are referred to the school physician or health agency for screening or complete examination.

Follow-up conferences between the teacher, nurse, parents and school physician, family physician, and community health agencies.

The Health Department and Board of Education also conduct in-service training for physicians, teachers, nurses and other health workers.

In New York City, school health services encompass both medical and educational functions. Detection, referral for treatment (but not treatment), cooperation in supervising a plan of care, and guidance are the chief elements.

The staff of the Health Department's Bureau of School Health consists of 6 full-time pediatricians and 250 part-time physicians, including 5 supervisors.

Nursing service, furnished by the Bureau of Public Health Nursing of the Department of Health, provides the equivalent of 375 full-time registered nurses, about three-quarters of whom have completed special public health training. Almost 50 per cent of the available nursing time of the Department of Health is given to health service for children of school age.

The Bureau of Dentistry of the Department of Health also participates actively in the school health service, primarily to provide free dental service at 165 clinics for children who cannot afford private care. In 1958–59, some 51,125 children received such care. The Bureau also offers rehabilitative care for children suffering from seriously handicapping conditions of the teeth, face and jaws, and maintains a preventive orthodontic service. The Board of Education supplies transportation for more than 1,000 children daily who receive free service from the Murry and Leonie Guggenheim Dental Clinic (supported by a foundation established in 1929), which cares for children who are unable to pay for private care.

A comprehensive program for handicapped children, including services for those with heart disease and rheumatic fever, orthopedic defects, vision defects, hearing impairment, speech disorders, convulsive seizures, and mental disturbances, is maintained by the Bureau for Handicapped Children (of the Department of Health) and the Bureaus for Education of Physically and Visually Handicapped (Board of Education). The Board of Education cooperates closely with the Department of Health in the educational placement of such children and provides appropriate instruction. Currently, about 326 special classes in the schools are attended by 5,000 children. Some 1,600 children are taught at home and 1,000 in hospitals.

The Bureau for Health Education of the Division of Child Welfare (Board of Education) is concerned with screening and other routines, for health counseling, and for the behavioral and emotional aspects of health. This division supplies equipment to public and parochial units and, through its staff of district counselors, conducts courses in health routines for teachers, and supervises local operations.

The principal agency concerned with the social and emotional problems of children in the schools is the Bureau of Child Guidance, assisted by the Bureau of Vocational Guidance. The Bureau of Child Guidance is staffed by psychiatrists, psychologists and social workers, acts as the diagnostic agency and child-family counselor for the public schools, and provides referral and pretreatment service. The Bureau accepts children whose conditions have been noted by the school authorities and whose current or potential condition warrants professional attention. During 1958–59 the Bureau gave some service to more than 18,000 pupils (kindergarten through junior high school), or about 1.7 per cent of the school population.

The nonpublic schools are responsible for conducting the same health activities as the public schools—vision and hearing testing, and growth measurement—and for recording results and comments on medical record cards. They cooperate with Health Department physicians, dentists, and nurses, and obtain equipment and instruction from the Board of Education for the screening work.

Recently, the parochial schools initiated their own classes for mentally retarded children who are screened by their own evaluation center. The Catholic Charities Guidance Institute now functions for many of the Catholic institutions in the same fashion as the Bureau of Child Guidance. The Jewish Education Committee is currently adding personnel to develop its counseling services.

PROGRAM DIRECTION

Policy-making for school health is the responsibility of the NYC School Health Coordinating Council, a permanent joint committee of representatives of both the Department of Health and the Board of Education. The Council considers new programs and revisions, reviews proposed directives and bulletins, and recommends institution of studies and research projects by these departments or others. The Council has no operational functions, but since its membership consists of the administrative heads of the units which carry out school functions, decisions may be quickly translated into action.

A Study of Case-Finding Methods in Elementary Schools*

I. Methodology and Initial Results

ALFRED YANKAUER, JR., M.D.; RUTH FRANTZ, R.N.;

ANNE DRISLANE, M.D.; AND SELIG KATZ, M.D.

WHAT ARE the most efficient and economic methods to discover children in need of medical attention in a school population? Acute infections are self-evident phenomena, discoverable on a day-to-day basis. Dental caries is so universal that its "discovery" is redundant. Impairment of vision and hearing are discoverable by simple specific screening technics which are, in general, satisfactory. Screening technics for children with deficiencies in intellectual or personality function also exist. Most other adverse conditions in middle childhood require, in the present state of our knowledge, some assessment of the "whole child" and his environment before a sound decision can be made as to whether he needs medical attention. This assessment requires medically trained judgment to a varying degree. At one extreme is the obese or emotionally disturbed child, the meaning of whose appearance or behavior is obvious. At the other, is the pale apparently listless child or the child with an asymptomatic cardiac murmur, both of whom require medical examination before the decision can be reached. Regardless of the nature of the condition itself, its "need of medical attention" is also contingent upon whether such attention is already being given at the time the condition is first recognized in the school situation.

Case-finding methods for the kinds of adverse conditions just discussed are few and difficult to evaluate. Frequent periodic medical examinations of an entire elementary school grade are generally considered an inefficient and uneconomic use of medical time and several studies in the United States and the United Kingdom have tended to confirm this impression.[1-4] The other existing case-finding methods seek to screen out of the total school population children with "pos-

* Reprinted, with omission of three tables, by permission, from the April 1962 issue of the *American Journal of Public Health*, Vol. 52, pp. 656–662. Copyright by the American Public Health Association, Inc., 1790 Broadway, New York 19, New York. The authors are, respectively, Regional Advisor in Maternal and Child Health, Regional Office of the World Health Organization, Washington, D.C., formerly Director of the Bureau of Maternal and Child Health, New York State Department of Health, Albany, New York; Health Educator, East Orange Health Department, East Orange, New Jersey, formerly Public Health Nurse, Albany County Health Department, Albany, New York; Assistant Director, Bureau of Maternal and Child Health, New York State Department of Health, Albany, New York; Assistant Director, Division of Special Health Services, New York State Department of Health, Albany, New York.

sible" adverse conditions for appraisal and judgment by the school physician. The best known method is teacher observation with or without teacher-nurse conferences. Other suggested technics are selection by height-weight growth chart analysis, by review of absenteeism, and by parent questionnaire.

The present study was undertaken to assess the relative values of these various methods of case finding. Although it has operated for only the first five years of a contemplated 10–12-year period, some of the preliminary findings and lessons already learned seemed of sufficient importance to justify a preliminary report.

METHODOLOGY

The study population consists of children attending two parochial schools serving a middle and lower-middle class section of the city of Albany. The parents of all children entering these schools are seen at the time of spring registration for kindergarten. The health program is explained to them and they are urged to have their child checked medically during the summer in preparation for school. Nine out of 10 families follow this advice, and the family physician's report is mailed to the school before the fall opening date in a stamped, self-addressed envelop given to the mother at registration time.

The following year all children in the first grade (whether or not they received the prekindergarten examination from their family physician) are given a careful pediatric medical examination in school. Before the examination the parent completes and sends to the school a health history form. As part of the appraisal, she is interviewed by the Public Health nurse who has worked in the project since its inception, and one of the several examining pediatricians who have been, for the most part, staff members of the Bureau of Maternal and Child Health of the New York State Department of Health. In 98 per cent of the examinations performed to date, the parent has been present. As a result of this initial appraisal, the child may be considered healthy, one or more adverse conditions[5] may be diagnosed, or the physician may wish to reevaluate the child at a later date. This base-line examination has now been given to all children in the first five grades of these two schools.

No periodic medical examinations are planned throughout the eight years of elementary school for this group of children. In the eighth grade, all children will be reexamined by a pediatrician unassociated with the project and without access to the school medical records.

During the intervening years, reliance for discovery of new adverse conditions was to be placed on four case-finding methods: (1) Referrals by the classroom teachers at any time during the year but stimulated by a semi-annual teacher-nurse conference with a systematic review of the class enrollment; (2) deviant growth chart records based on height-weight measurements taken on all children three times during the school year using standard equipment and procedure. Plans were made to utilize three kinds of charts in this analysis—the Wetzel grid, the Physical Growth Record of the Joint Committee on Health Problems of the NEA and AMA, and the growth curve charts of the Institute of Child Welfare of the University of California; (3) a questionnaire completed by parents each fall when the children returned to school which asks for intervening illness history and gives the parent an opportunity to request consultation or examination from the school health service. We have combined this questionnaire with an administrative device requesting exact information on how to reach the parents and their physician and what to do in case of medical emergency. The form is printed on a 5" x 8" card. With the active cooperation of principals and teachers there is a 100 per cent return. (4) A systematic review of the absenteeism records of each child twice a year by the nurse with follow-up to determine the reason for any continued absence of more than five days or a total absence of 20 school days per year.

Children selected by any one of these four case-finding methods are reappraised. Some are reexamined by the school physician and again classified as healthy, as having one or more adverse conditions, or as needing to be reevaluated at a later date. The medical care status of a condition at the time of its "discovery" is also recorded. In this way the results of each case-finding method can be evaluated in terms of its yield of new adverse conditions and the extent of its overreferral. The final examination in the eighth grade is planned as a means of checking the underselection of case finding, i.e., as assurance that no new condition has developed and been overlooked during these eight years. In order to reassure ourselves that we were not missing children in need of care, a sample of 18 fifth-graders with no known adverse condition who had not been medically examined in school since first grade were selected during the school year 1959–1960. They were reexamined by a pediatrician unassociated with the project, and all were found to be healthy. This interim, fifth-grade check-up will not be repeated in future years.

RESULTS OF FIRST-GRADE EXAMINATIONS

By the end of the 1959–1960 school year, 630 first-grade examinations had been completed. There were 484 of these children still attending the same school and the remainder had transferred to other schools.[6] It will be recalled that 90 per cent of this group had been examined by a family physician prior to school entry, i.e., one year before the base-line school examination in first grade. Adverse conditions found at the first grade school examination of these 630 children were as follows: emotional 39 of 6.2 per cent of all children examined (N = 630); allergy—36 or 5.7 per cent; orthopedic—20 or 3.2 per cent; nutritional—20 or 3.2 per cent; ear, nose, and throat— 12 or 1.9 per cent; genitourinary—9 or 1.4 per cent; and all others —21 or 3.3 per cent. Their distribution and prevalence in the group transferred and still attending the same schools did not differ significantly. The over-all prevalence figure is comparable to that reported by one of the authors in previous studies,[1] but the distribution by diagnostic category is dissimilar. Fewer orthopedic and ear, nose, and throat conditions, and more allergic conditions were found in the present group, a difference probably accounted for by variations in medical judgment. More emotional conditions were found, a difference probably accounted for by the fact that the nurse and doctor in this study worked in close continuing association with school staff.

Although 21 per cent of the children examined were found to have one or more adverse conditions, the majority were already receiving medical care, 92 of a total of 157. Most of those not receiving care were suffering from emotional or nutritional disorders (largely obesity). These conditions were already known to school and parent. Nine children of the 630 examined were found with adverse conditions not previously known to either school or parent. In seven of these children, no preschool examination by a private physician was recorded. One of the two children who had been examined previously was found after the school examination to have a mild iron deficiency anemia which responded well to treatment. The other was a girl with a tight imperforate hymen. These findings and their implications are substantially the same as reported in previous studies.[1]

The essentially negative case-finding features of this base-line examination, together with the excellent responses to preschool promotion of family physician examination and to requests for health information on initial and interim questionnaires, raise the question of whether the base-line school examination itself is necessary to our study. We plan to study this question more thoroughly and, if indicated, modify our original plans by examining in the first-grade only those children for whom no record of a family physician examination is available or where review of such examination and the parent questionnaire return indicates that special problems exist.

SUBSEQUENT MEDICAL EXAMINATIONS

The fact that no routine periodic medical examinations are performed after the first grade on this group of children does not mean that they are neglected by the school medical service. Almost all their records contain notes by the nurse, and many of them are examined again by the school physician because of selection by one or more of the case-finding methods in use. At the end of the 1959–1960 school year, there were 86 fifth-grade children who had received a base-line examination in first-grade. Excluding from consideration the special interim fifth-grade check-up previously referred to as well as children selected for medical examination by absenteeism review or growth chart analysis (see discussion later), 40 per cent of these 86 children had been examined one or more times after the first grade by the school physician. Children with adverse conditions present in the first grade were more likely to have been seen again.

CASE-FINDING METHODS

Our experience during these five years has convinced us that a systematic review of absenteeism is not a fruitful case-finding method in these two schools. Precise information about the cause of absence periods of more than five consecutive days was too often elusive or insignificant. Significant factors related to prolonged periods of absence or excessive absence days per year were more easily elicited through teacher-nurse conferences or through the annual parent questionnaire. For these reasons we have discarded absenteeism review as a case-finding method although we plan to continue to keep attendance records current for later analysis.

The systematic use of growth charts also appears at this time to be of questionable value as a case-finding method, although further exploration may disclose values not presently apparent. With the AMA-NEA and California charts, criteria for the selection of cases for reappraisal could not be firmly set. With the Wetzel grid, using the stated tolerance limit of one-half channel movement per 10 levels of growth or two to three developmental levels from own auxodrome per year, we found such gross overselection that reappraisal of entire grades at two-year intervals would have been a more efficient procedure. Thus out of 100 children with four or more years' growth data available, only five moved less than one-half channel per 10 developmental levels during the first two years of school. At the end of four to five years of school, only 33 of these 100 children were within one full grid channel of their starting point and almost one-quarter of them deviated by two or more channels from their initial channel. The auxodrome deviations were not so marked. However, they were also too frequent to be of practical value when the tolerance limit of two to three developmental levels per year was used as a cut-off point.

The grids of these 100 children appeared to fall into three general patterns during the first five years of elementary school: (1) growth remained more or less within the same or a neighboring channel but generally with much fluctuation in both directions; (2) a steady drift to the left toward obesity (although it should be remarked that half of the children who fell into the grid definition of obesity at any time were so classified on their first measurement); (3) a steady drift to the right signifying a chronic developmental lag.

The frequency with which spurts and lags in growth occurred in this group made it virtually impossible to rely on growth measurements as an "early" case-finding device. No doubt these spurts and lags are explicable. In some cases acute illness was an obviously related factor, but often no explanation was apparent and growth proceeded normally thereafter. A possible drift toward obesity appears to us to be reasonably apparent on inspection of the child and a simple calculation of increments between measurements, without the need of a chart as a case finder (although a chart may be useful as a teaching aid). The third group with its steady drift to the right of the grid needs to be studied further, and this we plan to do in the future. It is also possible that if the auxodrome cut-off point were set at five levels per year, the selections would be more discriminating. This screening level has been recommended by Deisher and Bryan[5] and we plan to study its application in the future. In any case we will continue to record the measurements of all children in the hope that retrospective analysis may shed some light on their usefulness in the school situation. We have no doubt of their contribution to the total medical appraisal of a growing child, but this is different from functioning in the school situation as a quick screening technic to select children in need of medical attention.

Both the annual parent questionnaire and the teacher-nurse conference with teacher referral appear thus far to be fruitful. Their full evaluation must await termination of this study.

RECOMMENDATIONS APPLICABLE TO
SCHOOL HEALTH PROGRAMS

We have no original recommendations to make, but can reaffirm certain accepted principles of operation on the basis of our recorded experience. These recommendations would apply only to elementary schools serving families of lower-middle class or higher social status.

1. A thorough explanation of the importance of a preschool check-up by the family physician can be combined with a brief account of the school health program at the time of school registration in the spring. Each parent should be interviewed individually but a group presentation would also be desirable. If the occasion of registration is given top promotion priority and supplemented by a convenient and confidential method of returning examination results to the school, it is likely to

yield a high dividend of admission examinations by the family physician who already has some acquaintance with the child, thus meeting the needs of the school and promoting the child's continuing health supervision, a goal of the National Congress of Parents and Teachers. Appropriate communication to promote understanding of such a program among the physicians of the community is also desirable.

2. The use of an annual health questionnaire to be completed by a parent each fall is a desirable addition to the standard school health service procedures. It can serve to keep the school informed of changes in health status, reinforce the importance of regular medical and dental health supervision, and let the parent know that the school medical service personnel stand ready to advise and assist the family at any time. Among junior and senior high school students such an instrument could be completed by the student himself.

3. Where relationships of health personnel to classroom teacher are close, efforts to review absences on a systematic basis, or to keep current growth chart records on all children, are not likely to be useful as case-finding methods, although growth charts may have other values in the school situation. Teacher referrals appear to be of key importance to case-finding in elementary schools.

SUMMARY

The plan of a projected 10-year evaluation of selected case-finding methods in two elementary schools has been described. Screening methods to detect refractive error or hearing loss and dental screening methods are not included in this study.

The findings from 630 children examined in the first grade are reviewed and compared with previous studies. Only nine children in this group were found to have an adverse condition unknown prior to the school examination and not to be receiving medical attention. Seven of these children had not been given the preschool examination by a family physician afforded to over 90 per cent of the remainder of the group.

Although no routine periodic medical examinations were made of these children, 40 per cent of those in the fifth grade had been medically examined in school one or more times since the first grade examination.

The use of systematic absenteeism review and the analysis of growth charts based on regular height-weight measurements did not prove productive as case-finding methods. Further analysis of the growth chart data is contemplated, however.

Recommendations for school health programs are offered as a result of the first five years' experience in this study. These include strengthening of an orientation and information system for parents, particularly at the time of school registration in the spring preceding entrance and the use of an annual health information questionnaire to be completed by the parent.

ACKNOWLEDGMENT: The assistance of the staff of the Albany County Department of Health and the pastors and school staffs of the Blessed Sacrament and St. Patrick's parish, Albany, N.Y., in organizing and carrying out this study is gratefully acknowledged.

1. Yankauer, A., and Lawrence, R. A. A Study of Periodic School Medical Examinations. I. Methodology and Initial Results. *A.J.P.H.* 45: 71–78 (Jan.), 1955. II. The Annual Increment of New "Defects." *Ibid.* 46:1553–1562 (Dec.), 1956. III. The Remediability of Certain Categories of Defects (with L. Ballou). *Ibid.*, 47:1421–1429 (Nov.), 1957. IV. Educational Aspects (with G. R. Wendt, et al.) *Ibid.*, 51:1532–1540 (Oct.), 1961.

2. Hubbard, J. P. Practices and Pitfalls in the Early Detection and Control of Heart Disease in Children. *J. Pediat.* 56:544–550 (Apr.), 1960.

3. Lee, J. A. H. The Effectiveness of Routine Examination of School Children. *Brit. M. J.* 1:573–576 (Mar. 8), 1958.

4. Withnell, A. The Value of the Routine School Medical Examination. *M. Officer* 99:31–36 (Jan. 17), 1958.

5. Acute infections, minor skin conditions, adverse conditions of the eyes and teeth, and loss of hearing were deliberately excluded from the study because they are capable of detection by other means than medical examination. When the term adverse condition is used in this report, it does not include the above conditions.

6. This is a fairly sizable loss of study population. However, it is due largely to the opening of a new parochial school. Further substantial loss by transfer is not anticipated.

7. Deisher, R. W., and Bryan, E. The Value of the Wetzel Grid in a School Health Program and Problems Related to Its Use. *J. School Health* 22:50–57 (Feb.), 1952.

5. The Armed Services

Research in Preventive Medicine*

THOMAS FRANCIS, JR., M.D.

PREVENTIVE medicine is at present a diffuse term meaning different things to different persons. At times it appears no longer to possess a central theme or philosophy. A change in name, as some have suggested, would bring little benefit since it might further obscure the intent. At times the field appears to be interpreted so broadly that care of the sick and disabled—that is, supportive and reconstructive medicine—occupies more attention than the primary objective. Of course, all of medicine, and I mean all sciences contributing to medicine, has a preventive aspect. But the virtue of preventive medicine lies in the concentration of attention on the maintenance of health and the prevention of disease. As Alan Gregg expressed it, "Preventive medicine has the charm and bewilderment and the opportunity of being virtuous, because applying preventive medicine is behaving as we should behave in the light of what we know of the vast capacities of medical science." Perhaps our complaints that preventive medicine is not fully appreciated tie in with the realization that virtue is not easily maintained and that we think as we live. Our problems of recruitment may relate to the fact that we spend more time in expounding virtue than in developing it.

CONCEPT OF HEALTH

Man's progress toward civilization has been closely intertwined with his development of measures to protect life. Some of the adversaries could be recognized even by primitive man, since they related to human behavior and aggression, but disease was understood only as a harmful effect of certain associations revealed by experience. The level of our current knowledge is not much more advanced. Descriptive information has increased tremendously, but we have gained only a slight foothold in understanding the mechanisms in-

* Reprinted, with omission of one table, by permission from the March 5, 1960 issue of the *Journal of The American Medical Association*, Vol. 172, pp. 993–999. This paper was presented at the meeting of the American College of Preventive Medicine, Atlantic City, New Jersey, October 21, 1959, during the tenure of the Third Annual Lectureship in Preventive Medicine. The author is Professor and Chairman of the Department of Epidemiology, School of Public Health, University of Michigan, Ann Arbor, Michigan.

volved in disease processes. The concept of a specific causative factor has been amply demonstrated but constantly challenged in cases in which the etiology of a disorder is yet unproved. We have derived empiric knowledge and procedures with which to limit the incidence or reduce the severity of some disorders, while others increasingly mount the walls of our ignorance. It is obvious that we have more effectively eliminated the buffalo, the whooping crane, and the trailing arbutus than we have obliterated the causes of disease. It is true that some regions of the world are gaining in this struggle; but in other areas unrelieved burdens still exist that constitute continued risks to health and peace in this mobile, shrinking world. Conversely, certain disorders of increasing damage to the longer-lived, more favored populations appear to be diminished by the conditions of life in crowded areas of economic want; this emphasizes the relativity of health, global or individual, and points out that we are scarcely on the threshold of understanding the problems of either health or disease.

Man is, above all, a biologic creature living in environments which expose him to an endless array of potentially pathogenic agencies. The effects of some of these are known, but new ones arise as our explorations of the universe enlarge, as we disturb natural adjustments, as we synthesize new products and new conditions of existence, and as we change our way of life. It cannot be expected now or later that a functioning community can be devised which is spared from all harmful exposures—like germ-free animals maintained in stress-proof isolation.

Health, then, may be considered a state of adequate structure and function, with adequate reserves. This state is being constantly bombarded by innumerable potentially pathogenic stresses, so that each person is in a state of potential disorder. The outcome depends on the ability of the person's reserve to absorb the stress without depleting his range of tolerance, or to respond with additions to his reserve to enhance health and resistance to the harmful influence. It is readily apparent that small shocks might be effectively buffered, while excessive insult or continued exposure might well break through. Variation in the threshold of tolerance among individual persons and at different ages is also easily pictured. Conversely, disease is a reaction to a stress which extends beyond the bounds of individual reserve and adaptability. (This can also be applied to a community.) In this sense, we would measure disease or disease potential in terms of health rather than defining health in terms of disease, and our efforts would be directed toward preservation of the norm.

Unfortunately, the available measurements of health are few. Despite bold efforts to proclaim a theme of "positive health," little information regarding the maintenance of health which has not derived from recognition that a certain procedure prevented disease exists today. Consequently, we have no adequate body of measurements of health that are not based on the absence of a disorder. In fact, we describe our present health activities as vaccination against smallpox, use of fluorides against dental caries, or something that is "good" for heart disease. Our current ability to detect and identify disorders depends largely on their severity; what we consider incipient is an already far-advanced biologic imbalance. Our so-called health statistics are commonly disease or death statistics. In fact, one of our most disturbing practices is to consider the importance of a disease in terms of resultant deaths, as if we were somehow to evite the inevitable. We split life and the family into convenient specialist categories to make the recording of a sequential, comprehensive view of the individual person's or group's experience difficult. We witness the tendency to move blithely under the cover of a slogan, or in response to the call of the huckster to realms of custodial care or administrative busyness with the end-stages of disorder, while we withdraw from profitable investigation and exploitation in the areas of their causation and prevention. It must be constantly repeated that research is the only hope for the development of preventive medicine—and now I am speaking of preventive medicine literally—namely, prevention of disease. Research offers a new face to the field of practice.

AREAS OF PREVENTIVE MEDICINE

The areas of true prevention now available may be summarized under three headings.

First, protection from chemical and physical exposure. This applies particularly to occupational health—one of the oldest and a continued area of interest.

Second, prevention by correction of dietary deficiency or excess. This area has a steady range of development as knowledge of the specific significance of various components becomes known and processing changes the character of natural foods.

Third, prevention of infectious disease by specific measures and sanitary social procedures. A limited number of severe, epidemic communicable diseases are effectively prevented by specific vaccination. A few bacterial infections can be prevented by drug or antibiotic therapy, if properly used. Some are limited by sanitary barriers under stable peacetime conditions or by environmental control. Entirely new agents of large epidemic potential are being recognized, and still others can be expected, but none has been eradicated.

Genetics is a field in which knowledge is increasing but which, as yet, is put to limited use in preventive procedures.

The tendency of preventive medicine to move away from unfinished business is nowhere more clearly emphasized than in the field of infectious disease. And nowhere is there a more precarious balance with respect to present preventive procedures. The return of the staphylococcus and other resistant organisms, the development of new antigenic strains, the reliance on sanitary facilities which can be easily disrupted, the ready possibility of importation of infections, the recurrence of epidemics when vaccinations are not thoroughly applied—all emphasize the narrow margin of safety in our safeguards.

The commonly repeated assurance that infectious disease is conquered is simply not in keeping with the evidence. This is emphasized in the compilations of incidence and death presented by Halbert Dunn in "Health and Demography" (1956). Up to 45 years of age, the 12 leading causes of illness are infections, with the exception of accidents, some "functional" digestive disturbances, and some of the disorders of the genital tract and breast in women aged 15–45 years. Beyond the age of 45 years, infection still constitutes a major factor as the immediate cause of illness, although an increasing amount of illness relates to disorders which are referred to as noninfectious.

The United States National Health Survey reports that in the year July 1957–June 1958 45 per cent of all bed-disability days, 36.5 per cent of work-loss days (for persons 17 years and older), and 67 per cent of school-loss days (for persons aged 6 to 16 years) were caused by acute respiratory illness alone. Respiratory disease was responsible for 60 to 66 per cent of the incidence of acute conditions recorded in every age group. In comparison with a total of 764 million days of bed disability caused by all chronic conditions in the United States in one year, there were 593 million from acute respiratory disease alone. The work-loss figures in days for the year were 219 million from respiratory disease and 226 million from circulatory, digestive, and arthritic disease, and impairments from injury or other origin combined. The average number of days lost by the usual working population from acute conditions was 5.98 and from all chronic conditions 6.52. These data represent the noninstitutionalized population of the country.

AREAS OF RESEARCH

The examples given clearly present to preventive medicine its continued responsibility in those areas of research dealing with the great body of day-by-day infections which repeatedly interrupt healthy, effective life. They probably are also significant factors in the etiology of other disorders whose origins and causes are as yet poorly defined. In addition, they are leading causes of death during the most vigorous periods of life, from the school years through 44 years of age. The point to emphasize, however, is that research must be increased and maintained in the area of the common, annoying disorders of health, in which the preventive promise is high. Human mortality is still 100 per cent; thus, while death is inescapable, these disturbances can be prevented.

The maintenance of effective health is nowhere in our scheme of life more actively required than in the military services. In the first place, the population involved is selected with care for its healthy status, and if it is to fulfill its functions in training or in operation, those disturbances most commonly disruptive of daily health must be controlled. As would be expected, they comprise primarily the acute diseases of young adult life and accidents. During 1958, the rate of total "excluded-from-duty" admissions to hospitals and quarters in the United States Army was 397 per 1,000 per year. The incidence of acute respiratory infections was 160, representing 46 per cent of all admissions for disease and 40 per cent of all nonbattle causes. Accidents were the next, with a rate of about 53 per 1,000 per year. But, in addition, the recorded incidences of 24 for the class of infective and parasitic diseases, 16 for gastroenteritis, and 15 for urinary and male genital disturbance, rheumatic fever, and others indicate another large group of infectious diseases. With its far-flung geographic dispersions and the increased risks attendant on wartime activities, the military services must also be constantly alert to other common disease problems that are largely avoided at home under conditions of peace and stability. Continued research into etiology, pathogenesis, and prevention of these ordinary diseases is essential, if effective manpower is to be sustained for military operations. It is an old saying that the medical lessons learned in one war are forgotten in the intervals of peace. There has always been a small body of devoted men who have sought to prevent this gap almost by individual effort, just as individual persons or small groups of investigators in civilian agencies have maintained progressive inquiry into specific infectious diseases. But the necessity for coordinated, continuing research which is directed toward prevention of these repetitive and persistent infective urchins has been realistically supported in few quarters.

U.S. ARMED FORCES RESEARCH COMMISSIONS

An outstanding example of sustained effort toward understanding and preventing common disorders is the Armed Forces Epidemiological Board. It was established in January, 1941, through the energetic foresight of the late Steve Simmons, chief of preventive medicine, with the aid of the surgeon general of the Army, Magee, and the guidance of the president of the board, Francis Blake, and the administrator, General Bayne-Jones. Expansion of the Army had been accompanied, as always, by an increase in the incidence of respiratory disease. The objective, as stated, was "to appoint and maintain a board for the investigation of the etiology, epidemiology, prevention, and treatment of influenza and other acute epidemic diseases in the Army" and to prepare in time of peace for exaggerated risks of wartime mobilization and operation. The organization was to consist of a central board, an additional group of expert scientists who could meet with the board, and investigative teams who could go to military stations for study and control of epidemics. It was emphasized that the organization should be flexible and not hampered by unnecessary administrative delays. The investigative units were termed commissions, and their major focus of concentration was respiratory disease, as evidenced by their names: the commissions on acute respiratory disease, on hemolytic streptococcic infections, on influenza, on mumps and measles, on meningococcic infection, on pneumonia, on cross infections in hospitals, and on epidemiologic survey. In addition, there were commissions on neurotropic virus diseases and on tropical diseases. Their personnel comprised 111 civilian medical scientists who were already engaged in research on these problems.

I recall the extended discussions at the early meetings about whether or not the commissions should serve only as fire-fighting units on call for emergencies in military situations. Although these sporadic excursions could be of aid, the need for continuity in the study of disease problems for fundamental research in microbiology and immunology and for supplementation of military facilities by university and other laboratories was clearly recognized. It was concluded that programs of intensive study must be sustained if the potentialities and the functions of the board were to be effectively met.

The contributions of the board and its commissions during World War II were such as to elicit the signal statement of one judge, that "No one ever got so much, buck for buck, in returns." By attracting and supporting the activities of groups of collaborating specialists, the commissions of the board became focal concentrations of expert knowledge and effective investigation of various diseases on a worldwide scale. It is a pertinent point, however, that it was the common infectious diseases of the area which required the concentrated attention of investigators—whether in the continental United States or in overseas locations.

The normal expectation was that the organization would be disbanded at the end of the war, but the demonstrated value of the commission's approach and the assistance thus available to the U.S. Armed Services was appreciated. It was redesignated the Armed Forces Epidemiological Board, as a Department of Defense agency, to serve the surgeons general of the Army, Navy, and Air Force for consultation of field problems, for field investigations, and for research in preventive medicine. While certain commissions have been discontinued or combined with others, new commissions have been formed, with an epidemiologic orientation toward special and persistent problems of preventive medicine.

At present there are 180 senior investigators officially attached to the board and its 12 commissions. In association with each responsible investigator, several more members of his staff usually participate in the research which the laboratory is pursuing.

ACCOMPLISHMENTS OF COMMISSIONS

I shall not attempt to recount all the accomplishments of the board nor to make expansive claims; they are not necessary. What is to be emphasized is that many of these accomplishments would scarcely have been possible had the studies not been made in military populations, with the aid of military scientists and physicians.

In the field of respiratory disease, major contributions in which the commissions have participated include the dynamics of meningococcic herd infections and their chemoprophylaxis; the spread and control of streptococcic infections and their sequelae; the development and application of an effective influenza vaccine, and the establishment of extended listening posts for detection and study of influenza viruses; the epidemiology of atypical pneumonia as a disease of recruits, basic demonstrations of its viral etiology, and later studies of adenovaccine effectiveness; further field demonstrations of immunization against pneumococcic pneumonia with polysaccharides; the demonstration of new respiratory viruses and their associated clinical reactions; studies toward development of vaccines against measles and mumps; the development of an effective vaccine against Q fever; intensive studies of the ecology and control of infection by Coccidioides immitis; and improvement in smallpox vaccine.

Major contributions have been made to the knowledge of and efforts to control infectious and serum hepatitis; to the identification of dengue and Phlebotomus-transmitted viruses and possible vaccines; and to identification of various encephalitic viruses, their serologic relationships, and vaccine development. Investigations into the principles of natural resistance; into the development, evaluation, and improvement of immunizing procedures; into mechanisms of infection; and into the disease process of such time-honored "old soldiers" as dysentery, typhoid, and cholera, which have not yet faded away, continue. In fact, the entire field of diarrheal diseases is under study, with attention to procurement of better information about the physiologic basis of susceptibility and the pathogenic capacity of the agent. Studies of cutaneous disorders—sensitizations, acne, itching, poison ivy, fungal infections, i.e., the ordinary ones—are yielding basic etiologic and prophylactic information.

Those studying rickettsial disease represent almost the only remaining nucleus of investigators in the United States, their activities continuing in fundamental research as well as in discovery of improved preventive measures or treatment. Their contributions to the knowledge of the milder form of epidemic typhus or Brill's disease, Tsutsugamushi fever (scrub typhus), and Q fever and to corresponding control measures have been outstanding. Much the same is true of the Commission on Parasitic Diseases with respect to malaria and schistosomiasis; they seek to maintain a corps of competent diagnosticians and scientific experts in the military services especially, but their work turns again to basic research for greater biologic information. Studies in environmental hygiene have provided data regarding pollution and the disposal of waste in Arctic areas, adaptation to warm climates, food control, and occupational protection. The influence of low-grade radiation on infection and resistance is being investigated.

The Commission on Accidental Trauma, adapting the epidemiologic approach to an important study of the role of the driver, the machine, and the environmental state has served as a focal point for interested groups who were otherwise isolated. They have had a definite influence on the consideration of safety features and on the search for measures to eliminate the hazardous driver. Although the military importance of accidents, both civilian and military, in motor vehicles is fully demonstrated, there are strong currents of resistance to the serious study of the institution of preventive measures. Nevertheless, the board has taken an important national leadership in creating an effective front of research into the problem of vehicular accidents especially.

One other area of known importance that has been sporadically studied is that of the relation of military housing to infectious and mental disturbances. With every increase in strength of military personnel, platitudinous surveys of the housing problem are made. Each change in barracks is made with little or no advice on the aspects of medical or health engineering. It is obviously a zone for extended study, but fatalism and jurisdictional authority interfere.

The research activities have been financed primarily through U.S. Army medical funds, although the other services have contributed to the support of certain specific investigations. Moreover, extended field studies have been conducted in U.S. Air Force and Navy installations. The individual investigators receive their funds on a contract basis after consideration and recommendation by one of the commissions, approval by the central board, and administrative concurrence by the service. At times, if funds are scarce, additional money may be sought from other agencies for a recommended activity, while affiliations and sponsorship by the commission are retained. The commissions do not propose to act as study sections or as granting agencies or to preempt control of an area of research. Their purpose is to gather into a mutual working relation military and civilian scientists with common interests and the dedication to work toward the solution of a given problem. By close adherence to the preventive medicine divisions of the three services, attention to the military needs can be steadily maintained. Disease situations which require investigation, difficulties in application of recommended measures, and future projections of the work accomplished can be brought forward for consideration by the appropriate commissions. But the areas of study are not laid down purely as military edicts; the scientific approach is largely devised by the scientific judgment of the experts in that field. In effect, each commission constitutes a research institute with a director, even though housed in laboratories of the affiliated investigators, in military installations, or in other institutions which may be sites of study.

Although the orientation is toward military preventive medicine, the entities under study are also the common causes of disability in the civilian population. Consequently, benefits are mutual and those who are benefited are our sons and daughters. Moreover, there is a great conviction among the participants in this work, as scientists and citizens, that the sustained studies are necessary if these problems of preventive medicine in the U.S. Armed Forces are to be met rather than ignored.

NEED FOR RESEARCH COMMISSIONS IN PREVENTIVE MEDICINE

The reason for this expanded discussion of the Armed Forces Epidemiological Board is (1) to emphasize the limited attention now given to coherent study of certain ordinary disorders and (2) simultaneously to point out how an amount of money, small in current terms, but invested in sympathetic support of a sustained united effort, can earn rich dividends. The "commission" plan of investigation recommends itself not merely as a source of expert opinion but as a unit of action research. It should not be an intellectually closed corporation but a collection of balanced judgment and study. It provides the means of encompassing, in a coherent fashion, research on numerous facets of a problem on which information is needed. This information can then be collated, critically evaluated, and projected in an environment of collaborating experts. Dictatorial or financial control of research is avoided by giving the direction of research to the researchers. It retains freedom for individual initiative within a framework of common purpose and objective. In fact, it can often provide support for new adventures which by themselves might wither. Flexibility and versatility permit a change in direction from the concentration on epidemiologic observation to fundamental study of reactions of the host or of the pathogenic agency, as indicated. The commission can provide continuity to research while deriving benefit from new or brief excursions into other areas and can buffer the disturbances of progress occasioned by hucksters and the promoters of expediency. An agency like the Armed Forces Epidemiological Board could well be expanded to deal with other problems and to serve more widely in the national need for research in preventive medicine. It can be a model for advance in difficult and little-understood problems of many kinds. It is my recommendation that, in the planning for future research, serious consideration be given to adoption of the "commission" plan.

FUTURE TASKS FOR PREVENTIVE MEDICINE

Preventive medicine has long been called the medicine of the future, but what is the future of preventive medicine? I repeat that its future will depend on acceptance, by those who uphold the philosophy of prevention in medicine, of the responsibility for research and the direction it takes and on its willingness to initiate and support vigorous, sustained research in preventive medicine in its literal sense, rather than to leave this to the now-and-then attention of other interests.

A dominant segment of medical research is directed toward the investigation of pathologic disturbances which have already become manifest. Clinical attention—and much Public Health effort—centers on the hope of restoring function or maintaining it at a level that will permit a useful life. Unfortunately, with the exception of certain infectious, toxic, or deficiency diseases, so-called therapeutic procedures do not commonly result in cures, for by the time the manifestations are recognized the defect is well advanced and not ordinarily reversible. This, in general, applies to diabetes, cardiovascular disease, chronic arthritis, cancer, including leukemias, major mental diseases, neurologic diseases, pollen sensitizations, and a variety of other disorders. Even with enhanced efforts toward detection of the asymptomatic stages of these disorders, the ultimate result is only slightly influenced.

Progress in our ability to deal with these currently irreversible disorders, or chronic states, calls for increased research, with preventive intent, to study the origins of a disease and the basis of susceptibility to it. It calls for a turn from preautopsy medicine to preclinical medicine. Epidemiologic investigations should be of prime value in identification of susceptible persons and in disclosure of pathogenic factors which convert the susceptible person, the potential case, into a frank case of disease. Beyond this, there is a need to determine the nature of susceptibility, of the defect or injury which depletes the protective reserve, and of the mechanism of the basic injury, to map out the setting. Knowledge should then lead to devising effective procedures of prevention.

Although there are mild stirrings in this direction, preventive medicine is essentially a neglected field. For its fruitful development, active employment of personnel and scientific methodology from all areas of medical science will be needed. In fact, it is an added facet, a necessary supplement to medical research generally. There has been an increase in the wealth of investigative tools with which to reach back into the beginnings of a disorder. But new perspectives, new ideas, and new modes of measurement will be needed. The epidemiologic, clinical, and laboratory disciplines must be merged into an operating philosophy of preventive research. As increased funds have permitted greater freedom of thought and greater boldness in the pursuit of medical research, there has been much wider extension of interest in the origins of these chronic diseases. It probably is evidence also of increasing maturity in research perspectives. Much of this is rising among those engaged in clinical investigation. But my recommendation is that preventive medicine, and especially epidemiology, take a position of forceful leadership in initiation and development in this area. "Grist is ready for the mill, the leaven is active, let's get cooking."

In the September, 1959, issue of the *American Journal of Public Health* there is a series of excellent and frank appraisals of prevention and control of chronic disease. Emphasis is given to the limited facilities now available despite much activity, to the still prevalent emphasis on detection of the disease, to the greater need to understand the problem confronting us, to the need for etiologic studies, to the study of susceptible persons, and to a discussion of the information necessary for primary prevention. The total effect is to point out the need for preventive research.

A further and more fundamental product of this research should be the development of adequate standards of health. In seeking information on susceptibility and reserve and protective mechanisms, new biological measurements will have to be developed before early deviations from health and recognition of abnormalities will be detectable. The normal physiologic responses to harmful stresses of various kinds will need to be established. The improvement in development and behavior of germ-free animals, despite exposure to varied hazards, is an example of how health may be studied in man. Since much of our present knowledge of health is primitive, the developments in biologic science at both the cellular and the molecular level may provide new dimensions for understanding the systemic and "organismal" state. With advancing knowledge a science of health may actually come into being.

This proposal is not intended merely as a declaration of virtuous ideals. Nor would I propose priority for any of the various entities, for in each of the disorders the need for research is great. The determining factor is the imagination and energy of the investigative group. Nevertheless, certain inferences and relationships suggest that atherosclerosis (especially coronary heart disease), diabetes, and rheumatoid arthritis may be more nearly ripe for picking than certain other diseases of a more diversified nature. But cancer and congenital defects are high on the list because of their probable association with infectious agents. It should be emphasized that the field of infection is wide open for study, for there is no adequate information about who, among a group of susceptible persons, will develop frank disease, inapparent infection, or no infection, when all are uniformly exposed, and that prevention of infectious disease is still in its early stages of development.

REPORT ON ONE STUDY IN
PREVENTIVE MEDICINE

The interest evidenced by the School of Public Health at the University of Michigan in the problem of preventive medicine has taken concrete form in the study of one total community—that of Tecumseh, Mich.—with a population of 8,500. The purpose is to study the health and disease and life and death of members of the population in relation to their biologic, physical, and social environment. The work was begun as a program undertaken by the faculty of the School of Public Health as a whole, with financial support from the University of Michigan for studies in "human resources." The community was mapped; the population was identified by individual persons, households, and genetic kindreds. Interviews and questionnaires obtained information about any of a series of diseases which the individual subjects and families acknowledged to exist among them. About 50 families gave histories of two or more cases of hypertension or of heart disease, and about 15 told of two cases of diabetes.

Our working hypothesis is as follows: A subject with hypertension or coronary heart disease, for example, serves as an index case. Whether related to environmental exposures encountered in the way or course of life or to genetic factors, the members of the household or of the genetic kindred, or both, are more likely to share those influences than other segments of the population. They are more likely to develop the disorder and hence to provide a focus of susceptible persons. Consistent study of the familial associates should then provide information on susceptibilty, the early stages of abnormality, and the course of development of the disease. A developing disease may be observed at different stages in the same unit. Moreover, since persons of all ages are included, observations on contributory factors may be made from early childhood on. That the origins of these diseases go well back into early life seems highly probable. At the kindred level, several generations may be kept under observation. Among those presumed susceptible, pilot studies in the development and evaluation of methods for detection of early aberration can be made. Relationships between the occurrence of different clinical entities can be studied in the same population. The continuing study may also be expected to provide some observations on the incidence of disorders and to suggest features for expanded study in larger populations.

At any rate, with support from the National Heart Institute, examination of the total population has begun, with Dr. Fred Epstein in charge. A comprehensive history, obtained from each family, provides special detail relating to cardiovascular disease, diabetes, arthritis, and chronic pulmonary disease. Each family is then examined clinically—a thorough examination being made, with supportive laboratory studies and again with special emphasis on cardiovascular disease. The population is examined in representative aliquots. In this undertaking we have had the warm support and assistance of the staff of the clinical departments, especially the medical staff, but including surgeons and psychiatrists. A special dental examination is being made of one sample of subjects. Surveys of spastic deformities, fertility, and respiratory disease by family distribution are being made. To date, nearly one-third of the population has had its examination, as requested, with an acceptance of 90 to 92 per cent. The data are being edited and recorded, and certain preliminary measures of uniformity have been made. Although no analyses have been made as yet, it is clear that interesting findings will be obtained. With establishment of the prevalence and selective distribution of various diseases by means of a thorough medical history and examination, the identification of the population will have been completed, and the foundations will have been laid for intensive continued study of special segments that harbor a given disorder or groups of diseases.

SUMMARY

New dimensions and postures are recommended for medical research. The guiding concepts should be (1) that research in preventive medicine in the literal sense be forcefully established, strongly supported, and effectively maintained; (2) that research in infectious diseases not be dissipated by deceiving slogans; (3) that research move toward prevention of the so-called chronic diseases whose scope is increasing; and (4) that preventive medicine will be the medicine of the future only if it accepts its proper responsibility, for the future is very near.

Our views of health, and its values, must, like our educational system, reflect our culture and our way of life. They must be projected as the image of our ideals. Freedom and democracy may seem like hollow triumphs if the hopes of life are submerged in a welter of disease. Security and longer life can be miserable acquisitions, if they mean only the continuation of unhealthy states. Preventive medicine can be our most progressive demonstration to all the world of our belief in human life and happiness. Peace, health, and security are of the same fabric. We should weave more of it.

6. The Voluntary Health Agency

The Role of Voluntary Agencies in Meeting the Health Needs of Americans*

ROBERT H. HAMLIN, M.D.

PRIVATE SUPPORT of health and welfare activities has been an important component of the American democratic tradition since the founding of the United States. The private citizen's and the private corporation's acceptance of public responsibility, expressed through the voluntary giving of time and money, is one of the major factors that has enabled this country to achieve such a high level of health and welfare services for its people.

Voluntary agencies have frequently provided the means through which private citizens and corporations have acted collectively for the betterment of their nation, their communities, and their fellow men. It has, thus, been possible for voluntary agencies to provide needed services, develop and pioneer new methods, and contribute significantly to the improvement of the well-being of the American people.

Voluntary agencies derive their ultimate sanction and direction from the supporting public. They are, in brief, a form of public trusteeship designed to give effect to the altruistic goals of numerous private contributors who wish to give of themselves principally for the benefit of others.

TYPES OF VOLUNTARY AGENCIES

In reviewing the contributions of voluntary agencies to the advancement of individual and collective health, it is unwise and, in fact, often misleading to consider voluntary health agencies and voluntary welfare agencies as separate, distinct entities. It is necessary, furthermore, in any fair and comprehensive analysis, to consider two other groups of agencies: the agencies which solicit contributions through independent appeals, the so-called "independent" agencies, such as national voluntary agencies with State and local affiliates, and agencies which obtain their funds through membership in a federation of agencies, usually a united fund or community chest.

The reasons for these views are manifold. Health and welfare services frequently cannot, and should not, be considered separately, for

* Reprinted with omission of two tables, by permission, from the September 1961 issue of *The Annals of the American Academy of Political and Social Science*, Vol. 337, pp. 93–102. The author is Roger Irving Lee Professor of Public Health, School of Public Health, Harvard University, Boston, Massachusetts.

impairments and improvements in the health status of an individual or group often have social and economic components which are of at least equal importance to the health factors. Numerous voluntary agencies and federations, furthermore, combine health and welfare activities. Many of the important problems now confronting voluntary agencies involve conflicts between national independent agencies and local federations. And, finally, much of the current debate and a number of the major problems of voluntary agencies can be resolved only at the local level, where both federations and independent agencies are found and where most contributors and volunteers personally involve themselves in agency activities.

GROWTH OF PUBLIC GIVING

Today in the United States, more than 100,000 national, regional, and local voluntary agencies, which provide health or welfare services or both as their principal function, solicit contributions from the general public on a wide scale to support a broad scope of activities. (If the 100,000 fraternal, civic, veterans, and related organizations that sponsor some health and welfare activities and the 300,000 churches, most of which provide some form of health and welfare services, are included, over half a million private nonprofit organizations, exclusive of hospitals, are involved in serving the health and welfare needs of the American people.) These agencies include individual organizations at the national, regional, and local levels, such as the American Heart Association and the American Red Cross on the national scene, and family and youth service, recreation and rehabilitation organizations, as well as local affiliates of national agencies, on the community level.

Public contributions to these 100,000 agencies exceeded $1.5 billion in 1958, or one-fifth of all philanthropic giving in the United States ($7.4 billion). Voluntary agencies with a primary interest in health received $570 million and private welfare agencies $950 million. On the assumption that the American public will continue to give at their current rate, contributions to voluntary health and welfare agencies can be expected to rise to $2.7 billion in 1970, or more than 14 times the $188 million contributed in 1940.

Since there is no satisfactory way of estimating the monetary value of philanthropy other than cash contributions to established voluntary agencies, the preceding figures understate the true value of American charitable giving. Examples of other forms of philanthropy are donations of food and clothing, cash contributions not made through organized agencies, and the countless hours of valuable unpaid services given by millions of volunteers acting as fundraisers, board members, or providers of services to the sick and needy.

Current contributions to voluntary agencies also understate total spending by voluntary agencies, since the agencies have other sources of income, such as accumulated capital, investment earnings, payments by clients, membership dues, and income from sale of goods, property, and publications. Current contributions, however, are the only form of income which can be estimated for voluntary agencies as a group.

THE GROWTH OF AGENCIES

The number and size of voluntary agencies have increased rapidly in the past two decades as the agencies have benefited from the great surge in charitable giving by the American people.[2]

National and regional voluntary agencies with a major interest in health grew from 15 in 1940 to approximately 100 at the present time. By 1958 these organizations raised at least $325 million compared with $15 million in 1940. They are expected to receive $460 million by 1965 and $575 million by 1970, if they continue to maintain their current proportion of total philanthropic contributions.

The growth of welfare agencies has not attracted so much attention as the increase in health organizations, partly because most welfare agencies are local, and not affiliated with a national organization. The $950 million raised by nonreligious welfare agencies in 1958 compares with $675 million obtained in 1945 and $150 million in 1940. Based on current rates of giving, their receipts from contributions will rise to $1.3 billion in 1965 and $1.7 billion in 1970.

United funds and community chests in the United States have expanded from 549 in 1939 to over 2,000 in 1960 and now contribute to the budgets of over 26,000 local, regional, and national member agencies. Their receipts from contributions have grown from $83 million in 1939 to over $440 million in 1960.

Participation in united funds and community chests varies widely among the national voluntary agencies, with some participating actively and others not at all. In 1958, united funds and community chests allocated $50 million to the American Red Cross—nearly 60 per cent of the $89 million it received—and $44 million to other national voluntary agencies. Exclusive of the Red Cross, national voluntary agencies with a primary interest in health received in independent public appeals approximately $175 million in 1958, or nearly three-fourths of their total income from contributions of $236 million.

PATTERNS OF GIVING

Donations from corporations and from individuals, both living and dead (death bequests), are the original sources of philanthropic funds. Of the total of almost $7.4 billion in philanthropic contributions from all sources in 1958, 85.6 per cent ($6.3 billion) was given by living Americans, 9.0 per cent ($669 million) in death bequests, and 5.4 per cent ($395 million) by corporations.

The proportions given for health and welfare purposes from these three sources vary considerably. Over 60 per cent of contributions by living individuals in 1958 went for religious purposes, while nearly two-thirds of all death bequests over the past two decades have been made for health and welfare activities. In 1947 two-thirds of the contributions of major corporations also went to health and welfare, although by 1955, primarily as a result of heightened corporate interest in education, this proportion had decreased to a little more than one-third. Corporate philanthropy, however, rose significantly during this period, so that a comparison of dollar values of giving for health and welfare does not present so drastic a picture as a comparison of percentages.

Corporations prefer, when making contributions for health and welfare, to give to united funds and community chests rather than to individual agencies, except for direct donations to Red Cross and hospitals. Forty per cent, or $77.6 million, of the contributions made to united funds and community chests in 1949 came from corporations, as compared with 35.7 per cent, or $152.5 million, in 1958. Excluding amounts given to the Red Cross, corporate contributions made directly to national health agencies are small, amounting to about $10 million in 1958.

AGENCY USE OF CONTRIBUTIONS

Despite the substantial investment in voluntary agencies, carefully evaluated information on their use of contributed funds is limited. The data generally available are those prepared by individual agencies or special groups of agencies in the manner each chooses. The result of the wide variety of reporting methods and categories of expenditures is a mass of information which does not readily lend itself to meaningful compilation and comparisons.

An attempt has recently been made to analyze the income and expenditures of 56 national voluntary agencies. Total income and expenditures reported by these agencies were, respectively, $292 million and $234 million. The large difference of $58 million between income and expenditures resulted primarily from the failure of several major agencies to report spending by their local chapters. In some cases, furthermore, agencies reported net proceeds rather than gross proceeds, thereby deleting information on fund-raising costs.

The data were derived from a review of financial reports prepared by the agencies and did not involve an evaluation of the internal decisions made by the agencies in originally allocating expenditures to various categories. Such a more detailed and accurately conducted study involving direct review of agency records might have significantly different results.

Although accounting and budgetary practices are generally better in united funds and community chests than in national voluntary agencies which raise their funds independently, the funds and chests still do not usually have, either on the national level or in local communities, an adequate breakdown of expenditures by different program activities. Only by extensive further research would it be possible at the present time to obtain reliable data which would permit national compilations and comparisons of expenditures among different groups of agencies.

Undoubtedly one of the greatest needs in the voluntary agency field is more standardized information which will permit a clearer recognition of the social and economic role which voluntary agencies play in the total spectrum of health and welfare services in the United States. The public could also use such information to assist in its decisions about contributions of time and money to the agencies.

COMPARISON OF GOVERNMENT AND
PHILANTHROPIC SPENDING

Although philanthropic support for health and welfare programs has grown immensely in the past two decades, government spending for these purposes has increased even more rapidly. The result is that many functions once largely performed by voluntary agencies have become joint responsibilities with government and, in some cases, assumed largely by government.

Government expenditures for welfare programs in 1958, for example, were $26.3 billion, or nearly 20 times the $1.35 billion in philanthropic welfare contributions. In 1940, government spending was $3 billion and philanthropic giving $200 million, or a ratio of 15 to one. Although private giving for welfare rose sharply during World War II, the increase from 1945 to 1958 was a modest 70 per cent— and it did little more than maintain 1945 purchasing power, because it was accompanied by a 60 per cent climb in consumer prices.

Government spending for health and medical care in 1929 was $513 million, or 14.2 per cent of the total spent by consumers, industry, government, and philanthropic organizations. By 1958 government expenditures had reached $5.8 billion, or 24.1 per cent of the over-all total of $23.9 billion. Philanthropic contributions for health and medical care in 1958 were $680 million, or 3 per cent of all private and government spending for these purposes, as compared to $80 million and 2.2 per cent in 1928. Nearly one-half of the $680 million in 1958, or $325 million, was given to some 60 national and regional voluntary agencies.

Medical research expenditures of the federal government increased some 70 times from 1940 to 1961, rising from $3 million (7 per cent) of total spending of $45 million for these purposes in 1940 to an estimated $496 million (55 per cent) of the total in 1961. Only 6 per cent, or $30 million, of all medical research expenditures in 1958 was made by national voluntary agencies—and more than half ($18 million) came from two agencies, the American Heart Association and the American Cancer Society.

This tremendous growth of government health and welfare activities has posed a major problem of adjustment for voluntary agencies. And, since there is every indication of a continuing pace of government program expansion, this process of adjustment may become even more acute. Federal government expenditures for medical research, for example, are conservatively estimated to rise to $1.6 billion, or 70 per cent, of the total in 1970. And health and medical care spending by government in 1970, based on a projection of only existing programs, will probably be at least two and a half times the dollar amount spent in 1958.

FUND-RAISING CONTROVERSY

Of all the controversies now surrounding voluntary agencies, certainly the most vocal and divisive has been the debate between advocates of independent and federated fund-raising. This debate is not, as many people seem to assume, merely one of fund-raising methods. Certainly the philosophic approaches to fund-raising by the independent agencies and the member agencies of united funds and community chests are distinct, with united funds and community chests conducting a single or federated campaign in each community for their member agencies and independent agencies seeking their funds in individual, separate campaigns.

The conflict, in general terms, is really a competition for public support between national agencies and local agencies, between health agencies and welfare agencies, and between special citizen groups and business and organized labor. The independent voluntary agencies usually have a national organization with a national health objective. They attract their citizen membership from a wide variety of individuals and professional groups interested in the particular disease orientation of an agency. The American Cancer Society and the American Heart Association are examples, with their national health objectives to eradicate cancer and heart disease and with their policies under the strong influence of physicians. On the other hand, united funds and community chests are predominantly composed of local agencies with local interests, principally in the welfare field. Businessmen and, to a lesser degree, organized labor have been the backbone of their efforts.

And the businessman has been in the center of the rising debate between independent and federated agencies. Probably the single most important factor originally precipitating this debate was the struggle between these two groups of agencies for the right to solicit funds, immediately and through periodic payroll deductions, in business enterprises. In most cases, the businessmen, with the support of labor, finally sided with the federations because, in their terms, federations are more efficient. The single, or federated, fund-raising campaign for a number of member agencies has, without doubt, been one of the major advances in the voluntary agency field. Efficiency in fund-raising, however, cannot be necessarily equated with efficiency in fund-spending—and federations have been, for the most part, far more successful in the former than the latter.

Nevertheless, the independent national voluntary agencies have generally been denied the right to make in-plant solicitations. Instead, they have sought funds through a wide variety of direct appeals to the public, often with greater success than the federations.

There is no good reason to presume that the conflict between the independent agency and the federation will diminish in the near future. In fact, it may become more strident, for there are indications that the rate of public contributions to both groups may gradually level off. With this leveling, and with rising costs of current activities and agency desires for new programs, the competition for funds may realistically become even more intense.

The major independent national voluntary agencies will not, of their own free will, join federations on the national or local scene, for they have been too successful in their separate efforts. And there presently are no compelling third-party forces—and probably should not be—to make them do what they strongly do not want to do.

United funds and community chests—dominated by local interests and faced with insufficient funds for their current member agencies—are not able, in many cases, to balance fairly the needs of national and local agencies. Federations are, after all, only human and respond more readily to the immediate, more vocal, and, therefore, effective demands of local groups, even though a national need may be more critical.

PLACE FOR DIFFERENT METHODS

Reasonable differences in philosophies and methods of fund-raising among voluntary agencies can be legitimate. There certainly seems to be a place for national organizations with national, State, and local affiliates which raise their funds independently to serve primarily national purposes. Just as necessary and important are the agencies which are concerned with the problems in each community and which obtain their contributions through joint fund-raising appeals.

Many people believe, however, that the interests of voluntary agencies and the growth of their health and welfare services to serve the American people are impaired, and perhaps threatened, by the increasing tempo and unreasonableness of the fund-raising controversy. The agencies, both the independent organizations and those in federations, have not themselves demonstrated an ability to deal satisfactorily with this paramount issue. In fact, they appear to be girding even more for battle.

There are indications that moderating third parties, such as government and private nonagency study commissions,[4] should be brought upon the scene, not to regulate directly the program of voluntary agencies, but to develop mechanisms for supplying better information to create a more informed, more discriminating contributing public. For example, uniform accounting and financial reporting for voluntary agencies, reasonably applied by the agencies and supervised in its application by accounting organizations and other interested groups, is potentially one of the most progressive, most illuminating steps which could be taken in this direction.

FUND-RAISING COSTS

The tremendous competition for the charity dollar has resulted in often uncertain and sometimes misleading statistics from voluntary agencies on their use of the public's contributions. In an attempt to present the most desirable, attractive image to stimulate the public's giving impulse, agencies are inclined to take unreasonable liberties in computing the various shares of their income which go for different purposes. The tendency is to overstate funds spent for services and to understate expenditures for administrative and fund-raising costs.

Agencies are in a position to do this, since, for the most part, they determine their own accounting policies and prepare their own financial statements. Audits by certified public accountants, who have no standardized accounting principles in the voluntary agency field to guide them, usually are only checks against fraud. These audits generally do not review the accuracy of allocations of expenditures by the agencies to their various program activities.

Voluntary agencies that participate in single or federated campaigns, for example, frequently state their fund-raising costs as that of the united fund or community chest, often said to be less than 5 per cent. A more accurate computation of individual agency fund-raising expenses in these federations would require the inclusion of the costs which are necessary to raise all contributions regardless of the source. Furthermore, united funds and community chests, which are basically fund-raising organizations—the member agencies individually spend the funds—do not generally include, as fund-raising expenses, the monetary value of the time spent on financial solicitation endeavors by member agency personnel. The separateness of fund-raising and fund-spending organizations in federations leads to these misleading figures.

Because independent agencies are both fund-raising and fund-spending organizations—and, therefore, must include in their financial statements both types of activities—they are not in a position to prepare as favorable statistics on fund-raising costs. There seems to be little doubt that accurately and fairly computed fund-raising costs of united funds and community chests, in many situations, would be larger than the amounts and percentages they usually state.

The uncertainty of factual data on expenditures is not substantially different with voluntary agencies which raise their funds in independent campaigns. Fund-raising costs reported to contributors by 10 major independent national voluntary health agencies,[5] for example, recently ranged between 7 and 15 per cent. The Board of Social Service Commissioners of Los Angeles, a government agency that audits and reports annually on organizations within their jurisdiction, reports fund-raising costs of 12.5 to 36.2 per cent for the local campaigns of these same 10 agencies. The wide discrepancy arises primarily from differences in allocation of costs between fund-raising and public education, with many agencies assigning part of fund-raising expenses to education.

Standardized accounting, applied equally to independent agencies and federations, appears to be the only feasible solution on the horizon for understandable, accurate statistics on fund-raising costs as well as accurate data on other disbursements by voluntary agencies. The present situation breeds nothing more than greater confusion.

ORGANIZATION

The vociferousness of the controversy over fund-raising methods has frequently misdirected the public mind from an equally if not more important issue. That issue is the capacity of voluntary agencies to fulfill modern-day, significantly altered responsibilities with an organizational and administrative structure that has changed but little during the past 20 years. The basic theme of the numerous questions now being asked with increasing frequency about voluntary agencies principally concerns the agencies' competence to carry out the roles which American society has assigned to them, not the need for the agencies' services.

The growing complexity of community health and welfare programs, the rapid multiplication of voluntary agencies, and the phenomenal increases in public giving all require much greater cooperative action by voluntary agencies, among themselves and with expanding government agencies, and in general community-wide planning for health and welfare services. Agencies in and out of federations need to demonstrate greater ability to terminate, modify, or consolidate programs when a better, more effective structure of agencies would result. It is to be seriously questioned whether over 100,000 voluntary agencies are required at the present time to provide private health and welfare services in the United States.

Regardless of the number, voluntary agencies, whether in federations or independent, need to give greater evidence of constructive cooperation in the development and provision of health and welfare services, if they are to fulfill these important functions:

(1) Determine new methods to improve the health and welfare of the American people.
(2) Demonstrate practical means by which these improvements may be made by both voluntary and government agencies.
(3) Inform the general public and the interested professions.
(4) Supplement government programs with personnel, facilities, and services.
(5) Protect the public interest by working for effective government agencies.
(6) Develop comprehensive, balanced community health and welfare programs.
(7) Promote and maintain legislation in the public interest.
(8) Support research into the causes of disease, deprivation, and inadequate services.

The responsibility for providing accurate data to the public, modernizing voluntary agency structure, and strengthening joint planning lies at present directly with voluntary agencies, for they have been given a unique, almost complete freedom to determine their own policies, even though they are clearly instruments of public policy supported by public contributions.

1. An additional $510 million was given to churches for their health and welfare programs within the United States. Thus, over $2 billion, or more than one-quarter of total American philanthropy, was contributed in 1958 for health and welfare purposes.

2. The significant growth of philanthropic contributions reflects not only rising personal and corporate income in the United States, but also the increasing share of personal income after taxes and corporate income before taxes given for philanthropy. The share of personal income has rather steadily increased, from 1.4 per cent in 1940 to 1.8 per cent in 1945 and 2.0 per cent in 1958. Each person in the United States in 1958 gave an average of $36 for philanthropy. Corporations in 1958 con-

tributed 1 per cent of corporate profits before taxes to philanthropy, as compared to 0.8 per cent for the span of years from 1936 to 1958.

3. *The Exploratory Study of Voluntary Health and Welfare Agencies in the United States*, Report of the Ad Hoc Committee appointed and financed by the Rockefeller Foundation, New York, 1961.

4. *The Exploratory Study of Voluntary Health and Welfare Agencies in the United States* (see footnote 3) recommended in July 1961 the ap-

pointment of such a commission of informed private citizens for a period not to exceed five years.

5. The American Cancer Society, American Heart Association, Arthritis and Rheumatism Foundation, Muscular Dystrophy Associations of America, National Association for Mental Health, National Foundation, National Society for Crippled Children and Adults, National Tuberculosis Association, Sister Elizabeth Kenny Foundation, United Cerebral Palsy Associations.

Conventional and "Self-Organized" Voluntary Agencies: A Comparison*

ALFRED H. KATZ, D.S.W.

SHRYOCK[1] has laid down several general pre-conditions for the emergence of the usual voluntary health agency: the clinical identification and differential diagnosis of a particular disease; the discovery of causation and consequent means of prevention; the growth of a social reform psychology and the growth of public dread or fear of a particular illness. Regarding the tuberculosis movement, Shyrock makes the point "that the advent of the antituberculosis movement had to wait . . . upon the discovery of some means of prevention or cure."

From his study of the history of 14 of the major voluntary agencies, Cavins identifies "two definite steps in the almost conventional formula for the organization of a national voluntary agency. The first is the realization that a serious socio-medical problem exists . . . the second state is reached when a local society is formed."[2] While the self-organized groups shared some of these pre-conditions for their origination, *they differ sharply from the conventional agencies in the immediate motivations and objectives of their founders*, as well as in the personnel of the originators.

It is clear that the National Tuberculosis Association pioneered a pattern of lay-medical cooperation for public education and remedial action; it is equally evident that the organization neither stemmed

---

* Reprinted by permission from the author's book *Parents of the Handicapped*, pp. 74–80, 1961. Courtesy of Charles C Thomas, Publisher, Springfield, Illinois.

from the initiative nor offered any role for the parents or relatives of those affected.

Another typical health agency with a well established history is the National Committee for Mental Hygiene (now the National Association for Mental Health). Its origin is somewhat less complicated than that of the Tuberculosis Association. Its prime mover was Clifford Beers, whose experience and work are told in his autobiography, "A Mind That Found Itself." According to Dr. C. E. A. Winslow, well known authority on Public Health, "rarely has a great movement been so truly the shadow of a single creative spirit as in this instance."[3] It was of considerable significance, of course, that Beers himself had also suffered from a condition which he devoted his life to combatting. He had been institutionalized for psychosis for a number of years after suicide attempts, but he recovered completely and set about to organize a committee to improve conditions in the mental institutions, and to educate the public regarding the care of mental patients. In doing so, Beers interested some outstanding thinkers, Professor William James, Dr. Adolph Meyer, Dr. William H. Welch, and other psychiatrists and neurologists. In his famous book, Beers projected his aims for an organization in the following words:

> This improvement can never be brought about without some central organization by means of which the best ideas in the world may be crystallized and passed along . . . the methods to be used to bring about these results must be placed on (a) high level . . . let the thing be worked up secretly and confidentially by a small number of men who know their business, then when the very best plan has been formulated and men of money have been found to support the movement . . . announce to the world the organization and aims of the society.[4]

When the National Committee for Mental Hygiene was organized in 1909, there were 30 charter members including Beers, William James, Drs. Meyer and Welch, but only two wealthy and prominent laymen, Henry Phipps and Mrs. William K. Vanderbilt. Phipps made a founding gift of $50,000 to finance the first three years of activity. There was no indication that any persons who had been personally affected by the problem, other than Beers and his brother, were involved in the organization. Financial support was not sought from the general community for a number of years. In his *The Mentally Ill in America*, Albert Deutsch relates the emergence of the National Committee for Mental Hygiene to the widespread movements of social reform of the period, inaugurated chiefly by physicians who secured the support of philanthropists. *There is no indication of the "self-help" or mutual aid approach in this movement or of the participation of those directly or indirectly affected by the problem.*

Another important national voluntary agency, The American Heart Association, was organized solely by physicians. It came into being in 1922 when 46 physicians attending the annual session of the American Medical Association organized the American Heart Association primarily to forward public education and carry on research.[5]

Both Gunn and Platt and Cavins reviewed the history of almost all the important national health agencies in the United States. They stress almost uniformly that *the origin of these societies was to be found in the public spirited action of physicians concerned with particular diseases or health problems.* The physicians interested wealthy and influential laymen to help create and support specific organizations or committees, which later developed staffs, programs and structures.

The second major point of contrast between the self-organized groups and other voluntary health and welfare agencies is a corollary of the differences in origin. The self-organized groups typically are *membership* bodies or associations, and generally give their membership an opportunity to participate in determining the affairs of the organization. With the exception of the Muscular Dystrophy Associations the constitutions of the groups studied provide for individual or family membership of those affected by the problem, and of other interested persons, upon the payment of a membership fee.

Membership in the self-organized groups has some of the characteristic properties of membership in citizen groups as analyzed by Thelens:[6]

1. The membership can be defined. It is known who is in the group, either by name or by definition.

2. Members think of themselves as constituting a group. There is a shared image of the totality, which marks it off from other groups.

3. There is a sense of shared purpose among members. The members can state some reasons for their being a group, and the reasons include a concept of something striven for, some advantage to be gained through mutual efforts.

4. There is a greater ease of communications among members than between members and non-members.

As indicated in the data from interviews and as briefly presented in the case-history summaries, membership in the self-organized groups reflects these elements to a significant degree.

Such a pattern of membership involvement, both in their historical origins—and currently—is found among only one other type of voluntary social or health agency—The Young Men's and Young Women's Christian Associations. These bodies were organized by young people for varied purposes: to provide vehicles for carrying out the social purposes of evangelic Christianity; to provide specific self-improvement and mutual aid services for their members, and for other, less privileged members of society; and to provide opportunities for social fellowship for Christian young people who reside in urban centers.[7]

Prominent in the "Ys" from their earliest days unto the present has been their membership character. Thus, Sims writes:

> Members had a stake in the total work of the YWCA as early as the 1870's, and monthly meetings of local boards of directors were open to all, members being urged to come to listen to reports and to ask questions . . . Often a new Association was organized because young women simply wanted a place to which they could go for recreation, education classes or just to make friends. They saw the YMCA providing such opportunities for young men and wanted the same for themselves. The Association magazine, the *Evangel,* said in 1892 that "the same young women *by* whom the Association is carried on are those *for* whom it is organized and those *for* whom efforts are made are those *by* whom effective work will be executed."[8]

Membership in most other types of voluntary agencies, however, is of a different character and does not result in such significant identifications.[9] In one type of voluntary agency where there is a Board of Directors, plus a prescribed number of "invited," "appointed," or "honorary" members, membership is not open but limited to a specified number. In other voluntary agencies, nominal membership is granted to individuals who make financial contribution of a specific amount. Such members, however, are not granted privileges beyond the right to vote for officers; they are rarely if ever invited to work on Committees of the Board of Directors, to run for office, or to advise on policy. In the case of most agencies of this type, such "membership" seems to be clearly a fund-raising or a public relations device. *Policy making in these organizations is considered purely a function of the Board of Directors, and not of membership.* Annual business meetings of these organizations are usually of a routine character, without sizable attendance or participation by members.

This situation contrasts sharply with that of the self-organized groups, where members are persons directly affected by and often emotionally involved in the problem. In consequence, at least a minority of members participate actively and sometimes acrimoniously in policy discussions that may have a direct and immediate bearing on their own lives and welfare.

In order to allow for such participation, as well as for purposes of developing their programs and organizations, the self-organized groups have frequent meetings. In the Association for Help to Retarded Children (N.Y. State) and United Cerebral Palsy, New York City, meetings are usually held monthly, and have educational and organizational aspects. In the League for Emotionally Disturbed Children, the frequency of general meetings is approximately five or six times annually.

The comparative frequency of membership meetings, and of other activities for members, in the self-organized groups is in clear contrast with the situation in other voluntary health agencies. Gunn and Platt obtained information on the frequency of Board meetings in some of the organizations they studied (finding, for example, that a majority of State and local TB Associations had from one to five meetings of their Boards annually) but neither these authors nor Cavins give an account of *membership* meetings, for the reason that in this type of agency they generally do not occur, except as pro forma Annual Meetings to formalize the adoption of reports, and the election of officers.

We must conclude then that the self-organized groups resemble voluntary membership associations, such as social, fraternal, trade union or other special purpose groups, in respect to their membership and membership participation character, rather than other voluntary health and welfare agencies.

In concluding consideration of these broad differences between the self-organized groups and other social agencies, it is of interest to emphasize similarities as well. Gunn and Platt list the following as a broad description of typical functions of the voluntary health agencies:

(a) Exploring or surveying, in search of needs not being served and new methods of meeting recognized needs.

(b) Demonstrating practical methods for improving the Public Health, and for their wider application by official or other agencies.

(c) Educating in a broad sense, in which all agencies engage more or less energetically and effectively.

(d) Supplementing health departments with personnel or facilities not yet available through public funds.

(e) Serving as guardians of citizen interest in maintaining the effectiveness of health departments.

(f) Guarding and advancing legislation bearing on health.

(g) Coordinating efforts with those of other agencies and groups having related purposes.

(h) Developing well-rounded community health programs.[10]

It is of considerable importance to note that the self-organized groups also perform all or most of these functions. Although they are distinct as to origin, motivation, and in their structural membership aspects, the self-organized groups in total definition must be viewed as falling clearly within the framework of the voluntary health agencies. They perform many functions similar to those of agencies in the established field. They may be best viewed as sharing in the general purposes and functions of other voluntary health and welfare agencies, but as having some particular functions and characteristics that grow out of their origin and continuing character as self-help associations.

1. Richard H. Shyrock: The Historical Significance of the TB Movement, in *Past and Present Trends in the TB Movement*, National TB Association, 1942, p. 47.

2. Cavins: *Op cit.*, p. 94.

3. C. E. A. Winslow: *The Mental Hygiene Movement*. Published by National Committee for Mental Hygiene, 1937, p. 306.

4. Clifford Beers: *A Mind That Found Itself*, 29th Edition, Doubleday and Company, 1953, p. 217.

5. Cavins: *Op. cit.*, p. 138.

6. Herbert A. Thelens: *Dynamics of Groups at Work*. University of Chicago, 1954, p. 231.

7. Cf., for a compact history of the YWCA's, Mary S. Sims: *The YWCA—an Unfolding Purpose*, New York, Women's Press, 1950, 156 pp.

8. *Ibid.*, pp. 128–29.

9. Tsouderos, for example, writes of the Minnesota Division of the American Cancer Society, one of the ten voluntary associations he studied in detail: "the membership of the association can hardly be called a membership group in the sociological sense. There is no evidence that there is social interaction among the members as members of this association, and the attendance at the annual convention is extremely poor." Tsouderos, John F. *The Formalization Process of the Social Structure of Voluntary Associations*. Unpublished Ph.D. dissertation, University of Minnesota 1953.

10. Gunn, Selskar M., and Platt, Philip S.: Voluntary Health Agencies —an Interpretive Study. New York, The Ronald Press Company, p. 55.

7.   Cooperation among Agencies

Cooperation Between Departments of Health and Welfare*

JONAS N. MULLER, M.D., M.P.H., AND PEARL BIERMAN, M.A.

IN 1952 the Joint Committee on Medical Care of the American Public Health and Public Welfare Associations posed the thesis that the interests and practices of Public Health and public welfare were bringing the agencies concerned closer together.[1] This was not a new thesis but a restatement that was especially timely in the light of the Social Security Act amendments of 1950.[2, 3] These amendments made possible federally matched direct payments to the providers of medical care for certain needy persons and established the Federal-State program of aid to the permanently and totally disabled.

During the past few years, through a field survey in eight States and 10 local areas, the APWA and the APHA have sought to determine what cooperative activities are conducted in some official health and welfare departments.

METHOD OF THE STUDY

The States and localities selected for study were among those in which we might expect to find an optimum potential for close working relationships between the departments. These were:

California: Alameda County, City and County of San Francisco, San Mateo County; Maryland: Carroll County; Massachusetts: City of Quincy; New Jersey: City of Newark and Essex County; New York: Ulster County; Oregon: City of Portland and Multnomah County; Washington: City of Seattle and King County; Wisconsin: Rock County and the Cities of Janesville and Beloit.

In each State, we arranged meetings with personnel in the State health and welfare departments, and in at least one local area. Occa-

* Reprinted by permission from the September 1956 issue of *Public Health Reports*, Vol. 71, pp. 833–848. The authors are, respectively, Professor and Chairman of the Department of Preventive Medicine, Flower and Fifth Avenue Hospitals, New York Medical College, New York, New York, formerly Staff Director, Subcommittee on Medical Care, Committee on Administrative Practice, American Public Health Association, New Haven, Conn.; and Assistant Chief, Medical Care Administration Branch, Division of Community Health Services, Department of Health, Education, and Welfare, Washington, D.C., formerly Medical Care Consultant, American Public Welfare Association, Chicago, Illinois.

sionally some State personnel accompanied us on local visits. The meetings were informal and frequently led into topics which heretofore had not been considered jointly by the health and welfare staffs.

The typical meeting found top representation from administration, medical social work staff from both departments, medical directors or consultants of the welfare departments, supervisors of Public Health nursing, and, especially from the welfare department, staff responsible for development of policy and standards. In one area, only two administrators appeared. At the other end of the scale, the chiefs of practically all operating units in both departments met with us.

Open-ended, but directed, questioning was used. Each agency was first asked to describe its overall program, with particular attention to the provision of health services to needy persons. Questions were then directed at relationships in regard to referral of patients, exchange of information, followups, and continuity of service. An attempt was made to call for illustrations of specific problems such as services to tuberculosis patients and to their families; preventive services to mothers and children; the determination of incapacity in aid to dependent children and aid to the permanently and totally disabled, and the application of preventive and rehabilitative services once such a determination was made. Case histories often were used to illustrate relationships or the lack thereof, particularly by the local agencies.

This more or less clinical approach was followed by questions designed to bring out interdepartmental relationships arising out of service responsibilities. Since this was generally the most successful method of achieving information, the present report is organized under service titles.

In the preparation of this report, we have drawn upon the meager literature on health and welfare department relationships and also upon the knowledge of agency operations gained in work with such departments.

PATTERNS OF COOPERATION

There are many patterns of cooperation between health and welfare agencies which differ in form and degree. Most of them relate to activities somewhat remote from the recipient of service, and few are vigorously directed at the prime goals of health. Moreover, cooperation is practiced relatively seldom and is rarely explicitly defined as policy.

This is not to say that there is noncooperation between health and welfare staffs. There is often simply no relationship on the administrative level. In this connection, Dr. Palmer Dearing, Deputy Surgeon General, Public Health Service, said before the Conference of State Public Welfare Directors in 1950:

"It is conceivable that an effective program might be developed without any formal provisions for cooperation." However, he went on hopefully to say that, "if health and welfare staffs work closely and congenially together and consult spontaneously whenever they deal with interrelated problems, they will inevitably make plans together and define areas of responsibility . . ."[2]

Unfortunately, we have found that many health officers specifically avoid the responsibilities arising out of the fact that disease is most prevalent among persons known to welfare agencies. We were told frequently that the health department feared being labeled as an agency for the indigent if it made any special provisions for health services to the needy.

Public welfare departments—dedicated to the prevention of abnormal dependency and to the achievement and maintenance of normal, secure, and productive social living—have the same objectives as public health agencies.

To help clients realize these goals, the welfare department will require professional help in the administration of a medical care program. The definition of medical care is a broad one and includes many of the personal health services which may be provided by or through the health department.[1]

> "Medical care is essential for individual well-being. Its objectives include the promotion of health, the prevention of disease and disability, the cure or mitigation of disease, and the rehabilitation of the patient. Medical care for needy as well as other persons must be geared not only to treatment of disease but also to preventing its occurrence or progress. For those needy persons who are already disabled, all possible use should be made of rehabilitation services so that individuals may be restored to productive living, may cease to require the continued services of other members of the family, and may be enabled to live as useful and happy lives as possible within the limitations of their disabilities."

If preventive services are not known to the welfare program, if they are difficult to obtain, or even refused, then the welfare department will have to establish them. This need has been acute for some time in regard to child welfare and may soon be as acute in other welfare programs, such as services for the aged.

Welfare departments are acquiring medical administrative machinery, knowledge, and skill. They have long been concerned with long-term illness and disability and with the aged. Services for unmarried mothers, for dependent and foster children, for the aged, and for the prevention of delinquency all involve extended health responsibilities. The alert health officer is interested in all these areas and will help the welfare department find efficient methods of providing the required services. The cooperative efforts of health and welfare agencies will improve the health of the entire community.

PUBLIC HEALTH NURSING

Public Health nursing services are the most widely used of the health department services available to clients of public welfare agencies. Extensive field relationships between caseworkers and Public Health nurses, for the most part, appear to revolve around episodes or cases. These relationships are generally informal and unplanned, often the result of an accidental joint visit to a household. In only one of eight States was there evidence of State policy directed at promoting such relationships except in the limited field of institutional inspection. This lack of definition of responsibility generally applies to local agencies as well.

In a number of communities, however, the services of Public Health nurses have been made available systematically to people served also by the public welfare agency. In Ulster County, N.Y., nurses from the county health department provide bedside care, including injection of medications, as an extension of the teaching program, for welfare clients who are homebound. Staff nurses obtain information concerning the family and home from the welfare caseworker. Case conferences are organized by field workers of the two departments on the initiative of either staff. Informal conferences, apparently more common, also are reported in the regular work sheets.

Some nursing services also are available at local nursing stations and at health department headquarters. The increasing caseload among the aged has increased the bedside care functions of the nurse although the number of patients is not great. Staff representatives of the health and welfare departments have met to consider methods of meeting the need for home nursing service without disrupting the Public Health nursing program.

The Ulster County Public Health nurses bring advice on nutrition to welfare families. Nutrition consultation from the State health department thus serves the local welfare agency indirectly. Public Health nurses also survey health care of children in foster homes.

This county has a well-developed orientation and inservice training program for staff nurses which draws upon the welfare staff. Much of the teaching is carried out in case conferences which involve all of the community agencies related to the particular case. At the time of our visit, there was no such use of health department personnel in the public welfare agency.

SERVICES FOR CHILDREN

State Public Health personnel participate actively in both administrative and clinical services for child welfare. Standards for child care facilities and programs of all types are often developed jointly. In several States, the maternal and child health division of the health department provides medical administrative and clinical consultation to the division responsible for child welfare in the welfare agency. In Maryland, a good deal of time has been spent on how, and by whom, health supervision should be provided in foster care and adoption programs. In Wisconsin, requests for consultation have been limited to problem cases, but the board of health participated in establishing the standards for medical care in the foster home program, as well as the standards used by the division for children and youth of the department of public welfare in licensing children's institutions and day care centers.

Locally, the health department is likely to be engaged only in direct clinical services—child health conferences, crippled children's services, and, to a lesser extent, child guidance clinics. Occasionally these services are operated jointly, and the crippled children's services may be under the local welfare department. Relationships are probably developed most extensively in the crippled children's program.

In many States, services for handicapped children engage both State health and welfare agencies, and sometimes, other State and local agencies as well. Primary State responsibility for the State-Federal program is in the health department in 32 States and Territories, in the welfare department in 8 States, and in a combined health and welfare agency in one State. In the remaining 11 of the 52 States and Territories reporting in 1954, the program is administered by special commissions (four States), by departments of education (three States), and in four States by the State medical schools.[4] Where cooperation is practiced, relationships may extend to case finding, organized referral systems, case conferences, foster home placement, acceptance of responsibility for payment for care, the determination of eligibility, and clinical services.

In California, the State program of crippled children's services is administered by the health department, but in about half of the counties the welfare department has been assigned responsibility by the local board of supervisors. On request, consultation may be provided by either State agency whose field workers maintain an active relationship to determine the best ways of providing consultation.

In Massachusetts, the public assistance and child guardianship divisions of the department of public welfare have agreed to pay the costs of care for their clients when crippled children's service funds are lacking in the department of Public Health.

In New York State, case finding for the crippled children's program is an accepted responsibility of welfare workers, as well as of health department staff. As long-term custodial care for children who cannot be rehabilitated is difficult to locate, problem cases are discussed by staff members of both agencies. In practice, most of the relationships in New York's program are between the State health department and the local welfare departments. The active support of this relationship by State welfare department policy is important. The welfare departments aid in finding foster homes for handicapped children. For children who are not found eligible for the Medical Rehabilitation Program (the crippled children's service in this State), welfare resources are occasionally called upon to provide services such as certain forms of orthodontic care.

In North Carolina, financial eligibility for care under the crippled children's program of the State board of health is determined by the State board of public welfare. This service, based upon a written agreement, is part of the State's policy of applying a uniform standard of eligibility for health services at State expense. In addition to investigation and certification of eligibility, the State board of public welfare agrees to assist with case-finding, to provide transportation for patients to and from clinics and hospitals, to help in locating special equipment and services when crippled children's funds are limited, and to provide casework service to the patient and family in the adjustment to long-term treatment. These services are provided through the county welfare departments under instructions prepared by the State board of public welfare and reviewed by the crippled children's department of the State board of health.[5] Similar agreements define the responsibilities of the board of public welfare in relation to the cancer program of the State board of health; tuberculosis sanatorium care provided by the North Carolina sanatoriums; correction of defects under the school health program of the board of public instruction.

TUBERCULOSIS CONTROL

The association between tuberculosis and economic deprivation calls for vigorous measures to prevent infection and to treat patients served by welfare agencies. In this area of communicable disease control, interdepartmental cooperation is highest, particularly between local agencies.

In their 1950 reports to the Public Health Service, 11 State welfare departments reported some type of tuberculosis control or hospitalization responsibility[6] although major responsibility rested with the State health department. It would be reasonable to expect some kind of relationship between these two State agencies concerning their responsibilities for certain tuberculosis control activities. Nevertheless, the annual report on State tuberculosis control programs for fiscal years 1954 and 1955[7] notes as one of the continuing administrative problems "lack of coordination of program activities among all interested State and local agencies."

Cooperation in disease control by State agencies was not evident during our visits. One agency head feared that any notification to welfare clients of the availability of preventive services could be considered coercion and therefore was not an appropriate public assistance activity. A welfare client, he thought, should have the normal opportunity to find out that a chest X-ray survey was due in his neighborhood and any action by the public assistance agency concerning the survey might make the client feel that he had to have an X-ray.

In Wisconsin, however, where the State antituberculosis association and the State board of health cooperate in sending mobile X-ray units around the State, each county welfare department is informed, through the State welfare department, when the unit is coming. All possible channels are used to encourage county agency clients to use the service. The latest tuberculosis control report of the Wisconsin State Board of Health notes that nursing homes are receiving special attention. Oregon also reported special efforts in regard to nursing homes with indigent residents. In this State, representatives of both State boards confer to arrange care for tuberculosis patients.

We found that few local health departments have encouraged the welfare departments to give new clients a chest X-ray. A somewhat larger number of departments, State and local, notify local welfare agencies of chest survey schedules and help them achieve a high level of client participation. A few health departments have conducted campaigns to find tuberculosis among residents of nursing homes, homes for the aged, and lodging houses for single men. Health departments not infrequently provide X-ray facilities, as well as tests for syphilis, for screening possible foster parents or operators of child care facilities. Routine health examinations for personnel of other care facilities, or for health or welfare department staffs are relatively rare.

After diagnosis, coordinated services are needed to help a patient to recover. The patient and his family need to understand the disease and the treatment program. The patient requires knowledge of his family's status and assurance that they will not be neglected. With the patient under hospital care, there should be periodic reports to and from the community agencies concerned with the patient and his family. Case conferences to set rehabilitation goals and make appropriate predischarge plans smooth the path back to active life. When care on an ambulatory basis becomes possible from a clinical point of view, social, economic, and Public Health problems which stand in the way of such therapy must be solved by coordinated efforts.

The integrated service of a combined local department of health and welfare, as in San Mateo County, Calif., has pioneered in meeting the needs of patients with tuberculosis. This department is responsible for the county institutions as well as for the full range of Public Health and public welfare services.

The entire tuberculosis control program is under the medical director of the sanatorium, to assure continuity of service from case finding and diagnosis through followup. A full-time Public Health nurse at the sanatorium keeps liaison with the field staff. Problems relating to the treatment plan for a patient are usually worked out in the district by frequent and informal meetings between the Public Health nurses and caseworkers.

If difficulties require administrative consideration, the family is brought to the attention of the supervisors. Medical consultation is immediately at hand. The staff confers on patients under care twice each month. A representative of the social service division participates whether or not the patient receives public assistance.

Planning two to three months ahead in anticipation of discharge from the sanatorium applies to every public patient in San Mateo County. The sanatorium itself has a rehabilitation program in which a representative of the district office of the State bureau of vocational rehabilitation shares. Psychiatric services also are provided. Thanks in large part to the relationship established by the department in this program, an unusually low proportion of patients leave the sanatorium against medical advice.

SERVICES FOR CHRONICALLY ILL AND DISABLED

In most communities, unfortunately, relationships in regard to chronic diseases and adult rehabilitation are not strikingly different from relationships in regard to disease control, with a few possible exceptions.

Basic Studies for Program Development

In two States noted for their chronic disease programs, California and New York, departments share actively in basic studies for program development. New York State studies have been concerned with the extent of chronic illness and disability. In California, the director of the State department of social welfare served on the advisory committee for the chronic disease investigation conducted for the legislature in 1949 by the State department of Public Health. Welfare directors of 38 counties contributed their experiences as well. Welfare officials contributed also to the 1954 health survey conducted by the chronic disease service of the State department of Public Health.

Mutual Support of Legislation

Cooperation on legislation, though somewhat rare, was noted in several States. Development of the Lemuel Shattuck Hospital in Boston, operated by the Massachusetts Department of Public Health, may be credited to the joint planning of the health and welfare departments and to their mutual assistance in preparing and supporting legislation required for its construction. This hospital for persons with chronic diseases is a base for both service and research.

Case Finding

Case finding is not widely practiced in welfare departments except in relation to communicable disease. For example, no State welfare department in 1950 reported to the Public Health Service responsibility for diabetes control;[6] only seven State welfare departments reported contributing to heart disease control; only eight to cancer control. This listing, however, does not cover "unofficial" responsibilities. Massachusetts, for example, is not included although the State health department's 26 tumor clinics regularly refer to the welfare department cancer patients who require and are unable to afford long-term care.

While welfare departments do play a part in case-finding for certain communicable diseases, most welfare staffs do not yet have sufficient knowledge to be an effective case-finding instrument for the non-communicable chronic diseases.

Determination of Disability

Health department clinics in orthopedics, venereal disease, rheumatic fever, chest diseases, and cerebral palsy often help welfare departments determine a client's disability. The general medical services, including clinics, of about 70 local health departments across the country are the major or sole source of medical care for welfare patients in these areas. A few of these departments, such as the Baltimore City Health Department, have attempted to work toward the prevention of disease, especially chronic disease, by offering physical examinations. A few, such as the health department in Newark, N.J., have disability evaluation units. And here and there, a local health officer serves as medical member of the welfare department's review team for eligibility for aid to the disabled.

Rehabilitation

Aggressive concern with rehabilitation is a relatively recent development in welfare work,[8] encouraged undoubtedly by the newest category of public assistance, aid to the permanently and totally disabled. Accompanying this new interest, however, is a certain feeling of frustration due, no doubt, to many long years of failure to obtain rehabilitation services for public welfare clients. Hence, a few welfare departments have developed their own rehabilitation programs.[9]

For most departments, this choice is neither wise nor possible. It ignores the resources of the local health department for the development, application, and coordination of rehabilitation services. Certainly the Public Health staff can help welfare workers concerned with rehabilitation problems by interpreting the social meaning of medical findings and acquainting them with the medical aspects of rehabilitation.

There are a few places, however, where health departments have put their long experience with habilitation and rehabilitation of crippled children to effective use for all age groups. We know of only one State where this is policy: Washington, where every local health officer serves as medical consultant to the district vocational rehabilitation counselor. Weekly meetings serve the day-to-day administrative needs of the vocational rehabilitation program. In addition, monthly conferences include any other local agency with an interest in a case on the agenda. The State health officer feels that this arrangement has been successful.

The California State Department of Public Health has been of help in the development of policies and procedures for improving opportunities for rehabilitation among the disabled parents of recipients of aid to needy children. The detailed story of the several interrelated projects involving the State department of social welfare, the bureau of vocational rehabilitation, and the department of Public Health is told in a series of publications.[10-14]

INSTITUTIONAL STANDARDS AND LICENSURE

Probably the best developed cooperative relationships at State level revolve around institutions, particularly their licensing. Information obtained from 44 States in 1953 indicated that in 30 States the health department had legal responsibility for the program for all institutions serving older people.[15] Six States assigned to the welfare department the accrediting program for all such institutions. And in eight States, responsibility was assigned to the health or welfare department according to the nature of the institution. The 1950 State health department reports to the Public Health Service indicate that, while health departments have major responsibility for licensing medical institutions in most of the States, welfare departments are responsible for most child care facilities in the States where there are licensing provisions; and in a few States, the welfare agency is responsible for the general or special hospital facilities.[16]

Expert guidance, consultation, and field service from personnel skilled in health and social services are required if programs of licensure or other forms of accreditation are to be more than perfunctory. Both health and welfare agencies know that licensing can be a "tool" to achieve a higher level of care and service. General health care, rehabilitation, the prevention of secondary disability, accident prevention, the use of nursing, nutrition, and social services, all call for their joint attention.

Cooperative efforts range from contractual agreements to informal but regular visits by field personnel of the licensing agency to the local health or welfare office for exchange of information. Joint action may include:

Definition and approval of standards.

Assignment of responsibility for various aspects of the inspection and licensing program.

Development of an educational program for the participating agencies, their local opposite numbers, and for the operators of facilities.

Exchange of information relating to the licensed facilities.

Coordinated efforts, when necessary, for enforcement of the licensing law and regulations.

These activities may be based on law or they may grow out of contractual agreements. In some places, the policy of each agency specifies working with other agencies to meet the responsibilities assigned by law or custom to one or the other agency. Most commonly, however, these joint activities, as do so many others, rest on the authority of custom.

One of the successful statutory requirements for sharing responsibility in an institutional licensing program is found in Kansas. "Adult boarding homes," which include proprietary skilled nursing, personal care, and simple shelter facilities, are licensed by the State department of social welfare. The law calls for the participation of the State board of health and the State fire marshal as well as county health and welfare departments and the local fire and safety authorities. Child care facilities are licensed by the State board of health in conjunction with State and local agencies indicated above. In each area, teams jointly inspect the homes. Their visits are supplemented by calls by individual team members to help the home administrator.

In Sedgwick County, interdepartmental meetings have grown out of the licensing program. At these meetings, boarding home management and care of their residents, and child welfare and child care facilities are discussed.

Even in this apparently well-planned development, however, a recent study of the attitudes of Public Health nurses in the adult boarding home program reveals complaints of overlapping responsibilities, difficulties with representatives of other agencies, slights to professional prestige, and administrative failure to heed their professional judgments. Nevertheless, this joint program has improved and increased agency services to recipients of public assistance and has certainly increased the quantity of preventive health services made directly available to these recipients.[17, 18]

In California, a tripartite agreement on standards and licensure responsibilities is observed by the State departments of Public Health, social welfare, and mental hygiene in regard to sheltered care for older people. The agreement results from a policy of working together to define the tasks that arise from responsibilities assigned by law to one or another department; to outline the knowledge, technical skills, and contacts of each department which could help the assigned agency to meet its obligation; and to agree on the use of all of the appropriate resources. Actually, joint conferences in this State preceded the writing of the law, to assist the legislature in preparing the requisite legislation. Such conferences are a regular feature of interagency relations in the California State Government. Mutual support of legislative programs and budget requests, based on understanding and an appreciation of common interests, is a natural outgrowth of this policy.

Oregon also offers interesting examples of interdepartmental institutional services. The State board of health licenses nursing homes and periodically circulates a list of licensed homes to the State and local welfare departments, a service that is by no means common, however elementary. The field staff of the licensing division visits the county welfare offices to learn what the staff knows about care in local nursing homes. This productive relationship, although found in a number of States, is often overlooked even in States with well-developed relationships in other areas.

The criteria for rates of payment to nursing homes were developed by the Oregon Public Welfare Commission with board of health consultation to relate payments to services needed and received.

Day care centers for children, a responsibility of the Oregon Public Welfare Commission, must have standards certified by the board of health to be eligible for monthly State aid. Group care homes for mentally and physically handicapped youngsters, licensed by the board of health, must meet standards set in part by the public welfare commission.

In Maryland, an interdepartmental committee sets criteria for rates of payment by the welfare department for nursing home care. A similar joint committee, with representation from health, welfare, and education develops standards for the licensure of day care centers in Maryland.

In Massachusetts, day care facilities for children, licensed by local health departments, use standards developed by a joint committee of the State departments of public health, public welfare, mental health, and education. Consultants of these departments are available to the local areas on request through the district offices of the State department of public health.

Illinois provides another "example of the way in which the health and welfare departments can work together to improve the service provided." The State department of public health, the licensing agency, sends to the public assistance agency copies of all letters to individuals operating or planning to establish nursing homes. This enables the State public assistance agency to exchange information with county welfare departments concerning nursing homes which have been or are about to be licensed. Observations of the public assistance visitor and of physicians who treat public assistance clients are transmitted to the health department. The two State agencies have cooperated, when indicated, in revoking or refusing a license. This close cooperative arrangement has helped to improve the quality of care in the commercial and other nursing homes in the State.[19a]

Local departments of health usually have limited relationships with State institutional licensing programs whether they be administered by the State health, welfare, or other agency. The local department may serve as a source for a sanitarian. On the other hand, county welfare departments are often prime sources of information on nursing homes and similar facilities, even when the State licensing program is administered by the health department. Unfortunately, there is rarely a two-way flow of information to enable the local agencies to know what recommendations have been made to institutions, what disciplinary action is pending, or which facilities are currently approved.

New York provides a notable exception to this generalization. Here the State department of social welfare administers the "approval" program for nursing homes and in addition some county health departments license these institutions. To help maintain the positive direction of these parallel accrediting programs, a working agreement has been developed between the respective authorities.

The report of a recent APHA study of the chronic disease activities of selected local health departments states that 72 departments (of 187 selected for study) license institutions caring for persons with long-term illness or disability. Seventy-one said that they participated with other community agencies in establishing standards of care in these institutions. Few indicated a solitary role in standard-setting.

NUTRITION CONSULTATION

Nutrition consultation is a popular and useful institutional service which crosses departmental lines.[20] The APHA study reported that, of the departments selected, 70 offer such consultation to institutions caring for the chronically ill and disabled. Forty of these departments employ a professional nutritionist; the others presumably draw upon a State consultant or upon their Public Health nursing staff.

The Nassau County (New York) Health Department has a unique feature of teaching nutrition in a program directed generally at improvement of service in nursing homes. A local licensure provision assigns to the department responsibility for setting standards and licensing nursing homes. The consultant services of a nutritionist from the State department of Public Health are available to the local department and there has been some direct service to nursing homes from the State health department personnel. Medical consultation relating to diet is available within the county department. Results of the Nassau County program with respect to food practices, safety, and nursing care confirm the usefulness of this educational approach.[21]

The Illinois Department of Public Health also maintains a nutrition consultation service in its licensing program.[22] In Maryland and Wisconsin, nutrition consultation is offered not to institutions but to the welfare department staff concerned with standards and licensure for children's institutions.

PAYMENT FOR INSTITUTIONAL SERVICES

Although public agencies have a growing responsibility for payment for institutional services, no one of the agencies is likely to have a staff adequate to ascertain that the public monies are well spent for institutional care. In many States, each agency purchases such services separately, with resulting annoyances and inequities to the institutions, and duplication of effort. It is an unfortunately common practice to pay higher rates for the care of bed patients than for patients who get out of bed with or without aid. (We do not recommend decreases in such payments. Rather, in view of the generally low and unrealistic rates of payment to nursing homes, we would call for the eventual application of the principle of payments based on the costs of care.)

There are several examples of cooperative action relating to the rates of payment to hospitals and related facilities, such as the joint committees for nursing homes in Oregon and Maryland mentioned above. Rates paid by the New Hampshire Department of Public Welfare also are based on a classification of nursing homes by the State board of health.

In two States, interdepartmental committees representing the major purchasers of general hospital care have agreed upon methods of establishing hospital payment rates. In Illinois, such a committee has operated successfully for the past 11 years.[19b] There the State Department of Public Health, the public aid commission, the division of services for crippled children of the University of Illinois, and the

State division of vocational rehabilitation use the same Technical Advisory Committee on the Purchase of Hospital Care. Members are hospital administrators representing the Illinois Hospital Association who meet periodically with representatives of the four participating agencies to advise on a cost formula and payment agreements. The State Department of Public Health provides staff, collects and analyzes the cost reports, certifies the cost figures, and classifies the hospitals. Each agency then agrees to pay hospitals on the basis of the certified costs.

In New York State, a similar plan is coordinated by a Hospital Rate Advisory Committee with representatives from health, welfare, education, mental hygiene, and the executive departments. The bureau of research and statistics of the department of social welfare makes the necessary statistical computations and certifies rates to each agency.

Rates paid to hospitals in Massachusetts by the department of public welfare are based on a formula and procedures for cost analysis worked out by the department of health and the State hospital association. In Virginia, the State department of health reviews and certifies hospital cost analysis for the department of welfare and institutions and the division of vocational rehabilitation and advises on hospital administration and licensure.

Interdepartmental services related to institutions appear to demonstrate the only clear-cut and consistent collaborative use of the skills of State health and welfare departments. But their potential for improvement of institutional services to people has barely been tested. Nor have they been used sufficiently to bring the resources of the two agencies together to consider other areas of mutual concern.

CONSULTATION OUTSIDE INSTITUTIONS

Consultation services are by no means restricted to the institutional setting. In the APHA study already mentioned, 123 local health departments (of 187 respondents) said that they provide consultation to the local welfare department. And 125 departments indicated that they receive consultative services from the welfare department. Only 34 health departments of 187 with some kind of active chronic disease program employ their own social workers. But another 123 departments use social work services obtained through some other agencies.

Asked whether the health department had knowledge of the welfare department policy on food expenditures, four health departments said that the information was not available from the local welfare department. Forty-one of the 187 health departments did not have the information.

In Quincy, Mass., on the other hand, the health department nutritionist has been an active participant in public welfare programs, assisting in training caseworkers and consulting on special diets. She has visited with caseworkers at homes where large families with small budgets need advice on food selection.

The bureau of nutrition of the New York State Department of Health, in addition to providing consultation to the State department of social welfare, has helped to bring together local Public Health nurses and caseworkers for education on food budgeting and nutrition. State nutritionists have also served as consultants to local interagency conferences of Public Health nurses, caseworkers, and casework supervisors concerned with specific families and their diet.

GENERAL ADMINISTRATIVE SERVICES

The California rehabilitation project mentioned earlier[14] was designed not only to extend the use of rehabilitation services but also to demonstrate the advantages of regular medical consultation to the public welfare program, and to call the attention of local departments to one of the ways of obtaining consultant services. A contractual agreement between the State departments of public health and social welfare calls for the full-time assignment of a medical officer to the welfare department.

New York State also offers examples of effective sharing of professional personnel. A health department nutrition consultant prepared a special diet manual for the department of social welfare and is available for other services. A dental consultant is detailed from the health department to provide services on a part-time basis. And, in an instance that is still unique, a deputy commissioner of health has been assigned to the department of social welfare full time as director of medical care. He has ready access to the resources of both departments, attends staff meetings of both organizations, and acts as interpreter of the programs of both agencies. The background of Public Health administration has made itself manifest in the medical care program for the needy, notably in rehabilitation services, in nursing home care, and in physicians' services.

The State department of social welfare has vigorously supported requests of the health department for social work staff. It has helped to draw up standards for such staff and has invited health department medical social workers to participate in semiannual meetings of its own medical social workers. The medical social service chief has provided orientation sessions on the welfare program to the public health nurses of the Department of Public Health.

Many State agencies fail to provide staff orientation in programs of related agencies, not to mention their own. Everyone appears to agree on the need for such orientation and most ruefully admit there has not been time to carry out adequate orientation in their own program.

Among devices for achieving knowledge of programs of other agencies is the joint committee, such as the New York State Interdepartmental Health Resources Board with representatives from the departments of education, health, mental hygiene, correction, labor, and social welfare; the Workmen's Compensation Board; and the Joint Hospital Survey and Planning Commission. Committees of the board provide a machinery for joint planning, coordination, and consultation. Other interdepartmental bodies, not part of the State interdepartmental health council but with health and welfare participation, include advisory committees to the department of mental hygiene and to the State Youth Commission.

None of these bodies is simply a paper representation. All have been concerned with planning and consultation and with joint studies and legislation. The State plan for chronic disease and rehabilitation facilities was thus jointly developed, as was also the rehabilitation program for adult public assistance recipients at the rehabilitation hospital operated by the State health department.

Local services and activities affecting administration of both health and welfare departments have been mentioned above under program titles, such as the use of joint staff conferences concerning patients with tuberculosis, child care, or for the definition of rehabilitation objectives for a patient. Such conferences for the solution of clinical problems play an important part in administration per se. They are, in themselves, manifestations of administrative policy. Case conferences serve also to bring people and agencies together, to understand one another and to exchange ideas and information. Often, the conference results in the definition or clarification of broad policy.

A meeting of the Suffolk County (New York) Health and Welfare Department staffs showed how multiple demonstration case conferences in a workshop setting help achieve "more efficient interagency referral and communication systems"[23] and more direct contact among staff members. As a result, a joint committee was formed to interpret each agency's progress "and to develop further techniques for a better understanding of each agency's program," with consequent increase and improvement in referrals to both agencies.

Joint committees and active membership in community councils of social agencies are familiar methods of approaching common problems. They may be used also as the setting for joint planning. Joint committees on nutrition, aging, adoptions, mental health, rehabilitation, and nursing homes are among the usual ones. Council committees on housing, on determination of medical indigency, and on medical care for the needy are not uncommon in communities engaged in evaluation of health and welfare services.

In addition to their technical consultation services, health department representatives may serve on the advisory committees of the public welfare program and on the board itself to encourage a preventive approach in both health and welfare programs.

COMPARISON OF STATE AND
LOCAL RELATIONSHIPS

Relationships between State health and welfare departments, whether established by law, contract, or verbal agreement, are more likely to be in the administrative area than in the area of direct service.

In local departments, direct service produces the greatest evidence of joint effort although, for the most part, cooperation is personal rather than official. This relationship could be broadened and made more effective by formal State and local policy.

CONCLUSION

Five years ago, former Surgeon General Leonard Scheele,[3] speaking to the American Public Welfare Association, said:

At any gathering of health or welfare people, the need for a cooperative attack upon interrelated problems is likely to be discussed. Public Health people talked about it extensively at the recent American Public Health Association meetings in St. Louis There is an equal eagerness among social workers. Yet, after the meetings are over, a cold, analytical look at actual operations in local communities and throughout the Nation shows that the "trend" toward cooperation is painfully slow. From the standpoint of structure for cooperative action, these organizations seem to be almost as far apart as they were in the days when welfare meant an occasional coal or grocery order and when public health meant a red placard on the home of a scarlet fever patient.

Although our current report describes patterns of cooperation among our State health and welfare agencies, Dr. Scheele's statement still applies. It is our impression that we have yet to reach the following four goals of joint activity:

1. Application of the normal program of the health department to the welfare population through active cooperation with welfare departments.

It may be necessary to modify or extend services within the range of knowledge, skills, and budget of the health department in order to meet the health needs of the welfare population. Meeting these needs may, of course, result in establishing an effective program of disease prevention.

Since ill health and disability rank so high among the causes of dependency, there is a moral responsibility and, in many instances, a legal responsibility to make health services available to the population in need.

The role of the welfare department in achieving the full application of the program of the health department to the welfare population requires active encouragement of welfare clients to use health services, especially preventive services. Welfare agencies do not hesitate to offer advice on a family budget or the food content of the diet possible within that budget. The relationship between client and agency offers an equally good opportunity for advice on when and how to use health services.

2. The development of appropriate health promotion and disease prevention activities in the welfare program itself.

A major responsibility of the health officer and his staff is to aid the welfare staff in identifying and developing areas in the welfare program which can serve to promote, protect, and restore the health and social usefulness of the people who come to the department for help.

First and probably most important is intake. Intake offers the ideal opportunity to determine the health status and needs of the potential client. This is the chance, usually neglected, to make preventive health services available as well as to establish a medical plan for the person and family in need.

Once the welfare department has accepted the client for service, the avenues toward health services are many and the guide is usually the caseworker. The achievement of health by the client, therefore, depends in large part upon the caseworker's alertness to the client's health needs and the worker's knowledge of the community's health resources. The welfare department needs the help of the health department in providing the orientation and knowledge necessary to create a high level of health interest among its staff. In our experience, welfare departments rarely call upon their health colleagues for such help.

Surely it is important for the caseworker who enters the client's home to be alert to the health status of the entire household; to try to ascertain what hazards to health rise out of the physical environment of the home and out of the social dynamics of the life within it. The translation of this knowledge into constructive family action implies health education, for which trained personnel of the health department should be able to offer knowledge, skills, and materials, as well as assistance through staff development programs in the welfare department.

In each of the categories of public assistance administered through the local welfare agency, there are opportunities for health department participation in identification of needs, in planning, in consultation, in the provision or coordination of services. Identifying and planning to meet rehabilitation needs of parents of recipients of aid to dependent children, tuberculosis screening for recipients of old age assistance, and consultation on problems among recipients of aid to the permanently and totally disabled are examples of services now provided in a few places by State and local public health departments.

As to general medical care, every welfare agency has one or more opportunities to tell its clients about services available and to encourage their intelligent use. There should also be opportunities to define the objectives of the medical care program to the providers of service and to assure that the program can function so as to achieve its objectives.

A positive approach to medical care, as distinguished from preoccupation with disease treatment, will emphasize prevention, early diagnosis, prompt treatment, and active rehabilitation. Such an approach will encourage appropriate use of the physician's services rather than impress upon the client that "he must not seek the doctor's help unless he absolutely needs it." Health department representatives, serving among other members of a medical advisory committee, can help to develop and foster a positive approach to the medical care program.

In some instances, the health department's personnel and services may be all, or part, of the medical care program. Unfortunately, we have found that even when the health department is responsible for the general medical care program, a positive approach does not automatically ensue.

The current emphasis on extension of welfare department services beyond cash assistance implies a continuing increase in the health responsibilities of welfare agencies: services for unmarried mothers, for dependent and foster children, for the aged, and, in some communities, for families at large; and services directed at prevention of juvenile delinquency, control of alcoholism, or at the maintenance and improvement of standards of institutional care. In defining the objectives of these programs and in developing ways to attain their goals, welfare and health departments need to pool their knowledge. This is reason enough for getting together.

3. An increased awareness of the social and economic needs of persons coming to the attention of the health department and a clear

understanding of the responsibilities, the potential activities, and the limitations of both agencies in support of people with such needs.

The welfare department has a right to expect that the health department is prepared to make referrals appropriate in content and time. Conversely, the health department has the right to expect appropriate referral for the services it offers. But this right is not fulfilled automatically. Public Health nurses may have a hard time relinquishing part of their responsibility for patients, as caseworkers may for their clients. Successful referral progams provide administrative support and assurance through knowledge of personnel and operations, that the best interests of their patients or clients will be served by referral. Regular contact between the agencies concerned is needed to make this possible.

4. The development of the necessary policy and procedures to achieve improved health and welfare services without duplication when several agencies are involved.

Many functions of welfare departments touch those of the health department. And "touch" is often about as far as the relationship goes. This is true particularly when institutional inspection and licensure are assigned the welfare department and the health department is assigned responsibility for the sanitation inspection. This latter function rarely extends beyond the determination of technical compliance with the law and its regulations. The standards of nursing home care appear to have been markedly improved, however, in those States and counties where health and welfare department cooperation has been consciously organized. Crippled children's services, the tuberculosis control program, and rehabilitation services for adults likewise are improved where there are mutual responsibilities.

Examples of cooperative activities directed toward this goal range from organized referral procedures and a policy of using interagency case conferences to written contracts for the provision of specified services under stated conditions and to mutual study of long-range needs and support of legislation.

When these objectives of joint activity are reached, efficient operation will be assured, and the potential for better service, where responsibility overlaps, will be recognized. Each agency will be sensitive to the needs, and aware of the resources, lying outside of its own area of service.

To date, in the words of former Surgeon General Parran:[24] ". . . In the tremendous problem of providing [health services] for the indigent, the social welfare agencies have taken the lead, largely because health departments have been unwilling or unable to accept this as a direct responsibility. The situation, however, is somewhat analogous to the relation of the health officer to the public water supply. He must know the needs for an adequate supply of potable water. He champions the provision of such a supply. He sees to it that the water plant is properly operated, even though this may be done by another branch of the city government. This is the minimum responsibility which the health department should assume, both for the public water supply and for the public medical service needed by those unable otherwise to provide it. In fact, the health department should be instigator of and friend to all useful activities for the conservation of life and health. For if health officers do not recognize their responsibility, using all the methods given us by science, to organize community attacks upon the causes of ill health, the public health profession will revert to the ancient status of sanitary police, and other public medical agencies will be established to deal with the major health problems of today and tomorrow. We may be sure such problems will be dealt with."

1. Tax-supported medical care for the needy. *Am. J. Pub. Health,* 42: 1310–1327, October 1952.

2. Dearing, W. P.: Medical care for public assistance recipients. *Pub. Health Rep.* 66:89–97, Jan. 26, 1951.

3. Scheele, L. A.: Cooperation between health and welfare agencies: A health officer's view. *Pub. Health Rep.* 66:163–166, Feb. 9, 1951.

4. U.S. Department of Health, Education, and Welfare: *Annual Report, 1954.* Washington, D.C., U.S. Government Printing Office, 1955, p. 66.

5. Statement of understanding between North Carolina State Board of Public Welfare and the Crippled Children's Department of North Carolina State Board of Health, Sept. 9, 1947. Raleigh, N.C., 1947.

6. Christensen, A. W., Flook, E., and Druzina, G. B.: *Distribution of health services in the structure of State government, 1950. Part 3. Personal health services provided by State government.* Public Health Service Pub. No. 184, part 3. Washington, D.C., U.S. Government Printing Office, 1953, pp. 131–146; 159–171.

7. U.S. Public Health Service: *State tuberculosis control programs as planned for fiscal years 1954 & 1955.* Public Health Service Pub. No. 396. Washington, D.C., U.S. Government Printing Office, 1954.

8. American Public Welfare Association: The place of rehabilitation in the public welfare program—a statement of policy. Public Welfare 13: 47–84, April 1955.

9. Muller, J. N.: The rehabilitation program of the department of welfare, City of Chicago. *Public Welfare* 13:3–7, January 1955.

10. Lefson, L.: Rehabilitating public assistance recipients. *Public Welfare* 11:47–50, April 1953.

11. Lefson, L.: From public assistance to gainful employment. *Performance* 3:4–5ff., April 1953.

12. California State Department of Public Welfare: A medical study of incapacitated fathers receiving aid to needy children. Sacramento, March 1954. Processed.

13. California State Department of Education: Rehabilitation of disabled parents in the aid to needy children program. *Bull. California State Dept. of Education* 23, August 1954.

14. Freedman, D. K.: Medical consultation in the State department of social welfare. *California's Health* 12:113–115, Feb. 1, 1955.

15. Standards of care for older people in institutions. Sec. 2, pp. 77–112, New York, National Social Welfare Assembly, National Committee on Aging, 1953.

16. Mountin, J. W., and Flook, E.: *Guide to health organization in the United States.* Public Health Service Pub. No. 196. Washington,

D.C., U.S. Government Printing Office, 1952, p. 52.

17. Foote, R. E: The public health nurse in the adult boarding home program. A talk delivered to the public health nursing section, American Public Health Association, Nov. 15, 1955. Topeka, Kans., Kansas State Board of Health, 1955. Processed.

18. Tracy, L. E.: How public health nurses feel about the adult boarding home program. A report delivered to the public health nursing section, American Public Health Association, Nov. 15, 1955. Topeka, Kans., Kansas State Board of Health, 1955. Processed.

19. Bierman, P.: Role of the State public assistance agency in medical care. A series of reports. (a) VII. Nursing home care; (b) V. Hospital care. Chicago, American Public Welfare Association, 1955; 1954.

20. Nutrition services—a summary report of a study of public health nutritionist services to child care institutions and foster family homes. Children 2:236, November–December 1955.

21. Kinnaman, J. H., et al.: Attending the nutritional needs of patients in nursing homes—Theory and practice. Am. J. Pub. Health 45:627–631, May 1955.

Medical Care of Children in Public Programs*

LEONA BAUMGARTNER, M.D.

I WILL concentrate my discussion on two fundamental defects in our current work and planning for improving the health of children in the United States: (1) the lack of smooth-functioning and effective organization in the provision of services, and (2) the absence of a "we-will-do-something-about-it" concern for the quality of the care provided. Although similar problems exist in the provision of health services to people of all ages, their effects on child health are particularly dire, since the establishment in the early years of a good base for health is of particular importance.

The situation with regard to health services for children is uneven throughout the nation. There are many states where hardly any services are provided, or where services lag scandalously behind the levels reached in others. Even in the "advanced" areas like New York, where much money has been appropriated for many years

* Reprinted by permission from the October 1961 issue of the *American Journal of Public Health*, Vol. 51, pp. 1491–1499. Copyright by the American Public Health Association, Inc., 1790 Broadway, New York 19, N.Y. This paper was presented before a Joint Session of the Maternal and Child Health and Medical Care Sections of the American Public Health Association at the Eighty-Eighth Annual Meeting in San Francisco, California, on November 1, 1960. The author is Assistant Administrator, Agency for International Development (AID), U.S. Department of State, Washington, D.C., formerly Health Commissioner, New York City Department of Health, New York, N.Y.

(though never enough money or enough personnel to meet demands), we are not getting the most for the dollars we now spend because of fragmentation and lack of organization. In addition, chaos and confusion in the organization of services keeps us from obtaining the best quality of care and service that modern medical technology has made possible in the past 35 years.

FRAGMENTED CARE

American health services today are indeed "a many splintered thing." The person or family that needs medical care must often go from place to place, or from agency to agency and spend long hours sitting in shabby and uncomfortable waiting rooms. Most often the patient must do this at the very time he is ill, worried, under stress, and when his inner resources are taxed to the utmost. Preventive care is obtained from one source, therapeutic care from another; "well babies" are served in one place, sick youngsters in any one of several other agencies or institutions. For one of his ailments a handicapped child goes here, for another, there, while for some conditions there may not be any place from which to obtain what is needed for a particular child. This applies not only to tax-supported, but also to privately-supported agencies, to children in families receiving public assistance, as well as to children in self-supporting families.

Part of this complex lack of organization, this "jungle," arises from the way in which funds are provided. Both service and administrative costs are repeatedly duplicated. For example, federal funds for health services to children in New York trickle through the State Departments of Health, Mental Health, Education and Welfare, and in the city itself are distributed by the Department of Health, the Department of Hospitals, the Department of Welfare, the Comptroller's Office, the Mental Health Board, and a Vocational Rehabilitation Service of the state education authority; and this takes no account of funds coming via the armed forces, the Veterans Administration, or other special agencies. Each adds something to the administrative costs, and when summed up these administrative costs are no mere pittance. This chaos is not peculiar to one geographic area, or to one socioeconomic group, nor is it to be found only in the public sector of our health economy.

What does this chaos lead to? How does it affect the providers and the recipients of the services? As I see it, it leads to several undesirable results. First, it is a wasteful and inefficient way to use our health resources, and further depletes the already inadequate pool of professional talent available for health services. It raises the cost of care for everyone, and it makes medical care the prize of only the most persistent. When communication fails between different agencies caring for a single patient (and sometimes the patient's medical record does not even get from the outpatient clinic to the inhospital service when he is hospitalized), the results can only be unnecessary repetition of examinations and laboratory tests and the compiling of answers to questions already asked a dozen times. Such delays and failure to communicate can even have fatal results.

Too often the person or the family who needs care may not be getting that care, simply because he is lost in the red tape created by the very people who are trying to help. This is particularly tragic in the case of children, where the lack of proper care in the years of growth are almost certain to have lifelong effects.

Such lack of organization leads to confusion, hardship, and frustration for the patient and his family. Is it any wonder that families neglect the health of their members? Talk to some middleclass family with say, three children and an elderly, chronically ill relative and you will see the unproductive time they spend caring for their health needs, the time it takes away from their busy lives and jobs. The professionals keep wondering why these families become "uncooperative." Perhaps they just cannot face referral to another specialist! Even families that may be well able to pay for medical care are not able, nor should they be called upon to pay for waste.

PROBLEMS COMPOUNDED IN LOW-INCOME
AND PUBLIC ASSISTANCE FAMILIES

If this is true in middle-income families, consider the additional difficulties encountered by low-income families. Obviously the children in these families are at special risk with respect to adequate nutrition, physical and emotional illnesses and handicaps arising, in part, out of their overcrowded, unsanitary, and unstable living conditions. Possibly because of the special family circumstances which qualify them for public assistance—and this may be particularly true of the Aid to Dependent Children category—the children in these families sometimes are less likely than others in the community to receive continuing medical supervision through arrangements made by the adults in whose charge they are. And this can happen even where economic barriers to medical care are removed through the provision of free services.

There are those who deplore the state of affairs in which a family must depend upon public funds for its support. Are there also citizens who are equally indignant when the fragmentation of services makes it almost impossible for such a family to get the medical care which could put the family back on its feet? Needless delays in the detection of serious illness, in rehabilitating the chronically ill, in reaching a diagnosis and doing something about it, all add to the social burden of caring for the dependent family and rob the family itself of independence.

GAPS IN CARE

Lack of efficient organization invariably creates gaps which might otherwise not exist. For example, in New York City, until very recently, although we have a wealth of health resources, we lacked centers where the epileptic, cerebral-palsied and even the hard-of-hearing child could have all his needs met in one place. Without such coordinated, comprehensive service, rehabilitation for these children is often ineffective.

I shall focus a little longer on services in New York City where I am more familiar with medical affairs. New York City has been committed to meeting the health requirements of its needy children for almost half a century, many decades before any federal legislation was enacted. Today the gamut of services for children, who cannot pay for private medical services, is wide. We provide preventive programs, immunization against communicable diseases, diagnostic and treatment facilities, and along with this, counseling and education for the parents. Our school health program provides one million school children with minimum preventive and corrective health supervision, regardless of economic status. The conquest of communicable disease among the children of our city pays tribute to the extent of the commitment and its accomplishments. However, rather than being complacent, we are aware of the serious shortcomings which exist in the way in which the city's intent is presently carried out.

There are 180,000 children on public assistance in the city who receive all of their medical care through tax-supported services. There are many more thousands of children whose families pay some part of their own medical expenses. In fact, special studies show that for every family on public assistance, there are roughly four low-income families who cannot pay for all of their medical services out of their own earnings. This so-called "medically indigent" group depends upon publicly-supported services for a substantial part of its medical care. The degree to which local governments undertake to meet the need varies widely in different communities in the United States, but the picture of a mixed economy in medical affairs is characteristic of all areas.

For the children of public assistance families in New York City, funds are available for a physician to see a sick child in the home, for that child to go to a hospital clinic and to receive hospital care, home nursing care, free drugs, dental treatment, and rehabilitation services. In other words, in our city, programs of the Welfare, Hospitals, and Health Departments provide all the service any one child may need.

The fact that money and services are available, however, does not necessarily mean that the child obtains what he needs to keep him well, or that the service is an integrated, coordinated, or, for that matter, an adequate one.

If the lack of organization and fragmentation is such as to produce anarchy and to keep those who need services from using what is available, then we are not getting the most for the money spent.

EFFECTS OF SYSTEM

What are the effects of our present system? How well is our commitment to the city's children being carried out? This past summer we looked carefully at what was going on in one of our health districts where the city is engaged in a new venture called the Neighborhood Conservation Project. Here, through the cooperation of public and private agencies, the city is seeking to salvage neighborhoods, not only by physical rehabilitation of structures, but also by coordinated and stepped-up use of all the community services which may improve the physical environment and the social climate.

This gave an opportunity to get some picture of the utilization and availability of personal health services. In connection with a census of families in a "Pilot Block" area, we determined if the many services provided were getting to the people who needed them.

In the "Pilot Block" there were over 200 families. Three buildings alone contained 85 families. Two-thirds of these 85 families had children. Of these, 18 families were found to be on public assistance. The rest had a median income of $250 a month. There were 50 children in the study group of "welfare" families, and 45 in the "non-welfare" group. Half of each group of children are preschoolers. We decided to include this "comparison group" of nonwelfare families as a "baseline" (not necessarily an "ideal" or a "norm") to determine whether we were achieving some of the objectives of providing medical care in a public assistance program; in other words, to see whether this most disadvantaged group of children was using medical and preventive health services to no lesser extent than families of similar socioeconomic status. Furthermore, we wanted to confirm our impressions whether these services were organized and coordinated in such a way as to provide most efficiently the best quality of care, and what affirmative steps were being taken to prevent these children from growing up with medical handicaps which might contribute to future dependency.

What we found was that the public assistance group families availed themselves of child health station services providing "well baby care" to a greater extent than those not on welfare—66 per cent as compared with 44 per cent. Incidentally, in this low-income area, 75 per cent of all the children born on hospital ward service each year receive their pediatric care in child health stations operated by the Health Department.

Of the children three years of age and younger, all welfare children were under child health station medical supervision compared with only two-thirds of the nonwelfare children. The same situation exists in regard to the immunization status of both groups. During the children's most vulnerable years, it would seem that, in this neighborhood at least, we are adequately discharging our responsibility to the recipients of public assistance, although we are fully aware that this situation does not obtain equally throughout the city. In fact one of the developments of the Welfare-Medical Program in which our department is engaged, is a recent move to identify and bring to the attention of the child health stations all these welfare children under five throughout the city who are not currently under medical supervision.

In the case of school-age children—even though here, too, there are funds to pay for diagnosis and treatment—our findings were not so encouraging. In comparing the number of physical defects which were referred for treatment by school physicians, we found that welfare children showed both more referrable defects, and a higher proportion of defects not under treatment, than did nonwelfare children.

Coming to the adults, the neighborhood survey findings showed a tendency for pregnant women in welfare families to obtain prenatal care at a later stage than those from nonwelfare families, and in 25 per cent of the pregnancies among welfare mothers there was no record of seeking prenatal care at all. For both groups it was found that community resources such as visiting nurse, homemaker, or child guidance services had never been used. As for treatment services, every adult in the welfare group reported attendance at an outpatient clinic in the previous year compared with only 25 per cent of the nonwelfare group, the others expressing "no need" for such services.

This little study clearly revealed a glaring multiplicity, duplication, and fragmentation of the services. One of the study families on public welfare was a composite of this general problem. In the past six months, Mrs. M. and her three children had attended the outpatient clinics of three hospitals, had been treated at a tropical disease clinic in a health center, and had been visited by three different panel physicians at home, while a grandchild living in the home was under the supervision of the child health station, and also receiving treatment at a local municipal hospital.

It would appear, that although we are doing a reasonably good job in bringing to our children the benefits of modern medical knowledge through immunization drives, child health stations, and skillful medical treatment for gross physical defect when they come to us, the mesh in the case-finding net is not fine enough. And the lines of these many services often cross each other in such a way that the patient can be starved for good medical care in a land of technical plenty. This is true despite the unusually active cooperation between the Departments of Welfare and Health.

CONFIRMING EVIDENCE

When we drew upon some of the experiences of the district health officers of the Health Department who have been serving as medical consultants in welfare centers, these observations were confirmed. Case studies revealed, for example, a 14-year old boy with a congenital cardiac condition who appeared to be about half his age, remaining most of the time in a crouched position or carried up and down the stairs by his mother. He had never had medical treatment or home school instruction. The health officers found instances of children who were neglected to the point of requiring hospitalization for acute malnutrition; children of psychotic or tubercular mothers, or of a parent with diabetes, who had never been examined to see if they, too, had diabetes, tuberculosis, or were in need of medical care; a 15-year old pregnant girl receiving no prenatal care who was declared a "juvenile delinquent" through court action in order to be placed in a home for unwed mothers; a 30-year old disabled father of three children who had been seen by a score of doctors, nurses, and case workers in his visits to various health and welfare centers, none of whom had initiated inquiries, or made any provision to provide him with a prosthetic arm which might have helped him become a more independent wage earner and father.

I cite these examples (we call them our "atrocity" stories) only to indicate the extreme cases in which our built-in case-finding mechanism of direct contact with welfare recipients and the administrative responsibility for financial aid do not operate efficiently or even passably.

What do these illustrations mean? They confirm the conclusion stated in the beginning that despite the number of programs provided and despite the money appropriated—and we are relatively well off in New York City in the amount of money spent—health services are run in an inefficient, wasteful manner, and sufficient emphasis has not been put upon the quality of the care.

The present way of doing things violates innumerable principles of good organization and administration. It leads, and I am deliberately repeating, to reduplication of laboratory tests, physical examinations, and x-ray examinations. It takes up the time of doctors, nurses, social workers, and technicians. It is confusing and discouraging for the patient and his family. The patient himself in the meantime may be getting poor medical care, although the individual segments of it may not appear to be bad. It is easy to pick up in our records the patient who is attending a clinic for the treatment of his chronic sinusitis over a period of months, during which time his attack of rheumatic fever, his acquired tuberculosis, or developing diabetes may pass unnoticed. This is medical and social anarchy and chaos.

ORGANIZATION

It seems strange that America which has been so often characterized as having a genius for organization should have allowed its health services to grow up with such a conspicuous absence of organization.

With better organization we might even find the apparent deficiencies in dollars and health personnel not so large as they now seem. There are groups pushing for more financing and those calling for more talent. But few call for better organization. Changes in the organization, in the marketing, and distribution of health services are essential. We must find ways to bring together the people and the facilities, and to bring them together in the most efficient and effective manner. Certainly we do not produce automobiles or detergents, or put satellites in outer space, or build highways without using our genius for organization. Why not call on it to give people better health? This does not mean efficiency in terms of an impersonal factory; the job can be done and still maintain the intimate and personal relationship between doctor and patient, which is important to good medical care.

We have been more concerned, it would seem, with where the money comes from than what the money is spent for. It would almost seem as if more attention were paid to the right of the hospital or professional person to "sell his wares," or to the particular fiscal category into which the patient falls, than to the medical need of the patient himself. To some, "quality" of medical services merely means that payment shall be made to groups that meet the most minimum of licensing laws. Few voices have been raised to ask how the money is spent, what the money is buying, how to avoid the waste— human, professional, and monetary—involved.

The new amendments to the Social Security Act present an unusual opportunity for all welfare medical programs at least to initiate a series of new activties that may help to raise the standards and improve the quality of the medical care received by welfare clients. The new amendments empower the Secretary of Health, Education, and Welfare, and I quote: ". . . to assist the states to extend the scope and content and improve the quality of medical care and medical services for which payments are made to or on behalf of needy and low-income individuals . . . (to) develop and revise from time to time guides or recommended standards as to the level, content and quality of medical care and medical services for the use of the states in evaluating and improving their public assistance medical care programs. . . ."

It is to be hoped that the Secretary will make use of the past experience and skills found in all of the various divisions in his Department and of various private and professional groups in formulating these guides and standards. According to the legislation such guides are not binding on the States, but should be helpful in improving the quality of care that people will get if, and it is a large if, the States are creative enough to develop their own standards, make the decisions, and stick by them. This is a golden opportunity for those interested in improving the health of all Americans, and for those interested in saving tax dollars. The federal crippled children's programs have helped States operate programs which have raised standards of care everywhere, and so have shown that the job can be done.

The kind of care that in the long run is probably less expensive, and certainly gives the patient more, is the continuing and comprehensive care which brings the right service to the right person at the right time, and does not leave it to the patient to coordinate all the care for himself.

TRIALS AT COMPREHENSIVE CARE

In New York City we are experimenting with different ways of doing just that for the children and famlies who are the responsibility of the Welfare Department. Not only will these experiments have value to us; their findings may serve as models for other areas in the country. In one district, for example, a five-year program is under way in which 1,000 patients will receive comprehensive, continuous, and coordinated medical care through a teaching hospital and a medical school. The other welfare families will continue to receive care in the usual disjointed fashion. The project, financed by the Health Research Council of the local health department, will study utilization rates, costs, and the quality of the care, and compare these findings with the costs and quality of the present machinery.

In another district, we are trying still another way—that of pulling together existing community resources. The attending staff of a voluntary hospital will provide the preventive, diagnostic, and prenatal care in the district health center of the health department. Those indigent and medically indigent patients, who will be referred for more extensive care, will receive their care from the same physicians in the outpatient and inpatient services of the hospital, thus establishing a continuity of relationships. In addition, the hospital will expand its service to include a large nursing home in the same geographic area, where 80 per cent of the patients are welfare recipients.

Another helpful development has been the establishment of an Interdepartmental Health Council, composed of the heads of the municipal Departments of Health, Hospitals, Welfare, and Mental Health. Through its monthly meetings and the activities of its many committees composed of scores of departmental representatives, many conflicts are resolved, many problems solved.

Another significant development in this attempt at a more coordinated approach in health affairs for the indigent is the recent appointment of an extremely well qualified physician and Public Health administrator to a newly created job of director of medical care services in both the Departments of Health and Welfare. He can call freely upon the multiple assets of a health department with its medical specialists, while administratively the program remains in the Welfare Department.

Within a matter of months it has been possible with this system to have district health officers act as medical consultants to welfare centers, visiting nursing homes where welfare clients are being cared for, and setting up functioning referral systems to existing health department services for pregnant women, preschool children, and infants born on general ward service. This concern for the health of the welfare client is penetrating to all levels of welfare and health personnel, and has established, in most situations, a constructive working relationship between the representatives of the two departments. An extra dividend from having health officers serve the welfare centers is the different point of view developed by many case workers in the Welfare Department about health services, and vice versa. This has led to the spontaneous development of imaginative efforts, small projects to uncover and deal with special health problems of welfare clients. Without additional staff or funds, these efforts are leading to better medical care.

Several organizational steps have also improved the care welfare clients are getting. These include (1) the development of medical audit teams which visit outpatient clinics where welfare clients get so much of their care, (2) formation of an interdepartmental working committee on medical reporting to improve exchange of medical information on individual patients, so as to facilitate diagnosis and treatment and cut out waste, and (3) speeding up medical evaluation of disabled parents in ADC families. Steps to develop machinery for preventive diagnostic services for new welfare clients, so that incipient disease may be detected and dealth with promptly, and plans for better home care are next.

SUMMARY

I wish to emphasize again that although there remains a need to finance research and medical care, to recruit more staff, to train more health personnel—doctors, nurses, dentists, social workers —getting more money and personnel is not enough at this particular point in our national and local development. It seems only fair to point out that money by itself is certainly not as important now as it was two decades ago. We are socially and politically committed to the care of those who cannot care for themselves. We are fully aware that it is the low-income family with the large number of children, that has less insurance and less money to pay for care, and that has the greater need for it. But it is inconceivable that we can, or will be willing to, spend the dollars or find the people that it would take to provide the medical care adequate to meet the nation's needs or demands if we continue to conduct our health business (public and private) in the present unplanned, uncoordinated, haphazard manner, with little or no regard for the quality of the services which has evolved over the years. Our current inefficiency is not only a matter of concern to those involved with the welfare or needy client; it affects the pocketbook and life of every American.

To reorganize health services, research is needed in a new way to finance studies on how to improve the organization of these services. Whether for aged persons or for children, whether financed privately by the family through out-of-pocket or insurance funds, by employers, or by government or private philanthropy, it is imperative that new methods of organizing and delivering medical services be worked out and applied at once.

Whatever we may agree upon as desirable next steps, nothing will have more far-reaching, more immediately valuable consequences than improvements which will flow from imaginative administrative revamping of our public programs. These improvements are not dependent on new legislation or new funds. They can be more easily planned because governmental units already direct what can be done. Perhaps the simplest and most practical step is to call a moratorium on the interdepartmental differences and jockeying for power, the bickering among the operating agencies, notably the Departments of Health, Welfare, and Education and the vocational rehabilitation services. The job is a big one—we can not waste time or personnel in feuding. We can also demand that the Federal government, from which so much money now flows, get its house in order so that the source of funds does not add to administrative confusion and waste.

Stressing these two points—the need for a new look and drastic action in organizing health and medical service in this country, and the need for putting more emphasis on the quality of care, that our money, particularly our tax money, buys—does not mean that I am unconcerned about the need to finance medical care. I am fully aware that I am speaking from one of the 12 states in the nation which has a form—even if disorganized—of a comprehensive medical program for public assistance recipients. In many parts of the country, it is true, federal funds which are available for such aid have not been drawn upon because the states have never appropriated money to match them. I have one word of warning for those working in these areas, from the sometimes bitter and uphill experiences in trying to revamp services which mushroomed too quickly. As new money becomes available, as the expansion of services becomes possible, as fought-for goals are achieved, we must take the additional time to set up desirable standards, to think through the most effective and coordinated way of doing the job, so that when it is done, it is done right. This is a job that can be done—this job of reorganizing our health services. Let us get on with it.

PART FOUR

The Sciences and Disciplines of Public Health

1. Preventive Medicine   428

2. Epidemiology and Biostatistics   431

3. Public Health Social Work   451

4. Public Health Nursing   466

5. Public Health Nutrition   474

6. Public Health Dentistry   482

7. Health Education   491

8. Occupational Health   508

9. Space Medicine   515

10. Radiologic Health   522

11. Genetics and Public Health   531

12. Public Health Laboratories   542

13. Public Health Psychiatry   548

14. The Behavioral Sciences in Public Health   567

15. Administration   583

"PUBLIC health has to do with persons of every rank, of both sexes, of every age. It takes cognizance of the places and houses in which they live; it follows the child to school, the laborer and artisan into the field, the mine, the factory, the workshop; the sick man into the hospital; the pauper into the work house; the lunatic to the asylum; the thief to the prison. It is with the sailor in his ship, the soldier in his barrack; and it accompanies the emigrant to his new home beyond the seas. To all of these it makes application of a knowledge remarkable for its amount, and the great variety of sources whence it is derived. To physiology and medicine it is indebted for what it knows of health and disease; it levies large contributions on chemistry, geology, and meteorology; it cooperates with the architect and engineer; its work commends itself to the moralist and divine."

From Public Health, a series of lectures by DR. WILLIAM A. GUY. *London, 1874*

An organism or a social institution grows through increasing specialization and differentiation of the functions of its component parts in interaction with its environment. So it is with Public Health. Its functions have become more numerous, complex, and varied in response to massive social changes, to scientific advances, and to its internal development. As new knowledge is gained from the laboratory or field, new applications of knowledge appear; when tested, they may require new kinds of specialists. The sweep of Public Health concerns and programs, its "target populations," as we have seen, are in steady change and flux, reflecting the play of social forces and of scientific progress.

As a concomitant, there has been a steady enlargement of the scope and number of the scientific fields and professional disciplines integral to Public Health. Physicians, sanitarians, and nurses are some of the older members of the Public Health team; biostatisticians, social workers, behavioral scientists, and psychiatrists are some of the newer.

In the articles presented here the chief features and attributes of the sciences and professional disciplines in Public Health research and practice are delineated. The order of these presentations is an arbitrary one, and implies no priority or hierarchy of importance.

ON GENERAL IMPRESSIONS AND STATISTICS

"GENERAL impressions are never to be trusted. Unfortunately, when they are of long standing they become fixed rules of life and assume a prescriptive right not to be questioned. Consequently, those who are not accustomed to original inquiry entertain a hatred and a horror of statistics. They cannot endure the idea of submitting their sacred impressions to cold-blooded verification. But it is the triumph of scientific men to rise superior to such superstitions, to desire tests by which the value of beliefs may be ascertained, and to feel sufficiently masters of themselves to discard contemptuously whatever may be found untrue."

> FRANCIS GALTON, *quoted by Jan Book in* Field Studies in the Mental Disorders, *published by Grune and Stratton, 1959, p. 400. Original source unidentified.*

1. Preventive Medicine

Preventive Medicine*

JEAN SPENCER FELTON, M.D.

PREVENTIVE MEDICINE is a broad group of activities directed toward the prevention of disease and the promotion of human health and well-being. It is not synonymous with Public Health, a branch of medicine concerned with safeguarding community health through a specific program directed by a health officer and a staff of specialists. It is more than a specialty; it is a way of practicing medicine with the long-term view of the patient's welfare the foremost consideration. The family physician, because of his knowledge of preventive techniques, plays a primary role in the practice of preventive medicine, but his effectiveness depends upon his being able to induce the patient to share responsibility for the maintenance of personal health.

HISTORY. Although interest in the prevention of disease dates back to the restrictive dietary codes of biblical peoples, the scientific aspects of preventive medicine did not develop until after mid-nineteenth century. With the establishment of the relationship between microorganisms and illness came the understanding of the infectious nature of many diseases. Late in the nineteenth century the control of communicable disease became a paramount concern. The discovery of the role of mosquitoes, flies, and ticks in the spread of disease made possible the elimination of great epidemics of yellow fever, cholera, typhus, plague, malaria, and typhoid fever. Comprehension of tularemia, Rocky Mountain spotted fever, and of viral- and fungus-caused conditions also was facilitated by extensive research, and work in serology led to the development of protective vaccines. Thus, a battery of immunizing injections became every child's introduction to contemporary preventive medicine in the United States.

The control of tuberculosis, as well as dental, mental, and social hygiene, was the major concern of various voluntary health agencies that arose just before and shortly after the beginning of the twentieth century. Later organizations were interested in the prevention and treatment of heart disease, arthritis, poliomyelitis, muscular dystrophy,

* Reprinted from *The American Peoples Encyclopedia*, © 1963, by special permission of Grolier Incorporated, Vol. 15, pp. 942–944. The author is Professor of Occupational Health, Schools of Medicine and Public Health, University of California, Los Angeles.

and hemophilia; and foundations created from sources of great wealth brought disease prevention to a worldwide level. Later, government health agencies through health education, Public Health nursing, well-child clinics, prenatal counseling, and industrial hygiene began making the individual more responsible for his own preventive medical care by giving him the necessary knowledge and guidance. Also, schools of medicine, in addition to teaching diagnostics and treatment, began to provide their students with a background of preventive medicine.

Areas of emphasis changed with medical advances. For example, interest in the prevention of the early onset of the degenerative diseases replaced in part the great attention formerly given environmental sanitation and communicable disease control. Alcoholism and other addictions, mental health, occupational health, home and highway accidents, air pollution, and cancer also became basic areas of concern to workers in preventive medicine.

Environmental sanitation, primarily the province of sanitary engineers, sanitarians, food chemists, and laboratory technologists, calls for constant monitoring of the water supply, swimming pools, methods and agencies of waste disposal, food preparation, ventilation, and housing facilities. Health education programs taught individual citizens the standards to expect in restaurants and markets, and what measures to use in their own homes with regard to food handling, refrigeration, sanitation, and environmental hygiene.

Communicable disease control is ordinarily a community responsibility, and continuing health education measures made the average person appreciate the need for vaccination, for the limited isolation of patients, the examination and immunization of contacts, the elimination of mosquitoes and ticks, the ridding of residences of rodents, and the importance of the early reporting of symptoms so complications could be averted. Established preventive inoculations in time became available against cholera, diphtheria, influenza, poliomyelitis, Rocky Mountain spotted fever, smallpox, tetanus, typhoid and paratyphoid fevers, typhus, whooping cough, and yellow fever.

It is in the area of child health that preventive measures were most energetically promoted. Emphasis on prenatal care reduced infant mortality and fostered early detection and correction of congenital abnormalities. Education of the mother in child care resulted in her seeking for her child preventive medical measures such as immunizations, early vision and hearing reviews, dental examinations, and psychologic testing. The prevention of accidents in childhood claimed the interest of insurance companies, safety engineers, poison centers, pediatricians, and health agencies; and much was done to instruct parents in the application of basic precautions that protect their children from physical impairment or loss of life.

The greatest growth of preventive medicine was in the area of chronic degenerative diseases. Studies of many different population groups yielded information relating to the cause and aggravation of degenerative conditions—information which could be profitably applied in the early years of adulthood. An impressive body of knowledge was developed regarding predisposing factors in heart disease, the emotional patterns which set the stage for alcoholism or obesity, the stresses which cause recurrence of acute arthritis, the physical states most likely to lead to diabetes (when a family tendency exists), the occupational groups in which cancer shows higher rates in general (or in which a selectivity for a special organ system is shown), and the external and internal elements most likely to cause allergic responses. This knowledge was put to use to defer the onset of heart or blood vessel disease.

Preventive medicine in the area of mental health entered the lives of people at all stages: as pre-school children, as pupils at the elementary or secondary school level, as college students, and as wage earners. Counseling and psychologic or psychiatric guidance received greater recognition, with the result that assistance by professionally trained persons was sought earlier than once had been the case.

Occupational health is an aspect of preventive medicine which received great attention. Medical teams in industry prevented illness among employees by means of frequent physical examinations and laboratory and X-ray examinations for early signs of tissue changes. Referrals were made to the workers' physicians for the institution of proper corrective care. Health education, control of potential occupational health hazards, and counseling and referral for emotional disturbances were also functions of those medical teams. This was prevention exercised in large groups, but the individual worker was instructed in mental hygiene and in the course for him to follow in order to maintain the peak in physical status for his years.

In addition to the areas of preventive medicine already enumerated there are programs in nutrition, medical social work, home nursing, school and college, health, and in space medicine—where prevention is the specialty in its entirety.

Practitioners who carry out the practice of preventive medicine are all those who are concerned with the elimination of disease and in the restoration and maintenance of well-being. The list of practitioners, then, includes the physician, the nurse, the sanitary engineer, the sanitarian, the health educator, the industrial hygienist, the biostatistician, the medical sociologist, the clinical psychologist, the social case worker, the rehabilitation worker, and most importantly—all responsible members of society.

2. Epidemiology and Biostatistics

Historical Epidemiology and Grid Analysis of Epidemiologic Data*

REIMERT T. RAVENHOLT, M.D.

MANY PERSONS think of death records as something inherently dull and uninteresting; but it was impressive to see the deep, active, and lasting interest in death records developed by the medical students who participated in this study.

There is a wonderful history contained in old death records; a mute eloquence of earlier days: of stormswept Puget Sound and falling Douglas Fir; of avalanche and cave-in; of the rush for gold in Alaska and the accompanying misery of diphtheria, meningitis, syphillis, and murder. The records bear witness that people die in many, many ways: of "execution by irate citizens"; of "lockjaw from a firecracker"; of "natural decay"; or by "lighting fuse of dynamite placed on head." The dead measured the quality of the water and milk, and tested each new means of transportation. As they recorded changing ways of dying they documented our changing ways of living. Few historical incidents escaped their mark.

* Quoted with omissions from the May, 1962, issue of the *American Journal of Public Health*, Volume 52, pp. 776–790, copyright by the American Public Health Association Inc., 1790 Broadway, New York 19, New York. The paper in its entirety was presented before the Association's Symposium (Chart I of the American Public Health Association at the 89th Anniversary Meeting in Detroit, Michigan, November 13, 1961). The author is Epidemiologic Consultant, Europe, Division of Foreign Quarantine, United States Public Health Service at the American Embassy, Paris, France. He was formerly Director of the Division of Epidemiology and Communicable Disease Control, Seattle, King County; Seattle, Washington.

Potentialities and Limitations of Epidemiology*

JOHN M. CASSEL, M.B.B.CH.

TO GAIN SOME understanding of the contributions that may legitimately be expected from epidemiology, it is first necessary to define what is meant by epidemiology and briefly trace the development of this scientific discipline.

To a newcomer the term "epidemiology" would seem most logically to be concerned with the study of epidemics, and epidemics are usually thought of as outbreaks of infectious diseases. Consequently, epidemiology is frequently considered as a science restricted to the study of outbreaks of infectious diseases. Historically this would have been an adequate formulation since, at the time of the development of this discipline, infectious disease epidemics were the most important and terrifying of the health problems afflicting mankind. These diseases therefore commanded practically all the attention and interest of all the health disciplines, including epidemiology. Today, however, as I hope to indicate, this would be inadequate as a definition.

HIPPOCRATES AND THE FOUR HUMORS

The origin of the science of epidemiology can be traced to the Hippocratic era in the Golden Age of Greece. Hippocrates was one of the first physicians to recognize that disease outbreaks were not happenstance occurrences, attacking unfortunate individuals at random. Different populations were subject to different types of diseases, and these occurred at different seasons. Furthermore, within any population were various subgroups with different degrees of susceptibility to these diseases. For example, some diseases attacked children primarily, others adults; some were most prevalent among the poor or among those who lived in a certain sector of the city.

From these beginnings two cardinal principles evolved which characterize and are central to the science of epidemiology. These are, first, that the unit of study of epidemiology is the group rather than the individual. By this we mean that the epidemiologic method is not the most appropriate technic for discovering why any particular person became ill when he did. More appropriately, epidemiology answers why people with a certain set of characteristics are more or less likely to become ill than other people without these characteristics. The sec-

* Reprinted, by permission, from *Public Health Concepts in Social Work Education*—Proceedings of Seminar held at Princeton University, Princeton, New Jersey, March 4–9, 1962. Published by the Council on Social Work Education in cooperation with the Public Health Service, Department of Health, Education, and Welfare, pp. 69–85. The author is Professor of Epidemiology, The School of Public Health, The University of North Carolina, Chapel Hill, North Carolina.

ond point central to epidemiology is that its major contribution has been in identifying those reasons for illness in aspects of the environment or way of life of the group under study.

As mentioned previously, the diseases of most concern to the Hippocratic physicians, and indeed to physicians for the next 25 centuries, were the infectious diseases. Furthermore, in this same period the aspect of the way of life of people of most concern to epidemiology was the relation of men to their physical environment. Thus, for example, in Hippocratic times the occurrence of disease was explained by the strength and direction of prevailing winds, the amount of rainfall and sunlight, the height above sea level, or the nature of the soil.

It is most important to recognize further that the particular aspects of the physical environment that were selected as explanations of disease were determined by existing theories concerning the causation of disease. This relationship between variables selected for study and prevailing theories of disease causation is equally true today and must be fully understood to appreciate the potential contribution of modern epidemiology. In Hippocratic times disease was thought to be caused by a disturbance in the balance of the four humors—blood, phlegm, black bile, and yellow bile—in the body. The proportions of these humors was in turn determined by the distribution of various attributes of living matter. These were categorized as wet or dry, hot or cold. The amounts of wetness or dryness, heat or cold were themselves determined by the proportions of what were considered to be the four elements making up the environment: earth, water, fire, and air. Thus, according to these concepts, the explanation for the occurrence of disease should be sought in those aspects of the environment which might influence the exposure of people to these four elements. It was therefore perfectly logical, given this theoretic framework, to search for an explanation for disease in the strength of winds or the amount of humidity.

MEDIEVAL MIASMAS

This concept of disease remained almost unchanged for more than a thousand years. The next major theory about the cause of disease occurred in the Middle Ages when the idea of miasmas was introduced. Miasmas were foul odors, or gases. According to this new theory, it was thought that many diseases, in addition to being produced by exposure to different proportions of the elements as defined by Hippocrates, could be caused by exposure to these miasmas. Many of our modern terms for disease derive from this theory. For example, the word malaria comes fom "mal" (bad) and "aria" (air); originally it was thought that malaria, or the fever of malaria, was caused by exposure to foul air or gases. As the idea of miasmas as a cause of disease became more accepted, the variables in the physical environment used to explain the occurrence of disease changed. Thus, many diseases were thought to be due to living in low marshy places or in areas of the city where excreta was thrown indiscriminately into the street. As you might expect, many people living in those circumstances did have high disease rates, but the reasons for the occurrence of such diseases given by the physicians of that day would be very different from those given today. Thus, once again the variables invoked as causes of disease were determined by existing theories.

PASTEUR, KOCH, AND THE GERM

The next major advance in our ideas about causation occurred with the discovery of microorganisms at the turn of the last century. The classical findings of Pasteur and Koch ushered in a new and important era in medicine which led to far-reaching results. On the one hand these discoveries led to tremendous improvements in our ability to treat many diseases and to a marked change in the factors in the environment studied to explain disease. Under the influence of the new microorganismal theory epidemiologic inquiries were now directed toward those aspects of the environment which might be envisioned as breeding places for bacteria. Thus, attention was (and still is) focused on exposure to contaminated water or food or polluted air.

Simultaneously, however, these discoveries tended to blind medical thought to other ideas about causation of disease. The new findings were so exciting that for many decades it was thought that knowledge about these microorganisms and how man came into contact with them was all that was needed to understand the cause of disease. This view is still widely prevalent in medical thinking, but gradually the realization has developed that the presence of a microorganism is at best only a partial cause, and sometimes not even the most important cause of a disease, even an infectious disease. This point of view can perhaps be best illustrated by some examples.

About the turn of the century the specific microorganism responsible for cholera was identified and it was found that people who had this disease excreted large amounts of the cholera bacillus in their stools. Despite this it has never been possible to produce cholera in human volunteers by feeding them cholera bacilli no matter how large a dose is given. At most a transient diarrhea occurs, but usually there are no symptoms at all. Apparently other factors besides the cholera bacillus have to be present before cholera can be produced, and these are sometimes more important for our understanding of the disease than is the bacillus. In fact, even with our extensive knowledge of the cholera bacillus today we cannot explain why cholera becomes transformed periodically from a minor pestilence in some oriental bazaar to a raging epidemic, and it is unlikely that further study of the bacillus alone will provide us with the answers.

As a second example we might think about tuberculosis. The cause of tuberculosis is said to be the tubercle bacillus. In a certain sense that is a useful formulation, but in another sense it is not useful. It is rather like saying, "The cause of automobile accidents is the automobile." This is undoubtedly true, but the automobile does more than cause automobile accidents, and accidents can be caused by more than the automobile. Intensive study of the tubercle bacillus does not tell us why it is that of a hundred people exposed to the bacillus in the United States only about three develop tuberculosis. Why do not the other 97 develop the disease? How do they differ, these 97, from the three who do get it? Why is it that in other countries of a hundred people exposed to the tubercle bacillus 10 or 20 or 30 will get tuberculosis? Why is it that in more and more people who are developing tuberculosis today we cannot find the tubercle bacillus? We find some other bacillus which we call "atypical" tubercle bacilli, but the disease seems to be the same. Thus, to consider the tubercle bacillus as "the cause" of tuberculosis is useful up to a point, but beyond that point it is not useful.

LIMITATIONS OF THE GERM THEORY

To understand the limitations of the microbiologic model of the cause of disease it is necessary to realize that the science of bacteriology, and from it most of the science of medicine, has developed in a peculiar fashion outside the mainstream of development of other sciences. Specifically this is the only science which classifies the object of study, bacteria, as good or bad. No physicist classifies his atoms as good or bad, nor do chemists classify their elements as good or bad. But we physicians classify bacteria as "good" (that is, bacteria that do no harm or are beneficial) or "bad" (that is, pathogenic).

One of the most eminent microbiologists in this country, Rene DuBos of the Rockefeller Institute, has advanced a rather ingenious theory to explain why this is so. He suggests that in nature man occupies the pinnacle of the pecking order; that is, he can eat anything on this earth and not be eaten by any other animal. In this he is different from all other animals who can eat some and be eaten by others. The one living species over which we have no control, however, are the microorganisms. In DuBos' view this lack of control has been responsible for microbiology's developing this pattern of classifying bacteria as good or bad.

Whether this explanation is adequate or not, it becomes necessary to consider the question of what makes a microbe good or bad. The particular bacillus that sours the French peasant's milk and makes delicious cheese is a good bacillus without which he could not make his cheese. That same bacillus sours your milk here in the refrigerator and therefore is a bad bacillus, an evidence of unsanitary habits. A hundred years ago tulip growers concentrated on a mottled red and white variety of tulip that was the most prized type. This mottling occurred when a particular virus lived in association with the tulip. A number of years later mottled tulips were no longer the fashion and people demanded solid colors—reds, whites, yellows, and so on. Suddenly then this virus which had been eagerly sought after became a "bad" virus, and tulips were sprayed to get rid of it. The virus had not changed, but our ideas of what was good or bad had changed.

Or consider the virus which "causes" poliomyelitis. A hundred years ago it was neither good nor bad. Although people were exposed to the virus, poliomyelitis occurred infrequently and paralysis was rare indeed. In the course of a hundred years the virus so far as we know has not changed, but polio has become a major crippling disease of young adults and children. We have changed, not the virus. The same may be said of infectious hepatitis. Man has probably been exposed to the virus for many centuries, but only in the last 10 to 15 years have we started seeing major epidemics of this disease. We will not be able to explain these phenomena by studying only the virus concerned.

The development of the germ theory of disease had a further unfortunate consequence for epidemiology. Believing that the answers to the causation of disease had been found, epidemiologic investigators restricted their studies. Before this, epidemiology had sought to identify those factors in the way of life of people which increased their risk of developing disease. After the discovery of bacteria most studies sought only to identify the means and vehicle of infection in a specific outbreak in an attempt to control that outbreak. Epidemiology thus changed from a research or investigative science to an applied technology. As such, it performed some useful functions and doubtlessly was responsible for saving many lives, but it ceased, for a number of decades at least, to add to our knowledge of the factors responsible for disease. Unfortunately it is this infectious disease "epidemic fighting" function of epidemiology that has become the prevailing concept of the discipline. In my opinion, this is one of the least important of its potential contributions.

Over the last 20 to 30 years there has been a resurgence of interest in the contributions that epidemiology, as an investigative science, can make to an understanding of the disease process. Through such an understanding it is hoped that rational leads for intervention can be developed.

This reawakening of interest has occurred simultaneously with a growing realization of the limited utility of the rigid microorganismal model of disease causation. In addition to the factors mentioned previously that tend to cast some doubts on the usefulness of this model, two further developments in the field of health have occurred which make a more sophisticated theory imperative. The first has been the dramatic increase in the noninfectious chronic diseases as major causes of death and disability in modern industrialized society. This change in the nature of our major health problems has occurred over the last 40 to 50 years. During this period diseases which for thousands of years have been cripplers and killers of mankind have decreased to their lowest point in human history, and have been replaced by new diseases. Coronary heart disease, lung cancer, diabetes, arthritis, and mental disorders may have occurred before, but never to the extent that we are seeing them today. The microorganismal model of causation gives us little help in suggesting the factors we must search for to explain these modern "plagues."

The second development is that it is becoming increasingly clear that we cannot explain the occurrence of disease solely in terms of man's relationship to his *physical* environment. An important factor is his relationship to other people; that is, to his *human* environment. Here also the theory which postulates that exposure to a microorganism is the cause of disease is of little use in determining what social or cultural factors—that is, *human* environmental factors—need to be studied to understand disease occurrence.

THEORY OF MULTIPLE CAUSES

How then does this microorganismal theory need to be modified to make it more useful for our purposes; that is, for the prevention and treatment of disease? First, it is necessary to recognize that inherent in the microorganismal theory of disease is the idea that there is a *single* cause—a microorganism or some other agent—for each disease, that each disease has its cause and each cause has its disease. This concept of a single cause we no longer find at all useful in any disease.

The lack of utility of any single-cause theory can easily be illustrated with such a disease as cancer of the breast. This is a useful disease to study in terms of "cause," because we can produce it easily in certain experimental animals—mice. Breast cancer occurs infrequently in mice under normal circumstances, but by selective breeding a strain can be bred in which 60 to 70 per cent, sometimes as high as 80 per cent, of the offspring will develop breast cancer. Thus it is possible to postulate a genetic factor, something passed down through the genes as a "cause" of breast cancer.

It has also been found that if these genetically susceptible mice are taken from their mother's breast at birth and allowed to suckle from a mother who is from a nonsusceptible strain, they will not develop breast cancer. The explanation is that the susceptible mothers excrete a virus in their milk which has to be present for breast cancer to develop in their offspring. So a virus is implicated in the cause of breast cancer.

However, baby mice born of nonsusceptible mothers and allowed to suckle from susceptible mothers (that is, fed milk containing this virus) do *not* develop breast cancer. Furthermore, not all mice born of susceptible mothers and suckled by these mothers from birth develop breast cancer. This develops only in female offspring, not in males. If estrogen, the female sex hormone, is injected into these male offspring shortly after birth, however, they too will develop breast cancer. Thus a third factor, a hormone, may also be thought of as a "cause" of breast cancer. Finally, mice in which all three factors are present— that is female mice bred and suckled by genetically susceptible mothers and then placed on a restricted caloric intake—rarely develop breast cancer.

Now in terms of a single-cause theory, what is "the cause" of breast cancer in mice? Genetic transmission? A virus? A particular hormone? Diet? Obviously no single factor is the cause; all four factors have to be present for breast cancer to develop. Any attempt to say *the* cause of breast cancer in mice is genetic or viral is not particularly useful.

Thus we have to change our thinking from a single-causal theory to a multicausal theory. Many factors can cause any particular disease, and what may be causal under certain circumstances may not be causal under others.

QUESTIONS OF HOW AND WHY

Even the acceptance of a multicausal theory, however, is not sufficient for our purposes in trying to understand the causes of any disease. We have to pose the further question: why do we want to understand causes? Are we concerned with the causes for the onset of the disease or with the causes for recovery? These factors, those causing onset and those causing recovery may be, and frequently are, different.

An elementary illustration may make this clear. We have many theories about the causes of coronary heart disease: the amount of fat in the diet, the amount of exercise taken, the number of cigarettes smoked, the level of blood pressure, genetic factors, and so on. Whatever the particular causes, let us consider two men each of whom has a heart attack as a result of the same causes and let us assume that each suffers the same amount of damage to his heart. Despite these similarities, we know from clinical experience that one of these men may be an invalid the rest of his life and the other may be like former President Eisenhower, completely capable of undertaking the strenuous task of directing a country. Although identical conditions may have led to the onset of their disease, different conditions determine their recovery.

One further aspect of "cause" must be taken into consideration for a fuller understanding of the disease process. For both types of causes, those responsible for onset and those responsible for recovery, we should be concerned with questions of "how" and "why." *How* does a person develop diabetes? "Some disturbance in insulin metabolism" would be the answer. *Why* does a person develop diabetes? Our knowledge of the relationship between disturbed insulin metabolism and the disease we call diabetes does not tell us *why* this patient at this point developed this disorder. If, however, in addition to knowing about the relationship of insulin metabolism to diabetes, we knew that immigrants develop the diabetes rates of their new country to the same extent that they absorb its customs, and if we knew what these customs were, we would be getting some clues that could help us answer these "why" questions. These customs might bring changes in diet and exercise and in the amount and types of emotional strain. These causal factors would tell us something about why or under what circumstances people develop diabetes and thus increase our knowledge about what needs to be changed to prevent new cases from occurring. In the identification of this category of causes epidemiology makes, in my opinion, its major contribution.

MODERN EPIDEMIOLOGY

Perhaps the relevance and importance of these points can be made more clear by an illustration. To do this I would like to present data from a modern epidemiologic study of a disease traditionally explained on the basis of one cause. It will become evident how much more can be learned about this disease if the questions are posed and the results interpreted within this broader theoretic framework.

The disease is tuberculosis and the "cause," using the traditional model of causation, would be the tubercle bacillus. Knowledge of the role of the tubercle bacillus has been helpful in telling us something about how people get sick—they get sick because of the tubercle bacillus—but it tells little about how they recover and nothing at all about why they get sick. As indicated above, the vast majority of people exposed to the tubercle bacillus do not develop tuberculosis. To determine why some do, it is helpful to know how people who do get tuberculosis differ from those who do not.

One relatively recent study in Seattle[2] gives some clues. This study started by dividing the city into four economic areas. Area 1 was the poorest, with the worst housing and the most overcrowding. Area 2 was a little better but also poor and overcrowded. Area 3 was about average for Seattle. Area 4 was the richest part of the city. The investigators examined the distribution of tuberculosis by area. As might be expected, the rates were highest in Area 1, lowest in Area 4, for both males and females. Examining the distribution by race, they found the same relationship for whites—but for nonwhites the pattern was almost reversed. The highest rates for nonwhites, both male and female, occurred in the richest area. The nonwhites in this area were not domestic servants but professional people—doctors, lawyers, business executives, and so on. The lowest rate for nonwhites occurred in Area 2, which in addition to being one of the poorer areas was that part of the city in which nonwhites lived in compact neighborhood groups and had many opportunities for interpersonal contact and friendships. The highest rates for nonwhites thus occurred in the area where they were a distinct minority without opportunity for warm personal contacts with other people. Conversely, for whites the rates were highest in those areas in which there were high proportions of nonwhite neighborhoods and where the whites had little opportunity for social interaction.

The next characteristic examined was residential and job mobility. Unlike the nontuberculous, those who developed tuberculosis had been highly mobile. They had moved from home to home about five times more frequently than does the average person in the United States, and they had changed jobs frequently. The third characteristic was marital status. Fewer of the tuberculous had been married and far more had been divorced or widowed than is true for the population as a whole. Finally, the fourth distinguishing characteristic was that a large proportion of the tuberculous lived alone in one room.

To summarize: At this point in time we find that the tuberculous are strangers in the neighborhood where they live; they often move and change jobs; if they marry, their marriages are frequently boken by death or divorce; and they live alone. People with these characteristics have been referred to by sociologists as "marginal men." They do not belong, they have few friends, few neighbors that they know well, no kin, and little contact with fellow human beings.

To determine whether the findings of this Seattle study had been observed elsewhere, I attempted to review as much of the recent literature as possible. No study was found that had specifically addressed itself to the question, but one accidentally provided corroborative evidence.[3] This was a study done in Britain in which the investigators addressed themselves to the relationship between overcrowding and tuberculosis. The authors selected some 14,000 or 15,000 families living in a city and used the living arrangements (less than one person

per room, one person per room, or more than one person per room)
as an index of crowding. All family members were x-rayed to find out
if those living in houses with more than one person per room had
more tuberculosis than those who were not crowded. (Before analyzing
the data, all lodgers in these homes were eliminated from the study
because the authors believed they would weight the one-person-per-
room category.) The families were also categorized by social class,
since it is known that tuberculosis occurs much more frequently in the
lower classes. The findings indicated increased tuberculosis rates in
family members as social class declined—but no relationship between
tuberculosis and overcrowding in any social class.

Fortunately the investigators included, as an appendix, their findings on the lodgers in these families. Although the lodgers lived under
the same general conditions as the families, their tuberculosis rates
were almost twice as high, particularly in the low social classes. The
major difference between lodgers and family members, of course, is
that the lodgers are more likely to be people without families or kin,
living alone, often single, and lonely.

STRESS AND THE SOCIAL ISOLATE

If the findings of these studies are accepted, they pose a
number of further questions. How is it possible that these factors can
increase the chances of getting tuberculosis? Obviously not all people
who are isolated develop tuberculosis even when they are exposed to
the bacillus; therefore, what are the differences between isolated people who develop the disease and isolated people who do not? What else
needs to happen?

A study of tuberculosis hospital employees sheds some light on
these questions. Each employee who had developed tuberculosis was
matched with a nontuberculous employee of the same race, age, sex,
date of employment, type of work, tuberculin test result at the beginning of employment, appearance of the first x-ray, presence or absence
of any other significant disease, marital status, income, and history of
alcoholism. So far as possible, the two groups were identical except
that those in one group had developed tuberculosis and those in the
other had not, although both had been exposed to the tubercle bacillus
as a result of working in a TB hospital. In each group the number of
situations likely to produce stress during the previous 10 years was
measured. These included economic factors such as financial worry
and loss of job, and social and personal factors such as marital stress,
social withdrawal, and personal crises.

The actual number of stressful situations did not differ in the two
groups, but the distribution of these stresses over time differed

markedly. In those who did *not* develop tuberculosis the stressful situations were distributed randomly, some years being relatively free of stress and some years having multiple stresses. In the tuberculosis group, however, the stressful situations mounted in a crescendo, each year being worse than the previous one. These situations reached a peak about one to two years before tuberculosis was diagnosed.

Thus it appears that people exposed to mounting life stress who are deprived of help and support from society, who have no friends or kin—that is, no one interested in them—have to handle these threats unaided. One of the consequences is the disease we call tuberculosis.

HORMONE BALANCE IN THE
TUBERCULOUS PATIENT

A question that would follow from such a formulation might be this: Why tuberculosis? There is evidence to show that tuberculosis is not the only deleterious consequence of such a set of circumstances. People who develop schizophrenia or who commit suicide, for example, have similar characteristics to those who develop tuberculosis. When a person develops tuberculosis, additional factors must therefore be present.

Some of these have been tentatively identified in yet another study from Seattle. In this, a group of tuberculosis patients in a hospital were investigated to determine the relationship between their hormone balance and their recovery from tuberculosis. The hormone measured is produced by the adrenal gland and called the 17-ketosteroids. It was found that the level of this hormone fluctuated widely from patient to patient, and that there was a close relationship between the emotional state of the patient and the level of his hormone. Those who had low levels of hormone tended to be apathetic, depressed, withdrawn—to feel hopeless. The closer the hormone level came to the normal for their age and sex the more the patients tended to be calm, contented, and well adjusted to their situation. Those who had high levels tended to show the classical signs of anxiety, restlessness, aggressiveness, hostility, fearfulness, and to refuse to stay in bed. Under adequate therapy those whose levels were nearest normal tended to recover the fastest. Those whose level was lowest tended to die and those whose levels were highest tended neither to recover nor die, but become chronic. If a patient's emotional state was changed, his hormone level would also change as would the response to tuberculosis. Thus, if an apathetic, withdrawn patient was made more calm and contented, his hormone level tended to rise and his chance of recovery from tuberculosis improved.

THE CAUSES OF TUBERCULOSIS

It is now possible to reformulate our concept of the causes of tuberculosis. Exposure to mounting life stresses in people deprived of emotional support from society will lead to their being overwhelmed, with a resulting increase in depression and apathy. This emotional state may lead to an alteration in hormone balance, which increases their susceptibility to the tubercle bacillus. If any of these factors are missing, tuberculosis is unlikely to occur. For example, people similarly exposed to mounting life stresses who are well integrated in society, who can get support from a wife or a husband, or from neighbors or kin, are not likely to become so depressed and apathetic and withdrawn as are the lonely, and thus would not have the alteration in their hormone level. Exposure to the tubercle bacillus would therefore not be followed by tuberculosis.

Tuberculosis was deliberately selected as a disease of traditional concern to epidemiology, namely, an infectious disease. I wanted to indicate, as dramatically as possible, that if modern epidemiology can increase our understanding of a disease about which so much is already known, it can make an even greater contribution to the study of conditions about which little at present is known. Not only can all diseases, noninfectious chronic diseases as well as infectious, be studied by epidemiologic methods, but many other states of health are amenable to such investigation. For example, epidemiologic studies have been conducted on accidents, industrial absenteeism, fetal survival, and growth and maturation. In addition, there is growing realization that various psychologic factors, including behavior development, emotional states, and intelligence, can be studied in a similar fashion. Finally, it is our belief that increased understanding of the various manifestations of social maladjustment—for example, delinquency, chronic dependency, and criminality—can also be gained through epidemiologic investigation. For all such conditions the major contribution of epidemiology will derive from its ability to elucidate the role of environmental factors, particularly factors in the human environment, in the causal chain.

The most important single factor which up to the present has limited the intelligent application of epidemiologic technics to such problems has been our inability to develop an adequate conceptual scheme indicating the relevant social and cultural processes. Whatever the present limitations of the bacteriologic theory of causation, for a time it provided a useful model which led to an intelligent selection of relevant variables in the environment. To proceed further and gain understanding of the impact on health of social and cultural processes we need a new model which takes into account the modern view of causation and indicates the types of social and cultural variables we need to study. To devise such a model requires the closest collaboration of the social and the health sciences and is a task of central concern to our Department of Epidemiology.

SUMMARY

Epidemiology is one of the sciences concerned with the study of the processes which determine or influence the physical, mental, and social health of people. It is with their health in relation to their behavior in social groups that epidemiology is primarily concerned.

Up to this point I have been concerned solely with the theoretical basis upon which epidemiology is, or should be, founded. Without such a basis epidemiologic investigation is sterile. The theoretic formulations should not be confused, however, with the methods and technics by which epidemiologic investigations are carried out. These methods, requiring considerable skill in execution, can be simply stated. Epidemiology is an observational science. The essential element in observation is comparison. In epidemiology we compare the characteristics of a group having a specific condition with the characteristics of a group without the condition. From our knowledge of the similarities and differences between the two groups, we derive hypotheses as to the processes which caused the condition. To carry out such studies, we collect facts concerning the state of health or condition being studied, the nature of the group in which the condition is being studied, and the habitat or environment of that group. Groups may vary in size from a single family unit to a whole nation; they may also differ in kind. But whether it is an informal, relatively intimate group or a formal organized group, the same general principles apply. Special indices, such as incidence and prevalence rates, have been developed to quantify these data and describe their distribution, taking into account the differing numbers of people at risk in various groups and the differing lengths of time they are observed. Various statistical procedures are required to determine the strength of any associations found to exist between the characteristics of the group or habitat and the state of health under study. Formal rules have been developed as to the generalizations possible depending on the nature of the sample and the way the data were collected. All these factors bear the same relationship to epidemiology that laboratory technics bear to, for example, bacteriology. They are essential tools without which scientific epidemiologic investigation is impossible. A knowledge of these tools without any grasp of the basic theory leads, however, to pedestrian studies of limited usefulness to investigation.

If social workers decide to apply epidemiologic methods to the study of social problems, I hope they will address themselves not only to the scientific technics required but to an even more challenging requirement: the development of meaningful conceptual models which can be made operational and tested. In this latter area I see great opportunities for fruitful collaboration between social work and epidemiology.

1. Dubos, Rene: *Mirage of Health.* Harper Bros., New York, 1959.

2. Holmes, Thomas H.: "Multidiscipline Studies of Tuberculosis" in *Personality, Stress and Tuberculosis.* Phineas J. Sparer, editor. International Universities Press, Inc., New York, 1956.

3. Brett, G. Z. and B. Benjamin: "Housing and Tuberculosis in a Mass Radiography Survey," *Br. J. Prev. and Soc. Med.,* 11, 1959, 7.

The City Health Department Statistician*

HOWARD WEST, M.P.H.

THE American Public Health Association's most recent "Directory of Public Health Statisticians" (1958) lists for 45 cities in the United States the names of one or more persons actively engaged in the "collection, processing, analysis or publication of Public Health statistics, including vital statistics and medical statistics." Superficial analysis of the directory indicates that for 19 of these cities "statistical" activities revolved principally around vital records, since only a registrar is listed. Apparently only 26 cities in the United States, nine of which are in California, have a statistician concerned with Public Health programs in addition to vital records.

These few facts clearly indicate that in most city health departments the statistician has no direct role. It seems fair to assume that, in general, data are available in these cities mainly as a result of State vital statistics tabulations, State requirements with regard to reportable diseases, Federal requirements with regard to grant funds, and as a result of counts of inspection, nurses' visits, clinic visits, and the like. While this array of data may add up to the kind of information which can occasionally be used effectively to justify budget in-

* Reprinted by permission from the November, 1961, issue of *Public Health Reports,* Vol. 76, pp. 995–998. This paper was presented at the 1960 meeting of the American Public Health Association in San Francisco, California on October 31 to November 4. The author is Director, Division of Research and Statistics, Group Health Association of America, Inc., Washington, D.C., formerly Chief, Program Planning, District of Columbia Department of Public Health.

creases, it is unlikely to be sufficient in scope or detail either to define the complex health needs of a community or to measure the effectiveness of the health department in meeting these multiple needs.

Although the great majority of cities apparently operate without benefit of the skills of the statistician, some, recognizing the importance and value of birth and death data, employ a registrar of vital statistics. A registrar increases the likelihood that the city can both gain maximum use of the information and carry on more effectively the unending efforts to improve the completeness and accuracy of these records.

THE LONE WORKER

The 1958 APHA "Directory of Public Health Statisticians" lists more than one statistician for only nine cities, outside California. While mere numbers are unrelated to the quality of work, they are related to the scope and quantity of work possible. In eight cities, the lone statistician has the entire burden of planning and directing the collection and processing of data as well as of analyzing results and making them available in usable form. The time needed to accomplish these fundamental statistical procedures as they apply to the regular programs of a city health department almost precludes statistical approach to other questions. While it is theoretically possible for one person to undertake both this basic statistical work and occasional field surveys or even sample studies, it is rather unlikely that he will. Aside from the factor of time, the solitary statistician would need for such a program not only well-rounded Public Health education but also broad experience coupled with resourcefulness and imagination. With such qualifications, it is unlikely he would long remain immune to the enticements of positions with a more promising financial and professional future.

With some exceptions, the solitary statistician probably will not be able to accomplish more than the development and maintenance of essential information describing health department activities, such as the number of various types of immunizations given, the number of venereal disease cases reported by sex, race, age, and the number of contacts brought to treatment. To be sure, the development of reasonably consistent, accurate, and timely data to describe the varied efforts of the average city health department is a feat greatly to be admired, even envied.

OPPORTUNITIES FOR SPECIAL PROJECTS

The health departments having more than one statistician are, with one exception, in cities of more than 500,000 population. Three of them are independent of a State health department, and thus are entirely responsible for the vital statistics and for the development of all other statistics necessary to the various activities of the health department. The struggle to provide useful basic activity data is not unlike that in cities having fewer resources. But efficiency is likely to be higher, not only because larger staffs provide an opportunity for some specialization, but because the tools are likely to be better. Such health departments usually have a full complement of punch-card equipment available to them. More advanced tools and larger staffs also provide some flexibility in the extent and scope of the statistical program. Although there is constant need to provide basic activity data and to refine and improve their meaning and usefulness, there may also be opportunity for nonrepetitive projects.

In the District of Columbia Department of Public Health, where we have had three, sometimes four, statisticians during the past six years, most of our time has been spent on development of valid and useful repetitive data. These efforts are never-ending, even for vital statistics, where experience is long and methodology well developed. We have strived also to gather a large variety of data useful for population estimates, to refine and further develop appropriate methodology, and to prepare annual estimates by age and race.

The statistician is needed also for a variety of nonrepetitive projects of surprising range and scope. In Washington, D.C., for example, income requirements for eligibility for hospital care had become out of date. How were the income scales to be adjusted so as to eliminate inequities and at the same time not make more persons eligible than could be cared for at city expense? A citywide income survey[1] with defined sampling error was determined upon; the necessary funds were obtained; criteria, content, and tabulation details were specified for the Bureau of the Census, which selected the sample, carried out the field interviews, and processed the results. The income tabulations were analyzed and used in developing and recommending adjustments in income requirements for eligibility which have proved to be within fiscal and facility limitations.

As another example, the neonatal mortality rate reached a low point in Washington about 10 years ago. Since that time it has risen somewhat. While the effect of changes in such factors as race and legitimacy can be accounted for, other factors which may have affected this mortality rate, such as changes in the amount and duration of prenatal care, require research. Revisions of the extensive medical items on the birth certificate will soon make available data of sufficient detail to provide useful measures of the effectiveness of the department's greatly stepped-up prenatal care program as well as potential clues for further research.

The rapid advances in the development of automatic data-processing equipment must in time have an impact on the larger city health departments. These powerful new tools make possible the development of much significant information not now available as well as more extensive use of existing information. The statistician must be prepared to participate, if not to lead, in evaluating the potentials for new program data as well as for data which may be available as a by-product of financial or other administrative information. He must also be prepared to develop the necessary procedures and programs for the equipment once it is available.

EFFECTS OF PROGRAM BUDGETING

Program budgeting, a concept developed about a dozen years ago and now filtering down to municipal governments, has begun to affect the role of the statistician in city health departments. In contrast to the traditional method of budgeting for each unit independently of the others, this new budget pattern recognizes the operational interdependence of the various organization units. It has also led directly to an entirely different perspective toward program operation and costs. These new approaches have in turn contributed to increased emphasis on program planning and evaluation.

In each of the three cities known to be using program budgeting, a statistician has been given the primary responsibility for program planning, evaluation, and research. And in each of these cities, these functions have been divorced from those of collection, processing, analysis, and publication of Public Health and vital statistics.

In this new role, all the training, knowledge, and skills of the Public Health statistician are being called upon as never before. He needs to be familiar with the numerous and complicated characteristics of his city—its people, its neighborhoods, its resources, both human and physical, its economy—in short, all its attributes, its problems, and its deficiencies. By one means or another data must be obtained which will provide the best possible statistical description of all of these. Against this backdrop, the health needs of the community must be fully determined in detail. In addition to health department, hospital, welfare department, and community agency data, the invaluable reports coming from the National Health Survey, as well as other nationally developed urban data, will need to be synthesized to reach a reasonably clear picture of community health needs.

The city health department is meeting various portions of some of these health needs. For almost none of them can or does it attempt to do the whole job. Numerous other agencies and the practicing private physician also are responsible for providing for the health needs of the community. The distribution of these responsibilities must be identified, and those segments for which the health department has responsibility and those which no group or agency has actively undertaken must be noted particularly. As the latter are identified, the question of whether the health department should begin to plan to fill these gaps will need to be answered.

STATISTICS IN EVALUATION

How successfully is the health department meeting its defined role in the community? Its statistical program should be able to provide data which will describe the extent to which the department is meeting the needs for which it has responsibility.

How do these accomplishments measure up to its budgeted and staffed plans to achieve projected goals? What are the gaps between accomplishments, plans, and needs? The effectiveness with which the department's programs are carried out must be differentiated from how well those programs actually satisfy community health needs. For example, is a significant increase in the proportion of women who are provided adequate prenatal care by the health department's prenatal clinics reflected by a significant increase in the proportion of women having adequate prenatal care who are delivered at the city hospital? Or did the increase at the clinics merely represent a shift in use of facilities?

The answers to such questions, as they apply to appropriate segments of the numerous programs of the department, provide an approach to evaluation of their effectiveness. And while careful evaluation may indicate the need for program modification, research is frequently required to provide the basis for valid modification. In the example just given, assume that the increase in adequate prenatal care provided by the clinics did in fact represent nothing more than a shift away from previous care patterns. What factors or combination of factors caused the shift? What combination of factors is needed to achieve a net gain in total prenatal care? These can be answered only by specific research. Program evaluation provides a means for defining problems, and research the means for attempting to solve them effectively. The statistician must inevitably play a major part both in the development of evaluation techniques and in the formulation of research projects to improve and enhance health department programs.

The APHA, through its Program Area Committee on Public Health Administration, will soon release for field testing a completely revised evaluation schedule for local health departments. This comprehensive document will require detailed definition of community health needs and program objectives, development and use of program measurements, evaluation studies, and identification of specific research needs. The hoped-for stimulation of local health department efforts along these lines will be difficult to accomplish unless the statistician is available and enabled to make his appropriate contribution.

FOUR STAGES OF DEVELOPMENT

The role of the statistician in city health departments to-day reflects four stages of development of statistical programs in the Public Health movement. Most of our city health departments are in stage one. These departments have recognized the importance of vital records and of the contribution that a registrar can make to the correct recording and use of vital records data. In stage two are those health departments which have accepted the concept that a statistician can make a contribution to the health program, but which apparently cannot afford to develop fully their basic statistical program. In stage three are found those larger cities which not only have greater resources, but which have also recognized the need for statistical staff in order to maximize the availability and usefulness of a wide variety of program data. Stage four reflects the recognition of the statistician not only in his role as a data producer and analyst, but as an objective and skilled interpreter of health problems and needs. In this new role, the statistician is assuming staff responsibility for planning, evaluation, and research in public health programs. The challenge of these broad responsibilities is great, but greater still is the potential significance of these developments to progress in Public Health.

1. District of Columbia Department of Public Health, Biostatistics and Health Education Division: *Income of families and individuals in Washington, D.C.,* July 1958.

3.   Public Health Social Work

Public Health Social Work*

ESTHER C. SPENCER

TWELVE YEARS ago, when I began to call what I was doing Public Health social work,[1] there was some controversy as to whether this label was justified. Even now there is disagreement regarding classifications of social work practice. Should practice be labeled according to where it occurs in terms of "fields," or should there continue to be differentiation of one kind of content from another through specialist-labeling of the individual social work practitioner as well? The profession is aware of its responsibility to clarify and define what it means by a "field of practice," the currently accepted means of distinguishing among the several areas into which social work is patterned; and whether this is an appropriate and enduring method of classification.[2] This writing represents one such effort.

That there is more than labeling involved in this determination goes without saying. For social work generally there is the fundamental question of a holistic approach to fulfilling the role society has ascribed to it: of preventing, controlling, and treating conditions adverse to the attainment of high level social functioning; and of enhancing conditions that foster and nourish personal and social equilibrium. To accomplish this there must be continuous "Articulation and refinement of the content of the various methods and fields of practice. . . ."[3] Decisions regarding the best means of "articulation and refinement" must be weighed against the danger of fragmentation and partialization that could be mirrored by divisiveness in organization of services—in the uses made of one kind of practitioner in preference to another. In the light of this, Public Health social work is undergoing scrutiny by the entire profession.[4]

ORIGINS OF PUBLIC HEALTH SOCIAL WORK

The origins of Public Health social work almost certainly lay in the recognition that problems of serious consequence to health involve multiple factors. Prominent among these are social stresses, also multiple in nature, but clearly identifiable in certain health prob-

* This original contribution was especially prepared for this volume. The author is Chief, Bureau of Public Health Social Work, State of California Department of Health, Berkeley, California.

lems. Initially the attack upon venereal disease as an undisputed health menace included social work personnel to assist in ferreting out sources of infection. Called epidemiologists, these early day disease control specialists represented one of the beginning movements away from total preoccupation with environmental measures. Though the "social diseases" might have been a natural springboard from which this young profession could demonstrate a skilled contribution, there is little to show for its presence in Public Health at that time.

The next, and for social work, more traditional functioning in Public Health began about 1927 in the Los Angeles County Health Department. With its 16 districts spread over a huge geographic area, this Public Health program was designed to give clinic services principally in tuberculosis and maternal and child health. Much as a hospital out-patient department might give help to a defined population group, the county health department district program carried out its public health commitment under centrally outlined policies. Staffs of physicians, nurses, and social workers were responsible to central office chiefs in their own discipline. Different from a hospital out-patient program, however, was the extent of medical care provided—a high percentage of service was based in classical Public Health responsibilities, such as tuberculosis case-finding and follow-up, and prenatal care. The social work program in this service derived from a well-established field of social work practice, in-hospital medical care, and defined its professional role almost solely in relation to illness. What took place in definitive program-planning and development remained almost exclusively with the central office, and was also mainly oriented to problems of illness.[5] Casework practice, and staff deployment were predominantly geared to "recalcitrant" cases in tuberculosis control, and to arranging for tuberculosis or maternal and child care elsewhere.

Rather than as a planned activity, consultation often grew out of casework services, and thus was not clearly defined as an essential characteristic of the job. Although it was usually included in job descriptions, the consultation role in medical social work was relatively shapeless and often confused with collaboration, case conferences, and supervision. While district staffs were encouraged to participate in community planning within their environs, rigidity of the line/staff relationships tended to weaken initiative. Data collection and evaluation of the kind expected of most Public Health workers today was absent; nor were personnel urged to participate in any of the department's research efforts.

Here, as in many beginning Public Health social work programs, was an almost intact transplantation of medical social work from its hospital base of operations to a setting that, while geographically different, functionally and ideologically retained many of the same approaches. Direct services to individuals was the chosen method of problem-solving. From an historic viewpoint this emphasis may well be regarded as progressive, with its stress on the importance of people, and the part played by the individual and family in disease control. The use of these data, however, was too fragmentary and not well enough related to practical problems in Public Health to make a notable impact.

Federal interest in State and local program developments was, at this time, becoming crystallized. Spurred by pressures arising from the plight of families and communities unable to meet the costs and demands of severe health problems, this interest began to express itself in Congressional action. Categories of illness involving high levels of cost, communicability, and emotion began to occupy the concern of individuals powerful inside and outside of government. Along with this came the economic crisis of the thirties, supporting the need for government assistance and leading to the Social Security Act.

Title V of the Social Security Act, with its appropriations to the states for services to crippled children, produced two phenomena of special note in Public Health social work. First, the intent and wording of the legislation legitimized not only the principle that handicapping conditions are expensive to treat; but, for our purposes more important: that there are vast potential social costs to be minimized by proper attention to the social needs of the children and their families as a feature of comprehensive medical care. Each state was thus nudged in the direction of establishing a social work program within the crippled children's services, and most states did so. Insofar as the services were developed in the health departments, widespread employment of social workers by State departments of health thus occurred. Congressional appropriations to the Children's Bureau for implementation of Title V enabled the second of the two phenomena of particular note: the development of a central medical social work section and a cadre of social work specialists deployed from Children's Bureau regional offices throughout the country as consultants.

The State health department social work programs that grew out of Title V legislation were extremely useful in providing a heretofore unavailable category of service; and in many instances they represented the inception of social work in State level health programs. It was the consultant service and all that it implied, however, that created the need to take a new look at social work's possibilities in such settings. An area of planning not hitherto apparent in social work program formulations now became explicit. Until this time social workers functioned by conscription in already patterned medical care services, which were based on the assumption that problems of harassing and handicapping illness had social meaning and consequences for the individual and the family. These problems were accepted as appropriate loci for the use of the characteristic skills of the social case workers. For the first time, by the deployment of consultants, social work began to say that direct service or one-to-one casework technic was not the most significant attack upon problems of social need.

CONSULTATION: A NEW SOCIAL WORK ROLE

The planned use of consultants thus brought another dimension to the social work role. Programming considerations different from those usually motivating staff assignments and functions began to be taken into account. Formerly, correlations between numbers of social workers and numbers of clients computed against the number of families one social worker could carry were employed to determine whether to expand or contract service. Now there was careful, detailed scrutiny of the legislative intent, and a greatly enlarged examination of the context in which the program was to operate. The background for this examination was far less specific in what the social worker had to offer numerically, and far more in terms of what the situation might require to meet social need. Before long, this exploration led inevitably to questions of who else, besides social workers, might be available for this purpose, and how might reciprocal changes in role and function be achieved.

Efforts to relate role to mandated program purposes and objectives broadened social work perceptions and moved them closer to Public Health values. Foremost among the latter was a concern for sound program planning; namely, that an objective assessment of needs included exploration of a comprehensive series of forces, with services scaled to an order of priorities in which prevention may stand higher than treatment, and factors of time and place are as significant as factors of personal need.

Selection of the consultant role demonstrated a dramatic shift both in knowledge and values for social work. Social workers who saw this as an improvisation, stop-gap, or dilution that could undermine the profession were resoundingly critical. Assisting others than social workers to understand and to make provision for psycho-social needs was described by first critics as an attempt to make "junior or surrogate caseworkers" out of nurses. Instead of defending their approach per se, consultants undertook to document what they were doing, and to analyze the relative advantages of their casework and consultation activities.[6, 7] Consultation they saw as a method by which social work values, knowledge, and insights could be transmitted selectively to others, to increase understanding and to strengthen case-management techniques.

Undoubtedly, this represented emergence of a new social work role. It tended to establish consultation as an important helping method closely related to casework, but with purposes, technics, and components of its own, and many of the principles of consultation today were thus formulated. No longer at issue was the potential application of social work skills to the solution of problems of larger segments of the population.

The success in extending attention to social need by transmitting to others their understanding, knowledge, and insights, stimulated social workers to define additional roles consonant with the operations, areas, and expectations of the Public Health setting.

It was again from the federal level that the consultant and other Public Health social work roles underwent further testing, shaping, and documentation, this time in tuberculosis control. In connection with mass, fast-tempo x-ray surveys of total populations above the age of 15 in large cities across the country, federal funds were given to health departments to provide staff for survey management and follow-up. Part of this program included special diagnostic clinics attached to local health departments. Funds were available for social workers to help patients and their families make the necessary adaptations to what was, for many, a changed and decidedly traumatic social situation. If social policy in the crippled children programs was largely responsible for social work in State level health programs, tuberculosis appropriations were certainly responsible for enlarging the scope of local health department social work. Where there were no State level Public Health social workers able to participate in tuberculosis programming, federal social work consultants gave assistance to the local administration in the establishment of services. This is exemplified by some early efforts in administrative or program-centered consultation, another currently well defined social work role in Public Health.

In the evolution of methods of social help and provision in Public Health, a good deal of thought has been given to consultation as an institutionalized procedure. Argument is often centered upon whether there is, or should be, any such role as that of a "pure" consultant— an individual who functions solely in this manner, presumably holding no other kinds of job responsibilities. If, as is supposed, there is such a role, social workers in the federal Public Health programs come closest to assuming it. They have no cases or clients as such; and the expectation of the agency is that they will spend a major portion of time, on a priority basis, giving administrative consultation to State level personnel. Though, as we shall see, there are many variations in the consultant role as practiced by social workers in State and local Public Health programs, this appears to be a fundamental characteristic of federal level social work.

But deliberations as to the possibility of a "pure" consultant are less useful guides to optimal Public Health social work than is the exemplary Public Health commitment to fashion role out of an objective assessment of the total situation consistent with rigorous problem solving. Significant as a model are the multiple and flexible constellations of activities involved in Public Health, with none regarded as central. Each method waits in the wings, as it were, to be summoned for use following thoroughgoing analytic assessment. For the most part these activities are not arrayed in any hierarchic order despite obvious differentials in salary scales among those who staff them. In part this is true because of the recognition that the constellation of factors outlined in these activities requires multiple methods and hence multiple disciplines. Each, therefore, demonstrates a gestalt of services in a special area of concern, e.g., control of chronic disease, control of communicable disease, or maternal and child health services.

SPECIALISTS OR GENERALISTS?

At the point of social work's entry into local health departments through tuberculosis appropriations an intermediate, though no less penetrating question was at issue: should the social worker in Public Health be a specialist attached to a single program category, or a generalist positioned administratively to move across the board, over all programs requiring this service? Seemingly, trends in governmental appropriations for health would continue to provide support through categoric fund distribution, and health department services would need to follow this pattern. Cogent factors can be marshalled in support of either approach: philosophic, practical, professional. These are of equal importance. Each must be given its appropriate place in any analysis of activities, objectives, and methods of operation—in a word—in program planning and organization of services.

As already noted, the sources of fiscal support make a profound difference as to patterns of staffing and service, and of course, as to when and whether objectives can be accomplished at all. Integration with specific categoric programs provides a structure for social work roles and services, and gives visibility attained only with great difficulty through other means. Functions in connection with explicit programs are more readily described and interpreted, and seem to have greater meaning to funding bodies than those involved generically with policy making, program planning, consultation, or community participation. It is relatively simple to justify need for social workers in program categories with already demonstrated significant social factors, i.e., tuberculosis, crippled children, mental retardation, and in those where social solutions have been tested and validated. Once the social work role is successfully established in a specialized program, it is possible to have other programs use the social worker as a consultant and thus spread knowledge and values over a wider area.

If there is a social work consultant in tuberculosis, in crippled children services, etc., then it is conceivable that several social workers would need to be deployed to the same agency, each to give consultation in a field of special knowledge. Lack of flexibility in maximum utilization of manpower, especially from a profession in short supply, constitutes an administrative obstacle inherent in highly specialized role assignments. Personnel employed continuously in one category of health usually function in team situations, and tend to be discipline-centered. In addition, there is a risk of becoming parochial in viewpoint, knowledge, and understanding of Public Health matters, since day-by-day preoccupation is with the category of illness or service. Where the entire agency social work activity consists of a series of individuals assigned to specialized programs, it is difficult for the department to develop consistent social policy, and to express a concerted opinion with respect to health-related social issues and concerns. No one is really in a position to speak for social work; and top administration has to select one or another spokesman according to judgments that are extremely difficult to make. Negotiations with outside agencies for interagency agreements and contracts, for coordination of service provision are piecemeal and without authority.

The State level Public Health social work program in California is an example of change from a highly specialized unit to more general integration with the mission and culture of the total department. Some of the ratiocination that went into this change will illustrate a thesis outlined earlier: that fundamental to optimal programming are skills in comprehensive assessment fully involved in the context in which the program operates.

Starting at the time of Title V in the conventional way, social workers were employed by the California State Department of Public Health primarily for casework services to crippled children. Although gradually there was assistance to the tuberculosis program, roles were essentially stereotyped to a carry-over from traditional in-hospital functions.

In California, State level leadership became increasingly pointed toward the goal of extended and improved services to people. Of notable interest to social work was the recurrence in legislative mandates of the phrase "services to people," as an expression of attitudes of responsibility toward the ultimate recipients of program benefits. With prodding from many sides—not alone by social policy makers— the scope of Public Health obligation to a total environmental viewpoint, including the social environment, became enlarged. Efforts to meet this obligation stimulated and supported increased recognition that social workers had reciprocal beneficial roles and should be mandated to act "across-the-board."

Some of the principles by which analyses and changes were accomplished have been mentioned. Abundant evidence provided by the setting through its vital data collection, surveys, studies, and research showed relationships between social phenomena and health at all socio-economic levels. Evaluation of social work practices gave clear indication that direct social services belong at the local level and that their development could be perennially deferred by trying to meet individual casework needs from the state level in a "drop-in-the-bucket" manner.

Services to specific programs which had been of major import in the past had to be examined to determine which of these was pertinent to new program objectives. On the basis of such evaluation, the State program no longer entered into direct casework services to crippled children's families, but gave assistance to local communities in finding ways of providing such services.

Similar trends were apparent in local health department programs. Health officers were recognizing locally a need for generalized social services in meeting a wide range of Public Health problems. Social workers who had been responsible for services to specialized programs began to move out into more generalized functions through the media of program planning, consultation, and community organization. Many health departments without social services looked to professional social workers for help in identifying social-health problems, and to demonstrate the areas in which casework was the specific need in problem solving.

Public Health social work was concerned with two strategic areas of its practice during this period. The wider profession was still focussed largely on the treatment of problems as identified by the client and by the client's willingness to take help. Public Health at the same time was placing challenging demands on social work to adapt its knowledge and competence to prevention, casefinding, diagnosis, and research. As a result there was an experimental development of social work program content oriented to the philosophy of community prevention and control. Of particular importance were the adaptations of social work skills to identification of community health needs; and positive, aggressive program planning and policy formulation aimed at groups of people at special risk, and sometimes sacrificing the individual in lower priority of need.

Major emphasis was placed, however, on the methodology of working with the already established Public Health services and programs, and particularly on learning the process of consultation and the consultant role. In this challenge, social work also had to develop new understandings of the roles and responsibilities of a wide variety of other helping professionals. It had to learn to adapt its skills to a new level of practice, and to develop a real conviction that other disciplines could be helpful through the use of selected social work knowledges and techniques. Experience and observation have indicated that the acceptance of responsibility in helping others to deal with social-health factors was not easily carried out by the social worker. The profession was grappling with the mastery of new techniques and at the same time with retention of a role in a professional climate where everyone has an interest in, concern with, and responsibility for social health problems.

In local health departments, the role of the Public Health social worker has substantially shifted to that of consultant and community planner. Because this is consistent with local program goals generally, several counties employ only one social worker. Though the ratio of social workers to other disciplines is, in total, considerably higher in California that in other States, local health departments may have fewer social workers than other types of personnel. Reciprocal influences govern this: special work, a comparative newcomer to this field has not yet, especially in the Public Health evaluative idiom, proved its value. Only recently has Public Health moved in the direction of explicit interest in social characteristics, personal needs, and services. Until now, Public Health philosophy lay more in identifying areas of service and methods of planning, staffing, supporting, and evaluating services rather than rendering them. With this as a primary motivation, the direct service role is more often exceptional.

Similarity in social work roles exists on the federal, State, and local levels in relation to the consultation function, though variations within this occur: federal and State level social workers give administrative or program-centered consultation; local staffs give case-centered consultation. Case-centered consultation in Public Health is offered chiefly to nurses and other care-giving personnel within and without the local health department.

This palpably workable distribution of Public Health social workers casts a different light upon the criticism raised earlier, and suggests a further answer to it: social work values should be elastic enough to permit limited numbers to figure significantly in program planning, priority setting, and methodology development. In fact, only as social workers are concerned to experiment with new problem-solving methods will they do more than simply survive in the Public Health setting. There is nothing arcane about Public Health's methods and activities. Its commitment to evaluation and replicability is such that if objectives are not clear and methods transferable, they are judged to be lacking in validity. This means that the setting provides designs, models, data, and mechanisms from which all may learn and copy. Using these examples, social workers discover that they can be inventive as long as their methods are appropriate, timely, clear, and susceptible to evaluation.

The Public Health social work picture at the State level should probably consist of a generalized program, strongly committed to development of local services; to training of social workers for Public Health; and to epidemiologic research which will more specifically identify the relationships between the social environments in which people live and their patterns of health.

NEW AREAS OF CONCERN

The rapid pace at which Public Health is moving into new areas of concern requires of social work a careful analysis of the effectiveness of patterns of organization and function in meeting goals. The sphere of Public Health responsibility for prevention and control of problems with major social elements has taken shape rapidly in the past few years—chronic disease, mental illness, industrial health hazards, juvenile delinquency, alcoholism, and narcotics addiction. The social elements in these categories of health have not been specifically spelled out. The attack on such problems is a double-barrelled one of epidemiologic study of causation and program development to implement knowledge now available. A crucial question is whether it is really possible with generalized social service organization and assignments to give enough content to specific epidemiologic study and program development. Some experimental alteration of the pattern of complete generalization has begun in California by assigning liaison workers to programs of ascending importance in the Public Health picture, in order to meet the needs for social work participation. To date, this assignment of liaison workers has not threatened, to a major degree, the conviction that social services should not be specialized, but should be rendered in the context of total health needs.

Within the framework of a continuing generalized responsibility, the ascending Public Health problems are making demands which necessitate decreased social service emphasis on older Public Health problems. Such need for continually changing patterns of disease control is not peculiar to social work. Program flexibility and changing of priorities is an inherent characteristic of all Public Health practice. For social workers, as for others, the criteria by which activities are decreased need to be spelled out. At the State level, the grouping of health problems into those of ascending and of descending importance offers some guides for limitation of service. In identifying, from the social work point of view, the problems of descending importance, one finds that these are not necessarily the problems of least magnitude but rather, as stated earlier, those in which much of the social content is known and the program needs are established. Goals for activity in such programs are, therefore, identified. All social service activities on behalf of single categories of illness need to be weighed in the light of the two primary identified objectives. Particularly needing examination are continued requests for case-centered consultation in areas where the movement toward program development is not evident, on the assumption that case-centered consultation may have reached a point of diminishing returns in accomplishing major goals. Satisfactions in working where people want social workers most must give way to a clear-cut use of the diagnostic process in studying problems and selecting courses of action which will have the greatest impact on development of services.[8]

In local health departments, certain distinct trends in the direction of program specialization are emerging. Major external influences operate in this changing picture. For two Public Health problems of ascending importance, namely, mental health and alcoholism, special funds are available to assist local programs. This trend is further stimulated by the availability of funds to local health departments for research and demonstrations in chronic disease, aging, and maternal and child health. In these categories of health need, the social content is often the major area for study and control, and the social worker is viewed as the key person in carrying out the direct service responsibility. Legislative mandates and special fiscal support are changing the organizational patterns of local Public Health social services at a time when social work has gained recognition as an integral part of overall program planning and operation. One must now examine again whether the responsibilities for identification of community social health problems, program development, consultation, and research can be accomplished less or more efficiently through a generalized or specialized social service focus; and how these responsibilities might be carried out by the individual social worker in the context of a clinical casework job.

Legislation, conditions of support, and public demand seem to make these clinical entities assume the form of circumscribed programs. In addition to this, the unknowns which surround the diseases themselves—unknowns of etiology, spread, and prevalence, and hence of social and psychologic impact upon families and communities, seem to make up a special field of forces that could isolate clinic members into a different set of personnel. Among these, the clinic social worker plays a deservedly responsible role. Increasingly, however, as these health problems yield to study, and their solutions become more comprehensible, other caretakers will be identified. While this is taking place, administration must not be crystallized into patterns of isolation and fragmented solutions such as were found in the early days of crippled children's programs. Patterns of organization and operation must be sought which will allow for rapid fitting of knowledge and experience into the total framework of Public Health. The very nature of these social health problems and the need for imaginative solutions make it important that there be social work involvement in the various functions.

Public Health social work draws from many basic social work methods for its comprehensive and dynamic understanding and promotion of social well-being, and for the perspective needed during the periodic reviews and restatements through which Public Health moves. Old charters provide adequate evolutionary data from which to proceed. Formerly applied as a series of more or less self-contained methodologic entities, these may be used at present as a springboard for mixing and refining skills according to new concepts of health need, with levels of practice worked out in a task-oriented value system.

SOCIAL WORKERS' SPECIAL CONTRIBUTIONS

To date, social workers have functioned chiefly in programs determined by others. The question to be faced is, "What is our program?" If one accepts the premise that social health is a valid responsibility of Public Health, social workers will take leadership in reaching this goal. Public Health social work is facing the same choice implied by Mary Richmond when she said, "I have spent twenty-five years of my life in an attempt to get social casework accepted as a valid process in social work. Now I shall spend the rest of my life trying to demonstrate to social caseworkers that there is more to social work than social casework."[9]

The "more . . . than social casework" is emphasized in the eloquent language of modern Public Health when it turns its attention to pathologic social changes; social distribution of illness; or the levels of social functioning as related to health levels. Experience points to the probability that though today's Public Health problems are engendered in a complex of psychologic and social factors, social solutions may arrive more readily than had been envisioned prior to the advent of the computer. Here are a few areas for immediate study and action:

1. It is probable that certain diseases cannot exist apart from the social patterns by which people live. Adequate epidemiologic studies will validate these hypotheses by convergence, if not by proof. The area for study is the social environment in which people live.

2. Epidemiologic research is a must in the identification of social health needs. More should be known about the epidemiologic method, and how to work with others who can help adapt social work knowledge to this method.

3. There is a need for development of tools for mass screening in

the field of social health. Ability to accept this, and to develop such tools, will determine whether any discipline can really have a place in the broad community programs of prevention and case-finding.

4. There is need for development of a system of classification of social pathology similar to that existing for the physical and psychologic. This lies within the expertise of social work.

5. Social health problems require a concern of social work with problem-solving from the general to the specific. This is not in conflict with the basic contribution of individualization, for the very uniqueness of social work lies in its being able to look at the whole person in the whole social milieu.

6. The basic concern for the intensive study of the individual in his social context can assist with development of an equal concern with the forces among individuals.

7. Clinical programs in Public Health need casework services, but it is also true that these services cannot be traditional. There needs to be a much more specific identification of the application of casework in a setting in which all professions are becoming increasingly competent to deal with social problems.

8. Consultation will probably remain a major process in Public Health practice. It is incumbent upon social work to continue to refine and systematize knowledge of the practice and teaching of this process.

9. Much of Public Health is done by other than health departments, particularly in the field of social health. Social workers should participate in the identification and documentation of community needs and the stimulation of others to accept responsibilities.

10. The program at all levels of Public Health social work practice needs to include explicit evaluation components, and formalized training responsibilities.

In recognition of three elements: (1) the need to provide greater education in Public Health to all social workers; (2) the fact that there are now data from this field amenable for teaching in schools of social work; and (3) that data from social work may profitably be fed back to the field of Public Health, the Council on Social Work Education, collaborating with several Public Health agencies, held a Seminar at Princeton, New Jersey, in the spring of 1962. In addition to demonstrating the readiness of social work educators to adapt and absorb new ideas and techniques, this seminar showed the vast areas of commonality of philosophy and values shared by social work and Public Health. Concepts of epidemiology, prevention, and community planning were models through which the what, when, and how of enriching social work curricula were discussed. "What impressed me the most at the Seminar were: the increasing rapprochement between Public Health and social welfare as chronic illnesses replace acute infectious diseases as the principal concern of Public Health; the effect on epidemiology of Public Health's concern with chronic illness and the significance for social welfare of Public Health's traditional concern with prevention."[10]

What of the future of Public Health social work in view of some of these major changes in health problems and their conceptualization in programming? While epidemiology and prevention may represent an important strand of traditional Public Health concern, their optimal expression in program is far from an undisputed operation.

Many social work roles obviously require further spelling out, but the following appear more and more commonly in health departments:

1. Standard setting and surveillance of quality of care in public institutions normally licensed by health departments; with emphasis upon restoration of patients to high levels of social functioning. Attention to availability, accessibility, comprehensiveness and continuity of service. Though there are pros and cons as to whether the health department itself should be rendering these services, there is little question as to its legal responsibilities for quality.

2. Development of tools for the measurement of social functioning of families and individuals, measurements to be applied in multiple health screening programs, and in a variety of social diagnostic procedures necessary for precise methods of intervention, realistic documentation of need, and ultimate evaluation.

3. Participation in the development of social data collection devices, action, and analysis. Data collection of this nature may be integrated with other forms of household sampling for correlation with physical morbidity data and for a more concerted drive to raise the community social health level.

4. Preparation of critiques of program plans and special projects that require skilled social content in their design.

5. Conduct, stimulation, and application of social research and demonstrations.

6. Participation in efforts to regionalize and distribute health services on a planned and realistic basis, making use of community organization techniques along with social diagnostic competencies.

7. Participation in the assessing and computing of social costs of illness and absenteeism vs. subsidies for specialized care and programs with high level specificity in prevention.

8. Planning and action for joint programming with related agencies in welfare and mental health.

In summary, there have been presented some ways the Public Health social work role has developed with reference to several traditional and historic methods and levels of social work practice. In presenting the influences upon this development, an attempt has been made to distinguish certain contributions by methodologic appropriateness as to purpose and reliability. Concluding with a series of emerging functions which require further elaboration and testing, is an open professional invitation to all practitioners to share in the great social adventure offered.

1. Unpublished Annual Report, Massachusetts Department of Health, Medical Social Training Project, 1951, by the author who was then in charge of this project to bring Public Health tenets, techniques and philosophies into the curricula of the three schools of social work in Boston. Page 24, ad seq.

2. Report of the Review of National Association of Social Workers Structure. Submitted by the NASW Board of Directors to the membership for action at the 1962 Delegate Assembly. National Association of Social Workers, 2 Park Avenue, New York 16, New York.

3. *Ibid.*

4. In 1961, the Board of Directors, NASW, appointed an ad hoc Committee on Social Work in Public Health to advise the Association regarding the place of this in the "fields of practice" action. The author is chairman of this Committee.

5. Unpublished Annual Report, Los Angeles County Health Department, Bureau of Medical Social Work, 1954.

6. Payne, Elizabeth: "The Role of the Consultant in Field Service," notes of a class in the graduate School of Social Work of the University of Southern California, Los Angeles, August, 1948.

7. Siegel, Doris: "Consultation: Some Guiding Principles," *Administrative Supervision, and Consultation*, New York: Family Service Association of America, 1955.

8. Spencer, Esther C., and Grass, Constance: Perspectives in Public Health Social Work—The California Picture. Presented at the National Conference on Social Work, Chicago, Ill., 1958, (mimeographed).

9. Richmond, Mary, cited in Hollis, E. V., and Taylor, A. L.: *Social Work Education in the United States*. New York, Columbia University Press, 1951, p. 145.

10. Chernin, M.: A Report on the Seminar in Public Health for Schools of Social Work. *Weekly Bulletin* (School of Social Welfare, University of California, Berkeley) April 27, 1962.

4.   Public Health Nursing

Public Health Nursing: Definition and Process*

RUTH B. FREEMAN, R.N., ED.D.

√

PUBLIC Health nursing cannot be differentiated from other types of nursing by its functions or activities. Virtually every activity undertaken in Public Health work will appear in some degree in other types of nursing. It is in the emphasis and configuration of activities, and in the degree of competence that is expected in certain areas of nursing that the difference arises.

Public Health nursing may be defined as a special field of nursing in which technical nursing, interpersonal and organizational skills are applied in appropriate relationship to the skills of other members of health and social professions for the conservation of community health. It includes comprehensive nursing care of individuals, families, and groups and, in addition, Public Health measures addressed to the community as a whole, such as epidemiologic investigations, law enforcement, or organization of the community for health action.

Nursing Care of Individuals and Families

Nursing care of families represents a major approach to community health conservation. A community cannot be in good health if its individual members are not healthy, and Public Health activities must be directed toward assuring for each individual the highest possible degree of physical, mental, and social well-being. In achieving this, the efforts of the family and of private medical practice must be supplemented by community action, to do those things which the family cannot do for itself.

More and more, the improvement of family health depends upon individual family service rather than environmental control or mass preventive procedures, and in this type of activity the nurse is the primary purveyor of health services.

Nursing of patients is based on helping through "doing for" and "doing with." Kreuter defines it as ". . . acting and interacting with the patient through physical and personal contact for his welfare, and

---

* Reprinted in part by permission from Freeman, Ruth B.: *Public Health Nursing Practice*, 2nd Ed. Philadelphia, W. B. Saunders Company, 1957, Chapter III, pp. 30–41. The author is Professor of Public Health Nursing at Johns Hopkins University, School of Hygiene and Public Health, Baltimore, Maryland.

intervening in his behalf between him and those stresses in the physical environment and in the social climate that impinge upon him."[1]

In distinction to nursing in other fields, the type and amount of care given to individuals and families must be related to community needs. The selection of those to be served, for example, must rest on the comparative impact on community health, rather than solely on the needs of the individual or family concerned. For example, a Public Health nurse could not serve a small proportion of the population needing her care, providing excellent and comprehensive care for a few, while ignoring the needs of others.

The unit of service in Public Health is likely to be the family rather than the individual. As the locale of the service is often the home, families are involved in the immediate situation, and observation of family members and of the climate of family interaction is facilitated. Furthermore, health needs of individuals in a family are so interwoven and interdependent that consideration of the family as a unit is often the only feasible approach.

Ferguson, in analyzing the service load of the staff nurse in an urban health department, found that the average number of health problems per nursing visit was 4.02[2]; this is exclusive of the social, emotional, and economic problems encountered in these visits. This would indicate that the presenting problem—or the primary reason for the visit—is seldom the only one in the family that requires nursing action.

The family case load in Public Health is also heavily weighted with well children and adults, and with minor or long-term illnesses. This gives unusual emphasis to the counseling and health supervisory phases of nursing.

Community-Focussed Services

Communities, like individuals, have a state of health. Such things as defective housing, fearful and resistant attitudes toward acceptance and employment of the mentally handicapped, and over-restrictive patterns of parental control may characterize a community and represent a health problem. The existence of disease carriers, accident hazards, dangerous water or milk supplies, or inadequately housed and staffed nursing homes are other examples.

Like individuals, communities also have differing levels of competence to cope with their own health problems. In some communities, unwillingness of different cultural groups to work together for slum improvement may deprive individuals and families of the chance for better environment which can be secured only through group effort. Lack of knowledge or indifference to the health needs of school children may lead to inadequate school health service. Lack of organization may fritter away the efforts of a few crusaders for health, which, if channeled into organized effort, might have a real effect on Public Health.

Public Health nursing involves the use of planning and community organization, of group and individual teaching, of epidemiologic procedures, of interpreting and helping enforce the laws and regulations the community has established for its own protection. The nurse's patient in this case is the community.

Whether directed toward family care or community action, the Public Health nurse works always in proper relationship with the many other individuals or agencies concerned. She may take leadership or serve in a supporting and participating capacity to other members of the health team, depending upon the situation and upon her own competence. She plans her own program and activities in relation to those of others, setting as her goal the improvement of community health through nursing practice.

PROCESS

Process in Public Health nursing may be considered in three general areas—use of technical and ministration skills, the use of self, and the use of group therapy. In practice, all three are interwoven and inseparable, and incompetence in any one area seriously affects the others. It is only for purposes of analysis that any separation is justified. No attempt will be made to identify areas that are unique to Public Health nursing, since few, if any, parts of the process can be separated from the general nursing base.

Use of Technical and Ministration Skills

The technical and ministration skills of nursing are closely bound to the expectations of patients and the community in relation to nursing. To the public, the nurse is one who helps, and these tangible helping skills identify her.

The skills of ministration—the homely arts of comforting the patient, of bathing and positioning, of making medicine acceptable, of supporting a paralyzed arm in a colorful scarf instead of a bandage—are important not only in themselves, but also because they may have a profound effect on the patient's feelings of security, his willingness to get well, his determination to help himself. They communicate to the patient a sense of wanting to help.

In a recent article a patient describes the discomfort and fear she felt when nursing skills were inadequate. She writes: "I sensed the nurses were uncertain about the irrigating procedure . . . I needed a nurse who had special training in the care of colostomies to give me specific instructions . . . had I been properly instructed my rehabilitation time would have been cut considerably."[3]

Ministration skills must be applied selectively and with full comprehension of their relationship to and dependence upon related physical and emotional factors. For example, bathing a patient when he should be developing greater capacity for self-care may retard his recovery, however skillfully done. Similarly, withholding such care or delegating it to someone other than the nurse at a point when the patient needs the security and warmth such attention can give, or an environment conducive to talking out his problems will also have a negative effect, even though the patient or helper may be perfectly capable of providing the necessary physical care. Simple ministration skills may also contribute to or delay physical restoration. The application of a good knowledge of body mechanics may help to prevent deformity in long-term illness, or help to restore arm motion following mastectomy.

The application of therapeutic procedures is based on knowledge of the procedure and its purpose, and also upon manual skills that permit gentle and assured performance. The nurse must be sufficiently familiar with the effects of medication or other therapy to foresee difficulties. The patient with hemiplegia and his family should know that some pain is inevitable with the physical therapy designed to restore motion to paralyzed limbs, and the nurse should be aware of and able to explain why this is so. The nurse supervising the tuberculosis patient taking medication at home should anticipate and prepare the patient for possible gastric distress.

Nursing also includes skills of observation. As in the physical care skills, the process of observation implies awareness of the interrelationship of various factors observed. Observation of the infant, for example, will be related to many factors such as maternal history of syphilis, or of extended or difficult labor, the possible presence of nitrates in the water supply, the competence of the mother, and the temperament of the infant himself.

Health counseling is also an integral component of nursing. Ranging from the giving of information to supportive listening, health counseling involves a sensitive balancing of expert consultation, guidance, and instruction adapted to the patient's physiologic state and to his needs as a human being. Through putting the knowledge and skills of nurse and family or group into a contributory relationship, the resources of both are applied to solving health problems. For example, in rehabilitative care of the postmastectomy patient, the nurse's knowledge of anatomy, of the effects of exercise and of the physiologic and pain responses that may be anticipated with exercise is combined with the family's knowledge of the patient's resistance to pain, the rhythm of the family day, the values that the patient holds dear and that will have a high motivational force. If these are applied so that each can and does contribute, a satisfactory program for exercises can be developed. If the nurse presents her knowledge in a way that makes the family feel she doesn't appreciate their problem, it will not be accepted and hence cannot be put to effective use. If the nurse avoids the family and is therefore unable to analyze the patient's potential for self-help, or to regard her tolerance for pain as a factor to be taken into account and made to work for rather than impede the therapy, the family knowledge cannot be put to work.

Use of Self

The process of Public Health nursing includes the extension of the nurse's professional self toward the family in such a way as to influence favorably its capacity for health, and toward co-workers in such a way as to permit free and productive use of one another's competence for the health program. Peplau says: "nursing is a human relationship between an individual who is sick, or in need of health services, and a nurse especially educated to recognize and to respond to the need for help."[4] This extension of one's self is essentially the communication of an aura of mutual confidence and trust, of valid personal example, and of recognition and strengthening of another's personal capacity.

Channeling Group Energy

In addition to the application of technical skills and personal relationships for the achievement of nursing purposes, Public Health nursing includes the channeling of group energy. Much of Public Health nursing is done with groups—families, classes of school children or school faculties, community groups, committees and conferences. Within each of these groups there is a great amount of potential helping power, which if released and channeled may have great value.

Participating in a Team Relationship

The emergence of the health team concept of care has been commented upon previously. The responsibilities of the Public Health nurse as a team member are set forth with great clarity by Coulter, who points out that team action characterizes every aspect of Public Health nursing practice.[5]

Someone recently said that working as a team member is "more than holding hands." It involves a process of balancing one's own goals with those of others on the team, of sharing as well as differentiating functions, of accepting as well as giving help. The additive services of the physician, the nurse, the teacher, the physical therapist and the parent provided separately to the convalescent poliomyelitis patient may result in fragmented rather than comprehensive care. The nurse must understand the objectives of the physical therapy regimen, and may share in providing treatment under the supervision of the therapist and supervise the parent in carrying out procedures. The physician must understand the nurse's concern and program for protecting the patient from strain, for developing maximum independence in the patient, and helping the teacher to avoid overprotection while at the same time making necessary adjustments in school routines. Each member of the team modifies his own contribution to conform to the whole.

The process of sharing professional responsibility involves clarifying the mutuality of respect and confidence that is basic to joint effort. The social worker must know that the Public Health nurse understands and respects the professional skills of social work, and that sharing certain obligations toward a family such as assistance with food budgets does not mean that either is "taking over" the work of the other. A fine balance between having each worker involved give the most comprehensive possible service while at the same time maintaining professional control by each of the several disciplines included on the team is the objective. This can be achieved only when the team is so organized that it is easy to exchange information, to develop plans and clarify mutual responsibilities and philosophy of service; when each discipline can and does interpret the functions and possible contributions of its field; when the security and confidence of each discipline can be maintained without rigidity in the lines of professional responsibility.

It is important in patient care conferences to be able to make clear to others the fundamentals of the nursing care involved, to report selectively and succinctly the critical factors that will affect the action of others on the team, to avoid professional jurisdictional disputes in favor of shared activity. The team should represent a multiple partnership rather than a hierarchy—with every member a full-fledged participant, and with the leadership shifting as one or the other members represents the greater competence in the particular area of decision or action.

Group Organization

In addition to membership and participation in team activities for health care, administrative or planning committees, and liaison relationships, Public Health nursing must concern itself with the organization of groups to facilitate self-help. One such activity is described by Bond in which she compares the effectiveness of lecture and of discussion group activity in which individuals were asked to make an individual decision or commitment in a group setting. In this situation, which compared matched groups of middle-income women, a significantly larger proportion of those exposed to the discussion-decision procedure sought a physical examination and established a habit of monthly self-examination of the breast than did those in the control groups.[6] To achieve the purposes of joint decision and action, group members are so selected that the individuals in it can help one another. For example, if a prenatal study group includes multiparous as well as primiparous patients, it may be expected that the experienced mother will be able to help the new one; families of bedridden chronically ill patients meeting together, sharing their experiences and perhaps their feelings may give to each a sense of not being alone, and also some very practical ideas for care. Conversely, if the composition of the group puts together people with such antagonism or conflicts of interest that they cannot work together on the problem, the benefits will not accrue. Manipulation of the conditions under which groups meet, and guidance directed toward encouraging each member to make his best contribution to the group are also essential in this process.

In such group organization the Public Health nurse shares responsibility with the health educator, who may in some instances organize the groups and in others provide consultant help to the nurse in her organizational efforts.

Strengthening Group Competence

In many instances—particularly in families—the Public Health nurse is working with ready-made groups. With these, as well as with groups organized for a specific purpose, continuing help is needed to identify and strengthen the capacity of the group to work out its own problems. It may be that there is need for factual information on which to decide what is to be done. It may be that differences in cultural background make it hard for some members to "talk up," even though they have good ideas and need recognition and support to free them of their shyness. Lack of understanding—or, in groups involving different kinds of professional workers, lack of common vocabulary—may create antagonisms and hinder action. Ways must be found through social activities or guided contributions to interpret one to the other, and to facilitate working together.

The process of identifying and strengthening group competence involves analysis based on sound knowledge of individual and group behavior, support and encouragement based on knowledge of the group members and their backgrounds, and leadership based on confidence in the group's ability to think and act wisely for itself, given the necessary facts and a favorable environment.

The process of Public Health nursing is a complex of doing for, of doing with, and most of all of helping others to do for themselves those things which contribute to optimum health, with each step of the process integrally related to the action taken by other professional or family members contributing to the total care of the family or community. It involves a synthesis of providing expert technical and instructional services, of using interpersonal skills better to understand, motivate and guide others in securing the best possible health care, and organizing groups to facilitate productive interchanges of skills and competence and maximum self-help. It borrows and synthesizes skills from many fields—from medicine, from social work, from education, from sociology, from psychology—adding those of nursing itself, to create a service which contributes, and, even more, stimulates and guides others to contribute to the conservation of community health.

1. Kreuter, Frances, "What is Good Nursing Care?" *Nursing Outlook*, 5:302–304, May, 1957.

2. Ferguson, Marion, *The Service Load of a Staff Nurse in One Official Agency*. New York, Bureau of Publications, Teachers College, Columbia University, 1945, p. 29.

3. No One Knows I Have a Colostomy. *American Journal of Nursing*, 51:703–704, December, 1951.

4. Peplau, H., *Interpersonal Relations in Nursing*. New York, G. P. Putnam's Sons, 1952, pp. 5–6.

5. Coulter, Pearl, *The Nurse in the Public Health Program*, Chapter I, "Team Relationship." New York, G. P. Putnam's Sons, 1954.

6. Bond, E., *Group Discussion Decision*. Minneapolis, Minnesota, Minnesota Department of Health, 1956.

5. Public Health Nutrition

New Dimensions for Public Health Nutrition: The Challenge of Chronic Disease and Aging*

DOROTHY M. YOULAND, M.S.

THE SHIFTING FOCUS and enlarging scope of health programs to meet today's changing health needs offer new challenges to nutritionists as well as other health workers. Since the turn of the century the United States population 65 years and older has multiplied four times in contrast to a doubling of the total population. Almost 9 per cent of the total population is now 65 years old or over and it is predicted that the proportion will remain constant in the next decade.

In addition to an aging population, we are faced with an unprecedented number of persons with chronic disease, impairment, or long-term illness. Reports from the National Health Survey[1] show that 70 million persons in the United States have one or more chronic conditions; this amounts to 41 per cent of the noninstitutional civilian population.

While chronic illness may occur in persons of all ages it is found with greater frequency among older persons, and about three of every four persons over age 65 are afflicted with one or more chronic conditions.

The concomitants of aging and the control of long-term illness are amenable to the Public Health method and there is evidence of increased concern and activity in chronic disease programs by official and voluntary health agencies. Today there are over 30 administrative units for chronic disease in state health departments compared to three such units in 1945. Visiting nurse associations report that up to 75 per cent of their total visits are made on behalf of patients with long-term illness.

NUTRITION, CHRONIC DISEASE AND AGING

Nutrition is the most important single factor affecting health. This is true at age 1 or 101, but too often this fact is overlooked in the development of new health programs. Nutrition is a

* Reprinted by permission, with omission of one table, from the March–April, 1961, issue of the *American Journal of Clinical Nutrition*, Vol. 9, pp. 211–216. The author is Nutrition Consultant, Public Health Service, Region II Office, Department of Health, Education, and Welfare, New York, N.Y., formerly Nutrition and Dietetics Officer, Area Office, Division of Indian Health, Public Health Service, Billings, Montana.

specific factor in the prevention and in the control of many chronic diseases.

Weight control is important in the primary prevention and control of certain diseases. Joslin[2] states that obesity is "the most activating factor next to heredity" in the development of diabetes, and he notes that 85 per cent of those persons with diabetes were overweight before the condition was diagnosed. A study of overweight and nonoverweight adults revealed twice as much chronic illness among the overweight group.[3] Persons with diabetes, arthritis, gout, and many forms of heart disease experience better control of these conditions and are more comfortable when they are of normal weight.

The therapy of persons with long-term illness often includes modifications in the kinds and amounts of food eaten. The Commission on Chronic Illness reported[4] that 43 per cent of the patients in general hospitals with long-term illnesses in one state were on some type of "special diet." From several sources[5-9] one obtains the estimated rates per 100,000 population of persons with chronic conditions in which diet plays an important therapeutic role: overweight (10% or more above "desirable weight" for persons 30 years of age or over) 200.0; arthritis and rheumatism (persons 14 years of age or over) 63.9; diabetes, 16.9; tuberculosis, 12.0; ulcers of the stomach or duodenum, 14.4; gallbladder disease, 8.0; and diseases of the liver, 3.8.

The economic status of the elderly is a factor that influences the nutrition of this group. Difficulties in obtaining adequate food loom large for three-fifths of the population aged 65 years and older who have a cash income of less than $1,000 annually[10] and many of these persons need help in learning which foods to select to obtain the most food value at the least cost.

Psychologic, social and physiologic factors also influence the appetite, food intake and nutrition of the aged.

WHAT IS BEING DONE

The majority of state health agencies employ one or more nutritionists and in most states they give some service to chronic disease programs regardless of their administrative placement. In at least ten state health agencies individual nutritionists are administratively responsible to chronic disease directors or give the major portion of their time to chronic disease activities. This is a beginning. Opportunities for nutritionists in new health programs are unlimited in variety and scope.

Public Health nutrition consultation at the Federal level is provided on a categoric basis from the Chronic Disease Program, the Heart Disease Control Program and the Division of Indian Health of the U.S. Public Health Service and from the U.S. Children's Bureau. Only the activities of the Chronic Disease and Heart Disease Control

Programs will be highlighted in this paper, however. Consultants from these programs are concerned particularly with the nutritional and dietary aspects of heart disease, diabetes, services for the aging, nursing home care and organized home care. They work through the Public Health Service Regional offices located in New York City; Charlottesville, Virginia; Atlanta, Georgia; Chicago, Illinois; Kansas City, Missouri; Dallas, Texas; Denver, Colorado; and San Francisco, California, to consult with and advise official and voluntary health agencies upon request. Consultation includes such topics as program planning and evaluation, recruitment and resource materials. Frequently program administrators are advised regarding the potential contribution of nutritionists to chronic disease activities and suggestions may be made about desirable qualifications and recruitment possibilities. The consultants also participate in such activities as educational workshops and conferences, and assist in planning and conducting research and study projects.

Recently one of the consultants assisted a state health department in developing plans for the nutritional aspects of a two-day educational program in diabetes. One health department was given assistance in planning and in carrying out a food service study in selected nursing homes. In another state help was given to the licensing agency regarding an educational program for nursing home administrators. Later the nutritionist contributed to the program by serving as a consultant during the conference.

The development of guide materials for use by the patient and professional worker is also an important contribution. Nutritionists from the Chronic Disease and Heart Disease Control Programs collaborated with professional organizations in the development of the standardized, simplified materials for use by persons with diabetes or who require sodium-restricted diets. The nutritionists have also participated in the preparation of filmstrips, records, and other material for patient and professional diabetes education. They are contributing to the development of recipe booklets for use with sodium-restricted diets and materials for physicians regarding fat- and cholesterol-restricted diets. A visual aid in the form of a flipchart has been developed to assist professional personnel with food service training programs for nursing home personnel. This teaching tool and an accompanying Instructor's Guide have been made available to state health departments.

The nutritionist at the federal, State or local level offers to chronic disease and aging programs her knowledge concerning food habits of the population served, the nutritional needs of specific groups, and how to plan and prepare food to meet these needs, the availability and cost of food in the community. The nutritionist's training in the dietary aspects of the treatment of medical conditions enables her to make contributions to professional and lay persons regarding the care of the chronically ill and aged. Her knowledge of quantity feeding and institutional management is useful in developing programs with nursing homes and other group care facilities. Skills in interviewing and nutrition educational technics enable her to work effectively in all of these newer programs.

Patient Education

Weight control projects by the "group method" have been conducted by a number of Public Health nutritionists who have joined forces with colleagues in medicine, agricultural extension service, nursing and health education for such ventures. Some states have developed cooperative programs which are continuing. In others, the Public Health nutritionist has been the catalyst to encourage and assist interested, qualified groups to sponsor group classes.

Persons with diabetes usually need assistance in following the diet plan prescribed by their physicians, and benefit from understanding food values. In several States, nutrition units have offered group diet instruction to such patients. Impetus for such programs and details of carrying them out may vary, but such activities should have the support and approval of organized medicine; they require individual patient referral by the physician. In a midwestern state, nutrition education for patients with diabetes was an outgrowth of diabetes case-finding programs. At the time persons suspected of having diabetes were referred to their physicians for diagnosis and follow-up, the physicians were invited to refer newly diagnosed diabetic patients to group classes conducted by health department personnel.

In an eastern State health department nutritionists conducted classes regularly for persons with diabetes at the request of the local medical society and in cooperation with the local dietetic association. Frequently, and preferably, nutritionists join forces with other professional health workers so that diet instruction is provided as part of an over-all guidance to the diabetic patient.

Public Health nutritionists are finding increasing opportunities to work with state and local voluntary associations on behalf of persons who require sodium-restricted diets. Classes similar to those for persons with diabetes have been held in a number of places.

Services to Institutions

One estimate[10] indicates that as a group persons over age 65 use two and a half times as much general hospital care as the average for persons under 65 years of age. According to Solon[11] nursing home beds are occupied by persons whose average age is 80, and

25,000 "homes" provide nursing or supportive services to chronically ill, convalescing, aged, disabled or infirm persons. These facilities, and approximately 3,500 small general hospitals (with bed capacities of less than 100), are focal points for service from Public Health nutritionists. Most of these institutions, because they are small, employ nonprofessional food service personnel. Administrators and staff need assistance with menu planning, food purchasing, therapeutic diets and other aspects of food service as well as with patient education. Nutritionists participate in training food service workers and offer consultation to administrators in a number of states. They also assist licensing agency personnel in their evaluation of food services in these facilities.

The nutritionist in one city health department assists the nursing home program in a number of ways. When the prospective administrator visits the health department to apply for a license, he meets with the nutritionist as well as other members of the staff. From them he learns the requirements he must meet to comply with the regulations and the services available from the department. With the cooperation of the nursing home association regular group meetings on nutrition and food service are presented for operators of existing homes. The nutritionist in this department, and a number of others from the East Coast to the far west, are responsible for periodic newsletters on food service which are distributed to nursing homes and other small institutions.

In a number of States, Public Health nutritionists have taken the leadership to develop, or have cooperated in the preparation of, diet manuals. These have been intended primarily to improve the quality of general and therapeutic diets in small institutions, but frequently they have served also to standardize and modernize diet therapy practices.

Assistance to institutions is provided in many other ways such as preparation of food service manuals; distribution of menu planning forms and nutrition guides; help in the selection and use of equipment; suggestions about kitchen layout and work simplification technics.

"Meals on Wheels"

"Meals on Wheels" is the name given to programs which deliver meals regularly to elderly, homebound persons who are unable or disinterested in preparing food for themselves.[12] Based on an idea originated in England, the programs have great public appeal and have been developed in about 20 localities in the United States. Nutritionists can assist in evaluating the community need for this type of program and in working out the details of preparing and serving attractive meals for a modest fee. In one state, nutritionists work with the sponsors to help insure menus of high quality and to assist in evaluating the service periodically. In another program sponsored by a voluntary agency, the nutritionist assumes all administrative details of the food service.

Organized Home Care

The role of the nutritionist in organized home-care programs has been delineated recently.[13] This is an area in which nutrition service has a great potential yet to be developed in most of the 60 programs in operation today. The nutritionist in one county health department gives regular service to an organized home-care program in her community; she not only attends all planning and evaluation conferences and consults with the professional staff on selected cases, but also gives direct service to some patients in their homes.

FUTURE TRENDS

What of the future for Public Health nutrition in new health programs? It seems inevitable that the amount and intensity of effort on behalf of the well and sick middle-aged and older adult will increase. Hopefully nutrition programs of the future will be geared to give adequate service to everyone throughout the span of life.

One group, which may well receive more emphasis in nutrition education programs, are middle-aged adults. Nutrition should be included in preretirement counseling programs that are becoming popular in industry. In one series in which this was done the nutrition session had the highest rating in the class evaluation. Also nutrition in its preventive and therapeutic aspects must be included more frequently in the health education programs of industry by such means as providing written materials, by working with industrial nurses and by giving individual nutrition counseling.

Dietary counseling is another field which holds promise for the future. Such counseling helps nonhospitalized patients understand and follow prescribed dietary regimens adapted to their individual needs. The Public Health nutritionist is in a unique position to see that such service is available. Depending on the local situation she may help to develop a referral system for exchange of pertinent diet information between the hospital and other community agencies, or she may assist in setting up a program to give individual counseling to persons referred by physicians. In any event she can assist Public Health nurses by providing them with necessary tools and technics to advise patients about diet.

There are about 5.5 million persons in the United States (or 3 per cent of the population) who have chronic mobility limitation.[1] Most of these persons can be restored to levels of self-care. Medical rehabilitation programs are organized to enable chronically ill, disabled or aged patients to maintain or recover functional capacity for the physical, mental and social demands of daily living. This requires the services and skills of all members of the health team. The nutritionist's role in restorative services has barely been touched, although she has much to contribute to professional staff and patients. Unless disabled persons are in a good state of nutrition how can they possibly have stamina to use crutches or to relearn the simple "activities of daily living" that spell the difference between a bare existence and a meaningful life? A nutritional history, taken on each person at the rehabilitation center or hospital, plus follow-up assistance to interpret and assist in making desirable diet changes, is one example of the service the nutritionist can provide.

What about the elderly person who is at home and is unwilling or unable to prepare food for himself? As already stated "Meals on Wheels" represents one method of providing food for such persons. The serving of hot meals at senior citizens' centers is being tried in a few places; one home for the aged offers noon day meals to nonresidents who wish to purchase this service. Other ways to provide food service to oldsters should be studied and nutritionists may need to stimulate such exploration.

SUMMARY

Public Health nutrition has specific and valuable contributions to make to programs focused on chronic disease and aging. In this new and challenging field the ways in which nutritionists can function are limitless. A few examples have been given to illustrate some ways nutritionists are serving and may increase services to their professional colleagues and the public in newer Public Health programs.

1. U. S. National Health Survey. Health Statistics. Limitation of Activity and Mobility Due to Chronic Conditions. United States, July 1957–June 1958. Public Health Service Publication No. 584–B11. Washington, D.C., 1959. U. S. Government Printing Office.

2. Joslin, E. P., Root, H. F., White, P. and Marble, A. The Treatment of Diabetes Mellitus, 10th ed, p. 94. Philadelphia, 1959. Lea & Febiger.

3. Hundley, J. M. In: Weight Control—A Collection of Papers Presented at the Weight Control Colloquium. pp. 11–12. Ames, 1955. Iowa State College Press.

4. Krueger, D. E., and Roberts, D. W. Characteristics of long term patients. Hospitals, 30, 15 (Pt. I) : 47, 1956.

5. Division of Special Health Services, P.H.S. Estimated prevalence of overweight in the United States. Pub. Health Rep., 69:1084, 1954.

6. U. S. National Health Survey. Health Statistics. Arthritis and Rheumatism Reported in Interviews, July

1957–June 1959. Public Health Service. Publication No. 584–B20. Washington, D.C., 1960. U. S. Government Printing Office.

7. U. S. National Health Survey. Health Statistics. Peptic Ulcer Reported in Interviews, July 1957–June 1959. Public Health Service Publication No. 584–B17. Washington, D.C., 1960. U. S. Government Printing Office.

8. Roberts, D. W. and Glasser, M. Chronic illness in an urban area. A progress report. Chronic Illness News Letter 6, November 1955.

9. West, M. D. and Altenderfer, M. E. Illness and Medical Care in Hagerstown, Md. I. The Prevalence of Chronic Disease 1955–57 as Measured by Household Interviews. Washington, D.C., 1958. Division of Public Health Methods, P.H.S.

10. Flemming, A. S. Hospitalization Insurance for OASDI Beneficiaries. Report submitted to the Committee on Ways and Means by the Secretary of Health, Education and Welfare, April 3, 1959. Washington, D.C., 1959. U. S. Government Printing Office.

11. Solon, J. and Baney, A. M. Inventory of nursing homes and related facilities. *Pub. Health Rep.*, 69:1121, 1954.

12. Keller, M. D. and Smith, C. E. Meals on Wheels: 1960. *Geriatrics*, in press.

13. Kaufman, M. and Bryan, M. S. The nutritionist in an organized home care program. *Pub. Health Rep.*, 74:873, 1959.

6. Public Health Dentistry

Trends in Dental Public Health in the United States and Canada*

DONALD J. GALAGAN, D.D.S.

DENTAL PUBLIC HEALTH PROGRAMS—if they are to have any meaning —must be a forceful expression of the interests and the needs of people. They cannot be planned, talked about, or judged apart from the social, intellectual, and economic context in which they exist. Over the last 15 or 20 years that context has been vastly altered. As a result, both the scope and content of dental programs also have changed.

The most important of the broader social trends influencing the dental and Public Health professions in both the United States and Canada is, without question, the gradual acceptance of increasing responsibility on the part of government for the health and welfare of its citizens.

Evidence of this social movement, which has found expression in a series of legislative proposals and actions, can be seen most clearly in Canada, particularly in its western Provinces. There, social legislation affecting health services has been broadened rapidly during the last decade. The Hospital Insurance Act and the Saskatchewan Medical Care Insurance Act are the best known examples.

In both countries the influence of community forces on the health professions is increasing steadily. Nothing which has happened in the last 30 years is of greater significance or of more importance to dental Public Health. This increasing influence of community forces clearly means that the public views good health care as a right, not a privilege. It means that on this continent neither the medical nor the dental profession can arbitrarily organize and control its practice without due respect for the wishes and the needs of the community. It means that, inevitably, there will be changes in the methods of organizing and delivering health services, including dental care.

These changes in social philosophy have altered the role of the Public Health dentist as well as the attitudes of the dental profession toward that role. Where once the Public Health dentist was looked

* Reprinted by permission from the August, 1963, issue of *Public Health Reports*, Vol. 78, pp. 649–654. This paper was given as an address at the American Dental Association Pan American Conference on Dental Public Health held in Miami Beach, Florida, on October 27, 1962. The author is chief, Division of Dental Public Health and Resources, Public Health Service, Department of Health, Education, and Welfare, Washington, D.C.

upon with some suspicion, now he is more likely to be seen by the dental profession as a friend and ally in a rapidly changing world.

Thoughtful leaders within the profession realize that the trend toward more formal planning for social purposes is not a plot fabricated by the Public Health profession but a reflection of a basic change in the attitudes of the people. The Public Health dentist, with his understanding of professional problems and his competence in community affairs, can be a decisive influence in the development of health programs which serve the best interests of both the public and the dental profession. That is exactly the role that today's Public Health dentists are trying to assume.

Against this background of major change in society's attitude toward government and professional attitude about Public Health, I should like to review some trends in dental Public Health on this continent in order to show what we are doing and why and how we are going about it.

PROFESSIONAL MANPOWER

The first trend in public health practice is the increasing concern by health agencies about the broad problems of professional manpower. A few years ago, when we spoke of manpower, we were referring to a problem whose outline was only beginning to emerge. Because population growth in both Canada and the United States was out of all proportion to growth in the number of practicing dentists, we knew that we were headed for trouble.

We recognized, however vaguely, that existing levels of supply were substandard. They passed as adequate only because the majority of those in need of treatment seldom saw a dentist. We believed it foolish to assume that future levels of dental demand could either be permitted or expected to remain unchanged.

The first efforts by health agencies to explore the manpower problem were designed to develop a realistic formula for long-range projections of the need for dentists. The formula was developed, and today we not only know approximately how many dentists we must train to pace population increases, but we also understand more clearly the impact which economic growth and such social changes as urbanization and higher educational levels have on dental demand and dental manpower requirements.

What we know is not encouraging. Simply to maintain current ratios, both Canada and the United States must increase markedly the number of dentists they train. Public Health agencies are therefore no longer concentrating solely upon the demonstration of a need for an increase in professional resources; they are actively engaged in the practical business of meeting that need.

There is, first of all, an intensification of effort in both Canada and the United States to build additional training facilities—the equivalent of some 20 larger-than-average schools for the United States, a near doubling of present capacity for Canada. With this expansion, Canada will be able to improve her supply ratios somewhat. The United States will be able to avoid any further decline in relative supply.

In the United States, the Department of Health, Education, and Welfare is sponsoring legislation which would authorize Federal Government grants for the construction of dental schools. The American Dental Association, the American Association of Dental Schools, and other professional organizations have testified before Congress in favor of this legislation. The Canadian Dental Association, in its brief to the Royal Commission on Health Services, has recommended the construction of four new schools and the expansion of several others. In each country the dental profession, in recommending and supporting Federal aid, has served notice that school expansion is not a need which should concern only the profession. The public at large must share this responsibility, a change the public seems willing to accept.

What else needs to be done? Obviously the available dental manpower will have to become more productive. One way of accomplishing this objective is to make greater use of auxiliary personnel. In the United States, the Public Health Service has been working closely with the dental profession and dental educators in teaching student dentists how to work with chairside assistants. We began with a few experimental projects because we had to learn what should be taught and how to teach it. These projects were eminently successful, and through a system of support grants, almost all U.S. dental schools now include in undergraduate programs training in the use of chairside assistants.

Yet we have never agreed on the nature or the extent of the assistant's role. What should we train these young women to do? The answer to that question cannot be given simply in terms of our own personal preferences and prejudices. What we say must be a measure of the future, not the past. The Commission on Survey of Dentistry puts it this way:[1a] "The full contribution of auxiliary personnel to dental practice will not be fully realized merely by increasing their numbers. A careful reexamination of the functions of the hygienist and the assistant is in order. However reluctant to do so, the profession should analyze the dentist's technical procedures and determine those that can be delegated to lesser trained personnel."

I believe that the profession is ready to support some significant changes in the functions of auxiliaries and this itself is a significant trend. Consider the fact that a little more than a decade ago, the dentists in this country abruptly terminated an experiment to evaluate the usefulness of the auxiliary that New Zealand calls the dental nurse. Yet, today it is the official policy of the American Dental Association to encourage experimentation with the duties of auxiliaries. There has been a parallel change in attitude in Canada, where the dental association, pointing to "the veritable impossibility of a major improvement" in the dentist-population ratio, regards an extension of the auxiliary's duties, particularly the hygienist's, as an important ingredient in manpower planning. These policies are an official and intelligent admission that there are tasks performed by the dentist which could be performed just as well by someone with less education.

In view of the legislation's authorizing experimentation with hygienists' training in Canada, with the formal training of assistants beginning here, and with the building of several new dental schools a real possibility in both countries, we should be acting more incisively upon that admission. For any significant redistribution of duties will obviously affect what we teach and where and how we teach it. Our future schools and their curriculums should be designed accordingly.

Because the definite trend toward a general manpower shortage is possibly one of the most serious dental health problems of our times, it has become, and rightly so, the focal point of a great deal of Public Health activity. But some particular shortages also demand careful attention. These shortages will not be automatically solved by an increase in numbers.

There is a shortage of dentists in rural areas. Some more remote sections of Canada and the United States have no dentists at all. Dental care may never be available in such areas unless special effort is made to attract a resident practitioner or to provide, as an alternative, the services of traveling dentists in mobile units.

The use of traveling dentists is standard in several Canadian Provinces. In the United States this practice has been given an interesting and valuable twist: in some areas, mobile units owned by the dental society are manned by private practitioners. But the best solution is obviously the resident practitioner. The question is how to recruit him for areas offering little in the way of cultural fringe benefits.

Canadian dentists propose a possible solution. They would have dental schools give preference to qualified students from rural areas. They also suggest bonuses for dentists who agree to locate in areas which currently have no practitioners. Intense student recruitment programs by local dental societies is another possibility, one that a Canadian society has tried with marked success.

Dental health programs, especially those at the State and local levels, have been hampered by shortages of both men and money. Canada also is faced with a similar situation. The people in each country pay a high price for this brand of economy. For many of the programs which could materially reduce the incidence of dental dis-eases and the pyramiding of unmet dental needs continue to be no more than modest miniatures of the real thing.

RESEARCH IN DENTAL PUBLIC HEALTH

This brings me to the second trend which can be identi-fied. Happily, it is possible to say that the people in both countries are far more aware of the problems in dental Public Health and more interested in seeing them solved than they have ever been before. The dental profession has played a leading part in arousing their interest and concern. Public Health agencies and the Canadian and American Dental Associations have pointed up the inequities which exist be-tween the budgets allocated to dental activities and to those of the other health sciences. In both countries, independent study commis-sions established to assess the status of dental health have strongly recommended that official health agencies at national and State or provincial levels expand and extend their dental Public Health programs.

One sobering aspect of current dental Public Health practice is the almost total neglect of research in methods of program operation and administration. In the last 10 years, there has been a tremendous increase in basic and clinical research in dentistry. In 1962, more than $17 million was allocated to the National Institute of Dental Research alone for support of intramural and extramural research and research training, more than 24 times its allocation in 1952. More than 140 institutions are receiving support from the National Institute of Dental Research for research, training, and fellowships. Yet almost none of this increased emphasis has been directed to research in Public Health practice.

This is not a problem to be dismissed lightly or excused on the basis of first things first. Our real reason for being in Public Health is to put the findings of basic research to work for the benefit of the public, to use knowledge with the greatest effectiveness in the shortest possible time. If we fail, then much of the point of learning is lost, and the public is less than well served.

As an example, through basic epidemiologic research we have the controlled fluoridation of public water supplies, a safe, economical, highly effective preventive for dental caries. Yet over the last few years, efforts to institute community fluoridation programs have failed more often than they have succeeded.

We do not really understand why this should be true. And though the future of fluoridation depends upon our knowing, we have not, as the Commission on the Survey of Dentistry points out, made much of an effort to learn.[1b] Only one university and one Public Health agency are engaged in any extensive research to discover the reasons for nonacceptance or how fluoridation can be effectively promoted.

Basic and clinical research will certainly continue to increase. We will be given new methods of prevention and control as a consequence. If variations on the pattern of acceptance of fluoridation are not to occur with each new discovery, then it is incumbent upon us to expend much more time and effort on research in program administration, community health practices, and the whole broad field of communication.

The absence of progress and the lack of a discernible trend in dental Public Health research in this instance is of real concern, and as significant as more desirable developments. A larger portion of all future dental grants must be devoted to research in Public Health. I would like to see the establishment of strong college courses, postgraduate and continuation training, and workshops in research methods in community health practice. I would like, in short, to see our ability to use knowledge keep pace with out ability to attain it.

The complexities of modern society are creating dental problems too big to be solved by any one group, too serious to be overcome by remedies out of the past. That is why public and private dental organizations are working together in planning coordinated corrective and preventive programs. That is why dental Public Health is committed to action—action which either supplements the efforts of private dentistry or strikes at problems whose solutions lie beyond the prevailing patterns of dental practice.

Once, in any effort to bridge the gulf between need and demand for dental services, the role of dental Public Health was largely that of health educator. We simply tried to improve our technics of teaching good health habits and of convincing people that adequate dental treatment was essential to their well-being.

Today we continue to be educators to the public, but this is only one facet of our responsibility—not its sum total. However well they learn the value of dental treatment, people cannot profit from learning if there is no care available to them. Many are sick, old, poor, or are emotionally disturbed. Dental care remains beyond their reach. Since there are people like this, there must be public agencies willing to accept the responsibility of providing dental care. Health agencies are already providing services to many beneficiaries of public welfare, although too often the majority receive only emergency care.

We have made notable progress in developing the treatment technics needed for the chronically ill and aged. We are conducting prototype programs for the care of handicapped children, the victims of cerebral palsy and the mentally or emotionally disturbed. There is a trend on the part of community and State Public Health agencies to offer continuing care programs for all such disadvantaged groups on a communitywide basis.

But millions of people in the United States are neither poor enough to qualify for public assistance nor yet able to pay readily for the dental services they require when they require them. It may be that the great majority of the financial in-betweens in this particular group can be brought within the pattern of private practice through one of the systems of prepaid insurance for financing health care. Hospital and surgical insurance are already an American commonplace, so much so that most people, whatever their income bracket, have coverage of one kind or another.

DENTAL PREPAYMENT PLANS

A last trend, barely discernible, is becoming clearer each day. Dental prepayment plans are relatively new, and they still lag far behind medical coverage both in the number of plans available and in the number of people enrolled. Ten years ago, coverage for dental care was almost unheard of. Today, 876,000 people are enrolled in private plans offering continuing services, and, in addition, 350,000 public welfare patients are being served through dental service corporations. Furthermore, it has been estimated that 15 million people will be under dental prepayment plans in another 10 years. Some estimates, looking to a mass demand from labor unions, run much higher, but the more conservative estimate is big enough to underscore the importance of prepayment to the future of dental health and dental practice.

In Canada, somewhat the same trend is evident. Dental care programs for about 200,000 public assistance beneficiaries are operating in five Provinces. Dental treatment is provided by private practitioners on a fee-for-service basis, the bills are paid from public funds, and the provincial dental society administers the program. The development of contracts with nongovernment groups has not yet materialized in Canada, although the dental profession has done some preliminary work in preparation for prepayment plans.

The development of dental insurance plans emphasizes the urgency of manpower planning. It most decidedly suggests that both dental Public Health and private dentistry have a stake in the future of these plans. If they are carefully constructed and administered, they can raise the levels of demand without any sacrifice in the quality of the care. They can raise the dental health standard of the general public without interfering in any way with the prerogatives of the dental profession. But it should be remembered that predictions of future growth in prepayment are in no way dependent upon the willingness of the profession to guide that growth. These plans will continue to increase if the people want them, with or without the assistance of the dental profession.

Both self-interest and the public interest can best be served if private dentistry and Public Health step up current studies of prepayment, develop prototype programs offering a variety of plans and approaches, and, at the same time, work closely with those private groups and organizations who are ready to begin a prepayment plan and are looking to the profession for help. To do less than this can only lead to chaos and a loss of professional prestige.

Neither these changes in approach nor the programs they produce are universally popular. Many dentists still consider any change in past or present practice arrangements as detrimental. They deny that prepayment dental care plans are necessary or even wanted. There are dentists who refuse even to consider the possible impact of insurance plans because they are opposed to them on principle. By opposing, they think, they end them.

Certainly life would be a good deal simpler if the public were committed to a doctrine of dental infallibility, if every problem dissolved beneath our disapproving stare. I doubt that either the public or the problems will be so obliging.

Consider the course of events in certain Canadian Provinces where, in the face of a strong professional opposition, dental mechanics have been licensed to make dentures directly for the public. The Canadian Dental Association diagnoses the probable causes as the shortage of dentists, the increase in the number of older people requiring appliances, "and perhaps the growing desire to buy everything at a discount—even health services."[2]

The problems which threaten dental health standards are no longer the exclusive concern of the dental profession; they are of deep concern to the general public as well. More importantly, the action needed to solve those problems is no longer the sole responsibility or right of dental professions. The public also has a decisive role to play in determining what the goals in dental health should be and in working to attain them.

The public has a responsibility to provide for the expansion of dental training facilities, a responsibility it proposes to meet through governmental aid to school construction. Effective public action can also bring into being the stronger dental Public Health staffs and activities that are so desperately needed. The marshaling of public interest and public action at the community level is the best hope we have of building the special programs which are necessary to care for the aged and the handicapped. Fluoridation can become a fact in hundreds of communities through incisive action by lay groups. With the advent of prepaid dental care plans, the public can finally and effectively bridge the financial gulf which separates so many people from the care they need.

In all of these areas, it will be the public's actions or the public's refusal to act which shapes the future of dental health. In none of them can the profession hope to exercise an effective veto. I see no reason why we should want to do so.

What we can do is to realize that growing public concern, far from being unwarranted interference, is one of the most valuable of our dental resources. Through the leadership of both Public Health and private dentists public interest and support can be translated into realistic, hard-hitting preventive and remedial action. Out of it we can hammer programs which serve the public's interest and protect our profession's standards. To do otherwise—to assume, in such an age as this, that dental Public Health and dental practice alone are mysteriously immune to change and alteration—is, at the very least, self-deluding. This assumption could be dangerous, a needless abrogation of professional prerogatives and an indefensible evasion of professional responsibilities.

1. Final report of the Commission on the Survey of Dentistry in the United States. American Council on Education, Washington, D.C., 1961, (a) p. 88; (b) p. 52.

2. Brief submitted to the Royal Commission on Health Services by the Canadian Dental Association, 1962, p. 17.

7. Health Education

Perception and Public Health*

GORDON W. ALLPORT, PH.D.

IN INAUGURATING the Dorothy B. Nyswander Lectures a year ago, Dr. Mayhew Derryberry prepared the ground for this evening's discussion. He made clear that during Dr. Nyswander's distinguished career of service—and partly through her leadership—the outlook and duties of health education have changed, and principally in the direction of closer cooperation with psychological and social science.[1]

At the time when Dr. Nyswander expanded her psychologic interests to include the field of Public Health, terror of infectious diseases was still uppermost. Since these specific scourges had specific causes, research in Public Health meant chiefly finding the antitoxin or antibiotic that would defeat the invading microbe. This work required little cooperation or knowledge on the part of the ordinary citizen. He was not deeply involved in sanitary engineering, water purification or rodent control. But he did develop, thanks to Public Health education, a "bacterio-technological perspective on illness."[2] He became vaccine conscious, as the recent rush of the public for Salk vaccine shows. Miracle cures he now understands; and his faith in them is still growing.

But where is the vaccine to prevent mental breakdowns, to lead people to early examinations for cardiac and cancer conditions, to abolish harmful practices of eating, sleeping and recreation, to control alcoholic and other addictions, to eliminate reckless automobile driving, to establish wholesome practices of child training? Health workers agree that we have now entered an era when the human factor—the whims, values, and perceptions of the ordinary citizen—must be considered before further progress can be made. Future advances will require the consent and cooperation of people. It is the public part of Public Health that will increasingly concern us.

It is not possible to review in a single lecture all the exciting ad-

* Reprinted with permission granted by the Society's Committee on Monographs, from *Health Education Monographs*, Number 2, 1958, pp. 2–15, published by the Society of Public Health Educators, Inc., 81 Hillside Road, Rye, New York. This paper was delivered as the second Dorothy B. Nyswander Lecture in Berkeley, California on May 23, 1958, a lectureship established in honor of Dr. Nyswander upon her retirement as Professor of Health Education at the University of California at Berkeley. The author is Professor of Psychology, Department of Social Relations, Harvard University, Cambridge, Massachusetts.

vances in social science that have potential value for future progress in Public Health. You are already familiar with many of these developments, perhaps especially those concerned with opinion and communication, with leadership and group process, with differing ethnic and regional requirements of Public Health work. For my assignment I have chosen to talk about perception and Public Health because I think it deals with a less well-known tie between your profession and mine. In practical terms the question I wish to examine is this: *Does the receiver hear and comprehend the health message as the health educator intends?*

THE PARADOX OF PERCEPTION

A traveler to Naples tells the following story. Arriving at his hotel overlooking the fabulously beautiful bay, his cab driver burst forth in rapture. Although the driver had seen the lovely view a thousand times he cried out, *"Come e bello, come e bello!"* The traveler agreed with his ecstatic driver and entered his hotel. There the inn keeper confided that he was having much trouble with a rich American oil magnate who had come to Naples to escape boredom in his retirement. But this American, after glancing at the view had merely sniffed: "Just trees and water and a city—I've seen them thousands of times." Hiring a taxi he drove to Pompeii and returned full of wrath. "I've seen enough good houses in my lifetime," he said, "without going to look at a lot that are in ruins." The oil magnate retreated to his only solace—a concoction made of schnapps and champagne. A few weeks later he developed delirium tremens and was shipped back to the United States.

The story illustrates our first principle: *environment may be less a matter of physical surroundings than of perception.* Two men in the same geographic spot do not live in the same environment. It is for this reason that a health worker, even though he does not alter his approach in the slightest degree as he goes from house to house, may be perceived as threatening or consoling, as a friend to be welcomed or as a pest to be avoided. The worker thinks that he plays a steadfast professional role; but he doesn't. Like the Bay of Naples, he is two things to two perceivers—and 10 things to ten perceivers.

But here we run into the prime paradox of perception: there *is* after all a Bay of Naples. Even while the process of perceiving is subjectively swayed it is likewise objectively anchored. Perception is governed by both outer and by inner factors; in the language of Plato, "the light within meets the light without." What we see and hear is, therefore, both veridical and distorted, both true and false.

The fact that we perceive the world around us fairly accurately is due to the evolution of sensory and brain processes well tuned to outer reality. Eyes perceive color, line, and shape with exquisite fineness; ears register accurately a wide range of air vibrations. The skin, less perfect in sensitiveness, still mediates evidence of shape and the finer gradations of temperature. The reason for this mirroring ability is undoubtedly its "functional usefulness." The organism has a better chance of survival if the sensory equipment is finally accurate. In a recent book, Woodworth rightly maintains that the first and foremost motive in life is man's pervasive need to handle his world competently.[3] For Woodworth the process of perception is the fundamental dynamism serving man's fundamental motive.

Yet by following the same line of reasoning we can say the perceptual process must likewise depart from true mirroring in order to be of maximum use to us. Not every tree in the forest comes into perceptual focus, but only the one we are chopping. Not every object on the dinner table is perceived with clarity, but only the bite we are about to put into our mouths. If you hear a babble of vague conversation how quickly *your* name stands out if it is mentioned. Selective perception is as much a functional necessity as is veridical perception.

In coping with our world it would not be enough to follow only "the light without." We have first to select what we shall see; in so doing we become hypervigilant toward some cues, and indifferent or actively defensive toward others. We perceive in order to cope; but coping means more than passive mirroring; it means the fulfilling of our needs; it means finding safety and reassurance, love and self-respect, freedom from worry, opportunities for growth, and ultimately a satisfying meaning for our existence. Thus it comes about that our coping may be best served by disregarding some stimuli entirely, by modifying our interpretation of others, and by blending incoming meanings with our past habits, present needs, and future directions.

The point is illustrated in a recent health investigation conducted by Dr. Dorrian Apple of the Boston University School of Nursing. Her problem was to determine when people "perceive" sickness, that is to say, what configuration of experience tells them that they, or someone else, is "sick." The answer is that the symptoms must be *actively present* now; they must be *acute and well-defined;* and they must lead to an *impairment of activity*. These criteria are additive; a really sick person will show all three conditions. Thus a man with fever and head cold, unable to go to work, is perceived as "sick." But a man with a vague and chronic discomfort in the chest who suffers no interruption in his daily duties is seldom seen as "sick."[4] From the health worker's point of view, of course, the latter case may be far more seriously ill than the former, and may need medical attention more urgently. But how shall the health worker deal with a sick person who perceives no sickness?

And when a person does perceive that he is ill, how greatly his perceptual field changes: objects previously of interest lose their demand; the health visitor is no longer perceived as a busybody but as an angel of mercy; bodily functions loom large; minor as well as major discomforts fill the horizon. Charles Lamb wrote, "How sickness enlarges the dimensions of a man's self to himself! He is his own exclusive object. Supreme selfishness is inculcated upon him as his only duty."[5] In illness the "bacterio-technological perspective" of which we have spoken melts away. The sick person cannot take the impersonal, aseptic view of the health worker even though he may pretend to do so. He is sensitized, as is the child, to his own fears, and to signs of love and support from those who care for him. Small matters arouse aggression or querulousness, ill humor or shame. An inadvertent frown on the face of the examining doctor or health worker may be perceived as a prophecy of doom.[6] A proud adult may even view his illness as a reflection on his heredity and therefore as a disgrace to his family. Verily the perceptual worlds of health and disease are not the same.

PERCEPT OR PROCEPT?

Before examining the application of modern perceptual research to health education may I invite your close attention to a current technical issue in the psychology of perception?

Up to now I have been employing the term *perception* broadly, as indeed many psychologists today do. There is good reason for this broad usage.

Psychologists have always known that perception is the process of adding meaning to sensory input. It is the process that creates a stable environment out of what would otherwise be a chaos of unsorted sensory impressions. Perception is the stabilizer of our mental life. While this fact has been known, psychologists' curiosity until recently was restricted to a few standard laboratory problems. Size and depth, localization and movement were studied on the assumption that somehow the structure of the outer world is cast in a veridical manner upon our sense organs—the few minor exceptions being known as "illusions."

Then, suddenly, less than two decades ago, psychologists grew excited by the discovery—though they should have known it all along—that perception is not merely the faithful translation of outer configurations into inner experience. Perception is profoundly influenced by two additional factors: by social and cultural custom, and by the personality of the perceiver. We sense what the outer world offers, yes, but we sense it through social and personal lenses.

So startling was the discovery that it became known as the "new look" theory of perception, deriving its nickname from the then current fashion in women's clothes. The theory has not yet been displaced by the "sack" or the "trapeze."

The theory says, in brief, that unless the external stimulus is unusually strong and compelling, what we perceive is a blend of the external message and of our own subjective meanings. Innumerable experiments have by now established the fact that the words we hear or the sights we see (at least if these are not compellingly clear and well structured) are influenced by subjective conditions. Among these conditions various investigators have identified the influence of hunger, thirst, fear, hate; likewise, the influence of deep-lying interests and values, traits of temperament, and of one's total character-structure and way of looking at life.[7]

The specific influence of social and cultural customs likewise shapes our perception of words, of time, and of worth. Examples of so-called *social perception* are to be found in Benjamin Paul's book, *Health, Culture and Community.* For instance, an American physician in a village in India will be perceived as a powerful and revered figure if only he pronounces the confident words, "The patient will recover." But in Chile the same degree of confident prediction may make the physician seem arrogant and hence to be distrusted.[8] In India a cow that falls sick on the streets of a city may be perceived as an object of compassion, whereas a dying man who falls down on the same street is avoided because to touch him would bring defilement.

To return to our technical problem: I have said that the enthusiasm of psychologists for the "new look" discoveries led them to use the concept of perception somewhat promiscuously.

Now a specialist is known by the words he uses carefully. Among the "careful" words for the psychologist should certainly be *perception.* But even if used scrupulously the concept inevitably covers the energy from the stimulus, receptor activity, a sensory core projected and organized through expectancy and intention, blended with subtle muscular adjustments, and capped by a lightning process of categorization made possible by bewilderingly swift associations with past experience—the whole baffling sequence occupying a split second, and resulting in a firm and well-configurated experience of objectified meaning. Yes, even the most careful use of perception must cover all these interlocking processes.

At the same time the term should not be extended to cover other so-called higher mental operations. It should not be stretched to include the judgment, reflection, evaluation or emotional response that follow rapidly on a percept; nor should it cover the subsequent trains of memory, imagination, and motor performance that ensue. Strictly speaking, a percept is a quasi-sensory organization—though involving central as well as peripheral processes—located "out there." It is a complex interpretation of sensory experience, but it is not coextensive with the whole of mental life.

To illustrate the point: suppose you ask a sample of people this question: *Would you agree that the world is a hazardous place where men are basically evil and dangerous?* If you do so you are likely to receive about half of your replies *Yes,* and about half *No.* Now, do those who reply affirmatively really *perceive* the world as threatening and *perceive* men as evil, or do they merely *judge* them to be so? Neither term is entirely satisfactory. To "judge" is to make an intellectual assertion, whereas a person who gives you an affirmative answer is likely to have such a deep-seated suspicious outlook that he actually *sees* malice in people's faces, much as did H. A. Murray's children after they had played a scarey game of "murder."[9] A person with such a deep suspicion might, on opening the door to a health worker, actually *see* the visitor as having a hostile face and menacing manner. At the same time not every distrustful attitude or activity is a perception. In his extensive analysis of research and theories of perception, F. H. Allport has shown that often what is called a percept is in reality the judgment of a percept or a response to a percept.

The truth of the matter is that psychologists today are in a predicament. While the classical account of perception is not adequate, it does offer us at least two concepts of direct pertinence to our problem. One of these is *apperception,* a recognition of the role of past experience and association in shaping a present percept. The second is the concept of *set,* a recognition of the incontestable fact that a person will for the most part perceive what he is at this moment "tuned" to perceive. But these concepts antedate "depth psychology." They seem a trifle intellectualistic and fail to allow for the fact that perceptions may be rooted in deeper layers of personality, in what Tolman calls our "belief-value matrix." Not long ago Postman helpfully proposed that the concept of "perceptual response disposition" (really a modern version of "set") may help us take care of all clearly identifiable factors that enter into the so-called "subjective" shaping of perception. And by distinguishing "perceptual response dispositions" from "mnemonic response dispositions" we can avoid confusing perception proper with the total process of cognition.[10]

Now this type of discussion is important for the psychologist who wishes to avoid terminologic promiscuity, and hopes for a model whereby he can distinguish one cognitive process from another. But what of the health worker? He too is a behavioral scientist—or, as Dr. William Griffiths has expressed it more accurately, he is a *practitioner* of behavioral science.[11]

The health worker, I suggest, needs a new concept that will bypass the fine distinctions so important for the psychologist, and enable him to deal all at once with the integrated disposition of a person to perceive, pay attention to, extract meaning from, feel, think about, and respond to a situation, and hold it in memory. It is this larger unitary process of the human organism that we seek to christen. For it is this more molar disposition of people with which the health worker must deal.

Borrowing from the philosopher, Justus Buchler, I propose that the term we need is *proception*.[12] The term recognizes the fact that each individual carries with him his past relations to the world, his cumulated experience, and at the same time is strongly propelled into the future. Every human being has "proceptive directions" which are his potentialities for seeing, hearing, doing, thinking, making, and saying. These potentialities are derived in part from his own temperament, and in part also from the culture and situation in which he has acquired his proceptive directions. The term designates the total process of personally relevant behavior from input to act. Unlike *percept* the term *procept* gives full weight to cumulative habit, emotional direction, and all others forms of "gating" that the complex psychophysical dispositions of the individual exert upon his behavioral sequence. It is wholly in keeping with modern research in neurophysiology to suggest that the procept "gates" (i.e., opens and closes pathways to) the percept.

Why do I deal with this terminologic issue in a lecture on public health? I do so partly to fortify the health educator in his future encounters with psychologists. If a critical laboratory psychologist says to you, "Look, you are using the term 'perception' too broadly and I find this a sloppy practice," the proper reply is, "Well, in the first place many of you psychologists are equally sloppy; but in the second place, if it pleases you better I'll speak when appropriate of 'proception' rather than of 'perception.'" This sophisticated reply will probably bewilder your critic, but it will surely shut him up.

But there is a still better reason for my terminologic digression. The point I am trying to make is that the health worker of the future cannot overlook the dynamic propulsion that causes one individual to accentuate, another to reject, and a third to distort the health message that is offered. Its reception will vary according to the nationality, the class membership, the ethnic group, and above all, the personality and present situation of the client. By suggesting the concept of "proception" I am hoping to fix your attention upon this variable of prime importance, and allow you no escape from it. "Perception" you might be tempted to shrug off as a problem for the psychologist; "proception" is clearly the concern of both pure and applied behavioral scientists.

PROCEPTIVE TYPES

We ask now, Is there such a thing as basic proceptive types? Without using this particular label many of the "new look" researches are in fact converging on precisely this problem. It is characteristic of these investigations that they first demonstrate some inner consistency among an individual's perceptions (considered in the narrow sense) and then discover that these ways of perceiving are in fact linked to the needs, the "directive states," the character structure, or to a whole "cognitive style" of the person.

Thus, for example, Witkin and his collaborators describe two basic and contrasting proceptive types (admitting, of course, that many people fall between the extremes). One type they label *field-dependent,* and the opposite *field-independent.* First they study certain elementary perceptual tendencies by placing a subject in a chair that can be mechanically tilted. The chair is in a room whose walls, ceiling and floors can likewise be tilted. The subject is asked to adjust a movable rod so that it stands vertically. Field-dependent subjects tend to adjust the rod so that it remains parallel to the tilted walls of the room. Field-independent subjects, by contrast, are able to disregard the visual field, and take their cues from their own sensations of gravitational pressure, and locate the rod closer to the true vertical.

Thus far the experiment demonstrates nothing more than individual differences in a limited perceptual task. But studying the same subjects further it is discovered that field-dependent persons are limited in other ways by the perceptual context; thus they cannot easily analyze out a particular geometric design that lies embedded in a complex visual pattern. Field-independent people, on the other hand, seem more able to disregard the context and discriminate the needed detail.

Now these perceptual styles turn out to be merely a part of a wider proceptive syndrome. The field-dependent person is characterized usually by a general passivity in dealing with the environment, by a certain unfamiliarity and distrust of his own impulses, by a low degree of self-esteem. On the other hand, the independent or analytic perceptual performer is in general more active and independent in meeting the environment, is higher in self-esteem, and shows greater control and understanding of his own impulses.[13]

Briefly let me mention several researches broadly confirmatory of Witkin's. In a series of experiments Klein discovers what he calls "levelers" and "sharpeners," the former behaving much like Witkin's field-dependent cases, and the latter showing the more highly differentiated ability of the field-independent type.[14] Even before the advent of the "new look" Goldstein identified "concrete" and "abstract" styles of cognitive operation that have much in common with Witkin's and with Klein's.[15] Ericksen overlaps this typology with his conception of *repressers* and *intellectualizers.*[16] In California, Barron discovers that *simplicity* and *complexity* are basic proceptive dimensions.[17] Boldest of all is the work of our friend and neighbor, Else Frenkel-Brunswik, whose recent death has caused us sorrow. She has related a purely perceptual tendency (called "intolerance of ambiguity") to the deepest proceptive layers of character structure, showing that people whose emotional lives are filled with prejudice and rigidity concerning their relations with other groups are people who, by and large, must have definiteness and structure in what they see and hear in the outer world.[18] There seems to be a relation here to the work of Hastings who, using Dr. Knutson's *Personal Security Scale,* found that observers who are low in personal security tend to locate objects—if these objects have no firm anchorage in the environment—as closer to themselves than do people who have a high sense of personal security.[19] It is as though anxious people are distrustful, apprehensive, and insecure even in handling simple percepts. Postman and Bruner have discovered a kind of "perceptual recklessness" among persons under stress.[20] Such persons seem to jump at premature hypotheses and demand a definiteness in the outer world that it may not in fact possess.

All this varied work, I am well aware, is not yet firmly collated and it is true, as Postman and other critics have pointed out, some researches are imperfect in design and in execution. But one cannot help feel that important knowledge is emerging, establishing beyond doubt the dependence of perception upon broad underlying proceptive directions.

Now for further applications to public health. The health worker himself is a selected, well educated, highly specialized person. In terms of these types, he is likely to be field-independent, an intellectualizer, a sharpener, an abstract thinker. But the people with whom he deals are likely not to be so. Particularly are they likely not to be so in times of illness, anxiety and strain.

For example, the health worker calls on the distraught mother of a sick child. The mother almost certainly is not listening, in a field-independent way, for coldly rational instructions. She is listening in large measure for approval of what she is doing, for reassurance, and hope. She is field-dependent: the health worker is seen as a global agent of mercy. Unless the health worker somehow puts his instructions within this context they are likely to be unperceived, distorted, or repressed.

Every health worker knows too that the proceptive dispositions of some people lead them to over-react to the educator's message even to the point of hypochondria, whereas others turn a deaf ear and repress what they hear. Workers on cancer control will surely recognize the overvigilant and over-defensive types. Since the health worker dislikes both hypervigilance and defensiveness, his own proceptive directions may lead him to assume erroneously that his client is an intellectualizer like himself.

Physicians, like all other health workers, have their own proceptive tendencies to guard against. It is a known fact, for example, that in the field of mental health patients who most nearly approach the therapist's status, having similar proceptive dispositions, are likely to receive from him the best treatment and most sympathy.[21]

Such class-anchored procepts are of great importance. For example, it is said that the main goal of public health work is "the inculcation in each individual of a sense of responsibility for his own health." Now this is a pleasant, middle-class, democratic-sounding axiom. It resonates sweetly among our own proceptive dispositions. But to some people, especially among what we call the "lower classes," such a maxim may not resonate at all. To them it may be perceived as a slap at their cherished domestic values. To them individual responsibility is a kind of self-centeredness. What is important is to take care of one's family in times of trouble, and to be taken care of by them. Self-responsibility is isolationism; it is even disloyal.

And how is it with our middle class emphasis on preventive medical, dental, and child guidance work—all of which demands present sacrifice for future good? The message of preventive medicine is less meaningful to people who from economic necessity have to live from day to day, seizing present gratifications where they can and leaving tomorrow's evil, as the Bible admonishes, to the morrow. . . . And a word about cleanliness. You and I are likely to see in a dirty house an index of moral turpitude. But those who live in such a house may view *our* concern for cleanliness as compulsive and downright neurotic. In this case who is to say whose perceptions are correct?[22]

ETHNIC PROCEPTS

An exciting new field of research is the proceptive study of health problems in cross-cultural perspective. Take the case of pain. One might think that such an elementary perception would have no cultural variation. And it is true that the best scientific evidence seems to indicate that the threshold of pain is more or less the same for all human beings regardless of nationality, sex, or age.[23] Can we then conclude that people perceive pain in the same way? In a limited and literal sense, yes; but we can also safely assert that they do not *proceive* it in the same way. Dr. Zborowski shows that, by and large, Italians regard pain as a physical misery to be complained about, to be relieved immediately, and then forgotten. Jewish patients, on the other hand, often regard it as something to be complained about, but also to be worried about in terms of its significance for one's future and the future of one's family. Old-line Americans generally view it as something not to be complained about, but to be relieved scientifically with an optimistic expectation regarding the eventual outcome.[24]

Now it turns out that in our own culture, but especially in foreign cultures, health workers must learn how sometimes to circumvent proceptive rigidities. In South Africa I found myself admiring the resourceful strategies of public health workers who when confronted with cultural beliefs harmful to health invented artful detours.

At one health station in Zululand it was found that the nutritional state of expectant and nursing mothers was deplorable. Milk was badly needed in their diet. The whole wealth of a Zulu homestead is in its cattle, and so in most cases the needed nutrient is available. It is forbidden by taboo, however, to partake of milk from cattle belonging to another kin group, and the wife of course lives with her husband's kin group. Worse still, a pregnant woman who partakes of milk will bewitch the cow who gave it. Hence, of all people in the community, the married woman is most rigidly excluded from partaking of milk. The belief systems here are too deep for the health educator to combat. But his imagination comes to the rescue. Powdered milk, because of its texture, is regarded as a wholly different substance by the tribe; hence prescriptions of powdered milk meet no resistance, and the health of the mothers is, through this strategy, greatly improved.

Again, in Zululand, tuberculosis is rife. It is possible with tact to persuade acutely affected patients to go to a sanitorium for treatment. But if the educational effort goes further and explains to the tribesmen that those persons are carriers of the disease, resistance will arise. This explanation is perceived as an accusation of witchcraft—for a person who carries a disease must certainly be a witch. Hence a father will insist on keeping his sick daughter at home rather than accept the implication that she is an evil agent.[25]

A physician friend of mine found that Zulu mothers were giving their children an opium-laden nostrum as protection against bewitchment. Rather than counter the mother's fixed belief in witchcraft prophylaxis the physician persuaded them that the drug would be just as effective if it were poured into the child's bath water. He told no lie, aroused no resistance, and improved the babies' health.

Such deceptions are occasionally necessary to circumvent proceptive rigidities. But there is an ethical hairline between beneficent deception and mendacious condescension. And this is a matter requiring constant moral vigilance. Kutner reports that one of the commonest complaints of surgical patients is, "They won't tell me anything," or "I want to ask them a question but they are always too busy." And the research of Dr. Beryl Roberts concerning reasons women delay in seeking treatment for breast lesions has shocked me with evidence of indifference and intellectual patronage on the part of some physicians.[26]

While proceptive dispositions, cultural and personal, run deep they are, after all, incident to the one basic desire of all mortal men: *the desire for meaning.* The health and suffering, the life and death of each individual are his own existential concern. The health worker should help, and not hinder, the person's quest for meaning in this sequence of mystery. To assume that the patient's perceptions are those of scientific medicine is certainly an error; but to assume that he neither wants nor deserves the truth is intolerable condescension. There is no solution to this ethical predicament of the health worker excepting to develop sensitivity to each patient at each stage of growth, to respect him as a unique being-in-the-world, and to advance his quest for meaning with all the skill at one's command.

FURTHER EXPLORATIONS

I feel I have touched only the fringes of my assignment. I should like to trace an additional score of contacts between perceptual research and public health work, but shall content myself with a brief mention of two.

Modern laboratory work on sensory deprivation has particular relevance. Until recently we have not known how important for our lives is the perceptual flooding of sights, sounds, smells, touches and muscular strains, and speech that engulf us. Like the fish we live in an environmental water, and like the fish we are slow to discover this fact. Recent research has shown how profoundly disturbing it is for a subject—even a healthy college student paid $20 a day for his pains— to lie in a condition where this perceptual bombardment is almost excluded—any kind of perception. He also develops hallucinations and loses an integrated image of himself and his body. He perceives his body as one thing, his "self" as another. And most remarkable of all, if his hunger for perception is in a small way appeased by the voice of the experimenter, he seems to develop unusual receptivity to the message. If, for example, the experimenter tries to persuade him that ghosts exist, he accepts the suggestion and even after returning to normal life, the indications are that this planted idea has taken firm root.[27]

Obviously this finding has a bearing upon the macabre problem of "brainwashing;" but it also has implications for the health worker. It clearly relates to the phenomenon Spitz has called "hospitalism."[28] Patients who have suffered even mild sensory deprivation through a long illness may develop unusual perceptual disturbances and suggestibility. Extending the thought further: we may raise the question whether the apparent stupidity and deficiency in learning ability among some children and among primitive tribes may not be due to the relatively low level of perceptual bombardment from their impoverished environments.

Finally, there is the critical area of child and parental guidance, an area of profound concern to health workers. Probably all of us are convinced that future advances in the physical and mental welfare of our nation require improvement in the attitudes and practices of parents, especially mothers. But one cannot change the attitudes of a mother without realizing that she has her own proceptive biases, seeing her child and her world in her own peculiar way.

Take the case of the young mother who applies excessive discipline too early in a child's life. She almost certainly is not intentionally cruel. Rather she lacks the ability to perceive the child's destructive acts for what they are. Every exploring infant is destructive: he pulls off your eyeglasses, spills his cup of milk, and soils himself. A young mother may perceive these acts as aggressive on the part of the child, and forthwith start her scolding, spanking, and withdrawal of love. Some mothers perceive aggressive intent when the child is only two or three months of age, and punish him accordingly. At the other extreme there are mothers so patient or so blind that they do not undertake to socialize the child even when, a year or two later, his destructiveness does involve aggressive intent.[29]

The point here is that the health worker cannot expect to change the mother's socialization practices without correcting her perceptions of her baby's behavior.

FINAL WORD

Summing up, it seems that the alert health worker has no choice: from now on he must develop skill as an *oculist*, training himself to look *at* his spectacles and not merely *through* them, and training himself to look both at and *through* the spectacles of the client with whom he deals.

He will soon discover that his habit of viewing sickness and health in a sharpened, field-independent way is not often his client's mode of perception, especially if the client is ill. He will discover that culture, social class, and personality lay down stubborn proceptive dispositions that fashion what a person sees and hears, what he thinks and feels, and what he does. Since, in the last analysis, every percept bears the signature of the individual, no reliance on rules-of-thumb, routine curricula, or mass media can adequately guide health education. To sense and to nourish the growing edge of each individual in his present situation is the only formula for success.

There is one lesson that all of us who teach need to learn. We are habitually tempted to present to our students and clients a summary statement of our hard-won conclusions. We entrust our cryptic wisdom to a burnished lecture or to a polished pamphlet, hoping thereby to bring our audience rapidly to our own level of knowledge. I try in a single hour to give the gist of my conclusions respecting proceptive processes—and I largely fail. You, as a health worker, may, at the clinic or on a doorstep, present your client with a finely wrought sonnet on sanitation or child care—but you too will largely fail. The sad truth is that no one learns from having conclusions presented to him. Learning takes place only when there is a need, a curiosity, an interest, an exploring, erring, correcting of errors, testing, verifying—all carried through by the individual himself. In school, in college, in the clinic we cannot scamp the process.

And it is hard to know how to present our invitation to learning to students or clients who, because of their own proceptive directions, have a need for safety and from freedom of threat, a need for simple and gratifying rubrics to reinforce their own prejudices; who are untrained in following evidence or logic, who are emotionally fearful and cognitively self-centered. It is usually approval they want and not fact, reassurance and not alarm, certainty and not challenge. Even those who appear on the surface to be objective and responsive often are not so; for them too the message is darkened, blurred, and misshapen.

Discouraging as the outlook may be, it is still inescapably the moral duty of the health worker to advance the learning process, even in the most resistant cases, as best he can, so that the client may participate constructively in his own destiny and become creatively aware of factors making for sickness and for health.

The time has passed when we can impose a mere routine of sanitation, nutrition, and hygiene, leading to a controlled, calculated, technically efficient life of conformity with our antiseptic cultural ideal. Such mechanical regulation leaves untouched the client's future role in managing his and his family's affairs. However important it may still be in certain respects to impose hygienic practices from the outside, from now on our task increasingly is to win the participation of the public in seeking sounder personal, domestic, and civic values so that the physical and spiritual welfare of our nation may increase.

This modern challenge to public health is no doubt the most difficult it has ever had to face. The comfort I offer is that the researches of social and psychologic science will increasingly provide strategic aid, especially perhaps its discoveries concerning the logic of *percepts* and of *procepts*.

1. Derryberry, Mayhew: "Health Education in Transition," *American Journal of Public Health*, 1957, 47, pp. 1357–1366.

2. Parsons, Talcott and Fox, Renee: Introduction to "Sociocultural Approaches to Medical Care," *Journal of Social Issues*, 1952, 8, p. 2.

3. Woodworth, R. S.: *Dynamics of Behavior*. New York, Henry Holt and Company, 1958.

4. Apple, Dorrian: "Definitions of Illness," Unpublished research from the Boston University School of Nursing.

5. Lamb, Charles: "The Convalescent," in *The Essays of Elia*. New York, The Macmillan Company, 1905, p. 222.

6. Lederer, H. D.: "How the Sick View Their World," *Journal of Social Issues*, 1952, 8, pp. 4–15.

7. For a recent review of the "new look" literature see Jenkin, N.: "Af-

fective Processes in Perception," *Psychological Bulletin*, 1957, 54, pp. 100–127.

8. Paul, Benjamin D. (Ed.) *Health, Culture and Community*. New York, Russell Sage Foundation, 1955. Cf. pp. 112 and 340.

9. Murray, Henry A.: "The Effect of Fear Upon Estimates of the Maliciousness of Other Persons," *Journal of Social Psychology*, 1933, 4, pp. 310–329.

10. For critical discussion of this issue see: Allport, F. H.: *Theories of Perception and the Concept of Structure*. New York, John Wiley and Sons, 1955; Postman, L.: "Perception, Motivation, and Behavior," *Journal of Personality*, 1953, 22, pp. 17–31; and Tolman, Edward C., "A Psychological Model," in Talcott Parsons and Edward A. Shils (Eds.), *Toward a General Theory of Action*, Cambridge: Harvard University Press, 1951.

11. Griffiths, William: "Communication Problems Facing Our Profession," *Health Education Monographs*, 1957, 1, p. 27.

12. Buchler, Justus: *Nature and Judgment*. New York, Columbia University Press, 1955.

13. Witkin, H. A., et al. *Personality Through Perception*. New York, Harper and Brothers, 1954.

14. Klein, George S. "Personal World Through Perception," in R. W. Blake and G. Ramsey (eds.), *Perception: An Approach to Personality*, New York: Ronald Press, 1950.

15. Goldstein, Kurt and Scheerer, M. "Abstract and Concrete Behavior: An Experimental Study With Special Tests," *Psychological Monographs*, 1941, 53, No. 239.

16. Eriksen, C. W. "The Case for Perceptual Defense," *Psychological Review*, 1954, 61, pp. 175–182.

17. Barron, Frank. "Complexity-Simplicity as a Personal Dimension," *Journal of Abnormal and Social Psychology*, 1953, 48, pp. 163–172.

18. Frenkel-Brunswik, Else. "Intolerance of Ambiguity as an Emotional and Perceptual Personality Variable," *Journal of Personality*, 1949, 18, pp. 108–143. See also Allport, Gordon W., *The Nature of Prejudice*, Boston: Addison-Wesley, 1954, Chapter 25.

19. Hastings, P. K. "A Relationship Between Visual Perception and Level of Personal Security," *Journal of Abnormal and Social Psychology*, 1952, 47, No. 2, Supplement, pp. 552–560.

20. Postman, Leo and Bruner, Jerome S. "Perception Under Stress," *Psychological Review*, 1948, 55, pp. 314–323.

21. Redlich, Fredrick C., Hollingshead, August B., and Bellis, Elizabeth. "Social Class Differences in Attitudes Toward Psychiatry," *American Journal of Orthopsychiatry*, 1955, 25, pp. 60–70.

22. For a discussion of the "belief-value matrix" in relation to social class see Simmons, O. G., "Implications of Social Class For Public Health," *Human Organization*, 1957, 16, pp. 7–10.

23. Harley, J. D., Wolff, Harold G., and Goodell. H. *Pain Sensations and Reaction*. Baltimore: W. Wilkins Company, 1950, p. 122.

24. Zborowski, M. "Cultural Components in Responses to Pain," *Journal of Social Issues*, 1952, 8, pp. 16–30.

25. These instances are described by Cassel, John, "A Comprehensive Health Program Among South African Zulus," in Paul, Benjamin D., *op. cit.*

26. Kutner, B., "Surgeons and Their Patients: A Study in Social Perception," in Jaco, Gartly E. (Ed.), *Patients, Physicians and Illness*, Glencoe, Ill.: The Free Press, 1958. See also Roberts, Beryl J., *A Study of Selected Factors and Their Association with Action for Medical Care*, unpublished thesis, 1956, Harvard Medical School Library.

27. Hebb, D. O. "The Motivating Effects of Exteroceptive Stimulation," *American Psychologist*, 1958, 13, pp. 109–113.

28. Spitz, Rene A. "Hospitalism: A Follow-Up Report," *Psychoanalytic Study of the Child*, 1946, 2, pp. 113–117.

29. Sears, Robert R., Maccoby, Eleanor E. and Levin, H. *Patterns of Child Rearing*. Evanston, Ill.: Row, Peterson and Company, 1957, Chapter 7.

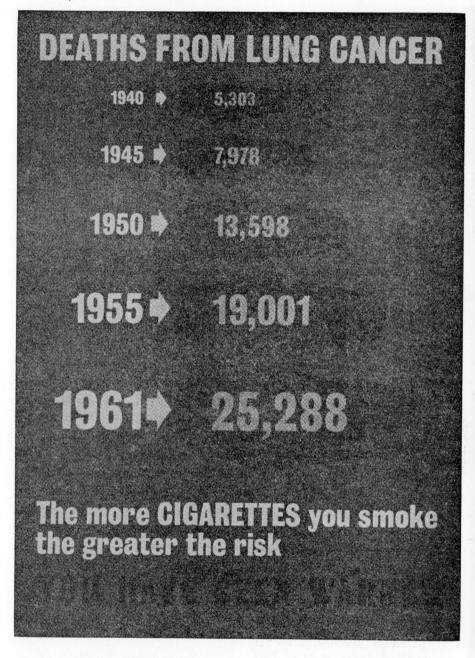

* These posters have been reproduced, by permission, by the Ministry of Health, London, England. They were issued May, 1962 by the Ministry of Education and Scottish Home and Health Department.

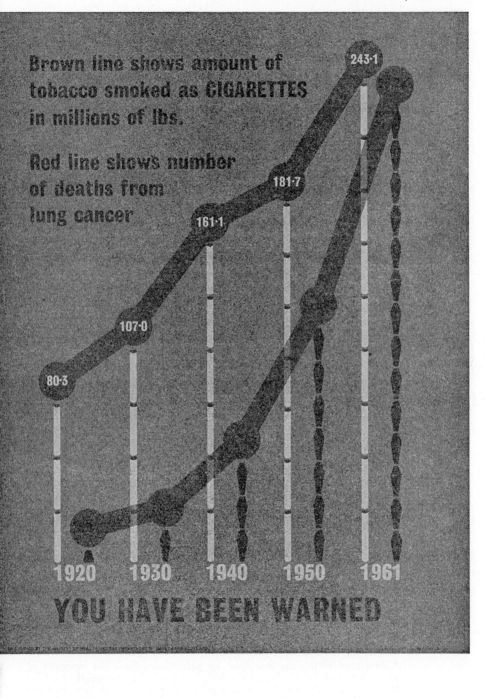

8. Occupational Health

Management and an Occupational Health Program*

N. H. COLLISSON

DURING MY MANY YEARS in industry, there has been much improvement in the human relations aspects of industry. The concept of industrial health, which started from practically nothing, has moved slowly from "post facto" medical care to the beginning of a concept of preventive medicine. It has expanded from the setting of fractures and the dressing of wounds to the more meaningful early diagnosis of irregularities, with corresponding better chances for early treatment and cure. During this period of progress, it has always seemed to be a strange paradox that the preventive maintenance of machinery and equipment was accepted and utilized well ahead of the concept of preventive medicine in the case of the plant workers and personnel. Certainly the major responsibility for this tardiness must lie with industry itself, but the medical profession is not entirely blameless. It is to this profession that industry must look for people, techniques, and the means by which we may achieve our objectives.

During this period of time, the human relations aspect of industry has undergone great change, a "bloodless revolution." It has changed attitudes and objectives and has, to some degree, met the issue of strife and misunderstanding. It seems worthwhile to examine this progress in some detail.

Medical men are familiar with the second industrial revolution in England and the United States in the early 1900's. It was this new concept of industrial production that first made mass production possible. It was a new and novel approach since it departed from the old "guild" concept of skilled workers and their own tools to the modern concept of high-speed production equipment financed by borrowed capital. It was almost a complete reversal of ideas and concepts, for originally, it had been the individual workers who, equipped with their tools, were their own bosses. The new concept placed them in the role of hired hands who were solely directed by management.

* Reprinted with some deletions, by permission, from the *Archives of Environmental Health*, Feb. 1961, Vol. 2, pp. 116–123. Copyright 1961 by the American Medical Association published under the Auspices of the Board of Trustees. This paper was an edited text of the talk given by the author at the American Medical Association 20th Annual Congress on Industrial Health, Oct. 11, 1960, and was titled, "What Management Expects of an Occupational Health Program." The author is Senior Vice-President, Olin Mathieson Chemical Corporation, New York, N.Y.

PIONEERS IN SCIENTIFIC MANAGEMENT

These important changes in the United States were brought about by two great men. Frederick Winslow Taylor, who once was a laborer and who died in 1915, increased industrial production by integrating men and machines. He was, indeed, the Father of Scientific Management. Elton Mayo was an Australian immigrant and later a Harvard sociologist, who died in 1949. He increased industrial production by humanizing it.

In his early studies, Taylor found that workers, not their bosses, actually set the production rates. He found they made funny wasted motions. Taylor increased production by the same men by breaking each operation down into its components. Taylor brought the stop watch and time and motion studies into industry. While there are many interesting stories about Taylor, it suffices to say that he made mass production possible, raised productivity, and at the same time raised the workers' wages. However, as a minus component of the equation, Taylor created a monster. He geared man's motions to machines, and, as a result, men or workers were thereafter soon regarded as machines. It was later demonstrated that there came a time when speed-up and attempted greater efficiency no longer produced a proportional improvement in production. In other words, the rising production curve flattened. In brief, in spite of its contribution, Taylor's philosophy had a tendency to degrade the importance of man, or the human element in industry.

Let us, for a moment, consider these consequences. We know today that all of the jobs in industry must seem important to each of us as individuals. The lowest-paid man in any industrial establishment must be convinced that his job is necessary and important. Its relative importance, i.e., one job versus another, is not nearly so important. On this point, Fyodor Dostoevsky said in his novel, *The House of the Dead,* "If it were desired to reduce a man to nothing, it would be necessary only to give to his work a character of uselessness." This was true then. It is just as true now. An employee's effectiveness, usefulness, and his entire attitude, fundamentally depend upon a conviction of his job's importance.

And so it was that Taylor's theory, which brought about so many marked improvements in production, quite naturally led to the myth that labor and management cannot get along, that their paths and objectives are different, and that therefore they must eternally fight.

Fortunately, there followed another man in this important cycle who introduced human relations into industry. Elton Mayo brought about realization that every worker must be convinced of the importance of his job. He must feel that his boss is interested in him and appreciates what he is doing. Mayo's work supplemented Taylor's work and thus brought realization that labor and management have many common interests. He brought about a better understanding that one cannot succeed without the other and that never-ending conflict, therefore, is not inevitable.

After many years the experience of industry has confirmed this theory. Industry can buy a man's time, a worker's physical presence at a given time and place; it can even buy a measured number of skilled muscular motions per hour or per day. It cannot buy enthusiasm, initiative, loyalty, the devotion of hearts, minds, and souls. These things must be earned.

Elmo Roper, of Columbia University, polled many workers over a period of 10 years. As a result of this poll, he found that their chief desires were (a) security (continuous work at good wages), (b) chance for advancement, (c) treatment as human beings, (d) dignity. Industry has learned that this is a reasonably accurate cross-section of the desires of the people who work in our plants.

OCCUPATIONAL HEALTH

Let us examine this thing called an industrial health program. Unfortunately, it is impossible to describe a model industrial health program that could be used by every industry. The program must vary with each industry. It must vary with its size, the product, the location, and the environment. It must, in brief, be tailored to fit the needs. In order to be as factual and as practical as possible, reference will be made to an actual plant of my corporation, located in the state of North Carolina. This plant employs about 2,400 people and is located in the open country about 30 miles from the nearest large city. It manufactures packaging materials and it has had an industrial medical program since 1950. In establishing and later administering this program, it was considered essential to have an intelligent and planned balance between equipment and professional personnel. The program must, perhaps even more importantly, have well-defined objectives. It must have the backing and support of all levels in management. It must have the confidence and acceptance of the individual worker. It needs the understanding and cooperation of the local medical profession. Without these, the best-planned program is doomed to failure.

The major features of the industrial health program at this plant are a medical center with facilities which are adequate, but not by any means elaborate. The facilities, however, carry a dignity commensurate with the objectives of the program itself. The use of some abandoned, ill-kept warehouse as a medical center will, in turn, most probably earn the same sort of evaluation for an entire medical program.

MEDICAL PERSONNEL

A competent medical director dedicated to the whole concept of improving the health and usefulness of the people in this industry was searched for and found. In industry we will not accept the cast-offs and failures, and we look to the medical colleges to prepare for us men skilled and competent in the large number of complex problems confronting a health program in industry.

The same ideals were applied in selection of a competent nursing staff of the highest caliber.

EXAMINATIONS

The program includes a complete physical examination for all employees once a year and more frequently for those in the older age brackets, as well as those with previously diagnosed or suspected abnormalities. It does not, by any means, overlook the supervisory or management group which represents management to the worker and as such demonstrates leadership ability. Of equal importance is the realization that top management of tomorrow is supplied from this group.

At the outset, it was established that all examinations and consultations were strictly confidential and patterned very much after the traditional and time-honored doctor-patient relationship. Management never invades this field of confidence.

Later the program was expanded to include special services emphasizing the early detection and prevention of chronic diseases such as hypertension, diabetes, cancer, arthritis, and emotional disorders.

On the theory that a sick man is often a careless man, and hence a hazard to himself and other workers, the industrial health program was carefully correlated with the plant safety program.

CONFIDENTIALITY AND SUPPORT

All of the data and records accumulated over the years of this industrial health program have been, and still are, regarded as confidential and the property of the medical director. Where an employee concurs, of course, records can be given by the plant medical director to an employee's personal physician. Otherwise, they are available to no one, including management.

It was found early that the program must have the understanding and support of local medical practitioners and the hospitals. This is not difficult to achieve if the program is explained in detail and the objectives or plans outlined to the local doctors in advance. Indeed, it was found that their support has been most meaningful to the success of this program.

Finally, it was soon found that of prime importance is the support and attitude of top management. This cannot be lip service. Given the best program and an able director with the best facilities, the program, nevertheless, will fail without this support. Management cannot buy a successful program by sheer capital investment. It takes dedication to the objectives and public knowledge of management's approval of the plan.

THE INDUSTRIAL OPERATION

Most of the Mathieson employees are, as a class, employed in what we term United States industry. It is therefore not only important to our national and individual security, but is the very foundation of our way of life. The United States is the greatest industrial nation in the world, with a gross national product of $482,-056,000,000 in 1959. Its industrial production has been an important factor in our growth and the key to our ability to defend ourselves. It has likewise been a major element in absorbing the world's excess population and determines our ability to help the less fortunate in the world. Finally, it has proved in the United States that with a rise in the gross national product, there comes about an automatic and proportional rise in our standard of living.

An industrial health program must be examined from the standpoint of profit and loss in precisely the same way any other undertaking of industry would be evaluated. In the first place, an industry is not designed to be a charitable institution. The terms of reference of any successful industry can be clearly defined in understandable language. An industry must make a good product at a competitive price. It should provide a safe and healthful place for workers. It is the responsibility of an industry to plan and do research in order to provide reasonably for the future employment of its workers and insure the continued security of the investment of its shareholders. It should compensate its workers adequately for their labor. It should provide a reasonable and adequate return to the shareholders who have invested their money in the establishment. Finally, it should start to maximize the dignity and importance of the people employed in its operations.

A GOOD MEDICAL PROGRAM

A good medical program creates a good atmosphere for the employee to work in. It reflects generally a better quality product and it influences the worker's entire attitude toward the plant and its management.

A good medical program persuades the worker that management is sincere in its concern for him. It promotes mutual respect between worker and management on an individual basis.

A good medical program convinces a worker that his job is important—that management must think his job is important, and hence that the worker is important—for, otherwise, industry would not trouble itself with his health and safety.

Finally, a good medical program increases the useful and gainful span of years of both worker and management. This means greater earning power for the worker and a longer period of his usefulness to the corporation.

These are highly important and meaningful to the worker and to management, and yet they cannot be evaluated directly into dollars of return or of cost.

A second question is, "Are the savings and returns solely the result of a medical program?" In this case, the answer is a categorical "No." To give all of the credit to an industrial medical program would ignore the plant safety program. It would ignore the planning and direction of management in these and many other related fields, and it would ignore the dedicated cooperation of management and worker in all fields. In other words, while a medical program, if it is a good one, is an important contributor to the results which I have previously discussed, it must only be considered as a coordinated contributor, working in planned harmony with all of the other aspects of good plant management.

A question which arises concerns the appropriateness of the inclusion of an industrial health program of this type in the field of labor negotiations as currently undertaken by labor and management: Is it an appropriate item to be included in collective bargaining? *Such a program has no place in collective bargaining discussions.* [Italics are the editors'.] Admittedly, it is the responsibility of management to provide a safe place in which its workers may pursue their tasks, but a medical program of this type invades the personal and confidential area of relationship between worker and management. It is an individual relationship peculiar to and differing with each individual. It is, therefore, foreign to the whole collective bargaining concept where an individual must, of needs, subordinate his own individual objectives and aspirations to the collective best interests of the entire bargaining unit. On the other hand, the union can be, and very often is, an important contributor to the success of an industrial medical program.

The importance of the complete cooperation of the local medical fraternity in the administration of an industrial health program cannot be overemphasized. It should be thoroughly familiar with the details of the program and, more particularly, with just what it is that management hopes to achieve. The individual industry will need and must depend upon the active cooperation of this group, and, indeed, if it is inaugurated under the proper auspices, there seems to be no conflict of interest.

STRONGER DEFENDERS OF THE PRINCIPLES

The visitor to the medical center may stop inside the little entrance foyer and read the dedication plaque which is hung there where all may see. It seems to set forth accurately the intentions and objectives then as well as now in building this facility. It reads, "The professional staff and facilities of this medical center are pledged to the task of achieving a healthier and happier life span for our workers through sound medical practices in order that by useful and gainful activity in their work, homes, and communities, they may become even better examples and stronger defenders of the principles and way of life which makes us a nation of free people."

9. Space Medicine

Recent Developments in Aviation and Aerospace Medicine*

WILLIAM F. ASHE, M.D.

IN THE HISTORY of the world's industrial development, no industry has grown more rapidly than aviation except numeric computation by electronic means. In 1903, the Wright brothers flew the first powered aircraft. By 1912, the first commercial airline, KLM, was operating between London and Amsterdam twice a week. In 1960, a total of 60 million tickets were sold to more than 10 million passengers who flew on United States owned and operated aircraft alone; the business air fleet far exceeded in numbers the entire United States Air Force, and the combined commercial and business fleets were fewer in numbers than the aircraft privately owned and operated for pleasure.

In October 1957, exploration of extraterrestrial space within our solar system became a reality. Only four years later, orbital traffic control is needed and man has gone into outer space and survived. Aerial mapping and surveying have almost outmoded the civil engineer surveyor. More than 4,000 companies seed, fertilize, and disinfect our crops. Forestry is dependent on aviation for both disease control and fire control, and few major airports can keep up with traffic growth. Every one of these situations has inherent medical problems. The study of these was called aviation medicine in the 1930–58 period and is now called aerospace medicine.

THE FEDERAL AVIATION AGENCY

From about 1926 until 1958, commercial aviation was controlled by the Civil Aeronautics Board, a quasi-judicial arm of Congress, and by the Civil Aeronautics Administration, a division of the executive branch under the United States Department of Commerce. In that period aviation grew so rapidly that adequate control, in the interest of public safety, was virtually lost. The medical criteria for certification of pilot and traffic control personnel changed virtually

* Reprinted by permission from the July, 1962, issue of *Public Health Reports*, Vol. 77, pp. 623–627. This paper is based on an address to the American College of Preventive Medicine, Detroit, Michigan, November 16, 1961. The author is Chairman of the Department of Preventive Medicine, College of Medicine, Ohio State University, Columbus, Ohio.

not at all in 20 years. Almost anyone could get a medical certificate to pilot a plane from almost any physician. If, by chance, a physician thought someone should not fly, his decision often could be waived by the Civil Aeronautics Board.

In 1956, President Dwight Eisenhower asked Edward P. Curtis, a former Air Force general, to take a critical look at civil aviation. He reported that all major airports were overloaded with traffic. Schedules were unrealistic. Medical control of aircrew personnel was almost non-existent, and there was no research seeking solutions to a multitude of problems. He recommended that a new set of statutes be enacted. In August 1958, by an act of Congress, the Federal Aviation Agency replaced the CAA, and the functions of the CAB were limited and defined more clearly.

In 1959, an adequate medical department was created under Dr. James L. Goddard, who reported directly to Elwood R. Quesada, the Federal Aviation Administrator. The physical requirements were stiffened for flyers and traffic control operators. Definite restrictions as to who might fly, when, and where were prescribed, and an upper age limit was set for pilots who carry passengers on the scheduled airlines. All pilots must now be examined by physicians accredited by the medical department of the FAA, and these certified examiners must show continuing interest in aviation medicine by participation in educational programs conducted or sponsored by the Agency's medical department. Adequate medical advisory panels exist to help the Civil Air Surgeon and the Administrator to arrive at proper medical decisions.

Medical research on a wide variety of projects is underway on a contract basis, and a new facility for intramural research has been built near Oklahoma City. Major accidents are being thoroughly investigated by trained teams, and pathologic examinations are made by trained personnel supplied by the Armed Forces Institute of Pathology. A recent FAA project is a study on medical requirements of airports of various sizes. Only a few airports have any medical facility of any kind; many lack even a first-aid room.

PASSENGER RESEARCH

While the Armed Forces have done exhaustive research on healthy flyers between the ages of 18 to 45, little concern has ever been given to the average passenger who buys a ticket. It has been tacitly assumed that if a situation is satisfactory for Air Force pilots, it is therefore safe for anyone. The fact is that from intrauterine fetuses of only hours' or days' existence to octogenarians of both sexes in all degrees of health, these assumptions may or may not be correct. For example, no one really knows what mild hypoxia for a few hours does to a 3-week-old fetus nor what such an experience does to the senile arteriosclerotic who can just get by at sea level.

With the sanction of the FAA, the National Institutes of Health is now supporting studies on passenger safety in jet travel at the Ohio State University Aviation Medicine Research Laboratories. Patients with various degrees of pulmonary disease and with various amounts of lung surgically removed are exposed to the simulated cabin altitudes of jet travel, given a meal, and are monitored for any untoward reactions. Patients with diverse types and states of heart disease, diabetes, cerebral arteriosclerosis, glaucoma, and arthritis will participate in similar experiments. Persons with colostomies also are studied.

In addition, healthy subjects are being exposed to the pressure changes associated with a window blowout or a failure of the pressurization pumps. This experience has its disturbing features when the subject passengers are sober and is extremely disturbing if they have consumed much alcohol.

FAA is carefully evaluating escape systems and escape gear. In another investigation by the Agency, pilots in the 45–60 age range are being exposed to potential hazards of a significant order to see how they react when compared with younger men.

MATS, the Air Force passenger carrier, has done postflight follow-up studies and showed that thrombophlebitis must be watched with care if passengers are going to fly long distances.

To learn whether flight affects mother or infant in any way, an epidemiologic study is contemplated by the Ohio State University group comparing 10,000 women who have flown in various stages of pregnancy with 10,000 who have not.

All of these studies are being carried out, not with the intent of restricting flying for anyone, but rather to provide adequate data for the engineers and designers of planes so they may make air travel totally safe for all.

BUSINESS AVIATION

The National Business Aircraft Association acts as the parent body to advise American industrial organizations about the use of aviation in business. United States corporations now own about 30,-000 planes, and fly executives and business associates an estimated 3 billion miles per year. Some companies have medical departments and prescribe flight standards far more rigid than those applicable to most commercial airlines. Others have little or no medical supervision. To assist them, one of my associates, Dr. Charles Billings, is preparing a medical manual to aid corporate personnel in handling the medical aspects of flying. Our goal is, of course, to provide the least restriction compatible with complete comfort and safety. This project is financed jointly by the FAA and the Ohio State University.

CROP DUSTING

One of the most hazardous of all types of flying is crop dusting. In a high-wing monoplane or an old biplane, crop dusters fly from 18 inches to 6 feet off the ground at 62 to 100 mph 16 hours a day for 5 months of the year. Every time they go above 100 feet or come down to reload, they lose money. Such flights are generally illegal, and for each one, special waivers must be obtained. These men fly back and forth through a multitude of noxious agents, the toxicity of which they rarely know, and not infrequently serious accidents occur.

The physical requirements and training standards for this sort of flying are not the highest in the land, and under certain circumstances a flyer can get by with only a class III ticket, or even none at all. Only two or three men in the entire 40,000-man FAA organization have had intimate experience with crop dusting, and none of these is a toxicologist or industrial hygienist. Only a few persons in the business know much about the toxic hazards to pilots, farm animals, and other forms of life.

This is also being corrected. A number of agricultural schools are testing better ways to seed, dust, and fertilize from the air. FAA is seeking better stall warning systems for the flyers. The seasoned experts are coming each year to the Ohio State School of Aviation to teach others how to dust crops safely. Courses in toxicology are becoming part of the training program, and medical supervision by experts is gradually being accepted. One cannot sell the seasonal crop duster pilot on physicians. He will say emphatically that he doesn't need one. But, if the physician is also a flyer and goes to this crop duster course, pretty soon the professionals begin to want to know how the physicians might help them. When told what their risks really are, they go all out to get help.

MANNED HIGH-ALTITUDE AND SPACE FLIGHT

At present nearly everyone is interested in space flight, and they should be because man will thoroughly explore space in part of our solar system, and he will do it within our lifetimes. However, he will not explore the stars in spaceships in the forseeable future. The nearest true star is so far away that at 25,000 mph it would take 80,000 years to get there, and if he went at speeds which could make the trip in 10 years, the laws of energy, mass, and velocity would change him into a nonliving thing.

For a thousand years or more in the universities of the world, students have been getting advanced degrees for research on what often seemed to be such obscure subjects as "The size of the penumbra of the moon in the various stages of earth and sun orbits" or "How many miles further away from us does the moon go each hundred years and why?" "What is correct time to the 10,000th of a second?" "How deep is the dust on the moon?" "Does the slight atmosphere of the moon contain only CO_2 or some water as well?" "Do the Moon, Mars, and Venus have active volcanoes?" "Where does the SO_2 go if there is no atmosphere?" "How much ozone is in the ionosphere?" "What and why are northern lights?" These Ph.D. dissertations, thousands of them, are now all important to successful manned space flight.

Studies of the medical problems of flight in our upper atmosphere, 10 to 100 miles up, are carried out largely with a research machine. Part rocket and part airplane and man controlled, it is called the X–15. A few studies in this area are also done in helium-filled balloons. True space studies are carried out with sealed capsules propelled by rockets.

The men who go up in these ships are exposed to vacuums which would cause their blood to boil if they were unprotected. Temperatures drop to $-60°$ or even $-100°$ F. and then rise to more than $250°$ F. as the air friction of reentry makes the plane's surface a dull cherry red. Astronauts must not only tolerate but function well in the presence of accelerations and decelerations of from 0 to 4,000 mph. The pilot is weightless for periods of from a few seconds to a few minutes. He is exposed to solar and cosmic radiations unknown on the earth's surface. Finally, as he returns to earth he is transiently exposed to serious low-frequency, high-amplitude vibration and buffeting. Is he frightened? Yes, he is, but no more so than the team of physicians who, on the ground, are electronically monitoring his every action and reaction.

A single example of a problem to be solved is this one: From the points of view of maximum tolerance to acceleration while in flight or with a blast escape mechanism and as a focal point from which to function effectively in a weightless state, it is highly desirable to have the pilot strapped fairly tight into a contour seat at a selected angle. However, when he is vibrated at from ¼ to 2 inches' amplitude at frequencies of from 4 to 30 cycles per second, he could stand the stress far better if he were free enough to allow his musculature to absorb the vibration. If the body is tightly bound, shearing forces develop which can easily tear mediastinal structures. Standing fluid waves may develop in the aorta and great vessels which hamper or transiently stop blood flow.

A great deal of discussion has been given to the question of why should man go into space, a totally hostile environment. Could we not learn just as much by nonliving sensors and avoid the risks?

Whatever one's philosophy may be on this question, man already has orbited around the earth, and will go into orbit around the Moon, land on the Moon, and perhaps also on Mars and Venus after a great deal more close-range study of these two planets.

The hazards of the environment of outer space provoke serious thought. Consider a few of them:

1. No one in this country knows anything about the physiologic and psychologic effects of prolonged weightlessness. We have not been able to simulate it on the ground. Air exposures to it have been measured in seconds. Water submersion studies have a number of drawbacks and, in fact, are not truly weightlessness as found in space. Most of what we think we know about the return of blood to the heart through the venous system suggests that it is mediated through muscular contractions or posture against the forces of gravity. What will happen in space? Since the presentation of this paper, Lt. Col. John Glenn's orbital flight has already told us much about weightlessness for a few hours. But no informed scientist is certain of the effects when exposures are increased to days or weeks.

2. Outer space is deadly silent. Man has never been able to build a room of zero decibels. Close approaches have caused test subjects to fall asleep. What will happen in a spaceship when man hears only radio signals from earth against a background of absolute silence?

3. Man on earth has never been able to look directly at the sun on a clear day without the protection of a smoked glass even though he sees it through 60 to 100 miles of air full of dust particles and water droplets. What will happen to rods and cones and to vision in outer space? Looking toward the sun, the astronaut will see blinding brilliance but, facing elsewhere, only absolute blackness except for stars thousands of light-years in the distance. It will be a colorless world of white and black with nothing to cause the spectrum and shades in between. He will be able to see a 3,000-mile segment of earth but will be looking from an empty atmosphere through 100 miles of air, dust, water, and clouds. What will he really be able to see? Consider the Snellen Chart. Then calculate the size of the object you could see from 200 miles of distance while traveling at 18,000 mph.

4. A fairly standard satellite day, based on our Vanguard orbits, is about 61 minutes and a satellite night about 33 minutes. What does this do to man's diurnal variations? What should be the astronaut's work, eat, and rest schedule?

5. How does one design a work area for an astronaut when the temperature of the external environment while in the shadow of the moon will be colder than −150° F. but which on reentry into the atmosphere may reach 3,000° F.?

6. Imagine the calculations necessary to shoot yourself in a rocket from the east coast of Florida at 2 p.m. on Tuesday to hit a certain

visible moon crater at 2 a.m. on Friday sufficiently gently not to break a single wire in your transistor radio. The takeoff must be slow enough not to exceed 10 g acceleration for more than a few seconds. The work environment must duplicate your office on earth plus a few hundred electronic gadgets. Water spilled from a glass floats around the room, as do you if you leave your desk, and when you try to step forward, you go backward or tumble end over end. Your secretary is soon a quarter of a million miles away, and the flicked ashes from your cigarette ignore the ashtray. One window looks like the inside of a furnace for molten glass and the opposite one appears to be painted black. Figure out how to maneuver food from a container to your mouth.

Be sure that you provide yourself with 70° F. temperature and 50% relative humidity throughout the trip, that O_2 remains at 20% and 150 mm. Hg, that there is no air pollution of any kind, and that the CO_2 stays at less than 0.05%. Don't forget Dr. Van Allen's little bands, for if you do forget you might as well walk past an unshielded cobalt 60 unit. Make certain you are able to provide us on earth with all of the capacities of the human brain while on your trip, else why should we send you? Design, make, and test all your gear. It had better be right because no one will give you insurance.

This is what the aerospace life science teams which include aerospace medical men are pondering.

EDUCATION IN AEROSPACE MEDICINE

Training for the specialty of aviation medicine in the military services is provided by the Navy and the Air Force but is limited to career officers.

In the civilian world, only the Harvard School of Public Health and Ohio State University have accredited programs, and only the one at Ohio is presently accredited for the three full years of academic, research, and service training. Many universities, however, contribute through contract research. The need for highly trained personnel in and out of the services is large and the supply is small. Few young men are interested in entering the field; yet those in it would do nothing else.

CONCLUSION

Aerospace medicine is the study of the hazards to health, safety, and productivity of all those concerned with human flight. Its purposes are entirely preventive in character. It is a legitimate specialty, much like occupational medicine, but in a highly specialized area, and, for the most part, much unlike Public Health administration.

10. Radiologic Health

Radiation Control*

SURELY EVERYONE is aware that radiation is a mixed blessing. But recent emphasis upon its fatal powers has caused some people to lose sight of its many benefits.

Some 17 years ago a Japanese city literally disappeared in a flash of light that shone as bright as any sun—and mankind entered the atomic age. From then on man was to learn to use radiation, to respect its power and to protect himself against its dangers. Radiation's potentialities are fearsome, wonderful, destructive, life-giving—and we are far from knowing all about it. However, we have learned two indisputable facts:

1. The use of radiation has already produced immeasurable benefits to mankind, and it is almost impossible to imagine the scope of benefits that might come from future developments. It would be most unfortunate if public hysteria, created by misunderstanding, would put an end to the use of this source of progress.
2. When it is necessary or beneficial to use radiation for medical, industrial, or research purposes, every effort should be made to avoid unnecessary exposure.

Its use as an instrument of national defense is not within the scope of this discussion, but the effect of radiation exposure will be examined.

WHAT IS RADIATION?

Webster's Dictionary says radiation is "the process by which energy is emitted from molecules and atoms owing to internal changes."

The most commonly used radiations are x-rays, gamma rays, alpha and beta particles, and neutrons. These are all classified as "ionizing radiations," because when they pass through any material, they pro-

* Reprinted, with omission of illustrations, by permission from the February, 1962, issue of the *Virginia Health Bulletin*, Vol. 14, pp. 3–11. The *Bulletin* is edited by J. Robert Anderson, Director of the Bureau of Health Education, Commonwealth of Virginia, Department of Health, Richmond, Virginia. Much of the background information for this article was obtained from Dr. Dade Moeller, Chief, Radiological Health Training Activities, Robert A. Taft Sanitary Engineering Center, Cincinnati, Ohio.

duce electrically charged bits of atoms or molecules which are called ions.

Io, the Wanderer, was a character in Greek mythology. The ion was named for her for an ion is a particle of matter or energy wandering free in nature, not attached to an atom.

Radiation can strike an electron orbiting around the nucleus of an atom and set it free, thus changing the nature of that atom. The radiation has "ionized" the atom. When a radioactive atom disintegrates, it may emit a combination of alpha particles, beta particles, or gamma rays. The first two are charged and are too large to penetrate far through solid substances. The x-rays and the gamma rays are the deep penetrators, but all of these rays are of concern to those whose job it is to protect us.

HOW RADIATION HARMS US

The penetrating ionizing rays emitted from radium, uranium, and other elements, and from man-made isotopes, x-ray machines, and nuclear reactors can harm us. They do this by entering our body and bombarding the atoms of which we are made, causing them to lose electrons, and thus changing their nature.

This change is slow and subtle, and its effect is cumulative. Only in the atom-bombed cities of Japan have there been instances of groups of humans receiving enough radiation at one time to cause quick death.

It is desirable to point out that we should have no fear of the ordinary radium dial watch or clock, or the face of a television picture tube in the home. These objects present no hazards in ordinary use.

Also, it is estimated that about half of the radiation a human being receives in his lifetime comes from x-rays. This is a diagnostic and therapeutic tool which need not be feared; merely respected and properly used.

Most scientists believe that ionizing radiation is always damaging to some extent, even the smallest amount causing harm to living cells. Humans have some 100 million cells—each with a predetermined task to perform. Depending upon the amount of exposure, ionizing radiation may destroy cells or seriously impair function. In addition, it is known that:

Lung Cancer was found in men who worked over long periods of time mining pitchblende, a source of radium.

Bone Cancer developed in watchdial painters who unknowingly ingested radium;

Leukemia is on the increase among survivors of the atomic bombings in Hiroshima and Nagasaki;

Radiation can cause alterations, or "mutations" in the genes of reproductive cells which determine the physical appearance and health of our children in future generations. These mutations (the great majority of which are harmful) may be hereditary;

Radiation accelerates the aging process which has been established by experiments on animals;

Radiation is capable of reducing fertility, the amount of loss being dependent upon the dose;

Irradiation of the eye may result in cataracts.

It must be emphasized that all of the above conditions have occured through an overexposure to radiation, and not from the day-to-day exposure common to the general population.

SOURCES OF ENVIRONMENTAL RADIATION

There are two sources of environmental radiation to which the human body may become exposed. One is natural or cosmic radiation which exists both in nature and within the human body. The second source is man-made radiation, and it is this that has caused the recent increase of radiation in our environment.

Industrial Radiation

Sources of radiation exposure associated with nuclear reactor operations include the reactor itself, its ventilation and cooling wastes procedures associated with the removal and reprocessing of its "spent" nuclear fuel and the resulting fission product wastes, and procedures associated with the mining, milling, and fabrication of new nuclear fuels. There are currently a great number of reactors in operation in the United States, with more in various stages of design or construction. Within the near future, it is expected that nearly all major colleges and universities will have reactors for research and instructional purposes. The use of reactors for the production of power is also expected to continue to increase, with a total of at least 23 civilian power reactors in operation by 1964.

Nuclear Testing

The world-wide total of nuclear detonations prior to the current Russian testing program numbered near 200. But more important than the number of detonations is their energy yield, which is a measure of the quantity of radioactive fission products released into our environment.

With regard to these radiation sources, all phases of our environment are involved. Although radioactive contaminants from our nuclear industry or from weapons test initially contaminate air and water, eventually these contaminants find their way into our food resources. Such environmental contamination results in radioactive materials being taken into the body, wherein they are potential "internal" hazards.

Man, therefore, is faced with a highly heterogeneous array of radiation sources—medical practice, cosmic radiation, nuclear industry, and nuclear detonations. Thus, this radiation released into our environment, in part, gains access to the human body through air, water, and food routes.

CONTROL OF ENVIRONMENTAL RADIATION

Control of radiation in the environment involves either source control or environmental control, both of which require an intimate knowledge of the radiation source and a continuous surveillance program.

Source Control

Source control is most easily applied in areas where the medical profession and nuclear industry are involved. Since we have said that at least half of the man-made radiation to which we are exposed comes from medical and dental x-rays, control of this source provides an excellent opportunity to reduce the total lifetime exposure of man to radiation.

Control of x-ray exposure is achieved by shielding, operating technics, and protection of personnel and patients. The proper location and shielding of an X-ray machine is extremely important. The machine must be so placed that its rays do not penetrate into areas where they might do damage. In a physician's or dentist's office, or in a hospital, care needs to be taken that rays do not go through the wall and into other places where people congregate.

To make sure that patients do not receive excessive exposure while undergoing diagnosis or treatment by x-ray, medical schools are teaching their students safe x-ray practices, manufacturers are building in filters and shields better to protect the operators and patients, and cones are being used to better focus the rays. In addition, both public and private practitioners are keeping the use of x-ray at the level of practicality and need.

Control of Industrial Radiation

Where nuclear industry is concerned, the major source of radioactivity contaminating our environment results from the waste materials which are discharged in the process of production. Criteria have been established for levels of radioactivity discharged which are judged safe, and a surveillance program established to ensure that the discharge is within these levels. Federal, State, and local governments have enacted regulations regarding the quantities of various radioactive wastes permitted for discharge and the concentrations permitted in air or public water supplies.

The nuclear energy industry, to date, has almost without exception satisfactorily met the waste discharge criteria adopted. The principal wastes discharged to the environment are fluid, and have contained comparatively low concentrations of radioactivity, although high in volume. Major atomic energy installations have, thus far, been located along huge water-courses in non-populated areas, tending to minimize the problem of waste disposal.

Environmental Control

Cosmic or "background" radiation and radioactive contaminations resulting from nuclear detonations are less subject to source control than radiation resulting from use by the medical and dental professions and nuclear industry.

Cosmic radiation has always been with us. Man has always lived with a certain amount of radiation, and has apparently thrived under these conditions. There is a great deal of radiation in outer space, some of which comes from the sun, but the earth's atmosphere is dense enough to prevent much of this cosmic radiation from passing through. In addition, the ground we walk on, the buildings we live and work in, and even parts of the human body are sources of radiation. This type of exposure is largely beyond man's control.

Radiation From Fallout

Fallout from nuclear weapons testing programs is currently the most important source of environmental contamination. It will probably continue to be a major source of long-lived fission products for many years to come, even if international control is achieved.

Fallout is tiny particles of dirt, stone, and other debris that become contaminated by the radioactive products of the bomb, and fall back to earth over a wide area. The closer to the earth the weapon is detonated, the more such particles rise into the atmosphere with the cloud, later to fall upon areas to which they are carried by the prevailing winds.

Control of the environment is at the present time the only method of protection that has been devised against fallout. This consists of treatment to reduce contamination, or curtailment of the use of the particular water or food media involved. Protection by shelter is the initial step of environmental control if subjected to extraordinarily large quantities of fallout.

PUBLIC HEALTH SERVICE ACTIVITIES

Public Health Service activities have been directed primarily toward broad environmental control, with emphasis upon a continuous and careful surveillance of our environment.

Working in cooperation with State and local health departments, the Public Health Service collects and analyzes, on a continuing basis, environmental samples from about 100 different localities in the United States. To facilitate rapid handling of these samples, laboratories are located in Las Vegas, Nevada, Montgomery, Alabama, Rockville, Maryland, Cincinnati, Ohio, and Winchester, Massachusetts.

Known as the Radiation Surveillance Network, this organization has measured fallout resulting from nuclear weapons testing, and immediately informed State health departments of significant findings. Also, in cooperation with State health authorities, the Public Health Service assays the total diet of selected population groups for radioactivity, analyzes samples collected from water supplies used on trains, airplanes, and other public carriers, and surface water samples from about 86 stations throughout the nation, and analyzes milk consumed by the public, for concentrations of radioactive elements of concern to public health.

RADIATION PROTECTION IN VIRGINIA

The bureau of Industrial Hygiene of the State Department of Health has been designated as the responsible agency for certain environmental and occupational radiation health hazards. The objectives of the State Department of Health's program in this field are:

To promote the reasonable use of radiation and radioactive materials in the State in such a manner as to prevent undue risks to the health and safety of the people of Virginia.

To inspect as completely as possible the sources of radiation in Virginia, and furnish valid recommendations for the correction of undesirable or dangerous conditions, using all available knowledge and means to secure compliance.

To serve as an information center on the subject of radiologic health.

To act as a liaison group between Federal agencies concerned with radiation and the people of Virginia both during times of normal activity and in case of emergency.

This is what the Bureau of Industrial Hygiene does now.

Assists the Atomic Energy Commission with inspection and installations and materials licensed for use in Virginia. This is done by providing personnel, transportation, special instruments, and technical assistance to the representative of the A. E. C.

Supplements the A. E. C. program by making periodic checks on agencies that use beta density gauges. These checks are required and involve making sure that radioactive material is not escaping the source.

Operates one of the stations on the National Surveillance Network of the U. S. Public Health Service. To do this, a high volume air sampler operates continuously atop the roof of the State Office Building. The filter on the sampler is examined for radioactivity. Rain and snow are collected, and used to measure the amount of radioactive fallout in precipitation. The Bureau keeps continuous records of the measurements.

Conducts a study on radioactivity in the Hampton Roads area, in cooperation with the State Bureau of Shellfish Sanitation. The study was suggested by the Atomic Energy Commission, U. S. Public Health Service, the Naval Bureau of Ships, and the Newport News Shipbuilding and Dry Dock Corporation, in anticipation of the arrival of the nuclear-powered ship *Savannah.*

In addition, the latter corporation has contracts for the construction of other nuclear powered naval ships. Also, an increasing number of nuclear ships berth and operate in the area. The Bureau is studying radioactivity levels of air, water, bottom silt, and shellfish, to determine if the presence of nuclear ships in the area increases the level of radioactivity.

Surveys x-ray equipment in city and county health departments. Such surveys are made to keep the x-ray and fluoroscopy equipment safe for patient use. Already these surveys have brought about the improvement of shielding, operating technics, and protection of personnel in many places. The Bureau tries to make repeat visits to these places to evaluate the initial recommendations made for the improvement of operations, even though the machines now are properly placed and protected.

Surveys, on request, the x-ray equipment of dentists and private physicians. This has been greatly expanded through the operation of the Sur-pak program, with the cooperation of the Virginia Dental Association and the United States Public Health Service. This program consists of mailing to each dentist a packet containing a film to be exposed to x-ray. The film is developed and evaluated. Any machine found to be delivering radiation in excess of that necessary for a satisfactory dental radiograph, such as that caused by excessive beam size, insufficient filtration, or leakage in the tube head, is remedied.

Again, the purpose of this program is to eliminate unnecessary patient exposure.

Ninety per cent of the 1100 machines in use by dentists throughout the State have been, or are in the process of being evaluated. The results are proving highly favorable. In fact, it is being discovered that a large proportion of the State's dentists operate at a greater standard of safety than is required.

Also, implements the recently enacted State law requiring the registration of all persons using x-ray equipment. Known as the Radiation Source Registration Act, its purpose is to locate sources of radiation, register the users with the Bureau of Industrial Hygiene, and obtain compliance with regulations designed to promote the utmost safety in the use of these machines. Where necessary, the Bureau has demonstrated ways in which the persons operating the machines may minimize their exposure to radiation. In many cases, changes in equipment and technics have been recommended to reduce the exposure received by the patient.

Reviews plans of x-ray installations, and examines installations under construction or renovation, for adequacy of shielding.

Also, personnel from the Bureau of Industrial Hygiene accompany, provide instruments for, and assist Atomic Energy Commission representatives whenever installations in Virginia are being inspected.

The Bureau hopes to expand its activities in the near future. The following areas are particularly in need of attention:

Many large radiation sources used for the inspection of welds, castings, and the like are brought into Virginia from other States. These sources are mobile, so that it is impossible to fix permanent shielding when they are in use. The Bureau cannot assure the safety of these machines unless they are required to be registered in Virginia, and notice given when they are moved from place to place in the State. There are other large sources of radium and x-ray used industrially in the State which should be checked periodically for proper shielding and safe handling technics. Other uses of radiation, such as static eliminators, may actually result in a leakage of radioactive material. Each user of such equipment should be required to follow a testing program against such a possibility.

THE NUCLEAR FUTURE

That the problem of environmental contamination by radiation will increase as the use of nuclear energy expands, is one of the major complexities developing in the field of Public Health today. One aspect of particular importance is the factor of TIME. The development of radiologic health programs must keep pace with the growth of our nuclear energy industries and other significant sources of radioactive contamination such as nuclear weapons. The rapidity with which these sources of radiation are evolving is probably the most significant aspect of the whole field of radiologic health. An informed public can make a valuable contribution to this endeavor to enable mankind to enjoy the fruits of the "flame of life" and not perish from its destructive forces.

11. Genetics and Public Health

Some Genetic Aspects of Public Health*

ROBERT W. DAY, M.D., PH.D.

INTRODUCTION

RECENT ADVANCES in genetics and in Public Health suggest that these two areas increasingly borrow from each other in methodology as well as tend toward mutually profitable and overlapping subjects for study. This is especially true in view of the trend of emphasis in Public Health, now more and more directed at the chronic, predominantly noninfectious conditions. The accompanying considerations of multiple etiologies, of complex interactions among environment, agent, and host, have served to emphasize the roles of the genetic material as determinants of disease.

As these trends in Public Health occur, so also have major advances in all phases of genetic studies. Notable is the newer knowledge of cell heredity, the nature and, to some extent, the workings of the code by which genetic information is transmitted with uniqueness and specificity to a protein product and thus to cellular activity. Although advances in cell genetics have come about largely through the use of relatively simple biologic systems the knowledge gained here will undoubtedly apply throughout the animal kingdom. The presence of DNA (deoxyribonucleic acid) as the genetic material is virtually universal, a logical consequence of the similarity of hereditary mechanisms in organisms varying greatly in other characteristics.

Many aspects of genetic study have direct application in Public Health activities; for example, increasing presence in the environment of radioactive materials is a cause of concern because of short-term (medical) and long-term (genetic) effects. Radiation, however, is but one of the forces capable of affecting the genetic material through mutation; others such as a variety of chemical substances, identified through their effects in animals, are also found in the human environment. Such substances are known to have immediate biologic effects on man, and may likely prove mutagenic as well. Use of genetic study in measuring and comparing mutation rates according to exposures is a necessary adjunct to control.

*This original contribution was prepared especially for this publication. The author is Assistant Professor of Epidemiology, University of California, Los Angeles.

HEREDITARY DISEASE

A long list of inherited diseases has been compiled (Gates 1946). The majority are rare conditions, although taken as a group, not inconsiderable. Several points, however, should be stressed at the outset. First, much more is known about genetic effects leading to abnormal conditions than about the inheritance and hereditary properties involved in biologic variables that fall within ranges currently considered as normal. Second, these diseases in which a clear-cut mode of inheritance is known, although extensive in terms of the total number of specific abnormalities, are outweighed in importance in comparison with the more frequent diseases for which an hereditary component is suspected. The latter do not conform to known patterns of inheritance but do show familial aggregations of disease not so far satisfactorily explained by common environmental conditions.

Genetic determination in a variety of diseases covers a spectrum somewhat analogous to that in infectious illnesses. For some conditions such as phenylketonuria a single locus and the appropriate abnormal genes are sufficient to produce the disease. In other cases, however, the presence of abnormal genetic material is apparent only in an appropriate environmental setting. Erythroblastosis fetalis is an example. Here the Rh positive fetus and the Rh negative mother are both needed to produce disease. The effect is also modified by parity and by the ABO blood group relationships between mother and fetus (Levene and Rosenfield 1961). Other diseases show some genetic component, but, as discussed above, not in the defined mathematic relationships implied by formal genetic theory. The contributions to etiology from a genetic investigation into any disease will depend, then, on how important heredity is in the abnormal mechanism leading to that disease, and, most importantly, upon the accuracy and completeness of methods for genetic analysis (Steinberg 1959).

Implicit in any discussion of genetics is an acknowledgment of the degree to which the field is subdivided. Those methods dealing with cells and well-controlled simpler cell systems contrast with, complement, and draw upon the technics of biochemical genetics. On the other hand, radiation genetics deals more with the effects of physical agents on the hereditary material. The recently introduced technics of tissue culture have found much use in genetic study, and are major methods in somatic cell genetics. A field of importance to the study of mass effects of disease is population genetics. Attention here is upon the movement of genes in well-defined interbreeding populations subjected to selection for favorable genes and selection against deleterious genes, meanwhile considering the consequences of the addition of new genes via mutation and migration. All technics of study are of course interdependent, and division into special groupings is arbitrary, but of both traditional and pedagogic significance.

EPIDEMIOLOGY AND GENETICS

The similarities between human genetics and epidemiology have been noted for some time. Neel and Schull (1964) devoted a chapter of their book to the subject, and recent reviews by Myrianthopoulos (1959), and another by Dublin and Blumberg (1961) cover some of the material presented here. An important discussion of certain methodologic problems relating epidemiology and human genetics is appended to recent papers by Morton (1962) and Lilienfeld (1962). Much of the genetic literature of interest in Public Health matters is scattered among more specialized publications. However, a basic approach to human genetics has been most recently presented by Stern (1960), and other additions to the list of general texts should include those of Fraser Roberts (1959), and of Neel and Schull (1954). Two recently published collections, one set edited by Steinberg (1961), Steinberg and Bearn (1962), and the other by Penrose (1961a) are valuable summaries of work of current interest.

The methodology of epidemiology, well known to those with Public Health training, consists largely of comparing disease patterns between different population groups. The major problems concern sampling of populations under study and ascertainment of cases. Much valuable epidemiologic evidence can be derived from the use of rather gross ascertainment practices exemplified, for instance, by death certificate data. Accuracy is not completely assured by such means of data gathering, but then the condition is usually common, coronary heart disease for example, and loss of some cases by misclassification errors is not serious, and may be sufficiently randomized so as to cause no problem in analysis and interpretation. A genetic study, however, is often more concerned with the accurate ascertainment of cases, and complete study of those families from which these index cases are derived. Such epidemiologic variables as specification or definition of a case, consistency of criteria, and search for missed cases are pursued carefully. This is especially true as genetic study has mostly dealt with diseases of low frequency, while epidemiologic studies have been directed largely at the common illnesses. Without a doubt, the growth of interest in a quantitative genetic approach to man, and the more widespread use of epidemiologic technics generally will do much to merge these traditional emphases and interests.

GENETIC DIAGNOSIS

The phenomenon of diseases completely determined by abnormal genes was mentioned previously. Generally, certain characteristics of a disease will aid in attributing to it an hereditary etiology: occurrence of the disease among related persons in definite numeric proportion; transmission from generation to generation, or vertical and *not* horizontal spread; failure to spread to nonrelated persons in the same generation; onset at some characteristic age without a specific precipitating event; greater concordance among identical when compared with fraternal twins; and others (Morton 1962). Those diseases or syndromes fulfilling the above criteria are then defined as genetically determined.

CHROMOSOMAL DISORDERS

Recapitulation of some of the properties of inheritance serves to underscore many of these features of inherited illnesses. Each new zygote, the product of a union of sperm and ovum, contains 46 chromosomes in 23 pairs, one member of each pair from each parent. The sperm and ova thus contribute equally 23 chromosomes apiece and the production of these gametes via the specialized process of meiosis is a unique property of the reproductive tract.

The normal diploid chromosome number of man, 46, was only recently confirmed (Tjio and Levan 1956), and the introduction of newer techniques has led to rapid developments in human cytogenetics. Most studies have utilized tissue culture of somatic (nongerminal) cells. Morphologic distinctions between chromosome pairs, or between groupings of pairs, have been established. The categorization so obtained is important because some diseases in man are consistently associated with losses or extra amounts of chromosomal material and, hence, fewer or more genes, thus resulting in an upset to the genetic balance.

In 1959, Lejeune and his coworkers (Lejeune, Gautier and Turpin 1959) described an extra small chromosome present in somatic cell cultures from four patients with mongolism (Down's syndrome). This finding has been widely confirmed. Shortly thereafter, two new syndromes of mental defect and variously related congenital malformations were reported (Patau, Smith, Therman, Inhorn and Wagner 1960; Edwards, Harnden, Cameron, Crosse and Wolff 1960). Techniques of somatic chromosome analysis are being widely applied especially in populations of the malformed and mentally defective where the frequency of chromosomal abnormalities is not only high, but also probably of considerable developmental consequence when compared with phenotypic normals.

The 23 pairs of chromosomes are divisible into 22 pairs of autosomes and one pair of sex chromosomes (Figure 1). The latter serve a sex-determining role in man. The male is XY and the female is XX. It has been shown that the Y chromosome is male-determining, for in those situations of X-polysomy, such as XXY, XXXY, the affected person is outwardly male. Conversely, in cases with abnormal numbers of X-chromosomes, and where a Y chromosome is lacking, the

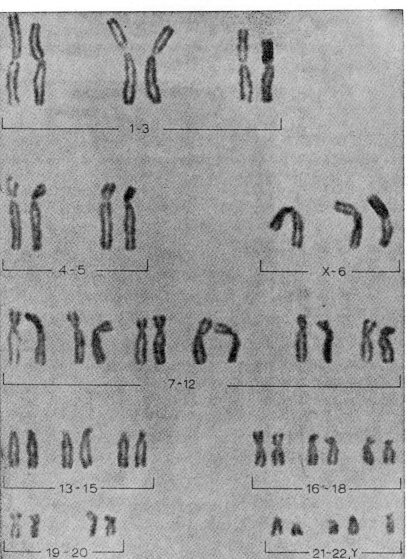

Figure 1. Normal male karyotype showing the XY sex Chromosomes and the 22 autosomal pairs.

patient is phenotypically female. Males and females with abnormal numbers of X-chromosomes are generally sterile, lack normal development of secondary sex characteristics, and may show some degree of mental defect.

The presence of 2 X-chromosomes in normal females, and but 1 in normal males might imply that for those loci that are sex-linked, the female would often produce two doses of a particular gene (allele) product while the male would be limited to a single dose (Lyon 1962). Differences in the magnitude of gene products, as predicted under this hypothesis, are not observed in the human. Rather, equality in gene action is achieved through inactivation of one of the X-chromosomes in the female. The inactivation, in turn, has consequences to both biochemical and cytologic behavior of the cell, and the latter has distinct importance in screening programs. The inactive chromosome forms a darkly staining mass at the edge of the nucleus, the sex chromatin body, observed in cells derived from many sites, perhaps most easily and appropriately in fixed and stained scrapings of the superficial epithelium of the inside of the cheek, or the so-called buccal smear.

To maintain equivalent sex-linked gene behavior in males and females alike, then, one member of the X-chromosome pair is inactive in the female and forms the sex chromatin body which provides an easy differentiation between the sexes. With abnormal numbers of X-chromosomes, X/O Turner's syndrome, the XXY male with Klinefelter's syndrome, etc., an anomalous sex chromatin pattern is observed when the expected nuclear sex (buccal smear pattern) is compared with the phenotypic sex. The buccal smear provides a simple, cheap, and rapid diagnostic test which has been widely applied as a screening method. Studies of populations of unselected consecutive births suggest a combined frequency of about one individual with anomalous sex chromatin per 200 live births (Maclean, Harnden and Court Brown 1961). The significance on outcome in terms of management instituted at birth through proper case finding, for patients with sex chromosome abnormalities, has yet to be assessed. However, certain defects associated with sex-chromosome abnormalities are no doubt susceptible to amelioration under favorable circumstances, and a yield from buccal smears taken on newborns of 1 in 200 when compared, for instance, with 1 in 10,000 estimated in phenylketonuria, gives ample grounds for intensive study as part of child health research.

METABOLIC DISEASES

A variety of metabolic diseases are also known to have a hereditary etiology. In genetic terms, the problems posed in these biochemical abnormalities are perhaps less complicated than the chemistry. However, the possibilities of treatment in these diseases are promising and in one in particular, phenylketonuria (PKU), a special diet essentially lacking the amino acid phenylalanine, when instituted sufficiently early in life (under six months preferably) permits normal development. The rationale for dietary management of this sort follows from an understanding of the genetic and chemical defect.

In brief, there are 2 genes (alleles) at the locus governing production of the enzyme phenylalanine hydroxylase. The common allele (P), when present in at least a single dose, and thus by definition a dominant, guides the production of adequate amounts of the hydroxylase; the enzyme, in turn, controls the orderly metabolism of phenylalanine. The recessive allele (p), when substituted at the two loci on the homologous chromosome pair, prevents synthesis of the hydroxylase, phenylalanine blood levels rise, alternate metabolic pathways are now utilized, and in some fashion normal intellectual development is usually impaired. The degree of defect is sufficient to prevent reproduction in affected persons. Thus, essentially all new cases result from matings between 2 carriers (Pp) and the theoretic expectation of any child from the appropriate mating having the disease is 0.25.

Of interest in Public Health programs are the problems of case finding in PKU (Centerwall, Chinnock and Pusavat 1960). As mentioned above, the dietary treatment is effective, but must be started at an early age. Therefore, a screening technic applied to all newborns would ideally indicate those few needing the special treatment. A major problem, however, is introduced by maternal-fetal interactions when the fetus is pp and a potential phenylketonuric and the mother is of the carrier genotype (Pp) and metabolically able to maintain normal amino acid metabolism while the child is *in utero*. The various tests available for screening out PKU cases in infants depend on a high level of phylalanine and the other abnormal metabolic products characteristic of PKU. Thus, any new procedure, when applied during the immediate post-natal period, while the child is still in the hospital and thus readily available for the screening, must be well tested against the possibility of yielding false negatives. The abnormally high blood levels diagnostic of PKU are often not achieved until the child is at least several days old. Wright (1962) has discussed this problem, and points out that a variety of case-finding technics need to be used because, thus far no test has been demonstrated with reproducibility to diagnose PKU among all newborns.

It has been suggested that special attention be given to later born offspring of couples both known to be carriers (Pp) through having had at least one affected child. The index or initial case serving to identify these high-risk families might profitably be sought among institutionalized retardates, those in special community programs as, for instance, special schools, and also in patients under observation because of developmental retardation. However, to register a couple as heterozygous (Pp) requires that they have already had an affected child (pp). Calculations suggest that somewhat more than one-half of the PKU children born in any given period will represent the first case in the family. Thus, case finding must be pursued in many ways if a high yield of patients is to be detected sufficiently early in life to benefit from the treatment.

Many suggestions dealing with follow-up of newborns are being made, and PKU screening is but one objective here. The over-all problem, however, will unquestionably have parallels in the future. Health departments will be increasingly engaged in screening programs, perhaps mainly because such agencies are repositories of vital statistics, and thus have available a complete enumeration of all potential cases. It should be stressed, however, that a PKU screening program means careful planning based on thorough understanding of the genetic and chemical problems involved.

DISEASE REGISTRATION

Implicit in the discussion of PKU screening, with careful attention to heterozygous parents discovered through the presence of affected offspring, is the idea of disease registration. As stated before, strictly inherited disorders are rare individually, but collectively are of considerable interest. Health agencies, responsible as they are for data collection, enjoy an advantageous position from which to assist in disease registration, both from mortality records and through the gathering of morbidity statistics. Examples of such data collection are the twin registers maintained in some states. Human twins present an excellent source for genetic study as the identical pairs are genetically similar at all loci, and thus present a method for weighing the relative influence of environment in modifying inherited traits, and vice versa. Twin registration is simple in that multiple births are noted on the certificate. Establishing zygosity, i.e., whether identical or fraternal, and follow-up are more costly and laborious. Extension of the registration idea to other conditions, however, is not impractical. For instance, the extensive insurance and other morbidity data already collected routinely could be sifted and possibly redesigned in form to yield information about heritable disorders; once a family carrying certain genes has been identified through an index case, the remaining pedigree is usually a good source of additional cases.

The discussion of PKU from a Public Health viewpoint may serve also to introduce the matter of prevention. Generally, primary prevention in genetics still takes the form of counseling. For those diseases in which genotypes can be diagnosed, information can be given, derived from basic theory, that indicates the relative risk for couples having affected children. PKU is something of a rarity at this time in that it is an inherited yet treatable disease, and thus is amenable to secondary preventive technics dependent on early case finding. A number of diseases appear to show heritable components, however, but not in the defined numeric relationships that are specified under genetic theory. Such conditions as coronary heart disease, diabetes mellitus, some forms of mental illness, malformations, including anencephaly and spina bifida, and many others all show a degree of familial aggregation. From studies of essentially an epidemiologic nature, many retrospective in design, series of empiric risk figures can be derived, and are useful in counseling. However, nothing is usually known in particular cases as regards *a* mode of inheritance—thus the reliance on empiric risks. With more exact knowledge of the hereditary mechanism involved in a given disease, theoretic values can be substituted. A good example of this is the current situation in mongolism (Penrose 1961b).

Another possible use of genetic knowledge may lie in identifying persons at increased risk for a variety of diseases. The association between the ABO blood groups and disease such as group A in gastric cancer, group O in peptic ulcer, etc., may be refined to the point of aiding in preventive programs (Clarke 1961). At present, these disease and trait (such as blood group) associations are empiric observations.

FREQUENCY OF INHERITED DISEASES

Finally, some assessment of the total impact of inherited diseases seems appropriate. Stevenson (1961) has recently published a breakdown, both by mode of inheritance and age and nature of onset, of genetically determined abnormal traits. The over-all value is 51 per 1,000 births, or 5 per cent. The two categories contributing most to this over-all frequency are designated as malformations and common disorders with some genetic components in etiology. These account for 20 per 1,000 and 10 per 1,000 births respectively. Chromosomal abnormalities are set at 4 per 1,000, a probable underestimate while malformations and diseases determined by genes at single loci (such as PKU) are valued at 5 per 1,000 for the former and 8 per 1,000 births for the latter. Finally, erythroblastosis is estimated for a North European Caucasian population at 4 per 1,000 births. This listing is not exhaustive, but does present important genetically determined diseases categorized very nicely for epidemiological purposes.

SUMMARY

In conclusion, this brief over-view of areas of genetic interest meshing with matters of epidemiologic and Public Health concern has emphasized some of the similarities of both fields in their approaches to problems. At present, giving priority to diseases in terms of extent and magnitude of disability, those conditions with a clear-cut hereditary etiology are not a major problem. Still, when diagnosis and treatment of a condition are available, failure to control is deplorable. On the other hand, most of the diseases of current major Public Health importance have some genetic components and more emphasis, certainly in the research aspects, is being given to heredity. Finally, the Public Health worker needs many skills, some more and some less specialized. The list of these skills and knowledge is always growing and always changing. Without a doubt, genetics is now on this list and will stay there for a long time, a result of the many mechanisms of heredity in disease determination, some of which have been discussed here.

1. Centerwall, W. R., Chinnock, R. F. and Pusavat, A. Phenylketonuria: screening programs and testing methods. *Amer. J. Pub. Hlth.* 50:1667–1676, 1960.

2. Clarke, C. A. Blood groups and disease. *Recent Progress in Human Genetics, Vol. I.* Ed. A. G. Steinberg; New York: Grune and Stratton, 1961. Chapter 4, pp. 81–114.

3. Dublin, T. D. and Blumberg, B. S. An epidemiologic approach to inherited disease susceptibility. *Pub. Hlth. Reports.* 76:499:505, 1961.

4. Edwards, J. H., Harnden, D. G., Cameron, A. H., Crosse, M. and Wolff, O. H. A new trisomic syndrome. *Lancet.* i:787–790, 1960.

5. Gates, R. R. *Human Genetics.* 2 Vols. New York: Macmillan, 1946.

6. Lejeune, J., Gautier, M. and Turpin, R. Les chromosomes humains en culture de tissues. *C. R. Acad. SCI.* 248:602–603, 1959.

7. Levene, H. and Rosenfield, R. E. ABO incompatibility. *Recent Progress in Human Genetics, Vol. I.* Ed. A. G. Steinberg; New York: Grune and Stratton, 1961. Chapter 5, pp. 120–153.

8. Lilienfeld, A. M. Sampling techniques and significance tests. *Methodology in Human Genetics.* Ed. W. J. Burdette; San Francisco: Holden-Day, 1962. pp. 3–16.

9. Lyon, M. F. Sex chromatin and gene action in the mammalian X-chromosome. *Amer. J. Human Genet.* 14:135–145, 1962.

10. Maclean, N., Harnden, D. G. and Court Brown, W. M. Abnormalties of sex chromosome constitution in newborn babies. *Lancet.* ii:406–408, 1961.

11. Morton, N. E. Segregation and linkage. *Methodology in Human Genetics.* Ed. W. J. Burdette; San Francisco: Holden-Day, 1962. pp. 17–52.

12. Myrianthopoulos, N. C. Genetics and public health. *Pub. Hlth. Reports.* 74:1098–1105, 1959.

13. Neel, J. V. and Schull, W. J. *Human Heredity.* Chicago: University of Chicago Press, 1954.

14. Patau, K., Smith, D. W., Therman, E., Inhorn, S. L. and Wagner, H. P. Multiple congenital anomaly caused by an extra autosome. *Lancet.* i:790–793, 1960.

15. Penrose, L. S., ed. *Recent Advances in Human Genetics.* Boston: Little, Brown and Co., 1961a.

16. Penrose, L. S. Mongolism. *Brit. Med. Bull.* 17:184–189, 1961b.

17. Roberts, J. A. F. *An Introduction to Medical Genetics.* London: Oxford University Press, 1959.

18. Steinberg, A. G. Methodology in human genetics. *Amer. J. Human Genet.* 11:315–333, 1959.

19. Steinberg, A. G., ed. *Recent Progress in Human Genetics, Vol I.* New York: Grune and Stratton, 1961.

20. Steinberg, A. G. and Bearn, A. G., eds. *Recent Progress in Human Genetics, Vol. II.* New York: Grune and Stratton, 1962.

21. Stern, C. *Human Genetics.* San Francisco: Freeman, 1960.

22. Stevenson, A. C. Frequency of congenital and hereditary disease. *Brit. Med. Bull.* 17:254–259, 1961.

23. Tjio, J. H. and Levan, A. The chromosome number of man. *Hereditas.* 42:1–6, 1956.

24. Wright, S. W. Mass screening for phenylketonuria. *J. Pediat.* 61: 651–652, 1962.

12. Public Health Laboratories

The Developing Role of Laboratories in Chronic Disease Programs*

WILFRED D. DAVID, M.D.

CHRONIC DISEASE and disability are the major health and medical problems facing our nation today. This is the premise upon which I base this presentation, and I do not need to defend the premise with a mountain of statistics. The size of the burden imposed today upon our people by cancer, heart disease, diabetes, arthritis, and a host of neurologic and other diseases is well known.

Not only are we faced with new impetus in the attack from chronic disease upon an older, more numerous, and more susceptible population; we are faced as well with the cases of chronic disability which accumulated while we were concerned first with the infectious enemy. In additon, we do not yet know the cause of most of the chronic diseases, much less how to cure or prevent them. Is it any wonder, then, that in dealing with such disease and disability we find ourselves running harder than ever before just to stay where we are?

In examining the role of health department laboratories in this struggle, I am not implying that the traditional services of the laboratory are becoming obsolete. There is the most urgent need to continue and to improve those services with which the laboratory has contributed so much to the control of infectious disease. Each day we gain new evidence that this war goes on, that the organisms we fight are fighting back.

What I do proclaim, however, is the need in the laboratory and all along the frontier of medical progress to focus more sharply upon the emerging problems of chronic disease. For medicine and science now fight upon two fronts—against infectious diseases on the one front and against chronic disease on the other. As a full member of the medical and scientific team the laboratory is committed. The only questions yet unanswered concern how far and how fast laboratories can move toward providing services for chronic disease.

* Reprinted by permission from the January, 1963, issue of *Public Health Reports*, Vol. 78, pp. 13–16. This paper was based on a presentation at the Sixth Biennial Planning Conference of the Association of State and Territorial Public Health Laboratory Directors and the Public Health Service in Atlanta, Georgia, June 15, 1962. The author is Assistant Chief, Division of Chronic Diseases, Public Health Service, Department of Health, Education, and Welfare, Washington, D.C.

On the basis of past experience I am confident that health department laboratories will take on new responsibilities in chronic disease just as fast as State and national action make this possible. I still recall with amazement, for example, the speed and efficiency with which State laboratories retooled to employ the new weapons of virology.

Unfortunately, retooling and retraining for chronic disease services are far more complicated and far less manageable than previous adjustments, from the administrative as well as the technical points of view.

In the first place the warrant of health department laboratories to deal with chronic diseases is not so well recognized as the traditional mandate to protect against infectious diseases. Nor is the background and training of laboratory personnel well oriented to demands in the chronic disease area. By and large, the emphasis in the past has been microbiology rather than biochemistry or pathology.

In addition, the chronic diseases are deceptive and complex. They have symptomless stages of development and are given to multiplicity. They involve the basic structure and behavior of cells, the chemical composition of the body and the effects of environment upon it. Before we are through we may be dealing with the most basic causes and chemistry of life itself. We indeed lack weapons against such an enemy.

However, we are not powerless. We may not have the best of all possible tests for uterine cancer, but we do have a good test. We may not be able with perfect accuracy to detect in infants the metabolic errors leading to mental retardation, but we are making progress.

As recently as January 1962, Congress authorized an expanded program with additional funds for neurologic and sensory disease control. Many of the hopes and plans for this new program in the Division of Chronic Diseases of the Public Health Service are firmly joined to progress in the laboratory. The strong belief exists that in the laboratory will be found, for example, the simplified and improved tests we need to detect phenylketonuria, galactosemia, glycine deficiency, maple syrup disease, histidinuria, Wilson's disease, and other causes of mental retardation.

Diabetes control is another field in which we are particularly encouraged and hopeful. Great strides have been made in developing improved laboratory methods and devices for case-finding. The number of States actively blood testing for diabetes is growing. At present, nearly a quarter million persons per year are screened for diabetes in programs reported to the Public Health Service by half the States.

Advances are being made in laboratory techniques to help the physician predict, diagnose, and treat disorders of the heart and circulatory system. The various laboratory techniques used in conjunction with anticoagulant therapy have been reviewed recently by the

Heart Disease Control Laboratory of the Public Health Service, and the results have been published.[1]

In our efforts against arthritis, we are beginning to move ahead. For example, blood uric acid determination holds the promise of being a practical method of screening for susceptibility to gout, a painful and crippling member of the arthritis family.

Also, we are following closely the development of tests to identify the rheumatoid factor even though we recognize that as yet little can be anticipated in the way of practical preventive measures.

Each day we can do more in the laboratory and in every other phase of medicine and science, if not to prevent the onset, at least to prevent the more serious complications of chronic disease and disability. The key to prevention in this secondary sense is early detection—finding the disease and referring the patient to his physician before overt symptoms can appear—and the key to early detection is the laboratory. More and more the scene is shifting from recognition of disease signs in the examining room to prediction of disease potential in the laboratory.

Clearly, services for chronic disease are an increasingly vital function of the laboratory, including the State laboratory. How well are laboratories prepared? What are the implications for laboratories in this changing emphasis? To my mind the answers all boil down to standardization and certification.

STANDARDIZATION

If the physician is to use the results of laboratory work for prediction, diagnosis, or therapy, he must know what the results mean and if they mean the same thing every time. All too often, however, when the physician seeks to interpret the results of laboratory tests he encounters a bewildering variety of techniques, often yielding different values and subject to different interpretations.

For example, numerous techniques are used to measure serum cholesterol levels in the blood. While measuring essentially the same thing, these techniques produce widely different ranges of test values considered normal. Furthermore, the results from a given technique may vary from laboratory to laboratory and even in the same laboratory from day to day. Obviously this is confusing, even to the physician familiar with laboratory procedures.

Naturally, physicians tend to mistrust work done in laboratories unfamiliar to them. At best the situation results in loss of time and energy and duplicate expense when the physician feels he must retest. At worst the physician can misdiagnose or order an unjustified change in therapeutic regimen.

Standardization does not mean regimentation. The latter is detrimental to the experimentation and initiative so vital to the improvement of methodology. Standardization means comparability or reproducibility of results. This problem is neither new nor strange to those familiar with the multiplicity of tests which so confused the early syphilis detection programs. In my opinion we are still plagued by such confusion in our testing programs for many of the chronic diseases. If the physician and the laboratory are to work effectively as the first team against chronic disease, this confusion must be overcome.

We are not without leadership dedicated to solving the problems of standardization. Dr. Gerald Cooper and his associates at the Communicable Disease Center in Atlanta offer an excellent example of such leadership. A number of State health department laboratories are actively cooperating in this and other standardization efforts. Much remains to be done, however, and no agency seems better qualified than the State laboratory for the task. Through guidance and direction to private laboratories the State laboratory can help immeasurably the medical profession and the public it serves.

CERTIFICATION

If proof is required of the need to certify laboratories, we have only to recall the recent accounts of unreliable work and doubtful practices in a few laboratories. In too many States there is neither licensing nor listing of the local private laboratories. In fact, a person totally untrained in laboratory science can often operate a clinical laboratory. Untold numbers of clinical laboratories now operate without adequate supervision or with only token supervision.

The laboratory, of course, has a responsibility to make as certain as possible that all its work is of uniform quality and reliability. But in the final analysis, certification and licensure are State and community responsibilities. Some method of assessing and assuring the quality of laboratory work is essential. In carrying out this responsibility the State or community must police the few. But for the many the need is more often for guidance, consultation, and training. Here again the State laboratory bears a heavy load of responsibility.

FEDERAL ASSISTANCE

In 1957, when the American Public Health Association's Committee on Laboratory Services in the Chronic Diseases made a survey, it was found that States most often cited lack of funds as the major reason for not expanding chronic disease laboratory services.

Today, this reason is losing validity. The trend favors financial and other assistance from the Federal Government to States for improving and expanding laboratory services, including services in chronic diseases. The Community Health Services and Facilities Act of 1961 is the latest and most important evidence of such a trend.

Two provisions of this act are of particular interest to laboratories. The first authorizes formula grants to assist States, primarily through public and private nonprofit agencies, in developing community programs aimed at the prevention of disability and the appropriate care of long-term patients. The emphasis is on out-of-hospital programs such as improvement of nursing home care, outpatient clinic services, rehabilitation services, and nursing care of the sick at home. The grants may be used by States to improve and expand activities of the State laboratory. The possibility of using grants to implement and enforce licensure or certification laws is only part of this picture. Through this mechanism we at the Federal level hope to encourage States to provide increased technical assistance and consultation to laboratory directors so that they may improve the scope and quality of their services.

In addition, the States may use grant funds to provide training and education courses to improve the competence of laboratory personnel. I see no reason why States cannot use these funds to contract for services from private laboratories and in this and other ways encourage and assist community screening programs.

The second provision of the new law of particular interest to laboratory directors is that authorizing grants for development of improved methods of providing services to the chronically ill. Whereas the formula grants generally seek to assist in initiating and expanding community services of established types, the project grants stress experimentation and demonstration to develop new and better methods of providing services. More than 160 applications for these project grants have been submitted, representing nearly every State. More than 70 applications have been approved and funded. Hopefully, the State laboratory will be able to share in this opportunity to investigate and experiment to benefit increasing millions of chronically ill and impaired persons.

Still another program with strong implications for the State laboratory is the new research grants program being developed in the Division of Chronic Diseases of the Public Health Service. The program is patterned largely after the research grants program at the National Institutes of Health. The difference is that we seek to encourage applied rather than basic research. We are particularly interested in:

1. Development, refinement, adaptation, and evaluation of screening and diagnostic tests which can be applied to large groups in order to simplify, accelerate, reduce the cost, or improve the reliability of early detection of chronic diseases.

2. Coordinating, organizing, recording, and providing care and related services, including laboratory services, to the disabled, aged, and chronically ill in a variety of settings.

3. Development and use of instruments such as electromechanical testing devices.

4. Development and use of new procedures and techniques in the detection as well as the management of chronic diseases.

SUMMARY

In Public Health, emphasis is shifting from the infectious to the chronic disorders. The laboratory has the responsibility to help physicians predict the implication of cellular and chemical change before symptoms appear and thus expose chronic disease before it causes serious damage. Present trends in legislation and programing indicate increasing support of laboratories from Federal-State activities.

1. U.S. Public Health Service, Heart Disease Control Laboratory: *Laboratory Techniques in the Control of Anticoagulant Therapy.* Prepared by Marguerite L. Chandler. Preliminary edition. U.S. Communicable Disease Center, Atlanta, Ga., revised May 1962.

13. Public Health Psychiatry

Action for Mental Health*

DIGEST OF THE FINAL REPORT OF THE
JOINT COMMISSION ON MENTAL ILLNESS AND HEALTH

THE MENTAL HEALTH STUDY ACT of 1955 directed the Joint Commission on Mental Illness and Health, under grants administered by the National Institute of Mental Health, to analyze and evaluate the needs and resources of the mentally ill people of America and make recommendations for the national mental health program.

The purpose of this report is to arrive at a program that would approach adequacy in meeting the needs of the mentally ill—to develop a plan of action, in other words, that would satisfy us that we are doing the best we can toward their recovery. The latter is not at present the case. We have not been able to do our best for the mentally ill to date, nor have we been able to make it wholly clear what keeps us from doing so. Attempts to provide more humane care for the mentally ill and to transform "insane asylums" into hospitals and clinics true to the healing purpose of medicine have occurred periodically during the last two centuries. While each reform appears to have gained sufficient ground to give its supporters some sense of progress, each has been rather quickly followed by backsliding, loss-of professional momentum, and public indifference.

Even if we can find the road to a substantial reduction in the human and economic problems of mental illness, we are obliged to remain in full view of certain intervening observations that provide little cause for hope except as we can dispose of them. We must note, for instance, the curious blindness of the public as a whole and of psychiatry itself to what in reality would be required to fulfill the well publicized demand that millions of mentally ill shall have sufficient help in overcoming the disturbances that destroy their self-respect and social usefulness.

Further, we must rise above our self-preservative functions as members of different professions, social classes, and economic philosophies and illuminate the means of working together out of mutual respect for our fellow man. We each have a responsibility that is common to all—our responsibility as citizens of a democratic nation founded out of faith in the uniqueness, integrity, and dignity of human life.

---

* Reprinted by permission from the March, 1961, issue of *Modern Hospital*, Vol. 96, pp. 109–124.

Why Has Care of the Mentally Ill Lagged?

The United States Congress, in the last 10 years, has given the American public a working demonstration of a new willingness to accept leadership and responsibility in active efforts to help citizens who are threatened by mental illness. The federal government's chief exemplifications of this demonstration may be found in the programs of the National Institute of Mental Health and the Veterans Administration. The good example has been followed in the efforts of State legislatures, governors, and their public health, mental health, and public welfare agencies in many States.

It is tempting to congratulate ourselves on the gains scored—in increased amounts of money spent for mental health research, in the increases in mental health personnel, in the beneficial effects of the new drugs. But the demand for public mental health services is still largely unmet, despite the gains.

One of the most revealing findings of our mental health study is that comparatively few of 277 State hospitals—probably no more than 20 per cent—have participated in innovations designed to make them therapeutic, as contrasted to custodial, institutions. Our information leads us to believe that more than half of the patients in most State hospitals receive no active treatment of any kind designed to improve their mental condition. This is the core problem and unfinished business of mental health. Eight of every 10 mental hospital patients are in State institutions. These hospitals carry a daily load of more than 540,000 patients, and look after nearly a million in a year's time.

Commonly, a clearly defined, well established public demand and need for a particular health program is sufficient to stimulate aggressive public action toward its support and progressive steps to organize whatever high-quality facilities may be needed. Quick responsiveness in meeting the demand is not characteristic in the mental illness field, however.

Mental illness, commonly regarded as America's No. 1 health problem, ranked fourth in the categoric interests of the National Institutes of Health in 1950, as measured by dollars spent; by 1960, it had risen to second, behind cancer. The gains of the voluntary campaign have not been commensurate, however. Voluntary mental health funds ranked eighth at the beginning and seventh at the end of the period, and were eighth in grand total.

Despite the "big push" in recent years to do something about major mental illness, the average proportion of general State expenditures and of State health expenditures going for the care of mental hospital patients actually declined.

The quality of care given these patients may be judged from the fact that State hospitals spend an average of $4.44 per patient per day compared with $31.16 for community general hospitals, and $12 or more per patient day both for tuberculosis and Veterans Administration psychiatric hospitals. Likewise, State hospitals have the lowest ratio of hospital personnel to patients, 0.32 per patient, as compared with 2.1 in community general hospitals.

For the last four years, there has been a net decrease in the number of patients living in state hospitals. This trend primarily reflected the benefits of tranquilizing drugs, the drugs making it possible to increase the number of patients who can be released from the hospital. However, since the number of patients admitted to these hospitals has continued to climb, the net decrease in the hospitals' population cannot be said to represent a reduction in the mental illness problem. What has occurred is an increase in the turnover and a shift in the whereabouts of mental patients. More are being maintained at home or treated elsewhere.

There are two ways to measure progress: from the standpoint of how far we have come, or from the standpoint of how far we yet have to go. By the first measure, we have made progress. By the second measure, we have little cause for self-congratulation and no cause for relaxation of efforts.

The first and pivotal question in appraising where we now stand and next should go is this: *Why have our efforts to provide effective treatment for the mentally ill lagged behind our objectives, behind public demand, and behind attacks on other major health problems?*

With Proper Treatment, the Schizophrenic Patient Has Three-in-five Chance of Leading a Useful Life in the Community

We began with the statement that we have not done so well as we know how for the major mentally ill, in terms of humane and healing care. This is to say that if all or most had the benefit of modern treatment, more patients would recover or show improvement.

Actually, the typical patient with schizophrenia or other functional psychosis (so called because no organic cause is known) has a much better outlook than do patients with some of the better known chronic degenerative diseases, such as cancer of the lung or stomach.

Treatment of mental illness stands on two rational pedestals, one social and one medical: humanitarianism and science.

Modern methods of treatment of major mental illness seek to systematize and capitalize on a historic trend away from punishment and toward "moral treatment," based on humane consideration for the patient as an individual and member of society. No longer does progressive psychiatry hold with the early dictum that "terror acts powerfully on the body through the medium of the mind, and should be employed in the cure of madness." We do still see residual manifestations of this latter approach in shock treatments.

To moral treatment has been added both psychotherapeutic and sociologic insight into how patients may be treated either individually or in groups, to bring about solutions of their problems of living with themselves and with others. To psychotherapy and social therapy (the "therapeutic community"), have been added the tranquilizing drugs, which may be described as "moral treatment in pill form." These drugs quiet the patient and make him more agreeable and easier to work with. In summary of what we know about the treatment of the major mental illnesses which fill our public mental hospitals, we may say:

1. The persistent attitude that schizophrenia is a hopeless, incurable disease requiring the patient to be removed from human society for the rest of his life is baseless.

2. The idea that the patient is totally insane is likewise without foundation. Medical psychology has consistently observed and generally accepts the fact that functional psychosis involves only certain of the components of the personality. The patient is sick in some ways and healthy in others. Rational treatment directs itself toward salvaging the healthy and reducing the sick parts of the mind.

3. Human beings regard loss of liberty, forcible detention, removal from the community, and imprisonment as punishment for wrongdoing; the mentally ill are no exception. It is generally agreed that the typical locked-ward State hospital, centering its interest on the physical rather than the mental welfare of the patient, increases the patient's disability by reinforcing rather than counteracting public pressure to reject the patient from the community. As the pioneer reformer, Clifford Beers, said, "Madmen are too often man-made." The open hospital, with unlocked wards, is one antidote to this disabling process. Another is treatment in mental health clinics of patients not actually requiring hospitalization. Many of the patients in State hospitals do not need to be there.

4. The insistent professional preoccupation with "cures" presents a blind alley. The present state of our scientific knowledge does not permit psychiatry as yet to formulate exact tests of cure. The outlook for the schizophrenic, the main source of the long-term accumulation of patients in State hospitals, is not poor but good under optimum treatment conditions. He has a one-in-five chance of spontaneous recovery without systematic treatment. Through proper treatment, he has at least a three-in-five, and perhaps as much as four-in-five, chance of improving sufficiently to lead a useful life in his community.

Many People—Including Physicians—Find it Hard
to Recognize Psychologic Illness as Illness

The way society handles its mentally ill has been the subject of scandalized attack many times. But, as already implied, repeated exposure of the shameful, dehumanized condition of the mentally sick people who populate the back wards of state hospitals does not arouse the public to sweeping humanitarian reforms, let alone stimulate widespread application of modern methods of treatment. Presumably, if we can answer why there has not been a strong public response (as there has been, for example, in the campaigns against tuberculosis, cancer, and heart disease) we then can determine why effective treatment for the mentally ill has lagged.

The answer, according to our analysis in the following pages, is that the mentally ill are singularly lacking in appeal. They tend to disturb or offend other people and, when they do, people generally treat them as disturbers and offenders and, of course, as if they were responsible for their behavior. In contrast, it has been the special view of the mental health professions that people should understand and accept the mentally ill and do something about their plight.

The public has not been greatly moved by this protest. People do feel sorry for the mentally ill, but, in the balance, they do not feel so sorry as they do relieved to have out of the way persons whose behavior disturbs and offends them. Patients with major mental illness come to be viewed as "impossible people," and mental institutions as places where they are sent when their families and communities "no longer can stand them."

The fact that society tends to reject the mentally ill is, of course, well known; little significance seems to have been attached to it, however.

We can name a number of processes, all of which add up to, or reinforce, the fact that the mentally ill repel more than they appeal. One characteristic of a psychotic is that he becomes a stranger among his own people. Since antiquity mankind has been prone to feel hostility toward the stranger, and this applies equally to any persons who behave strangely. A social system depends on order, and order depends on predictability in the behavior of one's fellows.

Normal persons for the most part want to do what they have to do to "get along." The typical psychotic does not. In consequence, society conventionally closes ranks against him. Identified major mental illness carries a stigma that cuts the bonds of human fellowship.

Many other diseases—tuberculosis, syphilis, cancer, for example—have at times stigmatized their victims. But the stigma of a disease recognized to be physical and lethal tends to disappear, or be offset, as it becomes better understood and publicly attacked. The reason, as we analyze it, is not that science has found causes and cures—the causes and cures of cancer and the leading forms of heart disease are still the subject of an intensive search.

Rather, the physically sick person fits society's deep-seated conception of a sick person. Feeling helpless, he turns to others for help and, receiving help, is responsive to it. He evokes sympathy. Commonly, the acutely ill psychotic does not appear to want help or accept help but, the reverse, thinks he is not sick and may interpret "help" as "harm." He repels sympathy. He is mad.

This lack of appeal has many dimensions. The rise of State hospitals and their persistence, despite all efforts to reform them, is the most outstanding example. Mental health authorities are in general agreement that society uses these huge institutions as dumping grounds for social rejects, rather than as true hospitals.

The mentally ill's lack of appeal as a public cause has been reflected in a lack of strong leadership and strong organization in the voluntary mental health movement, some State organizations excepted.

Several studies of public attitudes have shown a major lack of recognition of mental illness as illness, and a predominant tendency toward rejection of both the mental patient and those who treat him. There is a general agreement on these points in contrast to the lack of confirmation often characterizing parallel studies in the mental health field. (It is encouraging to note, however, that these negative attitudes are less among younger and better educated persons than the older and less educated groups.)

The circle of negligence and indifference becomes complete when we recognize that many members of learned professions are likewise inclined to turn their backs on the core problem of major mental illness.

General practitioners, as well as other members of the medical profession, have been found in a majority of instances to be both uninformed and unsympathetic when they are confronted with mental illness. The same observation applies, oddly enough, to many psychiatrists in private practice when we narrow discussion to the core problem of severe mental illness. The main concern of the popular psychoanalyst is with neurosis rather than psychosis; this is also true of other types of psychiatrists in private practice. Their major focus is on minor, and more easily treatable forms of mental illness. Even mental hospital superintendents themselves, it has been noted, may share the public's stigmatizing attitudes toward mental patients.

In summary, we need to become conscious, at the action level, of two points if we are to overcome the lag in the care of the mentally ill: (1) People find it difficult to think about and recognize psychologic illness as illness, or to see sickness as having psychologic forms. (2)

The major mentally ill as a class lack in appeal, which is to say that they are overburdened with liabilities as persons and as patients.

It should now be clear that one way around the impasse of public and professional attitudes that we appear to have erected would be to emphasize that persons with major mental illness are in certain ways *different* from the ordinary sick. With such an understanding and agreement, it might then be possible to proceed in the light of fuller reason to adopt more helpful attitudes.

The Mentallly Ill Usually Behave Irresponsibly; Society Usually Behaves Toward Them the Same Way

It is commonly stated that one in 10 is mentally ill or psychologically disturbed. When this estimate is limited to those with severe disorders that are socially disruptive or individually incapacitating, the ratio is perhaps one in 100. Society has organized itself and its handling of the one in 100 out of primary concern for the 99 who do not disturb their fellow men sufficiently to acquire the mental patient label. This does not mean, however, that we would long hesitate in modifying the system of exiling and thereafter dehumanizing patients whose illness makes them socially unacceptable, if we could be shown that a more desirable alternative is available.

The current trend, among more progressive mental health professionals and interested laymen, is to recognize and to pursue alternatives—to demonstrate that negative public attitudes are not insurmountable roadblocks; to show that it is possible to develop and practice friendly and accepting attitudes toward the mentally ill; to show that it is possible to work with them, to treat them as human being, and get good results. For example, during the last six years more than 1000 volunteer students from Harvard and Radcliffe Colleges and Brandeis University have worked regularly with chronic psychotics at Metropolitan State Hospital in Waltham, Mass. They have been active in ward improvement projects and as case aides—without harm to themselves or the patients. On the contrary, there has been a mutual benefit, in the notable improvement of patients and higher motivation of students, some of whom have chosen mental health as their career work. Many other examples of lay volunteers who work with mental patients could be cited.

It is a characteristic of the mentally ill that they behave in an irresponsible manner; it is a characteristic of society that we behave toward them in the same manner. The findings of the various projects undertaken as part of the Joint Commission's mental health study bear out our belief that this circle of rejection can be broken. Indeed, there are many signs that the process is well under way.

In all categories of service—hospitals, clinics, community agencies, schools, for example—we found a tremendous demand for authoritative information about mental illnesses and for access to available services. Waiting lists are the rule. It is a demand that we have not begun to meet. Only in the meeting of it will we have the opportunity for large-scale demonstration that public attitudes can be improved and mentally troubled persons can be helped.

In our nationwide survey of the American people's views of their own mental health, one in four adults disclosed he at one time had had a psychologic problem in which professional help would have been useful. One out of seven actually sought help—mainly for problems involving marriage, personal adjustment, or children. Forty-two per cent of those who sought help turned to their clergymen, 29 per cent to physicians in general, 18 per cent to psychiatrists and psychologists, and 10 per cent to social agencies and marriage clinics.

More than half of these troubled persons were sure that they had been helped—more in problems they saw as physical or external to them, than as psychologic or within themselves. But more were helped in making personal adjustments than in solving marital troubles.

The foregoing study together with our studies of community services, churches, and schools indicated the following: While the younger generation and better educated persons have greater recognition of the psychologic nature of many of their problems, and therefore see the need to deal with them psychologically, the demand for such services is not being met. Indeed, mental health facilities and skills are inadequate wherever one looks, whether to mental or general hospitals, clinics, counseling services, clergymen, family doctors, special rehabilitation services, or elsewhere.

Much information has been disseminated. Many meetings have been held. But the shortage of trained mental health personnel works totally against the purposes of mental health education. Increased mental health education only serves to tax already inadequate mental health services.

The Joint Commission made an intensive study of the demand for and supply of mental health professional manpower—particularly psychiatrists, psychologists, psychiatric nurses, and psychiatric social workers. This study made forcibly clear that the great shortages of manpower in these categories is inextricably related to the shortage of professional manpower in general—teachers, lawyers, physicians, scientists, technologists. And the professional manpower shortage is related to defects in our system of public school and college education. Most importantly, a large part of the nation's potential brainpower is being lost between high school and college. In fact, only about one-tenth of American youth become college graduates; only one-third of those of outstanding intelligence in high school go on to finish college.

Our manpower study concluded, with frank pessimism, that sufficient professional personnel to eliminate the glaring deficiencies in our care of mental patients will never become available if the present population trend continues without a commensurate increase in the recruitment and training of mental health manpower. The only possibilities for changing this negative outlook for hundreds of thousands of mental hospital patients would require a great change in our social attitudes, and a consequent massive national effort in all areas of education, including large increases in the number of persons engaged in mental health work, or a sharp break-through in mental health research.

A Sound Research Attack on Mental Illness
Must be Mounted on a Long-term Base

The demand for professional services for the custody and continuous care of patients with schizophrenia or cerebral arteriosclerosis could be greatly reduced by a major break-through in the prevention or treatment of either of these conditions with a biochemical or other technic that could be administered to large numbers by a single therapist. Together, these patients fill the great majority of mental hospital beds.

But even with maximum research support, we cannot count on increased purchasing power in the science market to produce the desired result within a given time. A characteristic of scientific research is that it ultimately produces results of potential benefit to us all, but we cannot predict when the result will come, or even that it will be the one we are looking for. There was a lag of 40 years between the time Karl Landsteiner discovered the cause of poliomyelitis, and when John Enders' group accomplished the tissue-culture break-through that made production of a polio vaccine possible. Sir Alexander Fleming was not looking for a penicillin when he observed its effects, and yet the antibiotics have made more difference in the control of infectious diseases than any other drug in medical history. It was research in anesthesia and motion sickness rather than mental health that brought us the tranquilizing drugs.

Our purpose here is not to be defeatist; only realistic. The enormous task of taking care of mental patients is matched by the enormous research lag in the study of human behavior. Only by making the research possible can we hope to overcome the lag. What we mean is that our total national investment in mental health research—in time, money, men and research and training facilities—simply does not measure up to the need for useful and reliable knowledge that could form the foundation of future progress.

The mental health sciences address themselves to the alleviation of a complex of biologic, psychologic, and sociologic problems that have plagued man through his history; mental health scientists face this task with an incredibly small fund of knowledge about causes and cures. It is a field where much-qualified guesses abound and general agreement is difficult to obtain.

A sound research attack on problems of mental illness and mental health can be mounted on no other base than a *long-term* one. The prospect of a crash program and a quick break-through is not realistic in the absence of a vast increase in basic knowledge. We have the examples in other fields, such as cancer and heart disease, where intensified research has been going on for some years in response to an earlier public focus of effort to solve these health problems. Hopes have been high and have remained so. Yet even in these areas the quick fulfillment of grand objectives is not yet at hand.

We can again illustrate our point via the major advance represented by introduction of the tranquilizing drugs, now used in the treatment of probably one-third of all mental hospital patients. Although these drugs quiet the patients, inspire hopefulness, and make mental hospital employment more interesting and attractive, they do not relieve, but rather increase, the need for professional experience and skills. The effects of the drugs must be closely watched and evaluated, for they are not without harm. At the same time, they make many more patients accessible to psychotherapy, rehabilitation and discharge from the hospital. Such drugs actually increase the need for trained therapists and helping personnel.

In making a statement of the aims and strategy for a more effective research effort in the mental health field, certain characteristics of the research enterprise must be taken into account.

One characteristic is the great *diversity* of persons, sciences, methods, and goals involved in "mental health research."

Another characteristic is the sharp cleavage in attitudes about *basic* and applied research: Basic research is defined as any scientific inquiry for the purpose of discovering and generalizing truths about the essence of nature, including man; applied research here refers to studies directed primarily toward the practical problems of preventing mental illness or treating mental patients. This cleavage leads to a neglect of basic research as impractical or unpromising, and to the false assumption that basic research should be done in universities; applied research, in hospitals.

Our study shows that the mental health research output is concentrated in a relatively small number of major universities and their medical centers. Smaller colleges and state mental hospitals account for an extremely small portion of the total research effort. There should be support for *flexible* and *experimental* programs of *stimulating* research in many different areas and settings.

The mental health sciences are preponderantly dependent on the federal government for their financial support, and becoming more so. The greatest single source is the National Institute of Mental Health. The federal percentage of total support for mental health research in 1958 was 57 per cent; the State percentage was 20 per cent. The pharmaceutic foundations supplied 17 per cent; private foundations and other sources, less than 6 per cent.

The above figures adequately demonstrate that federal government policies determine the shape, size, direction, and soundness of the over-all effort in mental health research. Current policy, emphasizing annual grants for specific projects by individual investigators, favors short-term research and applied research, as opposed to the long-term, more fundamental approach needed.

Science and Education are Resources that Must Have Adequate Support from Human Society, Whether Public or Private

The philosophy the federal government needs to develop and crystallize is that science and education are resources—like natural resources. They can meet an ends test, but not a means test or a time schedule. Science and education operate not for profit but profit everybody; hence, they must have adequate support from human society, whether public or private. The following recommendations are designed to help achieve this:

RECOMMENDATIONS

1. A much larger proportion of total funds for mental health research should be invested in basic research as contrasted with applied research. Only through a large investment in basic research can we hope ultimately to specify the causes and characteristics sufficiently so that we can predict and therefore prevent or cure various forms of mental illness or disordered behavior.

2. Congress and the State legislatures should increasingly favor long-term research in mental health and mental illness as contrasted with short-term projects.

3. Increased emphasis should be placed on, and greater allocations of money be made for, venture, or risk, capital both in the support of persons and of ideas in the mental health research area.

4. The National Institute of Mental Health should make new efforts to invest in, provide for, and hold the young scientist in his career choice. This recommendation would require that more full-time positions be supported for 10-year periods as well as some on the basis of lifetime appointments.

5. Support of program research in established scientific and educational institutions, as initiated by the National Institutes of Health, should be continued and considerably expanded in the field of mental health.

6. The federal government should support the establishment of mental health research centers, or research institutes operated in collaboration with educational institutions and training centers, or independently.

7. Some reasonable portion of total mental health research support should be designated as capital investment in building up facilities for research in states or regions where scientific institutions are lacking or less well developed.

8. Diversification should be recognized as the guiding principle in the distribution of federal research project, program, or institute grants from the standpoint of categories of interest, subject matter of research, and branches of science involved.

The Lag in Treating the Mentally Ill is Reflected in the Continued Existence of Custodial Care Hospitals

The patient care portion of our study centers on new patterns in the treatment of the mentally ill in the community and in institutions. These patterns, which together comprise the current trend in care of the mentally ill, involve:

Providing immediate help for the emotionally disturbed.

Extending the care of mental patients into the community via clinics and other agencies.

A broader conception of what constitutes treatment.

Individualizing of patient care in mental hospitals.

The breaking down of barriers between the hospital and the community—in effect, the open-hospital movement.

The development of a therapeutic milieu in mental hospitals— social treatment.

Development of after-care programs concerned with adequately supporting the patient so he can remain in the community or return there.

The practitioners who are developing new treatment programs believe in them and hope that they will result in better care and more effective treatment. The one constant in each new method appears to be the enthusiasm of its proponents, and most probably such enthusiasm transmits itself to patients in beneficial ways.

The salient characteristic of the best available treatment of psychotics, as we now understand it, is that some kind of relationship— psychologic or social—takes place between the patient and the helping person. This relationship can be formed by informed laymen working individually or in groups under the guidance of psychiatrists, clinical psychologists, or psychiatric social workers, as well as other classes of mental health workers—for example, nurses, attendants, and occupational and recreational therapists.

But programs reflecting newer concepts of treatment are relatively rare and unevenly distributed, with the large majority of State hospitals remaining custodial and punitive in their approach. Our thesis that the lag in the treatment of the mentally ill reflects a fundamental pattern of social rejection, is nowhere better evidenced than by the continued existence of these "hospitals" that seem to have no defenders but endure despite all attacks.

To achieve better care of patients, the mental hospital needs to be integrated into the community. This means keeping the hospital and its staff in closer touch with all the community's public and private service agencies. It means an end to the hospital's isolation from the community; in isolation, the backward, custodial system may thrive, whereas in the mainstream of community activity, a hospital's shortcomings may come to attention.

The State hospital must cease to be treated as a target for political exploitation. Patronage must end. These hospitals and their logical community extensions—clinics and after-care programs—must be manned in all cases by properly motivated career workers and not by hacks, professional or lay. These workers need to be well trained and well paid; they need the opportunity to do a good job and hence to demonstrate to the public what they can do.

The newer programs do nothing to solve the manpower problem, although they indicate the direction in which a solution may lie. This brings us to recommendations for improved care of the mentally ill.

A National Mental Health Program Should Avoid the Risk of False Promise in Public Education

RECOMMENDATIONS

1. POLICY. In the absence of more specific and definitive scientific evidence of the causes of mental illnesses, psychiatry and the allied mental health professions should adopt and practice a broad, liberal philosophy of what constitutes and who can do treatment within the framework of their hospitals, clinics and other professional service agencies, particularly in relation to persons with psychoses or severe personality or character disorders that incapacitate them for work, family life, and everyday activity. All mental health professions should recognize:

A. That certain kinds of medical, psychiatric and neurologic examinations and treatments must be carried out by or under the immediate direction of psychiatrists, neurologists or other physicians specially trained in these procedures.

B. That psychoanalysis and allied forms of deeply searching and probing "depth psychotherapy" must be practiced only by those with special training, experience and competence in handling these technics without harm to the patient (namely, by physicians trained in psychoanalysis or intensive psychotherapy plus those psychologists or other professional persons who lack a medical education but have an aptitude for, adequate training in, and demonstrate competence in such technics of psychotherapy).

C. That nonmedical mental health workers with aptitude, sound training, practical experience, and demonstrable competence should be permitted to do general, short-term psychotherapy—namely, the treating of persons by objective, permissive, nondirective technics of listening to their troubles and helping them resolve these troubles in an individually insightful and socially useful way. Such therapy, combining some elements of psychiatric treatment, of client counseling, of "someone to tell one's troubles to," and of love for one's fellow man, obviously can be carried out in a variety of settings by institutions, groups and by individuals, but in all cases should be pursued under the auspices of recognized mental health agencies.

2. RECRUITMENT AND TRAINING. The mental health professions need to launch a national manpower recruitment and training program, expanding on and extending present efforts and seeking to stimulate the interest of American youth in mental health work as a career. This program should include all categories of mental health personnel. This program should emphasize not only professional training but also short courses and on-the-job training in the subprofessions and up-grading for partially trained persons.

3. SERVICES TO MENTALLY TROUBLED PEOPLE. Persons who are emotionally disturbed—that is to say, under psychologic stress that they cannot tolerate—should have skilled attention and helpful counseling available to them in their community if the development of more serious mental breakdowns is to be prevented. This is known as secondary prevention, and is concerned with the detection of beginning signs and symptoms of mental illness and their relief; in other words, the earliest possible treatment. In the absence of fully trained psychiatrists, clinical psychologists, psychiatric social workers, and psychiatric nurses, such counseling should be done by persons with some psychologic orientation and mental health training and access to expert consultation as needed.

4. IMMEDIATE CARE OF ACUTELY DISTURBED MENTAL PATIENTS. Immediate professional attention should be provided in the community for persons at the onset of acutely disturbed, socially disruptive, and sometimes personally catastrophic behavior—that is, for persons suffering a major breakdown. The few pilot programs for immediate, or emergency, psychiatric care now in existence should be expanded and extended as rapidly as personnel becomes available.

5. INTENSIVE TREATMENT OF ACUTELY ILL MENTAL PATIENTS. A national mental health program should recognize that major mental illness is the core problem and unfinished business of the mental health movement, and that among those with severe mental illnesses the intensive treatment of those with critical and prolonged breakdowns should have first call on fully trained members of the mental health professions. There is a need for expanding treatment of the acutely ill mental patient in all directions, via community mental health clinics, general hospitals, and mental hospitals, as rapidly as psychiatrists, clinical psychologists, psychiatric nurses, psychiatric social workers, and occupational, physical and other nonmedical therapists become available in the community.

A. Community Mental Health Clinics. Community mental health clinics serving both children and adults, operated as outpatient departments of general or mental hospitals, as part of state or regional systems for mental patient care, or as independent agencies, are a main line of defense in reducing the need of many persons with major mental illness for prolonged or repeated hospitalization. Therefore, a national mental health program should set as an objective one fully staffed full-time mental health clinic available to each 50,000 of population. Greater efforts should be made to induce more psychiatrists in private practice to devote a substantial part of their working hours to community clinic services, both as consultants and as therapists.

B. General Hospital Psychiatric Units. No community general hospital should be regarded as rendering a complete service unless it accepts mental patients for short-term hospitalization and therefore provides a psychiatric unit or psychiatric beds. Every community general hospital of 100 or more beds should make this provision. A hospital with such facilities should be regarded as an integral part of a total system of mental patient services in its region.

It is the consensus of the Mental Health Study that definitive care for patients with major mental illness should be given if possible, or for as long as possible, in a psychiatric unit of a general hospital and then, on a longer-term basis, in a specialized mental hospital organized as an intensive psychiatric treatment center.

C. Intensive Psychiatric Treatment Centers. Smaller state hospitals, of 1000 beds or less and suitably located for regional service, should be converted as rapidly as possible into intensive treatment centers for patients with major mental illness in the acute stages or with a good prospect for improvement or recovery if the illness is more prolonged. All new State hospital construction should be devoted to these smaller intensive treatment centers.

6. CARE OF CHRONIC MENTAL PATIENTS. No further State hospitals of more than 1000 beds should be built, and not one patient should be added to any existing mental hospital already housing 1000 or more patients. It is recommended that all existing State hospitals of more than 1000 beds be gradually and progressively converted into centers for the long-term, combined care of persons with chronic diseases, including mental illness. This conversion should be completed in the next ten years.

Special technics are available for the care of the chronically ill, and these technics of socialization, relearning, group living, and gradual rehabilitation or social improvement should be expanded and extended to more people, including the aged who are sick and in need of care, through conversions of State mental hospitals into combined chronic disease centers.

It would be necessary to provide the intensive treatment services for the acutely ill, outlined in the preceding section, before large state hospitals could be converted to chronic diseases. It also would be necessary to make certain changes in federal and state laws.

7. AFTER-CARE, INTERMEDIATE CARE, AND REHABILITATION SERVICES. The objective of modern treatment of persons with major mental illness is to enable the patient to maintain himself in the community in a normal manner. To do so, it is necessary (1) to save the patient from the debilitating effects of institutionalization as much as possible, (2) if the patient requires hospitalization, to return him to home and community life as soon as possible, and (3) thereafter maintain him in the community as long as possible. Therefore, after-care and rehabilitation are essential parts of all service to mental patients, and the various methods of achieving rehabilitation should be integrated in all forms of services, among them: day hospitals, night hospitals, after-care clinics, Public Health nursing services, foster family care, convalescent nursing homes, rehabilitation centers, work services, and ex-patient groups. We recommend that demonstration programs for day and night hospitals and the more flexible use of mental hospital facilities, both in the treatment of the acute and the chronic patient, be encouraged and augmented through institutional, program, and project grants.

PUBLIC INFORMATION ON MENTAL ILLNESS

A national mental health program should avoid the risk of false promise in "public education for better mental health" and focus on the more modest goal of disseminating such information about mental illness as the public needs and wants in order to recognize psychologic forms of sickness and to arrive at an informed opinion of its responsibility toward the mentally ill.

How Can We Make State Hospitals in Fact What They Now Are in Name Only— Hospitals for Mental Patients?

Federal, State and local expenditures for public mental patient services should be doubled in the next five years—and tripled in the next ten.

Only by this magnitude of expenditure can typical State hospitals be made in fact what they are now in name only—hospitals for mental patients. Only by this magnitude of expenditure can outpatient and former-patient programs be sufficiently extended outside the mental hospital, into the community. It is self-evident that the States for the most part have defaulted on adequate treatment for the mentally ill, and have consistently done so for a century. It is likewise evident that the States cannot afford the kind of money needed to catch up with modern standards of care without revolutionary changes in their tax structure.

Therefore, *we recommend that the States and the federal government work toward a time when a share of the cost of State and local mental patient services will be borne by the federal government, over and above the present and future program of federal grants-in-aid for research and training.* The simple and sufficient reason for this recommendation is that under the present tax structure only the federal government has the financial resources needed to overcome the lag and to achieve a minimum standard of adequacy. The federal government should be prepared to assume a major part of the responsibility for the mentally ill insofar as the States are agreeable to surrendering it.

For convenience, the Veterans Administration mental hospitals can be taken as financial models of what can be done in the operation of public mental hospitals. *Congress and the National Institute of Mental Health, with the assistance of the intervening administrative branches of government, should develop a federal subsidy program that will encourage State and local governments to emulate the example set by V. A. mental hospitals.*

Certain principles should be followed in a federal program of matching grants to States for the care of the mentally ill:

The *first principle* is that the federal government on the one side and State and local governments on the other should *share in the costs* of services to the mentally ill.

The *second principle* is that the total federal share should be arrived at in a series of graduated steps over a period of years, the share being determined each year on the basis of state funds spent in a previous year.

The *third principle* is that the grants should be awarded according to *criteria of merit and incentive* to be formulated by an expert advisory committee appointed by the National Institute of Mental Health.

In arriving at a formula, such an expert committee would establish conditions affecting various portions of the available grant, including the following:

1. Bring about any necessary changes in the laws of the State to make professionally acceptable treatment as well as custody a requirement in mental hospitalization, to differentiate between need of institutionalization, and provision of treatment without hospitalization.

2. Bring about any necessary changes in laws of the State to make voluntary admission the preferred method and court commitment the exceptional method of placing patients in a mental hospital or other treatment facilities.

3. Accept any and all persons requiring treatment or hospitalization on the same basis as persons holding legal residence within the State.

4. Revise laws of the State governing medical responsibility for the patient to distinguish between administrative responsibility for his welfare and safekeeping and responsibility for professional care of the patient.

5. Institute suitable differentiation between administrative structure and professional personnel requirements for (1) State mental institutions intended primarily as intensive treatment centers (i.e., true hospitals) and (2) facilities for humane and progressive care of various classes of the chronically ill or disabled, among them the aged.

6. Establish State mental health agencies with well defined powers and sufficient authority to assume over-all responsibility for the State's services to the mentally ill, and to coordinate State and local community health services.

7. Make reasonable efforts to operate open mental hospitals as mental health centers, i.e., as a part of an integrated community service with emphasis on outpatients and after-care facilities as well as inpatient services.

8. Establish in selected State mental hospitals and community mental health programs training for mental health workers, ranging in scope, as appropriate, from professional training in psychiatry through

all professional and sub-professional levels, including the on-the-job training of attendants and volunteers. Since each mental health center cannot undertake all forms of teaching activity, consideration here must be given to a variety of programs and total effort. States should be required ultimately to spend 2½ per cent of State mental patient service funds for training.

9. Establish in selected State mental hospitals and community mental health programs scientific research programs appropriate to the facility, the opportunities for well designed research, and the research talent and experience of staff members. States should be required ultimately to spend 2½ per cent of State mental patient service funds for research.

10. Encourage county, town and municipal tax participation in the public mental health services of the State as a means of obtaining federal funds matched against local mental health appropriations.

11. Agree that no money will be spent to build mental hospitals of more than 1000 beds, or to add a single patient to mental hospitals presently having 1000 or more patients.

Our proposal would encourage local responsibility to a degree that has not existed since the State hospital system was founded, while at the same time recognizing that the combined State-local responsibility cannot be fulfilled by the means at hand.

Our proposal is the first one in American history that attempts to encompass the total problem of public support of mental health services and to make minimum standards of adequate care financially possible.

The outstanding characteristics of mental illness as a Public Health problem are its staggering size, the present limitations in our methods of treatment, and the peculiar nature of mental illness that differentiates its victims from those with other diseases or disabilities. It would follow that *any national program against mental illness adopted by Congress and the States must be scaled to the size of the problem, imaginative in the course it pursues, and energetic in overcoming both psychologic and economic resistance to progress in this direction.* We have sought to acquit our assignment in full recognition of these facts and judgments.

1. This Digest is a 10,000 word condensation of *Action for Mental Health*, a 100,000 word report made to Congress, the Governors, and the Legislatures of the United States. The Digest is provided as a convenience to public officials and the press, who require a quick impression of the findings and recommendations contained in the full report. Under no other circumstance, however, does the Digest constitute an appropriate substitute for the thoughtful and extensive analysis to be found in *Action for Mental Health*. For documentation of statements in this Digest, the interested reader is referred to the full work, published by Basic Books Incorporated.

14. Behavioral Sciences in Public Health

The Contributions and Limitations of Behavioral Science in Public Health*

LYLE SAUNDERS, M.A.

AT FIRST GLANCE it seems somewhat strange to make the relations of Public Health and behavioral science the subject of special discussion.[1] These two areas obviously have so much in common that it would seem as though it could be taken for granted that there is, has been, and should be some association between them. There has probably never been a time when those responsible for group health have not had to take account of a fairly wide range of behaviors; and also there has probably never been a time when those interested in learning about human behavior have not been concerned with those behaviors believed to be related to states of health and illness. The ancient peoples of Minoa, Crete, India, and Egypt left evidence that they were interested in understanding behavior, and in controlling it for the protection and improvement of community health. And one of the earliest codes of behavior, the Mosaic code of the Jews, formalized in explicit terms standards of conduct relating to health that must have been based on a long history of prior inquiry into the relations between certain types of behavior and subsequent states of health.

Looking back on the interests and activities of people before they were fragmented by specialization, it is sometimes difficult to tell whether a particular work should be considered a precursor of Public Health or behavioral science. The Hippocratic book, *Airs, Waters, and Places,* which George Rosen tells us[2] served more than 2000 years as the basic epidemiologic text and the theoretic source for understanding of endemic and epidemic disease, dealt with five factors—climate, soil, water, mode of life, and nutrition—as essential to the balance between health and disease. Mode of life and nutrition are of direct interest to behavioral science as are the social and technical

* Reprinted by permission from the *Behavioral Sciences and Public Health*, Continuing Education Monograph, No. 3, published by the Western Regional Office of the American Public Health Association, San Francisco, California, June, 1962, pp. 19–30. The author is Associate Professor of Preventive Medicine, University of Colorado, School of Medicine, Denver, Colorado. Recently he has been on a technical cooperation mission to India, in New Delhi, as part of the United States of America, A.I.D. program. The paper was part of an Institute on Public Health and Behavioral Sciences held April 9–11, 1962, in Los Angeles, California.

arrangements that must have been devised to cope with the others. John Graunt, tinkering with his bills of mortality in 17th-century London, in an effort to develop a statistical method applicable to problems of community health and welfare, was contributing to both Public Health and behavioral science. Edwin Chadwick's *Report . . . on an Inquiry into the Sanitary Condition of the Labouring Population of Great Britain* was both a Public Health report and a treatise on social science. The same could be said of Thomas Malthus's *Essay on the Principle of Population,* Lemuel Shattuck's *Report to the Massachusetts Sanitary Commission,* and a good many more of the health-oriented writings in the period that Rosen refers to by the phrase "Industrialism and the Sanitary Movement."

The historic association and the recent emerging convergence of interest between behavioral science and Public Health derive from two obvious, but fundamental, aspects of the nature of health and of Public Health activity:

1. Social and cultural behaviors are important factors in the etiology, prevalence, and distribution of many diseases. How people live, what they eat, what they believe, what they value, what technology they command are significant determinants of their individual and collective health.

2. Public Health is a social and cultural activity. Both its practitioners and the human targets of its services are, in their various interactions and transactions fulfilling socially-defined roles in culturally determined ways, and a good deal of their behavior is motivated, oriented, and constrained by the social and cultural contexts in which it occurs.[3]

Public Health thus must take account of certain types of behavior that are also of interest to the behavioral sciences, and Public Health activity itself consists of a complex of behaviors that is of intrinsic interest to behavioral scientists.

SEPARATE DEVELOPMENT OF PUBLIC HEALTH AND BEHAVIORAL SCIENCE

Despite their areas of overlapping interest and occasional points of convergence throughout a wide sweep of history, Public Health and behavioral science have, until recently, been relative strangers in modern times. Public health, for a century or more, has been emerging as a complex of related but distinct programs, organized and supported mainly as activities of government, and concerned mainly with practical problems of protecting and improving health. It has had much to occupy its attention and absorb its energies in the tasks of defining and legitimizing its status as a proper activity of government; finding and delimiting its area of activity; establishing working relations with private practitioners of medicine; achieving harmony and order in the internal relations among the several professions and sub-professions active in Public Health; dealing with epidemics and other health crises; improving the healthfulness of the physical environment; and making applications of the vast amount of new knowledge that has been coming from the physical and biologic sciences. Until recently, Public Health has had little time for, and less need to be aware of, behavioral science.

This course of events has perhaps been fortunate because, until recently, the behavioral sciences have had little that they could have contributed to Public Health. Although interest in and speculation about human beings extends far back in time—as can be demonstrated by reference to some of the earliest archaeological records—it is only within the past century that the search for knowledge in this area has shifted its dependence from authority and speculation to empiric research, and only in the past half century that knowledge about human behavior and human relations has begun to be something other than vague, impressionistic, and meager. It is true that, prior to the present century, there had been a great deal of theorizing and a considerable body of factual knowledge and practical wisdom has accumulated. But most of the theories were untested or untestable; the wisdom did not reliably provide guides to wise behavior; and the knowledge that existed was the knowledge of laymen, not of scientists.

Like Public Health, the behavioral sciences have been heavily preoccupied with their own development. They have had to establish themselves as legitimate academic disciplines entitled to a share of both public and scholarly support; they have had to come to terms with each other about the division of work areas in the broad field of human behavior; they have had to create the conceptual and methodologic tools that would enable them to apply the methods of science to human affairs; they have had to handle the organizational problems of developing sub-specialties within and between their disciplines; and they have had to learn to work in fields where issues are controversial, where new knowledge may threaten valued and deeply-rooted beliefs and practices, where any man could be a self-proclaimed expert, and where science-based knowledge has had to compete with common sense as a guide to conduct.

CONVERGENCE OF PUBLIC HEALTH AND BEHAVIORAL SCIENCE INTEREST

By a happy, and not altogether fortuitous circumstance, Public Health has come to a stage in its development where it is confronted with emerging problems involving social and cultural behaviors at a time when the behavioral sciences have developed to the point of having something substantial to offer and a disposition to help.

The needs of Public Health have been well stated by the editors of the *American Journal of Public Health:* "Health workers agree generally that we are now in a period when the human factor must be taken into account if Public Health is to handle its problems successfully. Many of the areas of health with which Public Health is today concerned involve individual voluntary action on the part of many people. There is also an increasing awareness that attitudes, beliefs, motives affect the willingness and readiness of people to take voluntary action with respect to their own health or that of members of their families . . . A central question of Public Health has become: Why do people behave as they do? Why do they behave like human beings? And for answers to this question Public Health workers are turning increasingly to those sciences whose central concern is human behavior and the conditions that affect and determine it—the social sciences."[4]

It has become commonplace in Public Health to talk of collaboration with behavioral science, and the major Public Health periodicals (as well as those of the behavioral sciences) are printing materials which indicate that a considerable amount of such collaboration is taking place. Public Health leaders, in their public statements, are calling attention to emerging problems of their profession that will require increased knowledge of the antecedents, conditions, and consequences of both individual and group behaviors.[5] Recent annual meetings of the American Public Health Association have included sessions on behavioral science, and the entire program of the 1960 Western Branch meeting was devoted to the topic, "Application of Behavioral Sciences in Public Health Programs." At that meeting each of the 10 professional sections considered separately how behavioral sciences might be useful in its field and all were able to single out current problems of some urgency in which it was felt that behavioral science could be of help. Behavioral scientists are now teaching in more than half the schools of Public Health in this country,[6] including California. For several years there has been in APHA an inter-disciplinary committee (of which Dr. Wellin is field director) concerned with the behavioral sciences in Public Health.[7] There is no doubt but that a considerable interest in the behavioral science has developed in Public Health.

For their part, the behavioral scientists have also shown an increasing interest in collaboration. The Society for Applied Anthropology, whose object is "the promotion of scientific investigation of the principles controlling the relations of human beings to one another, and the encouragement of wide application of these principles to practical problems," has had a long interest in behavioral science applications in health and its journal *Human Organization* consistently reports efforts in this area.[8] A review article, "Anthropology in Medicine," prepared by William Caudill for an International Symposium on Anthropology, held in New York in 1952, lists an impressive number of studies completed or in progress in which behavioral scientists were working on problems of interest to Public Health.[9]

For six years there have been sessions at the annual meetings of the American Sociological Association devoted to medical sociology. In 1955 a Committee of Medical Sociology was formed to permit an exchange of ideas and discussion of problems among persons interested in the meeting ground of behavioral science and medicine. This group, in 1959, was formally incorporated into the American Sociological Association as the Section on Medical Sociology with a membership of over 500 persons.[10]

From 1954 through 1960, the Social Science Research Council[11] had an active committee concerned with Preventive Medicine and Social Science Research. The Committee, which was composed of people from both Public Health and social science, defined its interest as lying mainly in the field of inter-disciplinary research, with a secondary interest in the teaching of behavioral sciences in schools of Public Health and medicine. It commissioned a number of original papers— six of which were eventually published—on such topics as medical institutions in sociologic perspective, intercultural health problems, community processes in relation to Public Health programs, the effects of stress on social and cultural systems, the implications of social class for Public Health, fertility control, the development of indices for appraising health department activities, the measurement of economic benefits resulting from improved health, and a sociologic analysis of the work role of the Public Health Officer. A major activity of the Committee was the organization of a Conference on Preventive Medicine and Social Science Research[12] that brought together some 30 leaders in Public Health and social science for a week of intensive discussion of collaboration between their fields of interest. Although the conference was designed to maximize free discussion and informal interchange, a number of papers, illustrating the wide range of existing and potential collaboration were read. Topics discussed included public attitudes towards polio vaccine; public participation in mass X-ray screening programs; field surveys of rheumatoid arthritis; fluoridation of water supplies; health beliefs and practices of California-Mexican-Americans; alcoholism as a Public Health problem; the relation of family culture to participation in a rheumatic fever clinic; and the development of a medical and Public Health program for Navajo Indians.

It is easy to document a growing convergence of interest between the behavioral sciences and Public Health and relatively safe to predict even more extensive collaboration than now exists. Behavioral science in Public Health is not a passing fashion; neither is it a universal panacea for all the ills that beset Public Health. With good will and understanding on both sides it can become a source of substantial—but limited—help with some aspects of some Public Health problems. There is, in the developing relationships a considerable potential for benefit for both groups. There are also some potential dangers and difficulties. The latter are not great, but they could be a source of disappointment and discouragement to Public Health people and social scientists who permitted their expectations of collaboration to become unrealistic.

LIMITATIONS OF COLLABORATION BETWEEN PUBLIC HEALTH AND BEHAVIORAL SCIENCE

One potential source of difficulty lies in the differing orientations of the two groups. Public Health is an activity of practicing professions. It is goal-oriented, program-oriented, and service-oriented. It draws scientific knowledge from a number of disciplines and seeks to make application of that knowledge toward the amelioration or solution of practical problems. It is concerned with action, and its success is measured in terms of changes it is able to induce in the environment or in the knowledge, attitudes, or behaviors of its target publics. Its basic value premise is "health is good," and its ultimate goal is to protect and augment that good.

The behavioral sciences, on the other hand, are disciplines, not professions. They are knowledge-oriented, theory-oriented. They are concerned with study and research, and their success is measured in terms of the scientific knowledge they produce. Their basic value premise is "knowledge is good," and their ultimate goal is to create more of that good.

These orientations are different, but they are not mutually exclusive. On the contrary, they are complementary. There is nothing in them that will necessarily prevent behavioral scientists and Public Health people from working fruitfully and harmoniously together. But their presence does suggest that it may be desirable, when collaboration is being arranged, to give some thought to the expectations each group brings with respect to methods and conditions of work and desirable outcomes. In some instances, effort and time may be required for each to understand the other, but these can be effort and time well spent if they come at the beginning of a collaboration rather than as a result of misunderstandings that crop up and have to be resolved after commitment has been made and work begun. "Know thyself!" is a fine, sound maxim. "Know thy collaborator!" may, at times, be equally sound.

To give some semblance of order, comments about limitations of Public Health-behavioral science collaboration will be grouped under three headings: limitations of the disciplines; limitations in the people; and limitations resulting from the nature of the collaborative situation.

LIMITATIONS OF THE DISCIPLINES

A first limitation in the disciplines arises from the relatively narrow range of human behaviors behavioral scientists are interested in or competent to deal with. No behavioral scientist, as such, is concerned with behaviors on the molecular, cellular, tissue, or organ levels of complexity. Rather, his interests are centered in those behaviors that derive from or can be identified with membership in social systems, the possession of culture, or certain psychic structures and processes such as personality, learning, and motivation. There are relatively few generalists in behavioral science. A given behavioral scientist may be competent in one, but rarely in several of these broad areas. And, given the fact of increasing specialization in the behavioral sciences as in other professions and disciplines, he may be competent in only some small portion of a single field. Since Public Health people are frequently interested in "total" behaviors cross-cutting personality, culture, and social memberships, the competence behavioral scientists are able to bring may not always be broad enough for the problem at hand.

A second limitation lies in the general inability of behavioral scientists to predict or control the behavior of individuals. Public Health people are, of course, interested in the behaviors of people in categories and groups, but when the chips are down they frequently want answers to such questions as why Mrs. Mezzamine doesn't get her children immunized? Why Juan Tortilla won't be hospitalized when he has been told he has TB and is dangerous to his family? Or how to get Mrs. Titwillow to leave that hovel she has lived in for 50 years and go to a nice comfortable nursing home (where she can rock on the front porch with her peers from two to four any warm afternoon). It is true that behavioral scientists can, and do, make pronouncements on these problems, but often after they have had their say, Mrs. M's darlings are still innocent of induced antibodies, Juan continues cheerfully to cough into the trusting face of little Jesus, Mrs. T. has a chair propped under the doorknob and a shotgun across her knees. It is a plausible hypothesis that in collaboration with Public Health workers the help available from behavioral science varies inversely with the specificity of the problem.

Another obvious limitation is the relatively undeveloped state of behavioral science knowledge. We have been observing people for much longer than we have been studying atoms, but we probably know more about the behavior of atoms than about the behavior of people. There are still some who think that human behavior is not amenable to scientific study. However, we are beginning to use in behavioral science the rigorous procedures and mathematic methods that have produced such spectacular results in the physical and biologic sciences. The best of behavioral science is now approaching a high level of conceptual and methodologic sophistication, and the quantity of output is exhibiting the same tendency toward exponential increase that has characterized other sciences. For all its recent gains, though, behavioral science knowledge is still limited. However, limited as it may be, it is the best knowledge we have in these areas and, as a guide to action, is more reliable than the rule of thumb, common-sense procedures we so frequently use in attempting to understand or control behavior.

A final limitation in this category arises from the relative rigidity of social and cultural behavior patterns. The "cake of custom," as Walter Bagehot termed it, is hard to break, especially in such institutional sectors as the family, government, the economy, religion, and health. As anthropologists have long known, social and cultural behavior patterns are interlocked into larger systems in such a way that change in one area often produces or requires change in another. Spontaneous social and cultual change is constantly occurring as a result of the dynamic interplay between people and their human and physical environments, but directed or planned change, such as Public Health is interested in inducing, is hard to achieve. Customs and habits tend to be rigid; other cherished values conflict with health values; powerful, organized efforts are often being made to bring about change in directions contrary to those desired by Public Health. It is relatively easy to dream up means that might lead to some of the ends Public Health would like to attain; the hard part is to hit upon means that are practical and in conformity with social norms—the rules of the game.[13]

LIMITATIONS IN THE PEOPLE

A second category of limitations on Public Health—behavioral science collaboration relates to some characteristics of the people who work in each field. As has been indicated, Public Health workers and behavioral scientists can be expected to differ somewhat in their orientation, their interests, methods, and goals. Public Health people want to *do* something about health; behavioral scientists want to *understand* something about behavior. Relatively few Public Health people have had extensive training in behavioral science, and rela-tively few behavioral scientists have had much professional exposure to Public Health. Thus each is likely to bring to the collaborative situation a lack of understanding of the other. Anderson and Seacat's 1957 study of about 200 behavioral scientists working in health[14] indicated that more than a third felt there was a lack of recognition of behavioral science as a legitimate scientific discipline in health, and about one in five mentioned encountering some misunderstanding of the behavioral scientist's role. Although only about a quarter of those responding indicated having had a considerable amount of experience with Public Health, the replies reflected an opinion that Public Health personnel have a better understanding of behavioral science than other types of health workers.

Russell Sage Foundation, whose fellows have had a considerable collective experience in health work, discusses problems of collaboration in its latest *Annual Report*. "Every country," the *Report* states, "has its own peculiar 'atmosphere' and culture; so does every professional subculture. The atmosphere of a hospital or a social welfare agency or a professional school is very different from the university department of sociology or a social research laboratory. Some initial recognition of the fact of difference, and early briefing in the manners and customs of the 'adopted country' will make for smoother and easier working relations. Neglect of these seemingly unimportant aspects may cause the newcomer sometimes to appear gauche, naive, and alien, and thus unnecessarily handicap him in establishing productive contacts."[15] For the behavioral scientist to work effectively on a Public Health team, George Foster has pointed out, he must see how his work makes a contribution to knowledge, but he must also be able to find satisfaction in seeing Public Health goals achieved and must have an understanding and appreciation of the values that orient the work of his Public Health colleagues. For their part, Public Health workers must know something of the values of the behavioral scientist and "must realize that he is judged by his associates by different standards than they, and that if these standards cannot be met, he will be a frustrated and dissatisfied teammate, however well prepared he is otherwise.[16] To help meet the problem of mutual lack of understanding, Foster urged that every collaborative effort include a reasonably long period of mutual indoctrination. The Russell Sage report emphasizes the same point in the comment that "while careful initial orientation can go far toward getting projects off on the right foot, nothing will obviate the necessity for sustained and systematic effort directed toward each party assimilating a working knowledge of the other's field."[17] On a more general level, the problem is being approached through such activities as courses in behavioral science in schools of Public Health, discussion institutes (such as this one), programs in behavioral science departments in some universities to train their graduates for work in health, and—in at least one university—through encouraging recent graduates in behavioral sciences to take additional degrees in Public Health.

LIMITATIONS RESULTING FROM THE NATURE OF THE COLLABORATIVE SITUATION

A final category of limitations are those that arise from the nature of the collaborative situation. Any multi-disciplinary or inter-disciplinary collaboration is subject to difficulties resulting from differences in concepts, language, working methods, and objectives. These general problems have been discussed at length elsewhere and need not be elaborated here.[18] Specific to the relationship between behavioral science and Public Health, however, are at least three problem areas that should be mentioned.

The first of these results from the relatively unstructured position of the behavioral scientist who works in Public Health. There is not much question about where physicians, nurses, sanitarians, health educators, nutritionists fit into the pattern of Public Health activity, but there is not the same consensus about where a behavioral scientist belongs or what he does. There is, as yet, no uniform, agreed-upon role for a behavioral scientist in Public Health, and one who goes into the field runs the risk of being himself confused and becoming a source of confusion for others. There are things a behavioral scientist is competent at, and things he is not. Unless these areas are clearly understood by both himself and others and used as the basis for fitting him into the organizational structure, he runs the danger of becoming anything from a general handyman to an esoteric hermit dealing in mysteries and speaking a language that no one else understands.[19]

Another limitation in this category centers in problems of the application of knowledge. Behavioral scientists, to use Graham Wallas's phrase, make butter; Public Health people spread it. The behavioral scientist who takes pride in being able to explain cogently and lucidly some aspect of behavior can be much deflated if the next comment of a Public Health practitioner is, "That is very fine and I think I understand it; now tell me how I can use it in this problem." Behavioral scientists, on the whole, have perhaps not been good at and not much interested in practical applications of their knowledge. Some may have given an impression of aloofness toward research problems growing out of practical needs. But if this has been true, the situation is probably changing. Behavioral scientists are coming to accept the idea that it is reasonable and legitimate for others to expect that the knowledge they produce will have practical applications. A respectable number are engaged in or have completed studies relating to immediate action problems. The Society for Applied Anthropology has a long history of interest in this area. The president of the American Sociological Society in 1954 pointed to a need for "middlemen" who would undertake to translate sociologic knowledge into forms in which it can be used by practicing professions.[20] And there is sufficient interest in the problem now to cause the Society for the Study of Social Problems to set as the theme of its 1961 meeting, "The Emerging Applied Social Sciences: Opportunities and Problems." There will continue to be a substantial proportion of behavioral scientists uninterested in practical problems and many also uninterested in health. But more, particularly among the younger social scientists, are coming to be concerned with both.

A final limiting factor is that arising from the fact that in collaborative efforts, Public Health people or programs become the object of study as well as an agent of study. Behavioral scientists who study efforts to influence behavior generally think that to understand their problem they have to look at the innovating agency or program as well as at the target population. They tend to see effective influence as something resulting from the interactions and transactions of two groups rather than as something that can be understood wholly in terms of the internal dynamics of one. Again to quote George Foster: "This makes the work more difficult, not just because there are twice as many variables, but because of the emotional element that enters the picture. The professional worker in an action program has little difficulty in seeing that the culture of the group with which he is working will determine how people react to him. He can see that patterns of authority and concepts of role in the client group will affect the way in which he must direct messages or ask for cooperation . . . It is not so easy for us to accept the fact that an understanding of our attitudes, values, and motivations—which we pretty much take for granted —is just as important in successfully bringing about change. It is sometimes painful to realize that we accept implicitly assumptions that have little validity beyond tradition, that much of our work is program-oriented, based on what we have learned and accepted uncritically, rather than problem-oriented, tailored to the job that faces us."[21] Behavioral scientists in health are sometimes faced with the obligation to observe, analyze, ask questions of and about their colleagues, and this is a difficult role at best. It requires of the behavioral scientist qualities of tact, sensitivity, empathy, honesty, and objectivity in the highest degree, and of the Public Health practitioner an equal degree of tolerance, trust, and forbearance. It is a tribute to the professional competence of both groups that co-operation under these circumstances frequently proceeds with smoothness, harmony and mutual respect.

CONTRIBUTIONS OF BEHAVIORAL SCIENCE
TO PUBLIC HEALTH

Despite these limitations—and the many that have not been mentioned—behavioral scientists can and do contribute to Public Health. The specific contributions are so numerous and varied that they cannot be summarized for brief discussion in any but the most general terms. Let me, therefore, simply suggest that the contributions come from two sources—the knowledge generated by behavioral science disciplines and the activities of people identified with them—and occur mainly in the three broad and similar fields of teaching, service, and research.

Perhaps it should be recalled that Public Health can benefit from behavioral science even if no behavioral scientists are directly employed in Public Health agencies or programs. Behavioral scientists presumably produce and have knowledge about certain categories of phenomena Public Health people are interested in, and the latter can (and do) use that knowledge directly just as they use that from such disciplines as biochemistry, pharmacology, and physiology. Public Health people may read behavioral science literature, attend behavioral science meetings, and use behavioral science concepts and methods as freely as they wish.[22]

Beyond the direct use of the knowledge they produce, behavioral science people can be used in a number of ways short of formal collaboration or employment in health agencies. Special gatherings can provide for the exchange of information and opinions; many social scientists are receptive to invitations to present their work or their ideas at Public Health meetings; many are willing, if asked, to review work being done in their fields of interest or to provide information or advice about substantive or procedural questions. Practically any behavioral science department in any college or university contains people who would respond eagerly to an approach from someone in Public Health with a problem.[23]

In the field of teaching there is much going on and more to come. As indicated earlier, at least half the schools of Public Health have behavioral scientists actively engaged in teaching their disciplines;[24] schools of nursing, particularly collegiate schools, are increasingly offering social science content in their curricula; and a number of schools of medicine, particularly in their departments of psychiatry and preventive medicine, use social scientists in their teaching. Public Health personnel thus have a triple opportunity to acquire some formal training in behavioral science as part of their regular study program: in their under-graduate course of study; during their primary professional training; and in a school of Public Health. One disadvantage at the professional school level is the necessity that sometimes exists for teaching a kind of general behavioral science at an applied level to people who have not had any previous training and are not familiar with basic concepts or behavioral science points of view.[25]

Behavioral science contributions to service programs are perhaps best made indirectly through research. There is little in the training of behavioral scientists that would make them adept at assisting directly with the giving of health services. Some fairly direct help can perhaps be given through studies of programs and evaluation of either processes or results. Slightly less direct are studies of the organization of Public Health agencies and the possible effects of internal structure on service programs. Contributions can also be made through research on the social, cultural, or psychologic characteristics of target populations, and on the relations of these populations with Public Health activity. An example of an approach that includes some of each of these avenues is a project now going on in New Mexico in which a group that includes Public Health people, anthropologists, and sociologists is studying the discourse that goes on between Public Health nurses and Spanish-American villagers in the area of orally transmissible disease in an effort to understand how what the nurse says can be reconstructed in such a way as to have meaning and motivational influence in the health belief system of the village people.

It is in the field of research that behavioral science has most to contribute. The availability of research funds, from private foundations—notably Russell Sage and Kellogg—and from the National Institutes of Health, has recently made it possible for a fair number of behavioral scientists to devote a considerable amount of time to projects of interest to Public Health. The 1959 edition of the Health Information Foundation's annual *Inventory of Social and Economic Research in Health* lists 841 ongoing projects, some 322 of which were new since the previous year. By contrast, only slightly more than 200 projects were listed in the first *Inventory* in 1952, even though an attempt was made at that time to include projects completed since 1945 and major projects completed as far back as 1940. The Index of the 1959 volume requires nearly 50 pages just to list the titles of projects, and the scope of research interest is as wide as the titles are numerous.

There is no effective way, in a few words, to give an adequate impression of the amount or range of behavioral science research of interest to Public Health that is now going on. One is tempted to list people and the areas they are working in, but there is just no way to make a representative selection short of an extremely long list. Perhaps the best that can be done is to repeat the list of what might be included in the field of social research on health as it was formulated at a multi-disciplinary conference at Chapel Hill in 1952. Included would be, said the conference report: "the study of the whole field of health and disease, of specific health problems, health personnel facilities and programs in terms of the disciplines known as the social sciences. Thus this area would include economic, sociologic, psychologic and political science studies of well and sick people, of the professions working in the health field, of cultural patterns, of institutions such as hospitals and Public Health agencies, of community structure and processes, and of interelations between the public, patients, and health personnel."[26] This is what needs to be done. And a fair start has been made.

1. The terms "Public Health" and "behavioral science" are used throughout this paper as if each denoted a distinguishable empiric entity. This, of course, is not so. Public Health is a complex of professions and activities of considerable diversity; behavioral science is a convenient term for referring simultaneously to several academic disciplines that concern themselves with social, cultural, or mental behavior. When Public Health is mentioned herein, it will refer to organized governmental activities that have as their object the protection and promotion of health among the population of a political unit. When behavioral science is used, the term will refer (as has become somewhat conventional) to the disciplines of cultural anthropology, sociology, and social psychology. Should a wider range of disciplines be indicated—e.g., economics, political science, social psychiatry—the term social science will be used.

2. Rosen, George. *A History of Public Health*. New York: MD Publications, Inc., 1958. pp. 33–34.

3. How much simpler and more certain of its results Public Health practice might be if the practitioner were not restricted to activities that are legally permissible, economically possible, ethically and morally proper, and in accord with the prevailing norms and values of the Public Health professions!

4. Unsigned editorial, *American Journal of Public Health*, 49:536, April, 1959.

5. See, for example, Dr. Thomas Parran Speech accepting the Leon Bernard Foundation Prize, 11th World Health Assembly, Minneapolis, Mar. 30, 1958, mimeographed; Dr. Leona Baumgartner, "Public Health in an Affluent Society," *American Journal of Public Health* 50:1521–1528, October 1960; Dr. Malcolm H. Merrill, "Implications of Behavorial Sciences and Social Changes for the Future of Public Health," Paper presented at the 1960 Annual Meeting, Western Branch, American Public Health Association, Denver, May 23–26, 1960.

6. A recent report indicates that in 1959–60 there were 29 people teaching behavioral sciences in schools of Public Health—12 full time in the school, seven full-time in the University, but part-time in the School, 10 part time. No school, however, had a major department of behavioral science. James L. Troupin, "Schools of Public Health in the United States and Canada: 1959–60," *American Journal of Public Health*, 50–1770–1791, November, 1960.

7. Among the committee's many activities was the organization of the New England Institute on Public Health and Behavioral Sciences that met at Winchendon, Massachusetts, September 9–11, 1959, to discuss "The Utilization of Behavioral Sciences in Official Health Agencies."

8. The Winter, 1958, issue was entirely devoted to the special topics of Mental Health and Preventive Medicine.

9. The article was published under the title, "Applied Anthropology in Medicine," A. L. Kroeber, Ed., *Anthropology Today*. New York: Wenner-Green Foundation, 1953, pp. 771–806.

10. The latest membership report of the American Sociological Association listed 291 members as employed in fields of health in 1959 (7 per cent of total membership) as contrasted with 65 in 1950. Some 188 members

(5 per cent) listed medical sociology as a "field of competence," and an additional 113 (3 per cent) claimed competence in the sociology of mental health. The percentage increase between 1950 and 1959 was 723% for medical sociology and 404% for the sociology of mental health, ranking them first and fifth among all fields of competence in rate of increase. Matilda White, "Membership in the American Sociological Association, 1950–1959." *American Sociological Review*, 25:914–926, December 1960.

11. An organization of seven scientific societies, set up for the advancement of research in the social sciences.

12. Skytop, Pennsylvania, June 22–28, 1958.

13. This point can be illustrated with some extreme examples. Dr. X's TB problems might be rapidly ameliorated if he could pay people with tuberculosis $500 a week to undergo treatment. But Dr. X doesn't have a budget that will permit such a course, and even if he did, he would be hooted out of his profession if he suggested such a thing. His venereal disease problems might be reduced if his health department could operate neighborhood brothels and establish prophylactic stations in all junior and senior high schools and colleges. The risk of lung cancer might be reduced if he had an $8.00 a pack tax on cigarettes, with the tax return earmarked for cancer research. These examples are ridiculous, but they illustrate the sound principle that behavior innovations are more likely to be acceptable if they are perceived as satisfying or rewarding and the point that health agencies are limited in terms of the means that they can use to achieve their goals.

14. Anderson, Odin W. and Seacat, Milvoy. *The Behavioral Scientist and Research in the Health Field: A Questionnaire Survey*. Health Information Foundation, Research Series 1. New York: Health Information Foundation, 1957.

15. Russell Sage Foundation, *Annual Report*, 1959–1960. New York: Russell Sage Foundation, 1960, pp. 10–11. Among the activities thought to be vital to the development of successful collaboration were: "1) de-

veloping an optimal initial orientation and level of expectation; 2) maximizing mutual assimilation of professional subcultural values, ideologies, technologies, and languages; 3) securing an appropriate structural position in the institutional setting for the social scientist; 4) clarification of the roles of the parties to the undertaking; and 5) increasing the interpersonal skills of the participants." pp. 8–9.

16. Foster, George, "Public Health and Behavioral Science: The Problems of Teamwork." Paper presented at the 1960 Annual Meeting of the Western Branch, American Public Health Association, Denver, May 23–26, 1960. Mimeographed.

17. Russell Sage Foundation, *op. cit.*, p. 11.

18. A detailed discussion of cross-disciplinary problems arising in collaboration between behavioral science and public health is to be found in Cecil G. Sheps and Eugene E. Taylor, *Needed Research in Health and Medical Care: A Bio-Social Approach*. Chapel Hill: University of North Carolina Press, 1954. Ch. 4, "Special Organizational Problems," pp. 94–138. Other references are listed in George Rosen and Edward Wellin, "A Bookshelf on the Social Sciences and Public Health," *American Journal of Public Health*, 49:441–454, April 1959, Section 8, "Problems of Interdisciplinary Work."

19. During the nine years that I was located in a Public Health agency, I found that I was regarded as a generalized wise man who was thought to be capable of providing sound counsel and effective help on problems ranging from administrative policy, staff morale, and intra-agency communication to such immediate practical questions as where to locate a mobile x-ray, how to get pregnant mothers in for prenatal examinations, and what skills are required in a health education department.

20. Young, Donald, "Sociology and the Practicing Professions," *American Sociological Review*, 20: 641–648, 1955.

21. Foster, George, *op. cit.* p. 11.

22. A considerable quantity of published behavioral science materi-

als on a wide range of topics of Public Health interest are now becoming available in both books and professional journals. Since there are good bibliographies (e.g. Rosen and Wellin, op. cit.) readily available, no attempt will be made to list any of these here.

23. The occasional use of social scientists as *ad hoc* consultants on Public Health problems could be a way in which members of the two groups in a given area could carry on the preliminary exploration of each other that Foster and others have insisted is so necessary to effective collaboration.

24. For a review of the situation with respect to teaching by one discipline, see Benjamin D. Paul, "Teaching Anthropology in Medicine and Public Health," paper prepared for the Conference on the Teaching of Anthropology, University of California, Berkeley, March 2–4, 1961. For a broader view see the series of articles under the heading, "Training for Social Knowledge in Medicine," in the *Journal of Health and Human Behavior*, 1:26–55, Spring 1960, and particularly James G. Roney, Jr., "Social Sciences in the Teaching of Public Health," pp. 47–52.

25. This is partly offset by the fact that some of the people who are teaching behavioral science in health professional schools have become highly adept at making their discipline meaningful in terms of Public Health problems and in stimulating and helping their students to seek more knowledge on their own initiative.

26. Sheps, Cecil and Taylor, Eugene, *op. cit.*, p. 17.

15. Administration

Some Substantive Limiting Conditions in Communication Between Health Officers and Medical Practitioners*

GEORGE ROSEN, M.D., PH.D.

COMMUNICATION is complex, difficult, and beset with pitfalls. Men talk, write, and gesture to themselves and to each other for many reasons and on innumerable occasions, yet not infrequently the result is confusion rather than clarity, nonsense not sense, misunderstanding rather than comprehension. Moreover, this recognition is neither new nor startling. Indeed, Cratylus, a friend of Plato, became so doubtful of the value of speech that in despair he decided to communicate only by pointing. Others have also noted and studied the same problem without necessarily resorting to such radical and desperate measures. Thomas Hobbes discussed the abuses of speech, pointing out among others that "men register their thoughts wrong, by the inconstancy of the signification of their words; by which they register for their conceptions, that which they never conceived; and so deceive themselves."[1]

Difficulty in communication arises, in short, from the manner in which an individual develops the meanings of a message. This development or interpretation of meaning, however, is generally correlated with and guided by the individual's perception, or more generally by the mode and degree of organization of his perceptual field. Thus, what a man sees and hears and feels in a given communication situation does not happen randomly; it is rather the result of a selection among certain choices of interpretation available to him in a given context. Furthermore, while each individual perceives and communicates out of a private world of his own, this world develops through social influences and processes. Whatever the individual's memories and experiences may be, they derive from the processes by which an

* Reprinted by permission from the December, 1961, issue of the *American Journal of Public Health*, Vol. 51, pp. 1805–1816. Copyright by the American Public Health Association, Inc., 1790 Broadway, New York 19, N.Y. This paper was presented before a Joint Session of the American School Health Association and the Dental Health, Food and Nutrition, Public Health Education, and School Health Sections of the American Public Health Association at the 88th Annual Meeting in San Francisco, California, November 3, 1960. The author is Professor of Public Health Education, Columbia University School of Public Health and Administrative Medicine, New York, New York.

individual becomes a member of and acts as a representative of one or more social groups. In these terms perception is essentially social perception, and as such is an aspect of the process of socialization. Even though communication, in the words of Margaret Schlauch, is "a compromise between the ultimate incommunicability of one person with another and the communication values attached to certain symbols,"[2] the fact is that we do communicate. That we succeed so well most of the time means that in becoming and acting as members of groups, in sharing experiences with others, we acquire a common store of associations, connotations, and other modes of interpretation. Thus, socialization is an essential factor in endeavoring to understand social perception and its relation to effective or ineffective communication.

SOCIALIZATION

Socialization is the process by which an individual becomes a member of a given social group, and it is by this process that cultures are transmitted to each new generation. In this sense, socialization has been recognized as a central facet of professional development. Merton has defined this process for medical students as one in which they "are engaged in learning the professional role of the physician by so combining its component knowledge and skills, attitudes and values, as to be motivated and able to perform this role in a professionally and socially acceptable fashion."[3] In other words, through the socialization process the physician is "trained" for the role he is eventually expected to fill in society.

As a result, despite significant individual differences, medical students at the end of four years exhibit a relatively high level of similarity. Eron points out that, "All of us who have been concerned with medical education for any length of time have noticed not only the profound changes taking place in students as they progress through four years of medical school, but how alike they all appear to be at the end of those years."[4]

INTERSPECIALTY RELATIONS

Despite this common basic socialization, however, and the generally strong orientation of health officers to the medical profession, relations between Public Health officials and medical practitioners have not been consistently good.[5] Conflicts between these two groups have occurred at various times ever since the establishment of modern health departments, and have varied in severity from simple disagreement to violent controversy. How and why do such situations develop? What factors are at work that lead clinical practitioners to accept or oppose the views, recommendations, and actions of Public Health practitioners? Does the process by which a physician becomes a health officer contain additional different elements than those to which other physicians have been and are exposed? It is likely that a review of a number of such cases will provide clues to answer some of these questions, and enable us to see in what sense inadequate communication can be considered an explanation.

The first case comes from the autobiography of Allen W. Freeman. In 1907, he was offered and accepted the position of medical inspector in the health department of Richmond, Va. Among his duties, he was to visit reported cases of diphtheria in order to be certain that the patients were properly isolated and that everything needful was being done. From Dr. Freeman's point of view, his visit to the first case seemed simple enough. "The family was well to do and the case was in the care of a graduate nurse. By the evidence of the empty syringes which the nurse produced the family physician had given antitoxin enough and in good time. The medical inspector had only to fill out his forms and take his leave. . . . But when he had finished his round of cases and reached the office he was told that Dr. Derby, the physician of the family he had just seen, had called up in hot indignation at his visit. He was not accustomed to having another physician visit one of his cases without first communicating with him. He considered it a serious breach of medical courtesy that the physician from the health department should have done so in this case." Recognizing that it was important "to go at once to Dr. Derby and explain why it had been necessary to visit his case and to apologize to him for any breach of professional courtesy," Freeman found the doctor in his office and "told his story as well as he could. Dr. Derby listened quietly to the story . . . , expressed himself as fully satisfied and gave his permission for similar visits to any other cases that he might report."[6]

The clue in this incident is provided by the behavior of the medical practitioner in terms of the concept of medical courtesy. Clearly, in his role as a practicing physician he had certain patterned expectations of how other physicians ought to behave toward him, and in turn how he should and would behave toward other practitioners. The code of behavior in terms of which the physician reacted to the medical inspector from the health department is part of the medical culture acquired by physicians in being socialized. It is part of the larger area of medical ethics, that aspect of the culture which is concerned with professional discipline, and which deals with such matters as advertising, fee-splitting, unfair competition, derogation of another physician, and other forms of unprofessional conduct. An important, if not basic function of this concern with the professional behavior of medical men toward the public and toward each other is to regulate access to the medical market, that is to patients. Furthermore, its function is to provide the medical profession with the means through which effective control can be exercised. In this sense, codes of ethics, or more accurately codes of behavior, institutionalize significant values of the medical culture, particularly those concerned with the economics of practice. Clearly, in 1907, the medical code of behavior took no account of the Public Health physician, who required access to a patient for noneconomic reasons.

THE ISSUE OF ECONOMICS

Other instances of conflict between Public Health practitioners and clinical practitioners reveal starkly the economic basis of the situation. For example, Josephine Baker, first director of the Bureau of Child Hygiene in the New York City Department, related that after child health stations had been established and were "doing well in the Brownsville section of Brooklyn, a petition was forwarded to my desk from the mayor's office, signed by 30-odd Brooklyn doctors, protesting bitterly against the Bureau of Child Hygiene because it was ruining medical practice by its results in keeping babies well, and demanding that it be abolished in the interests of the medical profession."[7]

In opposing the development of such activities by Public Health agencies, physicians in private practice were objecting to what they considered encroachment upon the area of medical practice. Linked with and buttressing the economic aspect are a series of prerogatives and values. These may be a part of the general value system of the society or may be limited to the medical profession. Thus, the compulsory reporting of communicable diseases, such as tuberculosis and the venereal diseases, was considered a violation of personal rights as well as a breach of the confidential nature of the patient-physician relationship.

On January 19, 1897, the New York City Board of Health adopted an ordinance requiring the reporting of cases of pulmonary tuberculosis by physicians. It did not take long for the storm to break.[8] An editorial on January 23 in the *Medical Record,* which took a leading part in opposing the action of the health authorities, clearly indicated the reasons for the conflict. "The real obnoxiousness of this amendment to the sanitary code is," according to the writer, "its offensively dictatorial and defiantly compulsory character. It places the Board in the rather equivocal position of dictating to the profession and of creating a suspicion of an extra bid for public applause by unduly magnifying the importance of its bacteriological department. . . . The profession as a whole has watched with jealous eye the encroachments of the Board upon many of the previously well-recognized privileges of the medical attendant." An editorial published by the same journal in

February, 1897, struck directly to the heart of the controversy. After pointing out that "there is no objection to the reports of pulmonary cases for statistical purposes," the editor continues, "it is, however, the extra missionary work assumed by the board which is the ominous and threatening quantity in the equation—the desire to assume official control of the cases after they have been reported, thus not only, by means of alarming bacteriological edicts, directly interfering with the physician in the diagnosis and treatment of the patient, but in the end, by the creation of a public suspicion of his ignorance, possibly depriving him of one of the means of a legitimate livelihood."[8] Other issues were also raised, such as the questionable value of bacteriological diagnosis, that the disease is not highly contagious, and that tuberculosis is so widely prevalent that any attempt at prevention is impractical. When it became evident that the health authorities in New York City would not retreat, the local medical societies made a determined but unsuccessful effort in Albany to deprive the Health Department of the power to deal with tuberculosis. Similarly, in 1912, when the reporting of venereal disease was made compulsory a new storm of opposition broke out. Eventually the opposition faded away.

Incidents of this kind have not been limited to New York City or to the United States. In 1876, when the health authorities of Greenock, Scotland, proposed to institute the compulsory reporting of cases of infectious disease, the medical practitioners of the town rose in a body to oppose such action.[9] Their opposition was based on the arguments that reporting would disturb the confidential relationship between patient and physician, that medical men should not be compelled to become spies, and that if reporting were made compulsory people would hesitate to call in a physician as this would lead to interference with their domestic concerns.

Around the turn of the century, the reporting of communicable disease in Chicago was impeded by a long dispute between the Health Department and the physicians of the city.[10] There were laws requiring the reporting of certain contagious diseases. Many physicians, however, refused to cooperate, insisting that the municipality pay 25 cents for each report. This stand was based on the provision of the state law remunerating physicians for the reporting of births. At one time physicians who did not comply with the law were prosecuted, an action which led the Chicago Medical Society to protest that "the principle at issue is whether our services can be extracted without pay." In reply the city health commissioner characterized this argument as "an excuse unworthy of any physician." The health authorities continued to insist on compulsory reporting without compensation, and even though the controversy dragged on for a few more years, the medical profession eventually accepted their responsibility.

COMMUNITY OR PATIENT ORIENTATION

For communication to be effective, those engaged in the process must in some degree share mutually acceptable frames of reference. Value patterns and ideologies serve this function by supplying axiomatic definitions of the situation within which communication takes place. Thus, physicians, whether health officers or private practitioners, generally share ideas concerning the scientific approach to the study of disease, the nature of disease, and, perhaps, ideas and methods of diagnosis and treatment. However, there are other ideas, areas of knowledge, and values which these two groups share only to a slight degree if at all. The tasks performed by various groups of physicians exhibit great diversity. The most common image of the physician is that he sees patients, and prevents, diagnoses, and treats illness. Actually, a large number of physicians fit this model only to a limited degree or not at all. Among these are radiologists, pathologists, anesthesiologists, and certainly Public Health administrators. Associated with this diversity are characteristic activities and ideas.

One point of divergence is in the approach to problems of disease. Josephine Baker phrased it well in her comment that the "field of Public Health was far removed from anything that had been comprised in any conventional medical training. Not that medicine was not an essential background—that was clear enough—but the mass attack instead of individual care began to come to the front. We were dealing with the problems of a community, and the individual became important only when he contributed to the problem as a whole."[11] While Dr. Baker's remarks concern a situation two generations ago, they are not irrelevant. Physicians practicing today were trained a generation or so ago, and even though some changes have occurred in medical education in the interim, the clinical practitioner is still basically oriented to the individual patient. Nor do medical students now being trained indicate much change.

VALUES IN CONFLICT

Furthermore, these divergent viewpoints are interlocked with other value clusters. An important cluster of this kind in American society is expressed by the emphasis on practicality. The definition of what is practical, however, will differ for the health officer and the clinical practitioner, and can be expressed in terms of three closely related factors: (1) the immediate goals for action; (2) the criteria used to determine which goals are more significant than others; and (3) the implicit framework of social concepts within which values are perceived and ordered.[12] The Public Health official may decide that prophylaxis is the most practical approach to the problem of controlling tuberculosis or venereal disease, and develop his program of action to achieve this end. On the other hand, the clinician may decide that such a goal is utopian because the most important task is to deal with the sick person, the person who already has the disease.

Such aims may in turn be affected by still other interests and value clusters. The important place of the economic interest in the relations between Public Health officials and medical practitioners has already been stressed. Moral issues can also play a significant role. Numerous observers of American culture have commented on its moralistic tendency. This dimension of community behavior may likewise align the practitioners of Public Health and clinical medicine on opposing sides of a health issue. Two examples illustrate the point, and can help us to tease out certain other elements that may be involved.

Dr. Herman Bundesen became Chicago's health commissioner in 1922 and soon initiated an organized attack on venereal disease. His goal was prevention, to be achieved through education, the distribution of prophylactic means at places where those likely to acquire venereal disease could obtain them (in drug stores, public toilets, and houses of prostitution), and by providing intensive treatment at public clinics.[13] This practical approach met with intense disapproval, not only in the press in general but as well in the medical journals. The "Medical Standard" denounced this "outrageous and unlicensed" use of the health commissioner's authority. For the *Illinois Medical Journal* the whole plan was "revolting." Nowhere, however, is the character of this moral indignation expressed with greater éclat than in the scrambled logic of this statement which the *Chicago Medical Recorder* quoted approvingly: "God forbid that above the Stars and Stripes any misguided, theoretical radical shall ever place the flag of Priapus and the bar sinister of the Phallic Symbol." Whether Bundesen's program could actually prevent syphilis and gonorrhea seemed of no concern to his medical opponents. It was more important to maintain the traditional moral code and the social mythology in which it was shrouded.

The introduction of such issues in opposing governmental action for the improvement of community health is strikingly illustrated by an incident related by Josephine Baker.[14] At a hearing before a Congressional Committee considering the appropriation of funds for the newly established Children's Bureau, a physician representing a New England medical society told the committee: "We oppose this bill because, if you are going to save the lives of all these women and children at public expense, what inducement will there be for young men to study medicine?" Senator Sheppard, the committee chairman, leaned forward and said: "Perhaps I didn't understand you correctly. You surely don't mean that you want women and children to die unnecessarily or live in constant danger of sickness so there will be something for young doctors to do?" "Why not," replied the physician, "that's the will of God, isn't it?" (One should note, however, that pediatricians as a group favored governmental action to improve the health of children, and specifically supported the Sheppard-Towner Act.)

MEDICINE AND THE STATUS QUO

The two instances just cited direct our attention to several other value elements that tend to produce a negative attitude to action by governmental agencies in dealing with health problems. One is the highly negative valuation of government and the expressed fear of centralized public authority evident in the statements and behavior of many medical practitioners. This is not surprising in view of the strong emphasis in our culture on individualism, and the associated view of health as a private matter. These attitudes derive not only from the earlier American experience, but even more significantly from the set of ideas known as Social Darwinism. In the terms of this philosophy, all life, and especially economic activity, was a moral struggle in which the strong flourished and the unfit succumbed. Any social measure concerned with welfare or health might interfere with the free play of market forces, and thus perpetuate the more vulnerable members of the community. The logical consequence therefore was to curtail government action as far as feasible. When coupled with a situation in which physicians develop and maintain a practice in a highly competitive context, any act by government which appears in some way to interfere with the access of physicians to the medical market is a hostile act to be condemned and opposed.

This does not mean, of course, that private practitioners will not accept measures intended to protect the Public Health. Any acceptance, however, tends to be hedged by conditions to safeguard the area of private practice. These attitudes and trends are of long standing. In their studies of Middletown, the Lynds noted these tendencies during the decade 1925–1935. They commented in 1939 that "the attitude of the majority of Middletown's doctors regarding private practice and Public Health facilities remains substantially that described in 1925. All proposals to develop clinical facilities of whatever type in Middletown still operate within the strait jacket of insistence by the majority of the local medical profession that nothing shall be done to make Middletown healthier that jeopardizes the position of the doctors."[15]

Nor has the situation changed very much up to the present. Evidence on this point is available in the studies by Rosenstock, Hochbaum, and their co-workers on the impact of Asian influenza on five communities. While the studies do not provide detailed information on the behavior of organized medical groups, there are several items which indicate that medical society officials tended to minimize the need for community measures involving governmental action, and that where they did act a major aim was as far as possible to maintain a business-as-usual situation. For example, in Hazelton, "the official policy of the local medical society was that vaccine should be administered by private physicians in their offices and further that the distribution of vaccine be left to the discretion of individual physicians."[16]

Clearly, the socioeconomic philosophy of most medical practitioners, the social logic within which they perceive values and behavior related to health, is widely at variance with the root ideas of Public Health. The latter have been so well stated by Gaylord W. Anderson that I can do no better than to quote him. Public Health activities derive logically from the fundamental social concept that "society has a responsibility to provide those necessities and protections which individuals cannot provide for themselves. . . . So long as we accept the concept of public responsibility, we must likewise accept the idea that people have both the duty and right to take those measures which will prevent illness or death from whatever cause. To deny this right of the people is to challenge the fundamental concept of democracy—a government by the people for the benefit of the people."[17]

VARIANCE OF ORIGINS

These divergent views derive also from the different origins of Public Health and clinical medicine. Public Health as a field of community action did not develop out of medical practice. The impulse to sanitary reform did not come from the medical profession, even though some physicians played a significant part in calling attention to the community problem of ill health and provided vigorous support in the development of action programs. Broadly speaking, what happened was that the builders of modern Public Health, accepting certain postulates of economic and social policy, established institutional forms into which accurate and effective medical knowledge could later be fitted. This institutional development did not arise simply from the growth of humanitarian sentiment or of social conscience. It resulted less from a concern for the welfare of the poor than from a growing realization that widespread disease in the community was not and could not be a problem only of the individual, that it was a problem of the entire community. Furthermore, there was an increasing awareness that the cost of disease in the community was a form of social waste that could be eliminated.

In short, from the beginning modern Public Health has taken a broad view of health in the context of community life.

This is not to disparage clinical medicine and the role of the medical practitioner. The central function of the medical profession has been and is to prevent, detect, and cure illness, thus saving lives and alleviating or palliating conditions that are not amenable to other treatment. This function, moreover, is performed primarily through service in a person-to-person relationship. Thus by the very nature of his activity the clinical practitioner tends to take a circumscribed view of the problem of disease. This tendency has been intensified by certain scientific and technical developments in modern medicine, and by the climate of opinion created by atomistic views of society, values such as individualism, and other related factors some of which have already been discussed. As a result, the social context and the community implications of the practitioner's work are much too often overlooked or ignored. Furthermore, the clinical practitioner tends to take for granted and thus to take little or no account of the fact that society provides the conditions which make his activity possible. There are physicians, of course, whose point of view is broader and who recognize the social, economic, and political factors that impinge on and are interlocked with community health institutions. Nevertheless, this group is at present a minority among organized medical practitioners. On the whole, clinical practitioners tend to take a narrow view of health problems in the community, to avoid involvement except where professional interests are potentially or actually concerned, and in general to remain magnificently insulated from the facts of community life. Again, this is a long-term trend. Hermann Biggs arrived at a similar conclusion in 1920. In an address before the New York County Medical Society, he said, "Now the general attitude of the medical profession is part of the kind of work they do; the fact that a physician is generally so absorbed in what he is doing, his own work and the work with his own patients, that he does not look out and get a broad view of the situation as it exists in the State, and his attitude, the natural attitude, is one of obstruction."[18a]

At the same time, the entire medical profession and its field of action are undergoing change. As an example, today, a large part of the profession, about one-third, works wholly or in part for salaries (in hospitals and medical schools, for governmental agencies, pharmaceutical companies, labor unions, and other physicians), and the proportion appears to be increasing. But while the position of the medical practitioner is being altered by changes in science, technology, and social organization, the ideology of individualism and competition still remains the uncompromising official creed. In relation to Public Health, the situation of the clinical practitioner has been well put by an editorial in the New England Journal of Medicine. "Organized medicine and the private practitioner," it states, "have questioned the aims and objectives of the Public Health physician, perhaps justifiably. How far should state-directed Public Health programs go? Should the tax-supported health programs be designed to encompass also citizens who are able to pay for their own care and treatment? Is continued encroachment by the state on the practice of the private physician in the best interest of the patient? Where does so-called 'public' health leave off, and where does 'private' health begin? Or vice versa? Is it possible for 'public' health to become so dominant that 'private' health, the private practice of medicine, will assume a less than secondary role in American medicine?"[17]

DIVERGENT "THEOLOGIES"

The divergent viewpoints of Public Health and clinical medicine continue to exist because they serve to create a consensus in each case for the different groups that maintain them, and because they are what the community as a whole or a particular group within it finds acceptable. However, such acceptability depends on the reassurance and support that the viewpoint and its associated ideas provide. "To a large extent," as Galbraith puts it, ". . . we associate truth with convenience—with what most closely accords with self-interest and individual well-being or promises best to avoid awkward effort or unwelcome dislocation of life. We also find highly acceptable what contributes most to self-esteem. . . . But perhaps most important of all, people approve most of what they best understand . . . economic and social behavior are complex and mentally tiring. Therefore we adhere, as though to a raft, to those ideas which represent our understanding. This is a prime manifestation of vested interest. For a vested interest in understanding is more preciously guarded than any treasure. It is why men react not infrequently with something akin to religious passion, to the defense of what they have so laboriously learned. Familiarity may breed contempt in some areas of human behavior, but in the field of social ideas, it is the touchstone of acceptability."[18]

Within a given community one would expect diverse groups to show differential readiness to accept or reject ideas and measures in terms of a group's self-image, of its interpretation of its interests, and in the degree to which they are congruent with the logic of the value system which prescribes and motivates the behavior of its members. The basic structure of any value system involves a set of interrelated though not always logically congruent principles. To the degree that such principles are employed to deal with reality and are altered in response to experience, the system may be considered more or less open and rational. However, no system of this kind is ever completely subjected to reality testing; in some measure the logic of the system remains autonomous and is accepted on faith. From this viewpoint, every value system has a "theology,"[19] to use the term in an expanded sense. Where a social group maintains a closed value system or moves to create one, this "theology" is even less subject to reality testing. The further such a process moves in this direction the more serious may be the consequences for the group, for the community of which it is a part, or for both.

Freedman has focused the point sharply in his statement that "Organized medicine has developed an almost obsessed suspicion of community organized health programs, particularly when administered by the government. Because Public Health agencies are the traditional operators of community organized health programs, Public Health physicians, who are agents of the government, have received the brunt of the private practitioners suspicions and have been tolerated with reluctance in organized medicine's circles."[5] One consequence of this situation is a considerable loss of contact between medical practitioners and the development and administration of community health programs.

This analysis helps to clarify further the attitudes of physicians in private practice and of Public Health practitioners. Lack of medical leadership in the development of new programs to meet the health needs of the community has been widely noted by various observers. A statement by Norton S. Brown, president of the New York County Medical Society, in 1959, explaining this situation supports our analysis. "The medical profession," he said, "is rapidly losing the initiative in health matters because we're not using diagnostic objectivity in economic and social problems. We're bemused by slogans and pat phrases that no longer have much to do with reality."[20] More recently Lindsay E. Beaton, president of the Arizona Medical Association, has commented in a similar vein. Endeavoring to explain the negative public image of the medical profession, he pointed to the fact, among others, that physicians have been "going steady" with their own false image of themselves. "We are," he said, "perhaps, more and more alienated from the common run of people by our altered relation to them. . . . We must not, with pious tongue in fat cheek, cry nostalgically for the old days and pretend that we are still nineteenth-century leeches and should be adulated as such."[21] And Dr. Beaton went on to point out the need for explicit programs that would be judged not in terms of the socioeconomic interests of a single group but rather in relation to the public interest. In short, what Drs. Brown and Beaton are advocating is that the medical profession break out of a closed system and begin testing its "theology" against the reality of current social needs and problems.

On the other hand, the Public Health practitioner by the very nature of his work must operate with a different value system. While it may in some respects overlap that of the clinical practitioner, its central focus derives from a responsibility to the public in matters affecting the health of the community.[22] Furthermore, a public health practitioner such as a health officer may be exposed to a greater degree of social visibility than the clinical practitioner. The duties of the health officer, such as community leadership, enforcement of laws and regulations, expenditure of public funds, or interpretation of Public Health activities to legislative bodies and community groups, require that he constantly test his ideas in terms of the reality situation which he faces. (The medical practitioner does this in the clinical situation.) In other words, the very nature of his role requires him to view problems in a community framework.

ROLE RELATIONSHIPS

The divergent value systems and self-images of the Public Health practitioner and the medical practitioner are buttressed and strengthened by the reference groups from which they derive the norms and standards for their professional behavior. Furthermore, these are also affected by the counter groups to whom they relate in the performance of their functions. Levine and Wellin, in an unpublished study of the role of the health officer, call attention to major functional areas which constitute his position.[23] He is a physician, a health administrator, a public official, and a leader or coordinator of community health affairs. In these capacities, the health officer becomes involved with greater or lesser frequency and intensity with other health officers, other nonmedical workers in Public Health, city officials and functionaries in other public agencies, members of the medical profession, representatives of voluntary agencies, consumers and the community at large, and extracommunity agencies, for example, a state health department. In the case of the medical practitioner, his position and its functions require him to relate himself to patients, medical colleagues, nurses, laboratory technicians, hospital and health plan administrators, and officials of medical societies. The relations with persons in each of these positions are by no means identical, and involve situations calling for differing attitudes and behavior. A useful tool for the analysis and understanding of these relationships is Merton's concept of the role-set, that is, the "complement of role-relationships in which persons are involved by virtue of occupying a particular social status."[24] This structure of role-relationships may be viewed as a framework for the organization of the perceptual field which practitioners need to perform their functions.

STATUS RELATIONS

To various elements already discussed one must add yet another, namely, status relations. It is no secret that Public Health is held in low esteem by medical practitioners. Those who enter this field are suspected of indolence, incompetence, timidity, lack of independence, being less interested in money, and more interested in helping people. This view is of long standing among medical practitioners. As Carey P. McCord describes the situation, a physician in the opinion of many of his professional brethren "may be in only four places—at the bedside, in the consultation room, in the hospital, at the academy of medicine. With a fair degree of tolerance these physicians accept the insurance doctor, the ship's physician, the medical Public Health officer, the medical teacher and the military surgeon, but rarely are they taken into the profession's bosom. Their enterprises are regarded as rather unfortunate happenings, though not entirely deplorable."[25] To a certain extent this attitude reflects the disdain present in our society for anyone who does not elect to follow the competitive pattern of the culture. The findings reported in 1959 by Coker, *et al.*, on Public Health as seen through the eyes of medical students tend to support this point.[26] At the same time these views probably also reflect the fact that Public Health practice as an area marginal to clinical medicine received a number of physicians of marginal status. Of their existence there can be no doubt. The portrait of Dr. Almus Pickerbaugh, health officer of Nautilus, Iowa, etched in acid by Sinclair Lewis, and the figure of Dr. George Bull, part-time health officer of New Winton, Conn., drawn with ironic compassion by James Gould Cozzens are indicative, and more routine evidence is available. It is impossible to say how representative such types have been of the health officer group as a whole. Nonetheless, such examples were sufficient to reinforce the low opinion in which Public Health was held. Furthermore, the recruitment and training of health officers on a professional basis is only a matter of the past 40 years or so. In 1921, there were 1,000 full-time medical health officers, of whom 225 were in the Public Health Service. The majority of health officers were appointed on a part-time basis and selected from the ranks of practicing physicians. Frequently these were political appointments. In 1921, Ferrell emphasized that "Capable men will not enter the Public Health field unless there is a reasonable prospect that their work will be recognized as professional rather than political, and unless they can have reasonable security of tenure."[27] Even though significant changes have occurred over the past 30 years in the recruitment and training of public health practitioners, the old stereotypes still persist and undoubtedly affect the relations of Public Health physicians and private practitioners today. To be sure, since 1949 Public Health has become a recognized specialty of medicine, and this may perhaps raise the status of the health officer. Yet one cannot overlook the fact that many of the areas of knowledge and the technics required by the Public Health practitioner today are nonmedical. In this sense, Public Health practice, even though a recognized medical specialty is probably becoming more and more marginal to clinical practice.

It should be clear at this point that difficulties in communication between Public Health practitioners and medical practitioners cannot be explained simply by calling attention to differences in perception and orientation. Beneath this surface lie conflicts based on real issues that cannot so easily be resolved. Hopes and wishes alone are insufficient to deal with real issues. The study of five communities by Rosenstock, Hochbaum, and Leventhal revealed that in all of them "the medical society appeared to be the one key group that could determine whether or not action of any kind would be taken and also the kind of action that would be taken." Indeed, the investigators were surprised at "the relative completeness of the authority of the medical society."[28] One may ask: What about the health officer and the local health department in these communities? Did they exist? Did the Public Health agency abdicate its role? Who is charged with responsibility for community health? The health department or the medical society? Clearly these are questions of political power, questions concerning the ability to make decisions and the authority to enforce them. From this viewpoint, communication is not the fundamental problem. Mutual appreciation between Public Health practitioners and medical practitioners may facilitate communication between the two groups, but only as long as the interests of private practitioners or of Public Health practitioners do not seem to be affected. One might also point out that the Public Health physician has often settled for limited goals in his relations with private practitioners, basing his adaptation on the premise that the boundaries of private practice must and will be little affected by his activities. To the extent to which he clearly separates his province of action (environmental health, vital statistics, etc.), he may be isolating his domain from that of the medical practitioner and minimizing the possibilities for conflict. Is there then, in this sense, a tacit decision on both sides not to communicate about certain matters? The problems raised here and previously in this paper all deserve investigation. Communication is affected by perception, and perception in turn by interests, values, status, and power relations. The issues in which these factors are involved will not be solved by goodwill or by better communication skills. Much more is needed. We need studies of the power relationships that exist in the community between the health officer, the organized medical profession, the political groups and others that affect his actions. What constraints (financial, political, social, personal) lead the health officer to act as he does? Only as such institutional questions are elucidated can we deal with the problem of communication in a truly meaningful way.

1. Hobbes, Thomas. *Leviathan or the Matter, Forme and Power of a Commonwealth, Ecclesiasticall* and *Civill.* Cambridge, England: University Press, 1935, pp. 14–15.

2. Schlauch, Margaret. *The Gift of Tongues.* New York, N.Y.: Viking, 1948, pp. 113–114.

3. Merton, Robert K. "Some Preliminaries to a Sociology of Medical Education," in *The Student Physician.* Edited by Merton, R. K.: Reader, G. G.: and Kendall, P. L. Cambridge, Mass.: Harvard University Press, 1957, p. 4.

4. Eron, Leonard D. The Effect of Medical Education on Attitudes: A Follow-Up Study. *J.M.Educ.* 33:25–33, 1958.

5. Following the preparation and presentation of this paper my attention was called to an article by Ben Freedman. Organized Medicine and the Crisis in Community Health Programs. *J. Louisiana M. Soc.* 112:231–237, 1960. This frank discussion touches the same problem as I do. Those interested in these matters should read Freedman's paper and the editorial comment on it—Public and Private Health. *New England J. Med.* 263:922–923, 1960.

6. Freeman, Allen W. *Five Million Patients. The Professional Life of a Health Officer.* New York, N.Y.: Scribner's, 1946, pp. 69–70.

7. Baker, S. Josephine, *Fighting for Life.* New York, N.Y.: Macmillan, 1939, p. 139.

8. Winslow, C.-E. A. *The Life of Hermann M. Biggs.* Philadelphia, Pa.: Lea and Febiger, 1929, pp. 144–146.

9. Ferguson, Thomas. *Scottish Social Welfare 1864–1914.* Edinburgh, Scotland: E. and S. Livingstone, 1958, pp. 402–403.

10. Bonner, T. N. *Medicine in Chicago, 1850–1950.* Madison, Wis.: American History Research Center, 1957, p. 189.

11. Baker. *Op. cit.,* p. 67.

12. Williams, R. M., Jr. *American Society. A Sociological Interpretation.* New York, N.Y.: Knopf, 1951, p. 391.

13. Bonner. *Op. cit.,* p. 193.

14. Baker. *Op. cit.,* p. 138.

15. Lynd, R. S., and Lynd, H. M. *Middletown in Transition, a Study in Cultural Conflicts.* New York, N.Y.: Harcourt, Brace, 1937, p. 395. See, also, id. *Middletown, a Study in Contemporary American Culture.* New York, N.Y.: Harcourt, Brace, 1929, pp. 443–444, and 451.

16. Rosenstock, I. M.; Hochbaum, G. M.; Leventhal, H.; et al. *The Impact of Asian Influenza on Community Life.* Public Health Service Publ. No. 766. Washington, D.C.: Gov. Ptg. Office, 1960, p. 14.

17. Anderson, Gaylord W. Public Health—A Mandate from the People. *A.J.P.H.* 42:1367 (Nov.), 1952.

17a. See reference 5. *New England J. Med.,* p. 923.

18. Galbraith, J. K. *The Affluent Society.* Boston, Mass.: Houghton Mifflin, 1958, pp. 8–9.

18a. Winslow. *Op. Cit.,* p. 354.

19. Broch, Hermann. *Massenpsychologie. Schriften aus dem Nachlass.* Zürich, Switzerland: Rhein-Verlag, 1959, p. 86.

20. Chevalier, Lois. You're Not Running a Private Concession. *Med. Economics* 36:100 (Jan. 5), 1959.

21. Beaton, Lindsay E. A Doctor Prescribes for His Profession. *Harpers Magazine* (Oct.), 1960, p. 150.

22. See Proposed Report on Educational Qualifications of Directors of Public Health Departments. *A.J.P.H.* 45:363 (Mar.), 1955.

23. Levine, S., and Wellin, E. "Role of the Health Officer: A Sociological Inquiry." Paper presented to the Committee on Preventive Medicine and Social Science Research, Social Science Research Council, New York, February 11, 1960. (To be published.)

24. Merton, R. K. The Role Set. Problems in Sociological Theory. *Brit. J.Sociol.* 8:106–120, 1957.

25. McCord, Carey P. *A Blind Hog's Acorns.* Chicago. Ill.: Cloud, 1945, pp. 24–25.

26. Coker, R. E., et al. Public Health as Viewed by the Medical Student. *A.J.P.H.* 49:601–609 (May), 1959.

27. Ferrell, John A. Measures for Increasing the Supply of Competent Health Officers. *J.A.M.A.* 77:513–516, 1921. 27a. See, also, id. Careers in Public Health Service. Ibid. 76:489–492, 1921. 27b. Rankin, W. S. Elimination of Politics from Public Health Work. Ibid. 83:1285–1287, 1924.

28. Rosenstock, et al. *Op. cit.,* p. 18.

PART FIVE

The Services:
Some Changing Emphases in Public Health

1. Medical Care   602
2. Rehabilitation   643
3. Poison Control   670
4. Epidemiologic Investigations   675
5. Nutritional Health   715
6. Home Care   735

NEEDED: A CONTINUUM OF HEALTH CARE

"TO make the best possible use of modern health knowledge, we need to devise measures for providing a continuum of health care to the individual. At present too much is left to chance. Whether a child is protected against the growing list of communicable diseases for which we have vaccines depends upon the kind of family he happens to be born into. Whether cancer, glaucoma, diabetes, and the other so-called silent diseases are discovered at their most treatable, and often painless stages, depends upon the degree of concern the individual has for his health. Relatively few apparently have enough knowledge or concern to seek and pay for medical checkups when they feel well. And the kind and quality of care the person with a chronic condition receives depends not only upon the alertness of his physician in keeping up with all the new developments in this field, but also on the availability of a variety of facilities and services, many of which are now lacking or inadequate in most communities. Because too much is left to chance, because care is so fragmented, we estimate that approximately 150,000 Americans die and more than a million are seriously disabled every year from conditions that could have been prevented."

THEODORE J. BAUER, M.D., in Public Health Concepts in Social Work Education, *New York Council on Social Work Education, 1962, p. 3.*

One of the operating bases of Public Health involves the development of flexible priorities in terms of which efforts are concentrated on one as against another health problem. The severity, frequency, and community impact of particular problems are weighed against the level of the technical knowledge and feasibility of mounting programs to overcome them. After considering the consequences of various courses of action, Public Health agencies reach decisions about desirable points of concentration and emphasis for their work. This Section is devoted to presentation of some fields of action and research which Public Health has recently established as important priorities.

Foremost among these is concern for the medical care received by the population. Public Health views the distribution, timing and quality of medical care as among the foremost determinants of health status for the individual and the group. To promote the latter, Public Health fights to remove institutionalized obstacles, maldistribution and inadequacies in medical care resources as described by Dr. Roemer, and promotes extension of the pre-payment systems reviewed by the Somers'.

Four papers discuss aspects of rehabilitation and disability prevention of significance to Public Health, Miss Switzer's presenting a comprehensive account of the important and expanding Federal-State program in vocational rehabilitation, and Lee stressing the often under-utilized resource of the community self-help group.

Public Health control programs—and the use of data derived from them for investigation and planning—are illustrated in the papers by Press and Buchbinder. Fruitful epidemiologic investigations into cardiovascular disease—our foremost cause of mortality—are found in the papers by Stamler, and Buechley, Drake and Breslow. A treatment approach to obesity—significant but often overlooked as a Public Health problem—is presented by Hillman.

Finally, Sheps and Kasten illustrate Public Health's current concern with care of the sick and disabled in their own homes in their discussion of the efficiency, psychologic benefits, and financial saving in bringing needed services to long-term patients through organized home care programs.

1. Medical Care

Medical Care Administration*

MILTON I. ROEMER, M.D.

THE PROVISION of medical care to any community is a varied and complex process. It is based on a wide range of methods of financing and a multiplicity of organized frameworks for delivering health services. The major portion of medical care for individuals in the United States is provided by private practitioners, usually on a fee-for-service basis. Medical care programs, however, involve many local agencies and groups, both public and private.

The local health department, in particular, can have a basic impact on the quality of medical care in the community, through the adoption and enforcement of health standards, through health programs under its direct administrative responsibility as well as for installations where medical care is rendered (e.g., hospitals, rehabilitation centers, outpatient departments), through its laboratory facilities and epidemiologic studies, and through its case-finding and follow-up in communicable and chronic diseases.

The chief administrator in a municipality or county will constantly find a facet of his job touching on medical care. He therefore needs some understanding of various programs, how they interact and affect each other, what governs the level of their expenditures, and the like. His responsibilities may encompass such seemingly widely separated functions as developing a health insurance program for city employees and supporting health department advocacy of a Salk vaccine program for women in the child-bearing years. This writing attempts to catalog most of the agencies that are involved in medical care, broadly or narrowly defined, and to indicate the population groups encompassed by the activities of these agencies. Only when the official sees the broad spectrum of services, the multiplicity

* Reprinted with omission of two figures, by permission from *Administration of Community Health Services*, published by the International City Managers' Association, and edited by Eugene A. Confrey, Chicago, 1961, Chap. 11, "Medical Care Administration," pages 221–246, and 516–517. The author is Professor of Medical Care Administration, School of Public Health, and Professor of Preventive Medicine and Public Health, School of Medicine, University of California, Los Angeles, California, and formerly Director of Research, Sloan Institute of Hospital Administration, Graduate School of Business and Public Administration, Cornell University, Ithaca, New York. At the author's request, the footnotes appearing in the chapter have been deleted. The selected bibliography on pp. 634–635 was the set of references appearing with the original publication.

of resources, and the nature of the funds involved can he function usefully in this vital area of community activity.

The discussion is focused on organized medical care activity involving groups of people. The relationships of private patients and private doctors recognizably are of continuing importance but are not the major subject of this chapter.

SCOPE OF PROGRAMS

Nearly all medical care programs in the United States are defined by certain limitations in the beneficiaries served, the diseases treated, and the technical services offered (which depend to a large extent on the availability of trained personnel and financial support).

Many programs of medical care are oriented to certain population groups that have been singled out for special protection or assistance. The indigent or recipients of public assistance are such a group. Military personnel are another such group, as are veterans. Local programs may be devoted to school children or industrial workers. Within these limitations, there may also be further restrictions on the illnesses treated (for example, medical office visits, but not home visits, for indigent persons).

Some community programs of medical care focus on the diagnosis and treatment of certain diseases occurring in any type of person. Such are the programs for tuberculosis, mental illness, venereal diseases, and cerebral palsy.

Still other medical care programs cope with any illness in any person but are limited with respect to the technical service offered. Such are programs for financing hospitalization or for offering high-cost drugs. A program of surgical services or one limited to nursing care in the home is in this class.

AGENCIES RESPONSIBLE

A useful way for the municipal or county administrator to view local medical care programs is by the type of agency sponsoring the activity. A variety of types may operate within a community directly or have impact on it from a higher jurisdiction, such as the state or federal level. Each of these forms of agency is of two classes: (1) where the health service is the central purpose, and (2) where the health activity is ancillary to some other purpose.

Governmental Health Agencies

A department of health, operating a medical care program, illustrates the type of agency in which health service is of prime importance. A special commission for mental hospitals—such as operates in many states—is another example. These governmental health agencies, whether local, state, or federal in origin, may be involved in medical care in a municipality.

Many governmental departments include health services as a support for broader objectives (i.e., health services are ancillary). Welfare departments which are concerned with total life needs of indigent persons often provide or purchase medical services for them. Veterans agencies do likewise. Departments of education often include medical care programs for rehabilitation as part of their general efforts to re-educate the physically handicapped, and also as an important part of school health.

Voluntary Health Agencies

A vast variety of humanitarian or charitable health agencies are primarily concerned with certain facets of medical care. The local cancer society may provide medical supplies, emergency medical services for cancer patients, or sometimes pay for radiation therapy. A visiting nurse association is a voluntary health agency engaged in providing a sector of medical care.

The Red Cross is a wide-spectrum voluntary agency which, among other things, provides certain medical services, such as the operation of blood banks. Many social casework agencies help their clients obtain medical care as an aspect of their wider objectives of aiding these persons with crucial problems.

Health Enterprises

Many agencies are in a business enterprise whose prime purpose is providing medical care, even though the activity is often nonprofit. It is an enterprise in the sense that individuals must buy their entitlements to specific services, unlike the usual arrangements of the governmental or voluntary agencies. Most important among these are the medical care insurance plans, such as Blue Cross, Blue Shield, or the consumer-sponsored programs.

Local industrial or other business enterprises, as a feature of their personnel programs, often conduct certain organized programs of medical care as an auxiliary or supporting service. These may vary from first-aid for on-the-job injuries to comprehensive medical care for the worker and his family. In this category also must be included the insurance companies that sell policies for medical care insurance.

Membership Health Organizations

Membership organizations such as Alcoholics Anonymous or societies of the blind, whose programs embrace a sector of medical care, have as their major purpose the joint health or welfare concern of their constituents. Such membership organizations as the professional societies of physicians, dentists, nurses, and others, which operate programs of education or research affecting medical care, would also be included in this category.

Finally, within the community is a variety of organizations of workers, farmers, women, veterans, religious groups, business men, and others that have broad objectives, among which may be some medical care. An example is a local medical care insurance plan of a fraternal lodge, or a women's club program to provide needed crutches and wheelchairs, or a local "meals-on-wheels" program to supply food to the home-bound chronically ill and aged.

ELEMENTS OF MEDICAL CARE ADMINISTRATION

The complexity of medical care administration depends on the nature of the program. Some programs of medical care are limited in scope, while others may be sweeping and complex. Administrative problems will vary accordingly. Whatever their complexity and extent, however, any medical care program can be analyzed internally by certain basic elements:

1. In any organized medical care program, there is always some type of agency responsible. Within the agency, there will be various systems of structuring, or delegating authority, of maintaining order by rules and regulations. There may be systems of securing advice and maintaining public relations that affect the service provided.

2. Funds for medical care programs are derived in many ways. They may come from tax revenues, from insurance contributions, from philanthropy, or from industry. Moreover, these funds are allocated to sectors of the program in different ways.

3. The persons entitled to care in the program must be specifically defined, and a system is usually necessary to assure such determinations efficiently. The eligibility may be predetermined, according to a person's status, or it may involve a fresh determination each time a medical service is obtained.

4. Since medical care is rendered by skilled personnel in special facilities, the community must arrange for providing these resources. Various contracts may be necessary between the sponsoring agency and the physicians, dentists, hospitals, or other providers of service. Specific standards are often stipulated as a condition for such participation.

5. There must, of course, be a clear definition of what services are offered, and under what conditions. Home calls by physicians for example, may be a benefit, but only on payment of a partial fee; or this fee may be levied only if the call is a night call. There are usually

specific exclusions of certain types of service or maximum limitations on certain categories of care.

6. The methods by which the local sponsoring agency pays for the service are of many types. Payments may be through indemnification of the patient who is then expected to pay the provider of service. Or it may be made directly to the provider by way of a salary, a capitation rate, a fee for each service, or combinations of these methods. Hospitals are reimbursed according to a variety of formulas.

7. The role of the local health departments in the promotion of the quality of medical care in the community has been mentioned above, as well as in other parts of this book. Many, if not all, medical care programs, both public and private, undertake special measures to assure the quality of service. These may involve in-service training, specialized education, medical research, or types of group discipline and professional review. An example of the latter technique is the perinatal mortality and morbidity committee established by the local medical profession or the local health council composed of professional, governmental, voluntary, and citizen groups. Even the absence of such deliberate measures is significant in any analysis of the characteristics of a medical care program.

8. Finally, every medical care program must have a mechanism to handle complaints and to protect the rights of both recipients and providers of service. There is generally a system for enforcing or at least encouraging compliance with the rules of the program.

PUBLIC MEDICAL CARE

To many municipal and county administrators, the concept of "public medical care" probably brings to mind the operation of the city hospital or the local welfare program. In most localities, however, public care is being provided for many groups in addition to the poor—for example, the medically indigent, veterans, migrant workers, the blind, school children, crippled children, totally disabled persons, and others.

Care of the Needy

Virtually every community in the United States has some organized arrangements for providing medical care to the poor.

ELIGIBILITY DETERMINATION. Since the basic test of eligibility is poverty, various forms of a "means test" are administered by welfare department personnel. The specific rules by which need is determined vary greatly among the states, and between localities within the states. Since the Social Security Act of 1935, however, a certain uniformity of definition has been achieved for four categories of persons who are entitled to public assistance with the aid of some federal funds.

These categories of persons come under the following programs: (1) old-age assistance (for persons 65 years or over found to be needy); (2) aid to dependent children (for children deprived of a family bread-winner because of disability, death, or absence of the father); (3) aid to the needy blind; and (4) aid to the totally and permanently disabled found to be needy. These categories are over-simplified, but if a needy person can be subsumed under one of them, federal financial assistance may be obtained.

A fifth category comes under a program often called "general assistance." It consists of those persons who are found by the local welfare department to be needy, but who do not fit into one of the specific programs listed above. This tends to be a much smaller group, but it has special importance for medical care since a common reason for this determination is the need for expensive health services. In other words, it is often medical need (usually hospitalization) that places a person on the welfare rolls, even though he is not otherwise entitled to either categorical or general assistance. Altogether about 3 or 4% of a municipal population is generally on the public assistance rolls, though the ratio obviously fluctuates with the business cycle and the community.

MEDICAL SERVICES. The specific medical services which these public assistance clients receive vary greatly among the states. They tend to be more comprehensive in the more prosperous jurisdictions. In some communities, however, they are virtually limited to the care of emergencies or severe disorders for which a "prior authorization" has been received from the welfare department.

The most common pattern for provision of medical care is a free choice of doctor by the welfare patient among a panel of doctors who have agreed to serve these people. There is a tendency, however, for only a small proportion of the doctors in a community to provide the great bulk of the service to these indigent persons. Outpatient clinics of hospitals are also used, for which the welfare department reimburses the hospital. Drugs are obtained only on a physician's prescription, and eyeglasses, dentures, or other appliances usually require a special authorization from the welfare agency as well.

ADMINISTRATION. The medical services, like the over-all financial assistance for welfare recipients, are usually administered by the local welfare department. There is often a part-time medical adviser—a local practicing physician—who helps in maintaining relationships with the various providers of service. At the state level, a full-time medical director generally formulates policies and procedures concerning medical care, supervises the program, provides consultation to local agencies, negotiates with medical societies and other bodies on fee schedules, and helps to prevent abuses. Most of the money for medical care comes from federal and state levels and is either granted to the localities or dispersed directly from the state level.

In two states, Kentucky and Maryland, administration of medical care of the needy has been delegated to the state health department— as well as to the local health departments in that state. In Florida, certain aspects of medical care of the needy are the responsibility of the state health department. About 40 counties or cities in other states have also assigned administrative responsibility for this program to the local health department, the latest being New York City.

PATTERNS OF PAYMENT. A large amount of care is provided free to the needy by the medical, dental, and other practitioners of the community. In organized programs, physicians and dentists are often paid for their services to welfare patients on a fee-for-service basis according to a specified fee schedule. This schedule has generally been negotiated with the professional society and tends to provide average reasonable fees (rather than low fees), the payment of which is guaranteed.

The major part of welfare department expenditures for medical care is usually referrable to hospitalization, because the welfare clientele is largely composed of aged persons (whose hospital needs are high), and because the poor living conditions of these people usually lead to longer-than-average hospital stays for any diagnosis. In recent years, hospital costs have risen more than other medical costs, largely because the heightened complexity of hospital service and the reduced work week have greatly increased the ratio of hospital personnel to patients. This combination of pressures has meant that in many states and localities, the welfare department has been unable or unwilling to pay hospitals the full costs of hospitalization for welfare patients. It has been commonplace for the welfare department to pay hospitals some flat figure such as $10 or $15 per patient-day of care, when the actual calculated cost per patient-day might be $25 or $30.

These practices force hospitals to make up their losses by higher charges to private patients or to Blue Cross insurance plans. The latter, however, object on the ground that the welfare patient ought to be the financial responsibility of the whole community, through government, rather than merely through the Blue Cross membership. Welfare departments sometimes allege that hospital cost accounting is unsound, that it is not suited to their patient load, and that the figures quoted often include factors (e.g., education of nurses or research) which ought not be added to the cost of patient care. In many localities, the arguments have been long and bitter and have arisen fundamentally from inadequate appropriations for the medical care of the needy.

In a few states, such as Connecticut and Massachusetts, state commissions have been established to make objective calculations of the costs of each general hospital in the state. It is thus recognized that costs differ among hospitals and that no flat figure could be equitable. Every state agency—not only the welfare department but others such as vocational rehabilitation or workmen's compensation—then abides by these established rates of payment. Such equitable payments to hospitals, institutions which are so important to the whole community, help to assure their solvency.

Medically Indigent

Although there is much discussion of the "medically indigent," arrangements for their medical care are far from clear-cut. The usual definition of a medically indigent person is one who is able to meet the costs of his general living needs but cannot cope with the costs of a severe illness. Precise identification of a medically indigent person depends, therefore, on the burden of his general living expenses (for example, number of dependents, debts pending) as well as on the extent of his medical need. In a sense, almost anyone short of the millionaire might be medically indigent if a disease of sufficient severity and duration strikes him.

Until recently, little was done by government to provide care to the medically indigent. Some of the wealthier states paid hospital bills for a small proportion of these people under local "general assistance" programs, as mentioned above, but seldom has care been extended beyond the hospital. The principal resource for medically indigent families has been the generosity of friends or relatives who lend them money and the willingness of physicians to treat for low charges or without charge. Hospital outpatient departments serve these patients at very low fees or entirely without charge, and inpatient care is often given by hospitals on public wards—at least in the larger cities—without any hope of collecting a payment.

VOLUNTARY AGENCIES. A variety of voluntary welfare agencies sometimes help the medically indigent. Family or children's social work agencies will often meet medical expenses for their clients who are of low income. The Salvation Army, in its program for helping destitute men, may cover medical expenses. Churches and fraternal lodges assist a disadvantaged member, as do some labor unions. The disease-specific voluntary health agencies, like the Cancer Society or the National Foundation (formerly for Infantile Paralysis), will sometimes help selected patients get needed medical care. A Public Health nurse or social worker who is well acquainted with community resources can advise a medically indigent family how to draw on several of these resources to meet the expenses of a particular illness.

MEDICAL AID TO THE AGED. A national program of care for the medically indigent was initiated in late 1960, when Congress amended the Social Security Act to increase funds for medical care under the Old-Age Assistance category and to add a new category: Medical Assistance to the Aged. In effect, this program provides Federal matching grants to the States, ranging from 50 to 80%, to help meet the costs of comprehensive medical care to persons 65 and over who are not receiving old-age assistance, but whose income and resources are determined by the states to be insufficient to meet such costs. The scope of medical services from which a state may choose includes hospital and home health-care services; outpatient and clinic services; skilled nursing home care; physician services; nursing, physical therapy, and related services; dental care, including dentures and prosthetic devices; prescribed drugs and eyeglasses; and diagnostic screening and preventive services. Services the state may choose must include one or more out-of-institution services.

The program is so new that its mode of operation is not yet clear. However, the law requires that it be administered by the agency which administers old-age assistance. In a few states, health departments are being called in under contract to provide medical and technical assistance or to act as agent of the welfare department in administering the medical assistance program. Aged persons who meet a test of "low income" will probably be certified as eligible and then be entitled to medical care from the usual personnel and facilities. Since a high proportion of the needs of this age group is care in nursing homes, large additional funds will probably be forthcoming to finance these institutions. This may help to elevate standards of operation in nursing homes.

Other Public Medical Beneficiaries

Aside from the indigent and medically indigent, who are found in every community, a number of other groups are entitled to medical care through governmental programs. Most, though not all, come under the federal government.

ARMED FORCES. Officers and enlisted men in the nation's armed forces are entitled to comprehensive medical care. A network of hospitals and field medical stations is located at military posts throughout the United States. Military personnel are also sent to medical centers concentrating on specialized problems, e.g., cardiac surgery. The medical and auxiliary staffs of these programs work in systematic medical departments, on government salaries. If a soldier or sailor is in need of emergency care while off post, he may be treated by local physicians and hospitals, who then are reimbursed by a military office.

DEPENDENTS OF MILITARY PERSONNEL.   At military posts, it has long been customary for the wives and children of men in uniform to obtain medical services from the military medical staffs. In 1955, this was made national policy, rather than leaving it to the discretion of each local commander. The entitlement was extended, moreover, to military dependents living anywhere and for medical services received from local civilian doctors and hospitals. The local services are financed in various ways, under contract with the Department of Defense. Hospital care in the East and West is provided by the National Blue Cross, in central United States by an insurance company. Physicians' services are provided variously by Blue Shield, the state medical society, or the same insurance company handling the hospital care. Service benefits are provided subject to a small deductible amount.

MERCHANT MARINE.   The Public Health Service operates a network of general hospitals, at principal coastal ports, which serve the medical needs of merchant seamen. The staffs of these hospitals, and their associated clinics for ambulatory care, are all salaried federal personnel. At smaller ports, however, local private physicians are engaged on a contract basis to give care to these men. The Public Health Service, whose hospital system was started in 1798, also gives medical care to members of the Coast Guard and the Coast and Geodetic Survey, as well as to the members of the Public Health Service commissioned officer corps and their families.

VETERANS.   Former members of the armed forces, whether engaged in actual combat or not, are entitled to a wide range of medical services from a system of medical facilities operated by the federal Veterans Administration. The 172 hospitals of this system are located in all major cities and are staffed by a corps of salaried personnel, supplemented by part-time private medical specialists who visit periodically.

A veteran is expected to go to the hospital nearest his home for care. If his illness or disability is "service-connected" (that is, arising during his time in military service or directly traceable to that experience), he is entitled to unlimited care of all types. Generally care given in Veterans Administration facilities, however, is for "nonservice-connected" conditions. To obtain care for such ailments, the veteran is only required to affirm that he is unable to afford this care privately. Care for nonservice-connected conditions, however, is limited to inpatient hospital service, and need only be provided if a bed is available. A large proportion of VA facility beds are occupied by mental and geriatric patients.

For service-connected disabilities, the veteran may also obtain care in his home town if it is more convenient and technically accessible there than at a VA facility. Physicians and hospitals are reimbursed under the "home-town programs," directly by the Veterans Administration according to established fee schedules.

INDIANS AND ALASKA NATIVES. The approximately 400,000 Indians and Alaska native citizens living on or near reservations, and regarded as Indians or Alaska natives in the community in which they live, may obtain free medical care through a system of federal hospitals and field health clinics now operated by the Public Health Service. In addition, the federal government serves the health needs of this group through contractual arrangements with nonfederal hospitals, private physicians and dentists, and other health agencies.

MIGRATORY WORKERS. To harvest the nation's crops, there are great streams of domestic migratory workers—over three quarters of a million, often travelling in families—who move into an area for a few weeks and then move on. During World War II, a federal system of organized medical care was provided through field clinics staffed by nurses and part-time salaried local physicians, but the program was discontinued at the end of the war.

In a few states at present, local health departments are extending some maternal and child health services to migrant workers, under federal grants from the Children's Bureau, and some services under the nation-wide venereal disease program of the Public Health Service, generally jointly with voluntary agencies and church groups.

The demonstration health programs in Fresno, California; Palm Beach County, Florida; and Mesa County, Colorado, are outstanding but not common examples of planned health programs for the migrant worker. These provide medical service through multipurpose clinics that operate at night and provide nursing services to the camps on a regular basis. Local physicians, hospital administrators, and public health and welfare workers are involved. However, with a few notable exceptions, the financing of medical care and provision of services is usually left to the domestic agricultural migrant workers themselves or to the farmers who hire them. The health care of foreign or off-shore workers is covered by law in the contracts under which they are hired.

PRISONERS. Medical care of prisoners is a responsibility of law-enforcement authorities at different government levels. The federal penitentiaries, under the Department of Justice, are staffed by Public Health Service medical officers. State and local prisons usually engage local physicians on part-time salaries. All but the smallest jails have an infirmary where sick prisoners may be hospitalized. The expense of these medical services is simply part of the cost of operating a prison.

OTHERS. Immigrants to the United States and incoming travelers from abroad are subject to medical examination prior to entry; in certain instances they are kept under medical surveillance when an excludable disease is suspected.

Disease-Specific Programs

Because of the high cost of care, the hazards of communicability, or the arousal of public pity, certain illnesses have been singled out by society for publicly financed medical care.

MENTAL ILLNESS. In all states care of the mentally ill in hospitals has been largely assumed as a responsibility of the state government. In metropolitan centers, mental hospitals may be operated by the city or county governments, but the vast majority of beds are in state institutions. For centuries the care of mental patients was primarily custodial, motivated largely by the desire to remove the "insane" from the community, but in the last few decades it has become increasingly therapeutic. Today the majority of patients entering a mental hospital are discharged within one year. The most difficult cases perhaps are the senile psychotic patients with organic brain damage, who are entering in increasing numbers because of the greater longevity of the population.

Mental hospitals are financed almost entirely out of tax funds, although some states require payments by those few patients whose families can afford it. The aggregate cost of operation of mental hospitals usually looms large in the state government budget, always exceeding that of the public health services, for example. Nevertheless, the expenditure per patient-day of mental hospital care is extremely low—typically under $4 per day—in comparison with average costs of $25 to $30 per day for care in a general hospital. It is these low expenditures that are fundamentally responsible for the grim and crowded conditions in many mental hospitals. Administration of these institutions is usually by a special state commission, a department of institutions (including prisons), or a mental health department; it is not usually the responsibility of the state health department. The latter agency, however, often operates mental hygiene clinics and other community psychiatric services which are a form of medical care for ambulatory patients.

DRUG ADDICTION. Two Public Health Service hospitals for drug addicts are available—at Lexington, Kentucky, and Fort Worth, Texas —to those eligible as defined by federal law, i.e., those who voluntarily apply and addicts convicted of an offense against the United States and committed by judicial procedures.

TUBERCULOSIS. Hospital care of patients with tuberculosis long has been a governmental responsibility, usually at the state level, although a number of local health departments administer municipal tuberculosis hospitals. In some states, the state health department supervises these institutions, along with the community services for case-finding and follow-up of tuberculosis patients, but more often other state agencies are responsible. With the great reduction in the tuberculosis death rate during the last 15 or 20 years, and the decrease in the incidence of the disease to some extent, many of these large tuberculosis sanatoria have been and are being converted to other purposes, such as chronic disease facilities, homes for the aged, or general hospitals. The community responsibility which has long been assumed for tuberculosis is now being gradually assumed for other chronic disorders. However, tuberculosis is still a problem in the United States. It was fifth among reportable diseases in 1959.

OTHER COMMUNICABLE DISEASES. Special municipal hospitals for the isolation and care of patients with acute infectious diseases used to be common, but most of them have now been closed or converted to other purposes. In a few cities, however, such institutions are still operated—usually as parts of a municipal general hospital system— and provide care to low-income persons. For the treatment of leprosy, a rare but serious disease, there is a federal hospital operated by the Public Health Service at Carville, Louisiana, and another in Hawaii.

CRIPPLED CHILDREN. The definition of a "crippling condition" varies, but in all states there is a program of medical care for children (under 21 years of age) with such handicaps. Orthopedic conditions, such as cerebral palsy or paralysis from poliomyelitis, are always covered, and in many states "crippling" is interpreted also to include deafness, cleft lip, or congenital heart disease. Federal grants for this program are provided to the states by the Children's Bureau. The program is usually administered by the state health department, but sometimes by the state welfare department or other state agency. (Arizona does not participate in the program.)

Services are given to crippled children through local physicians and hospitals that meet designated standards. Often special clinics are organized for periodic check-ups and for appraisal of new applicants. Surgical correction of defects is performed either in the home community or at a medical center away from the community when indicated. Some children may receive extended care in a rehabilitation center. While the federal law does not require limitation of this program to needy families, there is a tendency in most states for eligibility to be limited to children in low-income families. In 1959, there were 339,000 children in the nation aided by this program.

HANDICAPPED ADULTS. For adults with crippling conditions, there is another public medical care program in all states, aided by grants from the federal government. This is the vocational rehabilitation program administered ordinarily by the state departments of education since the medical aspects are considered auxiliary to retraining persons for employment. In 1959, about 280,000 handicapped adults received medical service under this program.

To receive corrective or rehabilitative therapy, a person must be suffering from a "static" physical defect which impedes his employment and for which he is unable to afford care privately. The regulations of the federal Office of Vocational Rehabilitation define the meaning of "static" defects, which generally include conditions which, if untreated, would remain essentially the same or slowly become worse. The definition is meant to exclude conditions like active tuberculosis or acute rheumatoid arthritis—which require general medical care—but to include conditions like paralyzed limbs or blindness which are no longer active but can benefit from rehabilitation. Services are rendered by local physicians and hospitals meeting specified standards. Payments are made on a fee basis. Many of the patients under this program receive long periods of care in rehabilitation centers. In Virginia and a few other states, the state vocational rehabilitation agency operates its own rehabilitation center.

HEALTH INSURANCE

Many self-supporting groups of persons use insurance to finance medical care. Through periodic payments into a fund, out of which medical and related expenses are paid, these persons are economically protected so that at time of sickness they have access to needed services without financial deterrents. With this fiscal mechanism, moreover, there are often associated various special arrangements for the organized provision of medical care in the community.

Blue Cross and Blue Shield

While they are by no means the oldest form of health insurance in the United States, the Blue Cross and Blue Shield plans have become the best-known and most influential. From a small beginning in 1929 in Texas, the Blue Cross plans have grown to an enrollment of about 57 million persons and Blue Shield to about 49 million persons. While the symbols of the "Blue" plans are nation-wide, the plans themselves are actually a network of independent organizations established usually on a state basis. In some states such as New York there may be several regional plans; in others, plans may cross state lines. There were 79 such plans in the United States at the end of 1959.

BLUE CROSS STRUCTURE AND ENROLLMENT. Blue Cross plans are designed to pay hospital bills, usually in semiprivate accommodations, for their members. Membership is generally based on groups of employed persons, such as the employees in a factory or a large store. The plans are spoken of as "voluntary," in that they are nongovern-mental and coverage is not legally compulsory, but most of members are enrolled as aspects of their employment in one enterprise or another. The insurance premiums are paid automatically through wage deductions, sometimes with an employer contribution as a "fringe benefit."

Each plan has a board of directors composed largely of repre-sentatives of general hospitals. The Blue Cross symbol was established by the American Hospital Association, and from the beginning the plans have been closely affiliated with the nation's hospitals. In recent years public representation on Blue Cross boards of directors has been strengthened. The staff of Blue Cross plans is much like that of insurance companies, but the plans themselves are nonprofit organiza-tions. Any earnings in excess of obligations are put into reserves or used for expanded benefits.

BENEFITS. A local Blue Cross plan will usually pay the full cost of a certain number of days of hospitalization in semiprivate room accom-modations per year. Thirty or 70 days are common limits, though several plans provide up to 120 days of coverage at full cost, and then an additional number of days at half-cost. These limits protect well over 90 per cent of all hospital admissions. Almost all in-hospital serv-ices are covered, although there are sometimes exclusions for certain expensive drugs or special diagnostic or treatment services. Other exclusions may relate to specific conditions (e.g., alcoholism, drug addiction) or illnesses for which there are programs with legal responsibility (such as mental illness, care in the armed forces, and workmen's compensation cases). There are sometimes waiting periods for maternity care, elective surgery, or care for chronic or certain specified conditions.

In recent years, several local Blue Cross plans have widened their benefits to include certain outpatient services, especially for accident cases, in order to eliminate unnecessary admissions. Some plans, e.g., in Buffalo, New York, include coverage for care in nursing homes—a provision of great importance in the light of increasing problems in geriatric care.

HOSPITAL RELATIONS. Blue Cross plans are spoken of as "service programs," implying that they provide their members guaranteed service, rather than cash indemnification for health expenses. This requires that the plans have contracts with the institutions providing the care. "Member hospitals" are ordinarily composed of all licensed general hospitals in the state or region encompassed by the particular plan. (In some States, e.g., New York, there are regional territories assigned among several different plans.) If a person is hospitalized in a nonmember hospital, he pays the bill and is then reimbursed by the plan for a fixed amount, which may or may not meet the total costs.

Contracts between the Blue Cross plan and the hospital usually specify an average "per diem cost" for which payment is made. Thus, all costs of room, board, nursing services, laboratory tests, physiotherapy, and other hospital services are averaged into the daily rate. In arriving at these rates, the Blue Cross plan must obtain a careful accounting of the hospital's expenses; individually calculated rates are usually computed for each hospital. It is easy to see how difficulties may develop between plans and hospitals on the computation of rates, particularly on whether such items as depreciation, interest on loans, nursing education, or medical research should be included in the calculation of the cost of a day of patient-care.

With the steadily rising costs of hospital service over the last 20 years, these per diem rates have had to rise, and Blue Cross premiums with them. These increases in the costs of hospital care are due to a large extent to increases in wages, costs of food and drugs, and to a great enrichment in the content of hospital service, including care, facilities, and medication. However, there has been some criticism of excessive use. Hospital personnel (which account for about 70% of total costs) have risen from a ratio of 1.0 to over 2.2 employees per patient in the last 25 years. Hospital admission rates in general short-term hospitals have risen greatly during this period for a variety of reasons, one of the major ones being the reduction in economic barriers because of health insurance. Meanwhile, the average lengths of hospital stay per patient have been reduced, so that the net rise of utilization rates (days of hospital care per 1,000 persons per year) has been, in fact, surprisingly small. The rising Blue Cross premiums necessitated by these rising costs of hospital care, however, have caused widespread public criticism.

PUBLIC SUPERVISION. Public reaction to the rise of Blue Cross premiums has been expressed in a number of states by protests to state insurance commissioners. The Blue Cross plans come under the supervision of the department of insurance in most but not all states. Where they do, the officials must approve of premiums as well as supervise the maintenance of reserve funds and other elements of plan operation. In order to ascertain the facts, they have held open hearings and launched special investigations in several states, such as Michigan, Pennsylvania, and New York. These proceedings have caused the Blue Cross plans to examine closely their whole operation and have put pressure on local hospitals to operate with maximum economy.

BLUE SHIELD. To complement the protection against the costs of hospital bills, Blue Shield plans have been developed to meet the costs of physician's services in hospitalized illness. Their enrollment procedures are similar to Blue Cross, but their membership is not so high. They are typically under the jurisdiction of appointees of the State medical society of each State. Many of the Blue Shield plans use the Blue Cross plan in their area for administration.

Most Blue Shield policies pay in part or in full for in-hospital surgical services, and some cover care for medical (i.e., nonsurgical) and obstetric conditions as well. The patient has free choice of doctor, and the plan pays the physician according to an agreed-upon fee schedule. Most plans, however, specify a family income threshold (such as $6,000 a year) above which the payment received from the plan may be supplemented by a private charge by the physician to the patient. Thus, these plans combine "service" and "indemnity" features.

There is great variety among the Blue Cross and Blue Shield plans throughout the country, with considerable adjustment to meet local needs. Protection tends to be low among rural people, the aged, and the lowest income groups—facts which present the most serious problems for voluntary insurance as a national movement. Benefits have expanded steadily but are still insufficient for long-term care of chronic illness. There are serious problems of premiums to groups with different illness experience, and controversies surround the use of unifom "community rates" versus "experience-adjusted rates."

Insurance Companies

The rapid growth of Blue Cross and Blue Shield led many insurance companies in the 1940's to enter the field of group health insurance. Individual "health and accident" policies have been sold by insurance companies for decades, but these have usually provided only cash compensation to the insured person for his loss of earnings during periods of disability. In recent years, the benefits have been greatly widened to include indemnification for hospital, surgical, medical, and other health expenses.

ENROLLMENT. Insurance company policies cover some 75 million people in much the same manner as Blue Cross plans, but the former have certain advantages for some groups which probably account for their national coverage now exceeding that of Blue Cross. One advantage is the provision of "package deals" to large industries, which include not only various forms of health insurance but life insurance and disability compensation as well. Fringe benefits based on such wider protection are usually attractive to both management and labor. Second, insurance companies engage widely in "experience-rating" of their coverage groups so that organizations with relatively lower hospital utilization among their members (e.g., groups with lower proportions of women or aged persons) are favored with lower premiums. This is a powerful enrollment inducement. Third, being unified nation-wide firms, the insurance companies can offer uniform national contracts to large corporations, such as the General Electric Company, without the complexity of different contract stipulations in each state in which the corporation has a local plant. Finally, since the benefits are cash indemnification, rather than services, all the energies of the insurance company can go into enrollment rather than into maintenance of relationships with hospitals and physicians. Moreover, the rise in costs of hospital and medical services are not reflected in commensurate increases in premiums; the difference between the indemnification and the increased costs can be passed on to the patient, at least for a while.

MAJOR MEDICAL INSURANCE. One of the important criticisms of insurance for hospitalization or in-hospital physician's services has been its failure to cover the costs of many elements of medical care, including hospital care beyond a set time. In a serious illness, the cumulative expenses of drugs, nursing care, physician's care in the home and office, physiotherapy, and other charges can be extremely high. To help cope with these costs, insurance companies began to provide, in the early 1950's, a new form of insurance to indemnify persons for "major medical expenses" of any type. Typically, however, these policies have a deductible provision, requiring the insured person to pay the first $100 or $200 of expenses in any illness; when the coverage takes effect, the insurance company then indemnifies for 75 or 80 per cent of medical and related expenses, with the insured person paying the rest. This form of insurance, with variations, has grown rapidly to an enrollment of 22 million persons in 1959.

HEALTH ASPECTS. The rapid extension of various forms of insurance company coverage for health services has helped millions of people obtain needed care and has also strengthened the financial support of essential personnel and facilities in the community. Despite the fact that the indemnification may be insufficient to meet full costs, it doubtless softens the economic impact of illness. On the negative side, however, indemnity insurance is a purely financial mechanism and does nothing to affect or control the quality of care received by people. There is no mechanism for directing people to the type of professional service they need, no surveillance over the technical quality of that service, no orientation toward prevention. Moreover, there is much evidence that the very availability of insurance has raised the over-all costs of medical care to the community, because the aggregate charges of doctors (i.e., the indemnity amount plus the supplemental fee commonly charged) tend to exceed what they would be to uninsured persons.

Consumer-Sponsored Health Plans

Another approach to medical care insurance has been taken by consumers in several parts of the country. In contrast to the plans sponsored by providers of service or insurance companies, these plans have usually set out to reorganize the patterns of medical care, as well as to prepay its costs. While the total enrollment of these plans is not high (about 5 million persons in 1960), their impact on thinking in this field has been great.

CONSUMER CO-OPERATIVES. One of the earliest of these plans was organized by a Farmer's Union cooperative society at Elk City, Oklahoma. The members paid not only for the costs of their medical care but also for the construction of a hospital. Instead of simply channeling the funds to individual physicians, paid on a fee-for-service basis, the cooperative engaged a team of physicians on salary. Thus medical care was given through a group practice clinic (see below), rather than in solo practice offices. Care was comprehensive—that is, it included physician's services in the clinic and home, as well as the hospital—and expanded gradually to include dental services, drugs, and other elements of health care. Costs to the patient, on this basis, tended to be lower and services more complete than under the usual private arrangements.

This pattern of health insurance, combined with group medical practice and comprehensive benefits, has been adopted in a number of communities where a well-knit membership group has taken the initiative. The Group Health Association in Washington, D.C., with a membership of about 46,000 as of January, 1961, is a well-known plan of this type. The Group Health Cooperative of Puget Sound in Seattle, Washington, with a membership of approximately 60,000, is another example.

COMMUNITY NONPROFIT PLANS. During World War II, the Kaiser Industries on the West Coast launched a health plan to cover its shipyard workers which has since expanded to include other employed groups in the community. The Kaiser Foundation Health Plan (formerly called the Permanente Health Plan) now operates 14 of its own hospitals and some 40 allied clinics, with teams of full-time doctors and others giving comprehensive prepaid medical care. Although it is administered by the Kaiser Foundation, it serves the community. Its membership in California alone is 600,000; its total membership 800,000 as of January, 1961.

The Health Insurance Plan of Greater New York (HIP) is another example of a community service plan under which its approximately 600,000 members receive a variety of medical services from about 35 medical groups. Treatment may be in the home, in the doctor's office, in the medical group center, or in the hospital. In return for a fixed premium with no additional charges, there is broad coverage of medical services. Originally established to serve the needs of New York City's municipal workers, it has been extended to include other groups. Membership through employment as a group is required initially, but coverage can be converted from group to individual contract if employment status changes. There are no waiting periods and no limitation on the number of services or duration of medical care. Community resources and facilities are used, both public and voluntary, on referral by HIP physicians and staff. Hospitalization insurance is required for membership and is provided by separate carriers.

LABOR-MANAGEMENT PLANS. Since the mid-nineteenth century, workers in certain isolated industries—e.g., railroad, lumbering, mining— have obtained medical care through local prepayment plans operated by the company. Typically there has been a periodic wage deduction which goes into fund used to employ one or more physicians to serve the employees. Often there is a management contribution as well. In the western railroads, these plans have been expanded to include the operation of large hospitals and clinics with staffs of full-time salaried physicians.

Labor unions also have become concerned with health insurance plans which provide direct medical service, since a beginning by the International Ladies Garment Workers Union in New York City in 1913. Some 60 "labor health centers" throughout the country are sponsored by unions or labor-management groups where ambulatory medical services are provided by salaried medical staffs to workers and sometimes to their families. The United Mine Workers of America has a welfare and retirement fund which has built a network of 10 general hospitals in the Appalachian region and which finances medical services both in these facilities and elsewhere. The Amalgamated Clothing Workers of America has its "Sidney Hillman Health Centers" in several large eastern cities, and the United Automobile Workers is launching a new program in Detroit.

A major share of ordinary Blue Cross, Blue Shield, or insurance company plans is of course financed through collective bargaining agreements made between unions and management. But organized labor has become increasingly interested in medical care programs which go beyond simple payment of bills to establishment of systematic clinics for comprehensive service. In some instances, as in the case of the street railway workers in Washington, D.C., and the longshoremen in Seattle, unions enter into contracts with existing consumer-operated prepayment plans to provide complete medical care to their members and dependents. The AFL Medical Plan of Philadelphia—a multi-union labor clinic—provides ambulatory services to its 75,000 members in over 30 affiliated unions. It is particularly significant in the community because it reaches a low-income group. Since it began operation there has been a marked decrease in the public welfare case load requiring hospital and clinic care.

Special Compulsory Health Insurance

Although often overlooked, a form of compulsory health insurance operates in every state that provides coverage for medical care required for industrial injuries and sometimes occupational diseases. In addition, seveal forms of cash-disability insurance on a mandatory basis have a close relationship to health services.

WORKMEN'S COMPENSATION. The laws of the 50 states, providing insurance protection for injured workers, have evolved one by one since 1910, and they are enormously varied and complex. Definitions of work-connected injuries and diseases differ, the conditions and amounts of cash compensation differ, and medical benefits vary greatly. The most common practice, however, is to require employers with, for example, three or more workers, to have insuance which will pay compensation for wage loss and medical expenses incurred by a worker who has been injured while on the job. This insurance is usually obtained from a commercial insurance carrier, although it may be provided by a state-government fund (especially where the employee group is a poor risk) or, in large corporations, on a self-insured basis. The injured worker ordinarily gets medical care from a local physician or hospital, and the expenses are paid by the insurance company; there may be a statutory limit on the amount or duration of such medical services.

To induce employers to introduce safety measures or take steps to reduce occupational diseases, such as improved ventilation to reduce dust hazards, compensation insurance premiums are usually experience-rated—that is, they are raised or lowered on the basis of actual accident experience. In most States, however, little has been done to assure prompt and effective medical care and careful rehabilitation after an injury has occurred. Arrangements are left to each employer or insurance company. A few of the latter—like the Liberty Mutual Insurance Company—have encouraged wide use of rehabilitation resources, but most have avoided "interference" with the provision of medical care. The state commissions or labor departments that administer this program seldom look beyond questions of coverage and fair cash settlement of claims by workers.

DISABILITY INSURANCE. In four states—Rhode Island, California, New Jersey, and New York—the compulsory unemployment insurance laws have been extended to include cash compensation for loss of wages due to disability. A somewhat similar system of disability insurance covers the nation's railroad workers under the federal Railroad Retirement Administration. This disability may result from sickness or injury of any cause, not simply from work-connected ailments. There is usually a waiting period of one week, and the maximum duration of benefits tends to be six months. Within these limits the disabled worker receives a cash benefit equal to a certain share of his usual wages from the state unemployment insurance fund.

The relevance of these programs to medical care is that they provide money which may help the disabled worker purchase needed services precisely when he needs them most and when his source of income would otherwise be cut off. In general, no governmental action is taken to encourage prompt and effective medical care which would hasten the return of the worker to his job and safeguard the insurance funds. The California program, however, supplements the cash compensation with payment for a share of the costs of hospitalization of covered workers.

Under the nation-wide social security system there is another form of disability insurance which is limited, however, to "permanent and total disability" cases. If a person covered by social security—that is, under old-age, survivors, and disability insurance programs—becomes totally disabled at any age for gainful employment, because of a condition estimated to be permanent, he then becomes entitled to cash benefits as though he were 65 years of age. This requires examination and certification by a physician. No funds are provided directly for medical care, but this social insurance coverage obviously can assist in the purchase of needed care by these seriously disabled persons. Many disabled persons who might otherwise constitute a burden to local welfare departments can be aided by these benefits.

MEDICAL CARE INSURANCE FOR THE AGED. In the late 1950's several bills were introduced in the United States Congress to amend the Social Security Act to provide insurance for hospital and medical care for aged persons receiving or entitled to receive old-age insurance. The best known of these proposals, the Forand Bill, emphasized coverage for hospital, surgical, and nursing home services, which are used heavily by aged persons. Great controversy was aroused by these proposals. As a result of these debates, the program for medical aid to the "low income" aged (discussed above) was enacted, but the problem of proper financing of the volume of health care needed by older persons, who tend to be meagerly protected by voluntary health insurance, has not been solved. As of March, 1961, the issue was still under active debate.

PATTERNS OF PROVIDING MEDICAL CARE

Thus far, there has been in this writing an attempt to indicate—to the city, town, or county administrator—the various programs that will be encountered at the local level for financing the diagnosis and treatment of illness as well as prevention and rehabilitation through insurance and public funds. These more or less collective systems of payment have important implications for the organizational patterns by which medical care is given to patients. Apart from the payment mechanisms, however, an understanding of medical care administration in the community requires at least a brief look at these patterns of service themselves.

Medical Practice

Physicians are licensed to practice medicine in the United States under the medical practice acts of the States. Ordinarily this requires a specified period of university training, an internship, and passing an examination. A psysician licensed in one State may be granted the privilege of practicing in another, if the two States have reciprocity (agreements cover about half the states). The National Board of Medical Examiners, a voluntary body, provides examinations which, if passed, are recognized as an adequate qualification by about 40 States. Once licensed, the physician has a permit to practice medicine in that State without re-examination and without limitation as to scope of service.

GENERAL PRACTITIONERS AND SPECIALISTS. The enormous complexity of medical science has given rise to great specialization through which the physician limits his work to a subdivision of the human body, a special age-group of patients, or to the application of special techniques such as surgery or radiology. These specialties are matters of voluntary determination, however, and are not embodied in the licensure law. American specialty boards prescribe requirements and certify physicians in some 20 subdivisions of medicine. Although the boards are nongovernmental, their certifications are recognized and often required by many public agencies (e.g., in workmen's compensation or crippled children's programs) for participation of doctors. Moreover, most hospitals base their medical staff organization on these specialty certifications; a physician's freedom to do certain types of surgery or other work in the hospital is often dependent on such ratings. In many instances, however, specialists such as internists do general adult practice, and pediatricians become family doctors as the children grow older.

Over the years the proportion of American physicians devoting full time to a specialty has steadily increased so that over one-half are specialists. They tend to be more heavily concentrated in the larger cities, but some specialists (especially surgeons) are found almost everywhere. The balance, of course, is composed of general practitioners, and much controversy surrounds their proper role in the increasingly complex field of medical care. It is often argued that no matter how specialized medicine becomes, every person still should have access to a "family doctor" who supervises his total health, cares for his minor ailments, and refers him to an appropriate specialist when necessary. Much waste and even error, moreover, can come from the frequent practice of patients going directly to a specialist without channeling through a general physician.

PRIVATE PRACTICE. Whether general practitioners or specialists, most American physicians are in private practice in independent offices. Patients have free choice of doctor and may or may not make wise choices in relation to the requirements of their illness. Within his office the physician is sovereign and is not subject to the various forms of group discipline found in the medical staff of hospitals. His income from patients must of course cover the overhead of running a practice, which tends to absorb about 30 to 40% of his earnings. There is great disparity among physicians' incomes, the highest earnings going to specialists and to those who have been in practice at least 15 or 20 years. The median net earnings of all male doctors in private practice in 1959 were about $22,000 a year (this is net income, after deduction of expenses).

This pattern of individual private practice yields great independence in the daily work of the physician, and this is an aspect of his life he tends to cherish highly. The extension of health insurance and many of the public medical care programs have not invaded this independence but have even fortified it by providing economic under-pinning to private solo practice, fee-for-service payment, and free choice of doctor. Many physicians believe that this independence is essential to maintenance of proper professional standards and a satis-factory doctor-patient relationship, even while recognizing that the finest quality of medical care is practiced in highly organized frame-works—e.g., in the great university medical teaching centers.

At the same time, a rising proportion of physicians in the United States is working in an organized setting and is paid by salary. This includes the young physicians in hospital training (interns and resi-dents); doctors in the armed services and the Veterans Administra-tion medical system; and physicians in Public Health work, medical and hospital administration, research, university health services, in-dustrial medical programs, pharmaceutic and insurance companies, and many others. Altogether, these salaried physicians constituted about 35% of the total in 1960.

MEDICAL SOCIETIES. The general professional attitudes of most pri-vate physicians on medical care programs tend to be expressed through their professional societies. These societies are found in almost every county and build up toward a system of State medical societies, and nationally, the American Medical Association. The medi-cal societies serve many purposes and have played an important role in elevating technical standards of medical education and per-formance.

There tends to be a high level of cohesiveness and protection of common interests among the doctors in a community, and this is expressed mainly through the medical society. Often therefore ad-ministrators of new programs of medical care in a locality seek approval by the medical society before proceeding. While formal ap-proval usually is not a prerequisite, it is generally good administrative practice to maintain liaison with the society and to seek advice and suggestions on personnel, procedures, and policies, particularly in a newly established medical care program.

Other Health Personnel

While the physician is the key member of the medical care team, many others are involved in modern health service.

DENTISTS. Patterns of providing and paying for dental care in the United States are essentially similar to those for general diagnosis and treatment, but with a much smaller role played by hospitals and much less impact from insurance financing. The private dentist may have two or three dental chairs in his office, he may be aided by a dental hygienist or nurse, and he may have a great deal of technical equipment which simplifies his work. But the predominant pattern is that of the independent solo practitioner, paid on a fee basis. There is an increasingly serious shortage of dentists in the United States, and persons knowledgeable in the field believe much can be done to increase the scope of dental service through the training of more ancillary personnel.

NURSES.   Unlike physicians and dentists, nurses tend to work mainly on salary in organized settings such as hospitals, health departments, or other medical agencies. Those doing private duty nursing at hospital bedsides or in patients' homes are a small minority. Although the number and ratio of nurses to the population have steadily grown, the increase has not kept pace with the increase in the number of hospital beds and the higher staffing standards in hospitals. Hence almost every local hospital and health agency faces a shortage of nurses. To cope with this, a number of auxiliary nursing personnel are being trained—practical nurses, nurses' aides, nursing assistants, ward clerks, and so on. The field of nursing education is undergoing change both at the level of the community general hospital, in which most schools of nursing are located, and at the universities, which are more and more training nurses with bachelor's degrees for positions of leadership.

AUXILIARY PERSONNEL.   Aiding the physician and dentist is a series of other technical personnel. The pharmacist may operate an independent drugstore, but his principal medical function is to fill prescriptions ordered by the physician. He sells, in addition, nonprescribed drugs, dressings, appliances, and an endless variety of commodities for personal hygiene and health. A variety of trained personnel—medical technologists, X-ray technicians, laboratory technicians, and many others—assist pathologists and radiologists in hospital and office. Physical therapists and occupational therapists carry out physicians' orders for rehabilitation of disabled patients. Some therapists operate private practices, but most are engaged in hospitals or rehabilitation centers. Medical social workers are attached to many hospitals to help bridge the gap between the doctor's orders and the patient's life situation in his community.

OTHER INDEPENDENT PRACTITIONERS.   Still other medical care personnel work not as auxiliaries to the doctor but as independent agents to whom patients may come directly for service. There are optometrists who refract the eyes and fit corrective eyeglasses. There are podiatrists who treat ailments of the feet. Some of these personnel work in organized clinics, under medical supervision, but most are in independent private practice.

Finally there are other types of practitioners licensed to practice in many states and to treat any patient coming to them with any ailment. Osteopaths are the most important of these. Although the historic origin of osteopathy is based on a narrow conception of disease as the result of maladjustments of the spinal column, it has steadily widened its outlook, and osteopaths are now trained in a manner similar to doctors of medicine. Chiropractors, on the other hand, are firmly wedded to a concept of disease causation which is similar to that of 19th century osteopathy, and they attempt to treat all ailments with manipulation of the spinal column. Where State licensure laws permit, both these types of practitioner are free to serve any patient; in some States, naturopaths are also free to treat all ailments by "drugless" means such as diet, water, and sunlight.

New Patterns of Service

With the variety of medical and associated personnel providing health services, it is not surprising that serious problems of coordination are found in every community. To provide this coordination, certain patterns of organized health service have evolved.

GROUP MEDICAL PRACTICE.   To bring together a variety of specialties in medicine, or to concentrate on one specialty, groups of physicians pool their skills and resources in group practice clinics. These teams usually contain three or more full-time physicians of different specialties, although about one-third of the existing group clinics concentrate on one field. With these pooled resources, the medical group is able to afford equipment and technicians that would be beyond the means of most solo practitioners. There can be exchange of ideas on individual cases so that better diagnosis and treatment can result. The number of group practice clinics has grown steadily, since the pioneering of the Mayo brothers in 1880, to some 1,800 units. They are most numerous in the urban centers of the midwest rural states.

Most group practice clinics are essentially in private practice, receiving individual patient fees for their services; some, however, are linked to prepayment plans. A small proportion operates their own hospitals, but the majority use community hospitals. Group practice clinics have sometimes been opposed by solo practitioners as "unfair" competition, but there can be no doubt that the pattern helps to coordinate diverse medical specialties.

HOSPITAL REGIONALIZATION.   Among hospitals, coordination is sometimes achieved through organization of regional councils. Thus several institutions in a geographic region work together through sharing of personnel (e.g., a pathologist), joint purchasing of supplies, common programs of employee recruitment and public relations, joint educational programs, systems of referral of patients or arrangements for consultations, and other cooperative measures. One program of this type is operated by the Bingham Associates Fund in Maine, and another serves the area around Rochester, New York. There are instances where a regional network of hospitals is actually under unified management, such as those hospitals operated by the Kaiser Foundation Health Plan, the United Mine Workers Welfare and Retirement Fund, and a special governmental project in Puerto Rico. Hospital regionalization has particular significance when it can elevate the quality of medical care received by isolated rural people.

OTHER NEW PATTERNS. Because they are discussed more fully in other chapters of this book, certain other coordinating schemes of medical care will only be mentioned. To bring together the varied skills required for helping the disabled person achieve his maximum potential, comprehensive rehabilitation centers have been developed in about 100 places. To provide high quality care to chronically ill patients in their own homes, and to free hospital beds for the use of more urgent cases, organized home-care programs have been launched by a few general hospitals in the larger cities. For the early detection of cancer and other insidious diseases, cancer detection centers have been organized, and a whole constellation of specialized ambulatory care clinics may be offered by the larger general hospitals. Mental hygiene clinics have been established under many public and voluntary auspices. The trend in the United States is clearly toward patterns of medical care which mobilize a variety of skills under one administrative roof.

FUTURE ISSUES IN MEDICAL CARE
Medical Care Problems

With the framework of medical care in the community as described above, what are the issues that the city or county chief administrator and the health officer will face in the decade of the 1960's? The key question in medical care organization is how a community, State, or nation can finance and provide scientific medical services in a way that leads to the maximum quality and quantity of service to all persons of the locality in proportion to their health needs. Where the government participates in medical care programs, its role is often one of financing services, with private practitioners providing direct service.

RECEIPT OF SERVICES. Despite the great progress made in public medical care and health insurance programs, virtually every locality will find serious inequities in the receipt of needed medical services by different sectors of the population. Physicians, hospitals, and clinics, provide much free medical care for the poor. However, those who are of low income but not indigent are usually not beneficiaries of such free services; what services they receive are generally fragmentary. Many studies have shown that the volume of disabling illness is higher in the lower income groups, while the medical services they receive are fewer. Medical and dental services still tend to correspond to income level rather than need; hospitalization appears to correspond more closely to need.

American communities are witness to corresponding disparities according to age level, with lesser financial access to medical and hospital care among older persons, despite their much greater need. Rural groups and minority racial groups also receive less medical care. There are great differences in cities and counties in the supplies of health personnel and facilities and, correspondingly, the volume of services the residents receive. These disparities remain, despite the great improvements that have been brought about by widening public support for health services—in voluntary charitable drives and in government—and the extension of health insurance. They serve to remind the city or county administrator of the need for much further community action to improve the distribution of medical care.

RISING COSTS. Another critical issue in medical care administration at the local level, as in so many other aspects of social welfare, is the steady rise in costs. Between 1936 and 1956, the percentage increase in medical care costs, on the 1947–49 base, was less than the "all-items" component in the Consumer Price Index. Since 1956, medical care costs, along with other items such as rent, have accelerated. It is the hospitalization sector of medical care prices, however, that has provoked great public reaction and has led to investigations into hospital and Blue Cross plan operations in some states. In countless localities there is much talk of "over-utilization" of hospitals associated with insurance coverage.

The rise in medical care costs, however, has not been great in relation to over-all national income. Between 1929 and 1959, national expenditures for health services as a whole rose from 3.6 to 5.4% of the gross national product (counting both private and public outlays). In the light of the vast extension of medical knowledge in this period, the aging of the population with the great increase in chronic illness requiring costly services (because of long duration), the heightened public appreciation and demand for medical care, and the expanded supply of technical personnel and facilities, this increase in outlay does not seem large. As for the hospital sector, the rise in costs can be explained to a large extent because many services formerly given in homes or offices (or not at all) are now given within the hospital, and the personnel-to-patient ratio in hospitals has more than doubled in the last 25 years. There is, doubtless, some wastage in hospital construction and operation, and especially in the pricing of drugs, but the predominant costs of medical care may be justified today by the rise in both quality and quantity of services being provided.

The task for the local administrator is not so much to hunt for ways of reducing costs—which could mean reduction in the delivery of services—as to find more equitable ways of distributing costs in the community (and in the nation); more efficient use of services, equipment, and personnel; and effective alternatives to hospital care. In all parts of the United States, this problem is being faced through organized community action in the private and public sectors.

PERSONNEL AND FACILITIES. Many serious problems surround the supply and distribution of medical personnel and facilities in the United States, some of which have been mentioned. Expansion of hospital construction has been aided by a federal subsidy program since 1947, and various proposals have been under debate for some years to subsidize the education of physicians and dentists. Some of this is being done indirectly through research grants to the universities. But more support is obviously needed from some source (regardless of auspices) if needs are to be met. In medicine and dentistry, the nation has actually been losing ground quantitatively, and a great expansion in training programs is needed to maintain the supply of personnel at the same pace as the growth in population.

At the State and community levels, there are needs for more systematic planning of hospital construction, including not only general hospitals but various facilities such as nursing homes for geriatric and long-term patients. No State or region now has any mandatory planning power except for that fraction (about one-fourth) of hospital construction aided by the federal subsidy program. Yet there is abundant evidence that the utilization rate, and hence the ultimate costs of hospitals, is determined by the supply and distribution of beds. Given insurance or public support of care, the beds that are built tend to be used, up to a limit that has not yet been reached in the United States. This is due to the constant pressure of unmet health needs in many communities and the absence of alternative forms of providing care.

HUMAN RELATIONS. A whole complex of problems is involved in the interpersonal relations of health personnel and patients in the large world of modern medical care. As specialization of functions has developed, both in institutions and outside, increasing concern has been voiced about loss of sensitivity to the total human needs of the patient. Conditions have long been particularly bad in overcrowded and meagerly financed mental hospitals.

The recognition of human needs is a first step to meeting them, and much progress has been made through education of personnel in human relations, increase in the use of social workers (who are specialists in this field), and institutional reorganization toward a more patient-centered focus. But much more remains to be done at the community level to adjust the administration of medical care programs to the needs of patients. There are also serious problems to be solved in the interpersonal relations of members of the professional health team itself (e.g., in the hierarchic structure of aides, nurses, doctors, and administrators in a hospital), not only for improvement of professional morale but also for the ultimate quality of patient care.

Medical Care Trends

The problems of medical care administration point up the significance of the trends that characterize the field.

ROLE OF COMMUNITY ACTION. There is a trend in the United States toward increasing community responsibility for the provision of medical care. In some areas, this action is manifested in the voluntary efforts of the leaders of the community, e.g., businessmen, professional people, medical societies, labor, and management groups. Elsewhere, the trend reflects increased government responsibility for this aspect of public interest. Measured only by dollars spent, the public share of health services has risen from 14% in 1928–29 to 25% in 1957–58, whereas the share from philanthropy has stayed more or less constant and the private share has declined.

The role of government is expressed not only in funds but in standards. At all levels, the scope of public medical care has widened to help assure minimal quality protection, supplementing the standards affected by private, voluntary, and professional organizations. This is seen in heightened standards for licensure of personnel and approval of hospitals and nursing homes. It is also seen in more exacting standards for participation of personnel in public medical care programs— criteria which tend to affect nonPublic Health services as well.

HEALTH INSURANCE. The impact of insurance financing on medical care is enlarging steadily. From less than 1% of the national expenditures for medical care in 1930, insurance meets over 18% of the costs today. Within the hospitalization sector, the impact is much greater, meeting about 35% of total costs in general hospitals. This change in the source of financing medical care has had important implications for medical practice and hospital administration. The shift, and the increase in tax-supported medical care, means that the costs are placed on the shoulders of a large population group, rather than just on that minority which in any one year is afflicted with serious illness. As a result, representatives of the total public, such as State insurance commissioners, or spokesmen for large subgroups, such as labor or management bodies, or consumer groups, can express a legitimate interest in how the public's money is being spent for medical services. The whole effect is to heighten public participation in and surveillance over the detailed provision of medical care in a community.

ORGANIZATION OF SERVICES.   Closely related to trends in public and insurance financing of medical care are the trends toward heightened organization of the technical provision of the services. Several of these new patterns of care have been mentioned. But in addition to the specifically new forms of program, there is a steadily increasing organizational structure to the old forms as well. The departmental structure and administrative process in general hospitals are certainly becoming daily more complex. The organized programs of medical care—for certain population groups, disease entities, or technical services—are becoming increasingly defined by systematic rules which replace subjective with objective standards of performance. Even the private practice of medicine, with office aides, record systems, and standardized clinical procedures, is a more orderly process than in the day of the horse and buggy and the little black bag.

Organization of both the economic and the technical side of medicine may create some human problems in our communities, but the evidence certainly is on the side of the human benefits of the organizing process—benefits in extended life, reduced suffering, and heightened productivity. Medical science, for its effective application, requires social organization, and the task is not to reduce the organization but rather to execute it in ways that respond also to the human needs of individuals.

Community leaders can help to achieve these forms of organization by seeing the whole medical care picture and taking the steps necessary to coordinate its many parts, particularly through Public Health education. Municipal government has a particular role to play in bringing together the numerous special groups involved in the provision and financing of medical care, so that efforts can be pooled toward meeting the needs of all.

1. American Medical Association. *Report of the Commission on Medical Care Plans*. (Chicago: The Association, 1958.) Vol. 1, 96pp.; Vol. 2, 179pp.

2. Anderson, Odin W., and Jacob J. Feldman. *Family Medical Costs and Voluntary Health Insurance: a Nationwide Survey*. (New York: McGraw-Hill Book Company, 1956.) 251pp. $6.50.

3. Bauer, Louis H. *Private Enterprise or Government in Medicine*. (Springfield, Illinois: Charles C Thomas, 1948.) 201pp. (out of print.)

4. Burns, Eveline M. *Social Security and Public Policy*. (New York: McGraw-Hill Book Company, 1956.) 291pp. $6.50.

5. Commission on Financing of Hospital Care in the United States. *Financing Hospital Care in the United States*. (New York: Blakiston Company, 1954, V. 1; New York: McGraw-Hill Book Company, 1955, V. 2 and 3.) V. 1, $4; V. 2, $4.50; V. 3, $2.50.

6. Committee on Medical Care Teaching. *Readings in Medical Care*. (Chapel Hill: University of North Carolina Press, 1958.) 708pp. $6.50.

7. Darsky, Benjamin J., Nathan Sinai, and Solomon J. Axelrod. *Comprehensive Medical Services Under Voluntary Health Insurance*. (Cambridge, Massachusetts: Harvard University Press, 1958.) 392pp. $7.50.

8. Davis, Michael M. *Medical Care for Tomorrow*. (New York: Harper and Brothers, 1955.) 497pp. $6.50.

9. Emerson, Haven, editor. *Administrative Medicine*.

10. Garbarino, Joseph W. *Health Plans and Collective Bargaining*. (Berkeley: University of California Press, 1960.) 301pp. $5.

11. Goldmann, Franz. *Public Medical Care: Principles and Problems*. (New York: Columbia University Press, 1945.) 226 pp. $3.25.

12. Greenfield, Margaret. *Medical Care for Welfare Recipients, Basic Problems*. (Berkeley: University of California Bureau of Public Administration, 1957.) 83pp. $1.75.

13. ———. *Medical Care for Welfare Recipients, State Programs*. (Berkeley: University of California Bureau of Public Administration, 1957.) 113pp. $2.

14. Health Insurance Institute. *Source Book of Health Insurance Data*. (New York: The Institute, 1960.) 80pp. Annual.

15. Jaco, E. Gartly. *Patients, Physicians and Illness*. (Glencoe, Illinois: Free Press, 1958.) 600pp. $7.50.

16. Jordan, E. P., editor. *The Physician and Group Practice*. (Chicago: Yearbook Publishers, 1958.) 238pp.

17. Kramer, Lucy M. "Drugs and Medicines." *Public Health Reports*, October, 1958, pp. 929–39.

18. Milbank Memorial Fund. Articles on medical care plans beginning with January, 1958 issue of the *Milbank Fund Quarterly*. A complete listing of publications on medical care plans may be obtained from Milbank Memorial Fund, 40 Wall Street, New York 5.

19. Moore, Norman S., and John Summerskill. *Health Services in American Colleges and Universities, 1953*. (Ithaca, New York: Cornell University, 1954.)

20. Mott, Frederick D., and Milton I. Roemer. *Rural Health and Medical Care*. (New York: McGraw-Hill Book Company, 1948.) 608pp. (out of print.)

21. Roemer, Milton I., and Ethel A. Wilson. *Organized Health Services in a County of the United States*. (Washington: Government Printing Office, 1952.) 91pp.

22. Roemer, Milton I., and Max Shain. *Hospital Utilization Under Insurance*. (Chicago: American Hospital Association, 1959.) 39pp. $1.75.

23. Rosenfeld, Leonard S., and Henry B. Makover. *The Rochester Regional Hospital Council*. (Cambridge, Massachusetts: Harvard University Press, 1956.) 204pp. $3.50.

24. Serbein, Oscar N. *Paying for Medical Care in the United States*. (New York: Columbia University Press, 1953.) 543pp. $10.

25. Sigerist, Henry E. *Medicine and Human Welfare*. (New Haven, Connecticut: Yale University Press, 1941.) 148pp. (out of print.)

26. Simmons, Leo W., and Harold G. Wolff. *Social Science in Medicine*. (New York: Russell Sage Foundation, 1954.) 254pp. $3.50.

27. Somers, Herman M., and Anne R. Somers. *Doctors, Patients, and*

Health Insurance. (Washington: The Brookings Institution, 1961.) 576pp. $7.50.

28. ———. *Workmen's Compensation: Prevention, Insurance, and Rehabilitation of Occupational Disability.* (New York: John Wiley and Sons, 1954.) 341pp. $7.25.

29. Stern, Bernard J. *Medical Services by Government—Local, State and Federal.* (New York: Commonwealth Fund, 1946.) 208pp.

30. Taylor, Keith O., and Donna M. Donald. *A comparative Study of Hospital Licensure Regulations.* (Berkeley: University of California School of Public Health, 1957.)

31. Terris, Milton, and Nathan A. Kramer. *General Medical Care Programs in Local Health Departments.* (Report to Subcommittee on Medical Care, American Public Health Association.) (New York: The Association, 1951.) 129pp. (out of print.)

32. U.S. President's Commission on the Health Needs of the Nation. *Building America's Health.* (Washington: Government Printing Office (5 volumes), 1952–1953.)

33. U.S. Public Health Service. Division of Public Health Methods. *Health Services for American Indians.* (Washington: Government Printing Office, 1957.) 344pp.

34. ———. Surgeon General's Consultant Group on Medical Education. *Physicians for a Growing America.* (Washington: Government Printing Office, 1959.) 95pp. 60 cents.

35. Yahraes, Herbert. *Making Medical Care Better—and Easier to Pay for Too.* (New York: Public Affairs Committee, Inc., 1959.) 28pp. 25 cents.

The Medical Care Program of the United Mine Workers of America Welfare and Retirement Fund*

WARREN F. DRAPER, M.D.

THE HOSPITAL and medical care program of the U.M.W.A. Welfare and Retirement Fund has been in operation since 1948. Its sole purpose is to make good medical and hospital care possible for about a million Fund beneficiaries, consisting mostly of bituminous coal miners, their wives, and dependent children under 18 years of age. They are located in mining communities in 26 different States and the Territory of Alaska.

The desperate plight of many of these people, resulting from inadequate or total lack of medical care prior to the Fund program, is revealed in various surveys culminating in a governmental publication, "A Medical Survey of the Bituminous-Coal Industry," issued in 1947. No State and county medical societies, no governmental nor

* Reprinted, by permission, from a pamphlet published by the United Mine Workers of America Welfare and Retirement Fund, Washington, D.C., and the July 1, 1958, issue of the *United Mine Workers Journal*, 69th Year, Issue #13, pp. 15–17. This paper was presented at the New England Hospital Assembly held in Boston, Massachusetts, March 25, 1958. The author is Executive Medical Officer for the Fund.

voluntary health or welfare agencies, nor any other group or organization had ever done anything which improved the conditions in mining communities in which the government report stated "the provisions for health are so very poor that their tolerance is a disgrace to a nation to which the world looks for pattern and guidance."

This is the reason that the hospital and medical care program of the Fund came into existence and this is the situation which it had to face. The location of the long-neglected patients in their homes, their removal on stretchers to medical institutions which could cope with the frightful condition in which they were found, and the months and sometimes years of skilled and costly treatment to restore them from a living death, are among the most dramatic stories of modern medical achievement.

Because of the hazardous character of coal mining operations, carried on for the most part in remote or mountainous areas extremely different from other industrial communities, our program is designed to meet the peculiar conditions that exist.

A primary objective is that the medical care shall be of the highest quality obtainable. This is ever uppermost in mind because of the gruesome results of the inadequate and sometimes total lack of medical care which have been seen at the medical centers to which the Fund has later sent these patients. Physicians in the coal mine areas are now encouraged to refer their cases to qualified specialists for consultation and treatment at Fund expense whenever this is in the best interest of the patient. Specialists also are brought to out-of-the-way localities to examine groups of beneficiary patients in consultation with their family physicians. Many thousands of patients and their physicians have been greatly benefited by the specialist services which the Fund has made available.

We have sent a number of our beneficiaries, 64 to be exact, to the Massachusetts General Hospital in Boston. Among other institutions to which we send our patients are the New York University Institute of Physical Medicine and Rehabilitation, the Kessler Institute of Rehabilitation, the Wisconsin Neurological Foundation, the George Washington University and Johns Hopkins Hospitals, the Medical College of Virginia and the University of Virginia Hospitals, the Vanderbilt University, Duke University and University of Pennsylvania Medical Centers, the Mayo, Ochsner and Cleveland Clinics, and the National Institutes of Health.

We keep fully informed of the quality of care that can be rendered at the hospitals in the mining areas. We have frequently assisted them in developing and maintaining higher standards. Great improvements have been made in these hospitals and a number have been accredited or are ready for inspection for accreditation, due wholly or in part to the incentive provided by the Fund. The hospitals we use are selected with due consideration to accessibility, the quality of service they provide, reasonableness of charges for the type of service rendered, and other advantages they may have to offer. The arrangements are made upon an individual basis and the government Reimbursable Cost Formula is the method of payment preferred.

There is no restriction upon the distance that a patient with an exceptionally difficult case may be transported at Fund expense, to insure the specialized medical care and services he needs. When the accumulated backlog of long neglected cases came to light during the first years of the program, hundreds of severely injured and diseased miners were sent all the way across the country because enough facilities were not available nearer home. Pullman cars were chartered for the purpose, with doctors and nurses in attendance. We still continue to transport many patients, with nurse escorts, to distant medical centers, although in smaller numbers as local facilities become available.

We stress the importance of rehabilitation. The inclusion in the medical care program of physical rehabilitation services to disabled miners and their dependents, and referral for vocational rehabilitation, has enabled many to become self-sufficient and largely self-supporting. We have received national recognition for achievement in this field. In brief, the hospital and medical care benefits consist of hospitalization for the length of time necessary in the opinion of the attending physician, physicians' services and drugs in the hospital, and specialists' services on an in-patient and out-patient basis. Some of the more costly drugs requiring long-continued use outside the hospital are provided in addition. This averts to some extent the necessity of hospitalization. The medical benefits are extended *in toto* to all eligible beneficiaries without restriction as to age. Not included are routine home and office care, long-term psychiatric care, routine tonsil and adenoid operations, general dental care, and services which the beneficiary is entitled to receive from public or voluntary agencies, through insurance, or third parties who may be liable.

One of our basic principles is to utilize the services of established physicians and existing hospitals, to the extent that they are available, to render high quality care at a cost that is reasonable and just according to accepted standards. In some of the coal mining areas in Kentucky, West Virginia, and Virginia, however, the number of physicians and acceptable hospitals were far from adequate to meet the needs.

The ratio of hospital beds was less than 2.5 per 1,000 beneficiaries. Early in the program many of the hospitals we had to use were so dilapidated and deficient in equipment and construction that they scarcely merited the name. It was often a question as to whether the hazards outweighed any possible benefits that might be derived by the patients who were forced to use them.

While many local physicians rendered the best service they could, under the conditions which existed, it was apparent that an adequate number of physicians trained in modern technics and specialist services could not be attracted to these areas until the necessary physical facilities were provided. This was the consensus of those who made inspections through arrangements initiated by the Fund, including high officials of the American Medical Association and State and local medical societies, as well as recognized authorities in medical education, Public Health, and hospital administration.

After broad consultation and thorough exploration as to other possibilities, the conclusion was reached that if better hospitals and medical care were to be provided in the foreseeable future, the Fund would have to take the lead.

Intensive surveys were conducted, and sites for the construction of a chain of 10 new hospitals were selected on the basis of greatest need of the beneficiary population. The chain, as constructed, consists of three central hospitals and seven smaller satellite hospitals, located in Kentucky, West Virginia, and Virginia. The central hospitals, which have 192 beds, 143 beds, and 199 beds respectively, are located in Harlan, Kentucky, and Beckley and Williamson, West Virginia. The satellite hospitals vary in size from 50 beds at Pikeville, Kentucky, to 92 at Whitesburg, Kentucky. These smaller hospitals, although well equipped with general care facilities, look to the appropriate larger central hospitals for assistance in handling the more difficult cases, either by specialists coming to them or by transfer of patients to the central facilities. A total of 1,045 beds is provided in the 10 hospitals.

The full-time specialists who joined the staffs of these hospitals came from some of the finest teaching centers in the United States. The hospitals were organized as open staff hospitals, and all the family physicians in the area who applied for privileges were accepted as members of the part-time staff. Non-professional personnel was selected from the large number of local people who had applied for jobs. These were given intensive in-service training and now, after additional months of on-the-job experience, have become experts in their respective fields.

Schools for the training of practical nurses have been established at our Beckley and Williamson hospitals. Already 159 men and women of mining communities are graduates of these schools, while 23 more are in training. A school for medical technologists is operating at our Beckley hospital and turning out limited numbers, who will soon begin to serve their own people in their own mountain regions. The latest move toward training personnel for service has been the opening, last September, of a school of professional nursing at Harlan, with a class of 25 men and women, now in their second academic college term at Morehead State College, Morehead, Kentucky.

All 10 hospitals are fully accredited. Graduate degree credit for field experience in the Memorial Hospitals is approved by the School for Nursing Service Administration of Teachers College, Columbia University, and residency programs in Medicine, Surgery, Pathology, and Radiology are now functioning in two of the central hospitals. Clinical conferences and symposia are conducted on a regular basis for our staffs and for physicians in the area, and groups of technicians and specialists in paramedical services are welcomed for regional and State meetings.

Philosophically, it is hard to estimate the impact on a medically impoverished population of 10 modern hospitals with highly trained and competent staffs, 150 full-time specialists and general practitioners, three schools wherein to learn careers, and medical care of a quality heretofore undreamed of in the mountains.

A program as liberal as ours, which provides the hospitalization necessary for adequate treatment, regardless of age of the patient or the length of time he needs to remain in the hospital, is expensive. It can be maintained only if the waste resulting from low quality care and unnecessary services is held to the minimum.

We assumed at the outset that every physician was competent in the field in which he claimed to be. We believed that if we permitted our beneficiaries to choose any physician whom they wished, organized medicine at the national, State and county levels would see to it that these physicians rendered services of high quality within their capabilities, and utilized specialist services at Fund expense when needed in the best interest of the patient. We believed that we could rely upon physicians generally to hospitalize only those patients whose illnesses could not be treated adequately in the home, physician's office or out-patient clinic.

We believed that an unparalleled opportunity was afforded for organized medicine and the Fund, working together, to develop a pattern of medical care that would serve the best interests of the patient, the physician, and the one who paid the bills. It seemed, almost, we might succeed. A commendatory editorial in the *Journal of the American Medical Association*, issue of December 11, 1954, concludes as follows:

> "Labor leaders, labor union medical administrators, and physicians everywhere can learn valuable lessons from the way in which organized medicine and the United Mine Workers have sat down together to iron out a host of difficult problems."

As data accumulated, however, it was evident that in many places surgical diagnoses and operative surgery for Fund beneficiaries were inferior in quality, and the amount of surgery was far in excess of that performed on others. This was confirmed by qualified surgical consultants who reviewed the records at our request or examined our patients at medical centers to which they were transferred. Furthermore, our rates of hospital admission and length of stay were far beyond the bounds of any experience in the United States.

These facts were discussed for several years with individual physicians, State and local medical societies, at meetings especially held for the purpose, at medical advisory committee meetings and elsewhere, but little change was brought about. It was clearly evident that county medical societies and hospital staffs are too often reluctant to supervise their colleagues and effect the drastic changes that should be made.

A few graphic examples will illustrate some of the problems encountered.

In one coal mining population group of 64,655, the hospitalization rate from January, 1955 to April 1, 1957 was 317 per 1,000 beneficiaries as compared with 190 per 1,000 in a similar adjoining group. Also, 2,411 persons were hospitalized more than three times, and one physician hospitalized 91 patients for an average of 4.8 hospitalizations each. He hospitalized one patient 27 times during this period of 27 months.

In one county group the appendectomy rate for Fund beneficiaries has been as high as 9 per 1,000 and the cesarean section rate 11% as compared with 5 per 1,000 and 2%, respectively, in similar groups in contiguous areas.

Nineteen per cent of the deliveries of Fund beneficiaries done by two doctors at one hospital were by cesarean section. After discussion and some education, cesareans were reduced to 6% in six months, and are now at the rate of 2%.

In one of the general hospitals with an average length of stay of eight days, we studied a series of 239 of our surgical patients who had an average length of stay of 21.3 days. One surgeon with 47 cases averaged 40.9 days for his patients. The surgeon had no special skills nor were his cases essentially different from those that his colleagues were treating.

A State medical society, after finding a member guilty of splitting fees and ghost surgery, decreed that his disciplinary suspension for 24 hours was to be kept confidential. This same individual successfully prevented accreditation of the local hospital by refusing to keep his records up to date. Review of his appendectomies revealed that nearly 75% were normal. He is an active member of his country medical society, which does not see fit to evaluate his activities.

With the State and county medical societies either unable or unwilling to exercise effective control over the quality of service rendered to Fund beneficiaries, and to prevent unnecessary hospitalization, the Fund was compelled to adopt procedures toward these ends.

In one area in which the quality of medical care, hospital admission, and length of stay were highly questionable, the Fund required consultation with an appropriate specialist as a prerequisite to hospital admission as far as this was practicable. It also stipulated that, whenever practicable, major surgery be performed by broadly competent and responsible surgeons according to criteria established by the American Board of Surgery or the American College of Surgeons. The results showed that we were able to effect 32.5% reduction in hospital admissions, a 36.8% decrease in hospital days, and a 7.0% drop in hospital days per patient. In studying rates of surgical patients, there was a 16.5% reduction in all surgical procedures brought about, and in appendectomies alone, there was a decrease of 59.4%.

These measures are still in effect in this area and the results have remained essentially the same to date.

The same measures were applied to other areas in 1955, and similar results were beginning to show when the American Medical Association House of Delegates passed a resolution disapproving our requirement for consultation on all patients prior to hospital admission. We discontinued this requirement to avoid an open break, hoping we could find another effective way of accomplishing the purpose to which the American Medical Association would not object.

The American Medical Association resolution did not disapprove of our refusal to pay individual physicians for services of inferior quality as judged by qualified consultants, nor to our unwillingness to pay physicians whose qualifications for surgery we are not in position to judge, when Board or College surgeons are available.

By these means we have effected reductions of up to 75% in gynecologic operations in some places, and in the reduction of the rate of hospital admissions from an average of 350 per 1,000 beneficiaries to 180 per 1,000 in one of our areas.

Violent objection to these measures was then launched by a number of State and county medical societies on the ground that the Fund is denying the right of free-choice-of-physician and thereby deteriorating the quality of medical care a beneficiary will receive.

In response to the urgent request of the Executive Medical Officer of the Fund that an A.M.A. Committee use its good offices in endeavoring to develop some sort of effective measures to which organized medicine would not object, a set of "Suggested Guides" was approved by the A.M.A. House of Delegates in June 1957, advising the Fund, among other things, that "Every physician duly licensed by the state to practice medicine and surgery should be assumed at the outset to be competent in the field in which he claims to be unless considered otherwise by his peers." This would place us back where we were 10 years ago, with a repetition of all the evils we have suffered in between.

In view of the foregoing and to serve the best interests of its beneficiaries, the Fund is now limiting its payments to physicians and hospitals whose services are necessary and essential in providing the hospital and medical care benefits which it has authorized. This provision has been in effect for the past four months. The results as compared with the same months in the preceding year are as follows; a decrease of 16% in the hospital admission rate; a decrease in 17% in days of hospital care; a decrease of 13% in total expenditures for medical care; and a decrease of 12% in the cost of medical care per beneficiary.

The reductions are on an industry-wide basis, and no beneficiary has been deprived of reasonable opportunity of receiving all of the medical and hospital benefits which the Fund has authorized.

This has been our experience to date. The only logical conclusions we are able to draw are as follows:

1. Every physician duly licensed by the State is not competent to perform any service that any patient may require, even if he claims to be.

2. Organized medicine, while insisting that it alone possesses the authority to judge and discipline its members, has thus far been unable or unwilling to establish and enforce effective means of doing so.

3. As matters now stand, the only way in which the Fund can insure the highest quality of care, and the maximum benefits that can be provided for the amount of money available, is through mutually satisfactory arrangements with physicians and hospitals whose services are necessary and essential.

2. Rehabilitation

The State-Federal Program of
Vocational Rehabilitation for Disabled Persons*

MARY E. SWITZER

AMONG THE MOST progressive and most rapidly growing public activities that bear the great significance on most Public Health programs is the Federal-State partnership program of vocational rehabilitation for disabled civilians.

In the 12 months ended June 30, 1962, the public program of vocational rehabilitation effected the rehabilitation of 102,378 disabled civilians into successful employment, thereby reaching the highest annual total in its 42-year history.

The public program encompasses the partnership in vocational rehabilitation activities between the Federal and State governments, operated under legislation that was first enacted in 1920, and modified at various times, as experience was gained and the philosophy underlying the public effort broadened. In 1954, Public Law 565 was enacted, amending the legislation to effect expansion and meet needs that then were apparent, and providing the means for much closer cooperation among the Federal and State governments, communities, and private organizations.

As it is operated now, the role of the Federal government is to provide national leadership and to administer several grant systems of Federal money for a number of purposes. The Federal function is performed by the Vocational Rehabilitation Administration, one of the constituent agencies of the Department of Health, Education, and Welfare.

The States perform the actual rehabilitation services for clients. Each of them, as well as the District of Columbia, Puerto Rico, Guam, and the Virgin Islands, has a specially constituted vocational rehabilitation agency, operating under a plan of services that meets Federal standards sufficient to give them eligibility for Federal grants that are available. In addition to the general agencies, 36 States have agencies exclusively for those who are blind or have severe visual handicaps.

The 1962 total of rehabilitations was not only the largest in the

* This is an original contribution prepared for this publication. The author is Commissioner, Vocational Rehabilitation Administration, U.S. Department of Health, Education, and Welfare, Washington, D.C.

history of the program, but was hailed as a significant mark in that it was the halfway point to a goal of 200,000 rehabilitations each year that was set at the time the 1954 legislation was enacted.

The goal of 200,000 rehabilitations a year was predicated upon estimates that 250,000 persons would reach the stage of disability each year that would cause them to require rehabilitation services in order to work—and with the prospect of benefiting from those services. It was assumed that the voluntary agencies which deal with various disabilities would be able to effect about 50,000 rehabilitations a year, thus meeting the annual incidence of need.

NEW AREAS OF SERVICE

This incidence probably will grow because of the progressive extension of rehabilitation services to groups that were being given scant attention in 1954. The mentally retarded were not receiving the attention in 1954 that they receive today on the basis of fairly recent demonstrations that most of them can be helped to become partially or fully self-sufficient through painstaking rehabilitative procedures.

Similarly, much more attention is being given now than previously to persons with speech and hearing defects. Also, there is continuing expansion of effort to rehabilitate the mentally ill. Advances in optics and lens-grinding have brought many persons who formerly were considered blind to the point where they can see well enough to function normally. In addition, the State vocational rehabilitation agencies are discovering that many more of the aging can be rehabilitated than was thought possible in earlier years. These factors and a steadily growing population soon will necessitate a considerable revision of needs.

The effectiveness of the public program is revealed in several ways. A disabled person is not counted as rehabilitated until his employment is verified as satisfactory to both the client and employer. Consequently, it is significant that about 4500 of last year's rehabilitants successfully entered the short-supply professional fields such as teaching, engineering, medicine, and related health activities. About the same number went into semi-professional work and most of the others have succeeded in skilled or semiskilled work, service occupations, and farming, while about 15% of the total became family workers.

Approximately 16,700 of the rehabilitants had been receiving public assistance payments of $18 million a year, and these were rehabilitated at a one-time cost of $17 million.

The total group will contribute about 150 million man-hours per year to the Nation's productive effort, and has increased its annual earning rate from $47 million, before rehabilitation, to $205 million.

SERVICES AVAILABLE

A considerable range of services is available to disabled persons. Provided in any necessary combination, one or more of the following services may be brought to bear upon any handicapped person's condition:

1. *Medical diagnosis to learn the nature and degree of disability and to help determine eligibility for services, the need for additional medical services, and the individual's work capacities;*
2. Medical, surgical, psychiatric, and hospital services to remove or reduce the disability;
3. Artificial limbs and other prosthetic appliances;
4. *Individual counseling and guidance, including psychologic testing, to help select and attain a vocational objective;*
5. Training, including occupational training and adjustment training, for the blind;
6. Maintenance and transportation during treatment, training, or any other phase of the actual rehabilitation process;
7. Tools, equipment, licenses, or initial stocks and supplies if these are necessary to give the rehabilitated individual a fair start;
8. *Placement in a job commensurate with the individual's physical and mental capacities;*
9. *Follow-up to ensure that the rehabilitated person is successful and that both he and his employer are satisfied.*

The services indicated in italics (Nos. 1, 4, 8, and 9) are furnished without cost to the disabled individual. Training (No. 5) is generally furnished without cost. Public funds are used for providing the other listed services to the extent that the disabled person is not able to pay for them.

In most of the States, the vocational rehabilitation program is administered as a division of vocational rehabilitation, under general supervision of the State Board for Vocational Education. The law permits the function however, to be lodged in a special agency that is primarily concerned with vocational rehabilitation. Several States operate under this arrangement. Most agencies for the blind are parts of the Public Welfare Department, but several State programs are operated by State Commissions or other separate agencies for the blind. Local offices are maintained in most important cities and services for individuals are provided through these.

The steady increases in vocational rehabilitation in recent years have resulted from a four-pronged attack on the problems of disability and dependency: (1) use of increased State and Federal funds for rehabilitation services, (2) training and recruitment of more professional rehabilitation workers, (3) establishment of increasing numbers of rehabilitation facilities and workshops, and (4) application of new knowledge and technics that have come from research in all parts of the country.

FEDERAL FUNDS AND STATE MATCHING

The Congress has been whole-heartedly cooperative in supporting vocational rehabilitation since the 1954 legislation set about expanding the program. There has been clear indication each year that the Congress has been willing to make available all the Federal money that the States are willing to match.

This, of course, is strikingly reflected in the growth of both Federal and State expenditures for the work. In 1955, for instance, the first fiscal year of operation under the new law, the Federal appropriation for the States was about $25.2 million, and the States made available $15.1 million for carrying on the program of services to individuals. These figures included $700,000 of Federal funds and $350,000 of State funds for "expansion," a temporary activity that was carried on for three years.

By 1962, the straight support and improvement of the State programs brought $64 million in Federal funds and the States matched this with about $40 million of their own funds. For the 1963 fiscal year, the Federal support appropriation is about $73 million, to be matched by $45.5 million in State funds.

Thus, it will be seen that the program of providing services to disabled individuals has increased in nine years from $40 million to $118.4 million—almost a three-fold increase.

SUPPORT FOR PROFESSIONAL TRAINING

Similarly, the effort to obtain adequate professional staff for a nationally expanding program brought strong action. The Congress, in enacting the 1954 law, recognized that more and better trained professional people would be needed. Consequently, for the first time, the Vocational Rehabilitation Administration was given authority to support such training.

The first appropriation was small—$900,000. This provided support for 77 teaching programs in several educational institutions, including 201 traineeships. In addition, it covered the cost of 16 short-term courses in varied subjects.

The training program has grown steadily. For the current fiscal year, the Vocational Rehabilitation Administration expects to support 325 long-term teaching grants in medicine, rehabilitation counseling, nursing, social work, occupational therapy, physical therapy, prosthetics education and orthotics, speech pathology and audiology, and psychology. Traineeships will be provided for some 2400 qualified persons in these long-term courses, and for more than 3000 persons in refresher and special courses.

About 175 educational institutions will be engaged in these activities, and the Vocational Rehabilitation Administration expects to expend about $13.3 million in this area, or $3.6 million above the 1962 level.

The distribution of traineeships gives indication of the emphasis being placed to obtain short-supply personnel. Of the approximately 2,500 trainees, 450 are now in medicine with accent on the rehabilitation aspects of medicine; 732 are in rehabilitation counseling; speech pathologists and audiologists number 421, indicating the seriousness of the effort to combat speech and hearing difficulties.

Through the other major training activities, the traineeships are distributed as follows: nursing 55; occupational therapy 255; physical therapy 187 (and here the need is so great that undergraduate trainees are given support); social work 239; psychology 47; and prosthetics and orthotics 18.

There are many reasons for the heavy emphasis placed in several areas of training. In allocating available training funds among the professional fields, the Vocational Rehabilitation Administration attempts to achieve a suitable balance related to the more acute personnel shortages, to geographic distribution, and schools' abilities to offer the kind of training needed to improve the work of State agency and other rehabilitation personnel.

In addition to these considerations, the training program offers encouragement to schools that have or will develop curricula to train specialists in rehabilitation of the blind, the deaf, the mentally retarded, and the emotionally disturbed. There is also support for training that is interdisciplinary in nature, and pilot projects in collaborative practices are encouraged.

The emphasis on training in medicine reflects the acute shortage of physicians qualified in the specialty of physical medicine and rehabilitation, one of the newer fields. The emphasis placed on this discipline is reflected in the fact that in 1963 almost $3 million of the $13.3 million in training funds is for teaching grants and traineeships in medicine.

By this emphasis, the Vocational Rehabilitation Administration hopes to fulfill the growing role of the physician in the national rehabilitation program. Physical rehabilitation is, of course, basic in the program. The growing categories of disabilities make it imperative that not only the practitioner of rehabilitation medicine keep abreast of rapidly appearing current developments, but that the physicians in general practice also be aware of those developments and of the rehabilitation potentialities of their State agencies.

Consequently, training grants in the field of medicine have as their major goals: (1) to give all medical students an understanding of rehabilitation philosophy and methods so that concepts of total health care may be incorporated in their future practice of medicine; (2) to stimulate interested medical students in future specialization in physical medicine and rehabilitation; (3) to increase the supply of physiatrists by support of residency training in physical medicine and rehabilitation; (4) to offer physicians in other medical specialties closely related to chronic illness and disability (psychiatry, neurology, orthopedics, internal medicine, urology, and Public Health) opportunities for learning about rehabilitation methods; and (5) to provide physicians now in practice with orientation or refresher courses in rehabilitation techniques in the major disability categories.

THE REHABILITATION COUNSELOR

The rehabilitation counselor is the key worker in the program. The counselor is the first rehabilitation worker who hears the story of the disabled person and who makes many evaluations and decisions of consequence. The counselor is the liaison between the realities of the public program and the individual needs of the disabled person, and a person of growing stature in private and public operations in rehabilitation. The counselor guides the client through the growing complexities and the many technical and social considerations that are involved in the rehabilitation process, balancing its operations with the personal problems of the disabled person, and, in many cases, his family.

The counselor must have a knowledge of social work, of psychology, of Public Health and welfare procedures, of medical, surgical and hospital practices in relation to physical and mental restoration, and of employment practices, especially in his own area. This last factor carries a special responsibility, for it is upon the success of the counselor in matching the abilities of the disabled person with work opportunities that the ultimate success of the public program depends.

There is another growing responsibility in the training program for counselors, brought about by a necessity for specialization. The enlarged category of disabilities with which the public program is concerned—mental illness and retardation are conspicuous among them—is stimulating the provision of training for counselors in the special implications of certain disabilities.

The rate of graduation of counselors has been about 250 a year. The need is almost three times as great, and VRA is attempting to make up this need.

OTHER PERSONNEL SHORTAGES

There are other shortages of critical importance. An estimated eight to nine millions of our people have speech and hearing difficulties. Currently there are about 10,000 clinicians to serve them, half the number needed to provide an adequate volume of services.

There are grave shortages in physical therapy, occupational therapy, in psychologists, in prosthetists, and in social workers. In occupational therapy the estimated need is for 16,000, the number in practice is about 6,000, and there are about 500 graduates each year. The shortage of physical therapists is acute. The present number of 8,400 in practice should be one-third more. Enrollments in approved courses are far below capacity. In consequence, the Vocational Rehabilitation Administration has initiated a system of undergraduate trainee grants to attract students, and in 1962 all but four of 40 approved schools had such projects in operation.

REHABILITATION FACILITIES

The third major factor in the continuing effectiveness of the vocational rehabilitation program is the growth in rehabilitation facilities and workshops, and in their use. The Association of Rehabilitation Centers, in a 1962 study and analysis, identified 131 rehabilitation centers, most of them of considerable size and function. In 1954 there was a bare handful of comprehensive centers, no matter how loose the definition.

The 131 identified centers probably are less than one-fourth the total if many smaller, single disability facilities were to be considered. Under the Medical Facilities Survey and Construction Act of 1954 (an extension of the Hill-Burton hospital construction program), 234 centers or parts of centers have been approved for construction at a total cost of $150 million, with the Federal Government supplying slightly less than one-third of the cost.

Under the 1954 legislation, construction grants could be approved only if the center were to be qualified as a comprehensive center, i.e., with medical, psychologic, social, and vocational services included within its program. Most of the new centers were strongly oriented toward medical services, although there is now a growing emphasis in many parts of the country on greatly increased vocational services in centers. Under amendments approved October 5, 1961, a center may be approved for construction if it provides medical services and one other.

The use of these centers, where concentrated services can be given for the more severely disabled clients of the vocational rehabilitation agency, has grown impressively. In 1955, the State vocational rehabilitation agencies spent $850,000 in rehabilitation centers for services for 2400 clients. In 1961, the last year for which reports are available, the expenditure was $6.5 million for services that benefited 17,000 persons. A severely disabled client can make better progress in a center where virtually all of his needs are met, than if he must receive his services piecemeal, and perhaps from sources less skilled or experienced than will be found in a center.

The opportunities to acquire work skills and tolerance, similarly, are considered greater in sheltered workshops than in the open market, where few business concerns are inclined or geared to part-time work under conditions where concessions must be made to the limitations of the workers. There is no record of the number of community workshops in operation in 1954, but most estimates run close to 250. So great have been the advances in this field, that the current number is thought to be about 800. Thus many more people have the opportunity to use the workshop as a stepping stone to competitive employment or, if need be, as a place where they can achieve permanently some degree of independence and self-reliance.

RESEARCH

The fourth great stimulus to progress in vocational rehabilitation lies in the research arm of the Vocational Rehabilitation Administration. Like the other major stimuli, this has its origins in the 1954 legislation. Before then, the Vocational Rehabilitation Administration had no authority to conduct research and demonstrations, but this legislation provided the authority and with it a small appropriation —$300,000. Activity in this field, as in all others, gained momentum rapidly and support grew. In 1962, for instance, funds for research amounted to $9,450,000, and for the 1963 fiscal year, $10.5 million was budgeted.

Almost 600 research or demonstration projects have been completed, are in being, or have been approved for operation since 1954. Some 200 projects have been finished. The research and demonstration programs represent a Federal investment of some $26 million through 1962. Projects are submitted by colleges and universities, medical schools, hospitals, rehabilitation centers, a broad range of private groups, and State rehabilitation agencies. They are considered by a statutory National Advisory Council on Vocational Rehabilitation, which makes recommendations to the Commissioner of the Vocational Rehabilitation Administration.

Amounts of grants are in the discretion of the Council and Director, and the basic criteria of a project's value lie in its promise of solution of common problems and improvement of services. As in all research of this nature, there are two parts to the total endeavor. One is the development of knowledge, the other its validation and translation into action. Some of the projects have produced dramatic results and these are being applied widely in many areas.

EXAMPLES OF RESEARCH

Seven years ago the Vocational Rehabilitation Administration was approached for a research or demonstration grant by a psychiatrist at the New York Psychiatric Institute, Dr. Franz Kallman. This man had learned the sign language and other means of communicating with the deaf. He wanted to determine, by clinical methods, whether it is possible to give psychotherapy and other help to psychotic deaf people. Approval was given for a five-year study project. Dr. Kallman, working with State mental patients, found some who had been in hospitals for as long as 20 years, with no communication with the outside —much less with the benefit of psychiatric treatment. No one could reach them. His study encompassed not only the effects of psychotherapy, but he also delved into the genetic aspects of deafness. He found, of course, some horrible results of "inbreeding" among the deaf population, some peculiar patterns of behavior. He concluded that the deaf who are mentally ill can be helped if psychiatrists are trained to communicate with them.

In consequence, he has trained a staff. The State has set aside a 30-bed ward at the Rockland State Hospital, and is bringing patients to these beds. These are chosen from a list of 500 deaf people in mental hospitals and schools for the mentally retarded. The State is supplying regular psychiatric treatment, and the Vocational Rehabilitation Administration is financing special psychotherapy by subsidizing Dr. Kallman's trained staff. The Vocational Rehabilitation Administration's commitment is $140,000 a year for five years—a total of $700,000. But it has been learned that help can be given to the deaf, and efforts are now being made to demonstrate that Dr. Kallman's methods can be applied effective in many States.

Another of the VRA's most dramatic and risky undertakings that has turned out well involves a series of surgical procedures used in alleviating the tremors and rigidity of Parkinson's disease.

There are many other areas of research in which the Vocational Rehabilitation Administration is active. For several years the Vocational Rehabilitation Administration has supported training programs to instruct mobility experts how to teach the blind to move about with freedom—a great asset to a blind person. From these training programs at Boston College and Western Michigan University have come enough qualified sighted trainers to enable the Vocational Rehabilitation Administration to consider demonstrations within the States. Soon there will be a constant flow of qualified experts available to serve in institutions, and elsewhere, to help the blind conquer one of their greatest obstacles to success.

At Case Institute in Cleveland, the Vocational Rehabilitation Administration has research under way to measure the amount of pressure exerted by disabled people on various parts of their bodies while in different positions. This, it is hoped, will contribute to the prevention or alleviation of decubital ulcers.

Also at Case Institute there is research under way to setting up electronic control boards which will provide the stimuli for paralyzed people to go through a whole series of guided and powered movements that will enable them to carry on a wide range of activity—from combing their hair, eating, and other activities of daily living to movements in occupational patterns.

Massachusetts Institute of Technology is engaged in research to increase the ease of written communication with and among the blind, while studying other means of improving the blind person's adjustment to a sighted world. One result, thus far, is the connection of a high-speed Brailler with an electric typewriter, so that an operator can type text in English and, through an electronic process, the text will be reproduced simultaneously in Braille.

Additionally, the Vocational Rehabilitation Administration is supporting 20 optical aids clinics in 19 States. Through advances in lens-making and optics generally, many who once were blind in the legal sense now work with relative ease.

Another area in which the results of a research or demonstration project are being applied widely is mental retardation. One of the first demonstration projects authorized under the new law was in support of the Association for Help of Retarded Children, in New York City, to train mental retardates to the point where they could achieve some degree of independence. So productive was this effort that 36 demonstrations, patterned on this prototype, have been initiated in 29 States.

A new development in research and training has been inaugurated with the establishment of vocational rehabilitation centers at four major universities, where rehabilitation research and training activities can be conducted in connection with their medical schools. With grants from the Vocational Rehabilitation Administration, new centers are in operation at New York University, University of Minnesota, University of Washington, and Baylor University.

The new centers are part of a plan calling for a limited number of such projects in universities having medical schools with comprehensive teaching and research programs in physical medicine and rehabilitation, as well as resources for research in other phases of rehabilitation.

PREVENTION OF DEPENDENCY

The evolving philosophy of rehabilitation makes the eradication of dependency from disability the prime objective of the public program. In this concept, those who plan the future of rehabilitation look at the disabled person in a constantly changing perspective. It is not enough to prepare disabled persons for jobs—they must be placed in satisfactory work, or made able to live with a minimum of dependence on families or institutions.

Accordingly, programs have been developed to screen disabled applicants for benefits from the Bureau of Old Age and Survivors Insurance for rehabilitation potential, and a growing proportion of them are being prepared for a return to work. And, in amendments to public welfare legislation in 1962, a new linkage was sought between the public welfare and the public vocational rehabilitation systems. President Kennedy outlined the objectives of the combined effort in these words when he signed the new legislation:

"This measure embodies a new approach—stressing services in addition to support, rehabilitation instead of relief, and training for useful work instead of prolonged dependency. This important legislation will assist our States and local public welfare agencies to redirect the incentives and services they offer to needy families and children and to aged and disabled people. Our objective is to prevent or reduce dependency and to encourage self-care and self-support—to maintain family life where it is adequate and to restore it where it is deficient."

The concept is not new, for it has been tried locally for many years. Now we have the job of making it work on a national scale, by looking at a family where disability has struck, and regarding an unemployed breadwinner along with dependent children as fit subjects for benefits under the enlarged concept.

Much of our research is being aimed at the roots and the prevention of dependency. Progress continues with the ingredients we find, and with the goal—in the Vocational Rehabilitation Administration, in the State agencies, and in the hundreds of cooperating agencies, institutions and facilities—of giving needed help to all who require it in order to achieve the dignity of independence and contributing citizenship.

A new and complicated aspect of the nationwide rehabilitation program is the doubled proportion of older people in our population in the past 50 years, which is bringing mounting concern to those who plan and prepare our health and rehabilitation programs. At the turn of the century there were slightly over three million persons, or 4.1% of the total population, who were 65 years old or more. Now, with a population expanding from a burgeoning birth rate and with an extended life span, there is also a great increase at the other end of the scale, and, according to estimates of the Bureau of the Census, in 1975 there will be a total of almost 22 million persons—9.3% of the population—who will have reached those years where chronic illnesses are most prevalent.

A more comprehensive view of aging among our people reveals that our population has 52 million persons who are 45 years old and beyond. A national estimate made in 1958 by the Public Health Service indicated that there were then more than five million persons in those years who had been disabled for more than three months, principally by such conditions as cardiovascular disease, arthritis, genitourinary disorders, and impairments of hearing, sight, or the extremities.

The Vocational Rehabilitation Administration has estimated that about 1.5 million of these 5 million long-term disabled persons of 45 years or more—among them 115,000 persons of 65 years and beyond—would be feasible for vocational rehabilitation through the nationwide State-Federal program, which emphasizes employment. This leaves some 3.5 million disabled persons of 45 years or older who probably cannot be rehabilitated in terms of work, but who could, in varying degrees, be returned to self-care and independence through appropriate services, lifting them from dependency on families, institutions, or public welfare, with consequent benefits to their dignity, relief of growing burdens on institutions, and reduction of public and private costs for their maintenance.

Here, then, are twin goals for rehabilitation of the disabled over 45 years: one for those who can be restored to employment, and another for those who can be prepared to live independent lives, caring for their daily needs—dressing and feeding themselves, getting about, and participating in family and community activities.

The expanded scope of the public program has integrated it well into the nation's health program. Now, in growing combination with those aspects of public assistance in which disability is a factor, it looms larger than ever as one of the major contributions to the strength of the nation.

Intensive Rehabilitation:
Recent Experience in a Chronic Disease Hospital*

JOHN E. AFFELDT, M.D., VERNON L. NICKEL, M.D.,
JACQUELIN PERRY, M.D., AND BERTRAND C. KRIETE, M.D.

THE CONCEPTS of patient care in acute and chronic disease hospitals have become fairly well established and fixed. Minor changes appear as knowledge, technics, and drugs improve, or as disease patterns change.

The acute hospital functions as the center for diagnosis and care, covering nearly all disease entities. The average period of hospitalization is less than two weeks. If, after diagnosis and definitive care have been accomplished, the patient has not recovered sufficiently to be discharged, he is transferred to a chronic disease facility, if such exists and if a bed is available.

The chronic disease or long-term illness hospital, whichever it may be termed, is usually prepared for a minimal or slightly higher level of medical care. Facilities for diagnosis and care of patients in acute phase of disease are minimal because it is assumed that the patients entering such units have passed that stage. If complications of an acute nature develop or new problems arise, the patient is returned to the acute hospital for care. The ratio of physicians to number of patients is relatively small because activity is minimal. The rate of discharge is low and the average length of stay is several years. Hence the admission rate is low.

At first glance this arrangement between acute and chronic facilities seems logical. However, experience with such an arrangement, or even a deeper look at it, points up some serious problems.

At the chronic disease hospital, the limitations of staff and diagnostic facilities make further diagnosis improbable. This is important with regard to cases incorrectly or incompletely diagnosed during the time of stay in an acute hospital. Treatable and sometimes curable conditions are missed, resulting in unfortunate and prolonged hospital care. The lack of diagnostic and treatment opportunities makes it difficult if not impossible to develop and maintain a stimulated and competent professional staff. These features minimize discharge possibilities.

The acute hospitals are so crowded with patients in critical condi-

* Reprinted with omission of four tables and one graph by permission from the October, 1959, issue of *California Medicine*, Vol. 91, pp. 193–196. This paper was presented before the Section on Orthopedics at the 88th Annual Session of the California Medical Association, San Francisco, California, February 22–25, 1959. The authors are respectively, Medical Director; Chief, Surgical Services; Orthopedist; Chief, Medical Services, Rancho Los Amigos, Hospital Department of Charities, County of Los Angeles, Downey, California.

tion that they can hardly handle the acute problems in their facilities, let alone give adequate attention to reconstructive problems in patients sent back to them from chronic disease hospitals, or even in patients on their own wards who need such care. Despite this situation, planning agencies are still advocating that general hospitals be the center of all active care.

The number of patients with long-term illness is increasing. This is due to improved acute care, which reduces mortality but does not always result in cure, and to increased longevity with additional time for degenerative diseases to develop. The result is an increasing demand for long-term beds, a trend that will continue as long as the prevailing attitude is that active care ceases when the facility for treatment of acute illness feels it has done all it can.

This demand can be met by building more beds, by increasing the discharge rate or by a combination of both. Building more beds is only a temporary solution as the number of these patients is cumulative. On the other hand, if some of the patients can be improved by more intensive care, and discharged, the present number of beds would handle more patients. In essence, the only way to meet the increasing demand without continually building more beds, is to increase the salvage or discharge rate.

The question is, can a sufficient number of these patients be salvaged by intensive rehabilitation to warrant the expense of such a program? Administrators will not seek the necessary funds for purely social benefits to the patients, but will do so if economy can be demonstrated.

It is the purpose of this paper to present the results of an intensive rehabilitation program at the Rancho Los Amigos Hospital. The results parallel those reported by Hilleboe[3] at the New York State Rehabilitation Hospital. We believe these results answer the above question in the affirmative.

FACILITIES

Rancho Los Amigos Hospital is the chronic disease hospital for Los Angeles County, receiving medically indigent patients from the acute hospitals. The bed capacity is nearly 2,500, plus over 700 nursing home beds under contract. Despite this size, there are between 300 and 500 patients occupying beds in the acute hospitals who are awaiting transfer to this hospital. These patients seriously clog and hamper the activities of the acute hospitals. Half of the patients at Rancho are over 65 years of age and the average length of stay is three and a half years.

In 1952 funds, staff, and facilities were provided to develop an active intensive rehabilitation program for the large number of severely paralyzed poliomyelitic respirator patients who had accumulated there over several years. The results were good,[1, 2] tempting the staff to extend the intensive methods to some of the other disabled patients with a myriad of other diseases. Consequently, in 1955 staff and facilities were provided for an intensive rehabilitation program for non-poliomyelitic patients in a 35-bed unit. This included, in addition to an increased medical and nursing staff, physical and occupational therapy, medical social service, psychologic and vocational services, bracing and splinting as well as a developmental orthotic shop, surgical, X-ray and clinical laboratory services. The results were better than expected, resulting in expansion of the program.

PATIENT SELECTION

The patients admitted to the 35-bed intensive rehabilitation unit were selected by physicians of the staff. There were two sources for patients. Initially selection was from patients already at the hospital, which limited the choice to patients who had already been there for years beyond their initial illness, and long since had become accustomed and adjusted to a quiet and protected hospital environment. Their vocational opportunities had disappeared, family contacts had diminished, and interest in outside life had dimmed. To some, there was no interest or desire to undergo a program of rehabilitation. They did not want their situation disturbed, unless there was something better to hope for and probability of achievement.

It was therefore important for the staff to search for those who had the physical and mental potential for successful rehabilitation, and then convince them of their potential in order to raise their desire for the program and make them willing to work hard for results.

The second source of patients was referral from surrounding acute hospitals, particularly the Los Angeles County General Hospital. Members of the staff of the county hospital who happened to know about the program would periodically refer from their wards patients who they felt were potential candidates. It soon became obvious, as others have reported,[4] that the sooner patients could be started in the program after the acute stage of disease passed, the shorter the time required for rehabilitation and the better the results. Despite this knowledge, priority was given to patients already at the hospital, in recognition of a feeling of first responsibility to them.

PATIENT CLASSIFICATION

In order to evaluate the patients before and after treatment we used a profile classification originally designed for our post-poliomyelitis rehabilitation program. The patients were classified with this system at the time of admission to the rehabilitation program and again at the time of final disposition of the case so far as the program was concerned. The classification was based on the status of the patients in four categories:

1. Physical dependence—meaning how dependent they are upon help from others to carry out their normal daily activities. They were permitted to use any devices available to them, as we are only interested in what they can do for themselves as against how much help they need from others.

2. Respiratory—need for mechanical respiratory assistance, such as the iron lung or other respirators.

3. Vocational—defined as their ability to provide for their financial needs at whatever level they are accustomed to. This included their family needs if they had the responsibility for such.

4. Motivational—defined as their desire to improve and their willingness or eagerness to work for such.

Each area was broken into one of three scales: I. Minimal or no disability; II. Partial disability; III. Full disability.

A patient could be a D-III (fully dependent on others for physical help), but be a V-I (financially independent) by virtue of mental skills and good motivation (M-I). On the contrary, a patient could be physically disabled in such a way that he is physically independent (D-I), yet be financially dependent (V-III) owing to poor motivation (M-III). We purposely used a gross three-scale classification limited to four basic categories in order to avoid detailed classification of many functions. The respiratory factor is obviously more important with poliomyelitic patients, yet quadriplegics may also have such involvement.

RESULTS

From November 1955 to November 1957 there were 85 patients who completed the program—69 adults with an average age of 38 years and 16 children with an average age of seven years. The age range was from two to 71 years. The duration of illness from onset to admission to the rehabilitation program averaged five years, with a spread of from three weeks to 32 years. The previous period of hospitalization ranged from three weeks to 12 years. The average length of stay in the rehabilitation program was six and a half months. Among the 85 patients there are 28 paraplegics, 12 with quadriplegia, 11 with various neuromuscular diseases, 10 hemiplegics, and the remainder with amputations, arthritis, arthrogryposis, encephalomyelitis, muscular dystrophy, miscellaneous orthopedic conditions, and rheumatic heart disease.

The profile classifications are of interest. On admission, 37% were completely dependent on others for physical activities. Another 42% were partially dependent, making a total of 79% who were dependent upon others for help. On release from the program the figures are reversed. Now, only 30% are dependent with 70% completely independent. The respiratory group showed only one patient with sufficient involvement to require partial use of a respirator. The low incidence was due to the fact that no poliomyelitic patients were included in this study.

The results of rehabilitation are seen in the fact that 68% of the adults released from the program were discharged to their homes, with over half going to employment, not counting the women who went back to housework. Twenty-six % remained at the hospital, and hence were transferred to the convalsecent wards. This was usually due to a social problem of some sort, such as having no home or family. The majority of those staying at the hospital were sufficiently improved that they needed less care; in fact, they were employed on the grounds of the hospital.

The social benefits of such a program are enormous. They include reestablishment or protection of a person's dignity and self-esteem, reestablishment or preservation of his home and family, and interest and participation in an active life. The economic benefits are equally great and from the standpoint of persons responsible for governmental budgets and taxes are of even greater importance. The benefits can be shown in three ways. First, in regard to financial status. Sixty-three % were completely dependent for financial help from others on admission, whereas on discharge the proportion had dropped to 26%. This is important with regard to taxes, for the bulk of financial help to these people and their families is from public welfare funds. Another important consideration is that over 50% of the patients discharged became employed and thus taxpayers again.

The second economic benefit is the savings in hospitalization costs per patient. The daily cost on the rehabilitation wards is $19 as compared with $9 for the convalescent wards, the difference being due to the higher staffing ratio and more intensive medical services on the active program. But the length of stay was so much shorter that the total cost was much less. Thus $19 times the 195-day average time in hospital under the intensive rehabilitation program (six and a half months) equals $3,700 cost for rehabilitation. The usual convalescent care at $9 for 1,260 days (three and a half years) costs $11,340. Thus the average savings per patient is about $7,640. From a purely budgetary standpoint this savings does not become apparent. The hospital's budget does not drop; it rises, for it is carrying a more active program. However, this does not in any way alter the fact that for every patient discharged earlier because of an active program, thousands of dollars are saved.

The third economic benefit is in the greater usage of hospital beds. It is obvious that shortening the period of hospitalization will allow more patients to occupy a bed in a year. Because the demand for chronic beds is greater than the supply, either more will have to be built or a greater turnover will have to be accomplished, or perhaps both. With construction costs averaging $10,000 per bed, the increased cost of an active rehabilitation program over a convalescent program that requires more beds will again manifest economic sense.

The job satisfaction and professional achievements by the staff in the program have been contagious to all the personnel in the hospital. Coupling this with the social and economic benefits already outlined leads one to appreciate the feeling that an intensive rehabilitation program is an important function of a chronic disease hospital.

1. Affeldt, J. E.: Concept of patient care in a respiratory and rehabilitation center. *Poliomyelitis: papers and discussions presented at the Fourth International Poliomyelitis Conference*, Philadelphia, J. B. Lippincott Co., 1958, pp. 618–623.

2. Affeldt, J. E., West, H. F., Landauer, K. S., Wendland, L. V., and Arata, N. N.: Functional and vocational recovery in severe poliomyelitis, *Clinical Orthopaedics*, 12:16–21, 1958.

3. Hilleboe, H. E., Levin, M. L., Brightman, I. J., Schlesinger, E. R., and Reynolds, F. W.: A pilot program for the rehabilitation of disabled welfare recipients. A preliminary report, *New York State J. Med.*, 57:1737–1741, May 15, 1957.

4. Whittico, J. M., Lawrence, M. S., Stauffer, D., and Elman, R.: Three-year pilot rehabilitation study in a general hospital, *J.A.M.A.*, 164:1633–1635, Aug. 10, 1957.

Alcoholics Anonymous As a Community Resource*

JOHN PARK LEE

"Alcoholics Anonymous is a fellowship of men and women who share their experience, strength and hope with each other that they may solve their common problem and help others to recover from alcoholism.

The only requirement for membership is a desire to stop drinking. There are no dues or fees for A.A. membership; we are self-supporting through our own contributions. A.A. is not allied with any sect, denomination, politics, organization or institution; does not wish to engage in any controversy, neither endorses nor opposes any causes. Our primary purpose is to stay sober and help other alcoholics to achieve sobriety."

AA PREAMBLE

* Reprinted with permission of the National Association of Social Workers from the October, 1960, issue of *Social Work*, Vol. 5, No. 4, pages 20–26. The author is Secretary of Health and Welfare, Board of National Missions, United Presbyterian Church in the U.S.A., New York.

ALCOHOLISM IS KNOWN to social work today as one of the most complex and baffling problems the worker faces as he attempts to help families solve their problems. Few are the social workers who have not heard of Alcoholics Anonymous and its great success in enabling tens of thousands of alcoholic men and women to win their way back to sobriety. Many have been curious to know how this group has succeeded when so many other individuals and groups have failed; to learn more about its workings; and finally, to discover how they can relate to Alcoholics Anonymous for the benefit of their clients.

Any social worker who is contemplating working with AA, as it is commonly known, would do well to read very carefully the statement that appears at the head of this article. This is AA as the members see themselves. This is a description of Alcoholics Anonymous which is read at the opening of virtually every AA meeting around the world. If the social worker who wishes to work with Alcoholics Anonymous will take the time to study the statement carefully, he can avoid many of the difficulties that are encountered in working with AA and have a better chance of securing the help of this fellowship for his client.

First of all, as the statement says, Alcoholics Anonymous is a fellowship. This is probably the best word that could be chosen to describe this unique group of men and women. It is not an organization in the commonly accepted sense of the word, with structure, charter, bylaws, officers, directors, executives, and so on. It is not an agency in any sense; AA members would strenuously resist being described as a welfare agency. It is not, of course, a church, although as we shall see later it has a deeply spiritual basis.

There is no executive with whom the social worker can consult and whom he can call in the way he might call the executive of another social agency. There is no board of directors whose interest must be solicited. Rather, it is a loosely knit group of men and women who have banded themselves together, as the Preamble says, for the sole purpose of helping each other stay sober, and to carry the message of how they did so to other alcoholics.

In the framework of AA—for it does have a structure of sorts—each group is completely autonomous. Each is organized as it sees fit; conducts its affairs in its own way; holds as many or as few meetings as it wishes; uses literature prepared by headquarters as it desires or, if it does not like this literature, prepares its own. It may have a committee directing its affairs, or merely a secretary charged with some of the basic responsibilities of providing a place to meet, getting speakers, providing for the coffee and doughnuts that follow the meetings.

In larger communities, there may be an intergroup association which correlates the services of all the groups in the area and serves as an information center for all concerned. AA also has a general service office in New York City which has no authority over local groups but serves them as they may wish service: with preparation of literature, publication of AA books and the monthly magazine, *The Grapevine*, and contact with groups and individuals around the world. It provides, however, no direct service to alcoholics; it is the AA central referral agency to put interested alcoholics or their families in touch with the AA group nearest to the inquirer.

If the interest of Alcoholics Anonymous is to be obtained in behalf of a client, the social worker must expect to be working with several people at first until the client settles down with one sponsor, to whom he will relate more closely as time goes on. The sponsor may change; AA is extremely flexible. The social worker must be constantly expecting that there will be changes in the AA relationship as it develops.

He should also note that the only qualification for membership is a desire to stop drinking. AA has none of the problems of membership present in other groups. There is no formal sponsorship, no admission committee, no potential blackball, no fees or dues for membership. Rather, if the alcoholic expresses any interest at all in maintaining sobriety, he is entirely welcome from that moment on.

It is important for the social worker to realize the absolute independence on which AA insists. The statement declares that "AA is not allied with any sect, denomination, politics, organization, or institution." Through sad experience, members have learned that their group can be utilized for ends with which all the members do not agree—that if the organization becomes involved with any particular sect or group or political organization, this will be divisive for its membership. Its strength and safety depend on committing itself wholeheartedly and solely to the program of helping its members to achieve sobriety, leaving to individual members to join or not join, to support or not support, to oppose or accept any group or cause they may see fit.

One of the "Twelve Traditions" of the AA movement reads as follows: "An AA group ought never to endorse, finance, or lend the AA name to any related facility or outside enterprise, lest problems of money, property and prestige divert us from our primary purpose."

This does not mean that AA is hostile to social work, or to churches or hospitals or doctors or psychiatry, or to any person. AA members have had difficult experiences with many of these agencies and groups and have their personal views about them, but the movement as a whole is not opposed to or in favor of anybody else— rather, it is glad of the interest and concern of any other group for the welfare of alcoholics. AA people work very closely and successfully with doctors, psychiatrists, clinics, hospitals, church groups, and others in helping alcoholics. There is no reason why a similar effective relationship cannot be established with a social worker in behalf of any client.

BASIC NEEDS OF AN ALCOHOLIC

There have been considerable discussion and speculation as to why AA has been able to succeed in helping alcoholics while other methods have been so lamentably ineffective. Various people have various explanations. This writer's is that it succeeds because it meets the basic needs of the alcoholic at the time he is confronted with the AA program.

1. The first thing the alcoholic needs is hope—hope that he can recover. No social worker who fears that alcoholics cannot recover can be of any assistance whatsoever to an alcoholic. No matter what the worker says, the alcoholic will sense his lack of hope and react to it. The alcoholic has heard for years from all sources—from his family, his friends; from doctors, nurses, and hospitals; sometimes from ministers and priests, sometimes from social workers—the word that he is "hopeless." As he hears this day in and day out, week in and week out, he comes to believe it himself. As long as the alcoholic believes he is hopeless, any program of recovery is bound to fail.

By merely introducing him to a group of recovered alcoholics, Alcoholics Anonymous automatically restores hope to him. As he looks at the AA group, he consciously or subconsciously says to himself, "If they can do it, I can." Hence, in the very first contact with this group one of the alcoholic's basic needs—hope—is met.

2. The second need is to be received as a member of the human race. The alcoholic's experience during his days of acute alcoholism is that of universal rejection. His life is a succession of closing doors. His friends' houses are closed to him because his behavior is such that they can no longer tolerate having him around. The doors of employment slam in his face and may be actually bolted against him through a blacklist. It may seem that the doors of his church are shut against him, and he has known for some time that entrance to most hospitals is firmly barred. Finally—and this is most tragic of all—the doors of his own home may be closed to him. Sometimes it seems that the only remaining open door is that of the jail or the mental institution, and this is closed and locked behind him when he is forcibly thrust in.

The alcoholic comes to think of himself as one who has no importance whatsoever to anybody else in the world; he suffers from a loneliness so intense that few nonalcoholics with the greatest power of empathy can appreciate. It is this feeling of utter despair, of complete loneliness, of essential meaninglessness to others, that produces a kind of frantic, hectic drinking to achieve forgetfulness and blot out the horror that life has become.

Here again, from the first contact when he is welcomed with open arms by the members of AA, the alcoholic feels that he is back in the human race again, no longer an outcast. No one asks him where he has been; no one asks him if he is sorry; no one suggests that he ought to be ashamed of himself; nobody points a finger of scorn. Rather, he is asked if he wants to do something about his drinking, and is told that he is entirely welcome. He learns that he has as much status from the day he joins the AA movement as those who have been in it for perhaps 15 or 20 years. The value of this acceptance is incalculable; it is one of the tremendous supports AA provides for its new members.

3. The alcoholic needs to accept his alcoholism. It is difficult for the nonalcoholic to believe that alcoholics cannot clearly see that drinking is the cause of their difficulty. The alcoholic, given perhaps even more to rationalization than the average person, points to explanations outside himself for his drinking. He will tell you that he got drunk because he was tired, or sick. He will tell you that he got drunk because his mother-in-law came to town, or because she left; that he drank because he was given a raise, or was fired; that he drank too much because the Democrats won, or because the Republicans won.

All these reasons that seem good to him are, of course, totally spurious. He is drinking because this is the nature of alcoholism: the alcoholic drinks in an uncontrolled fashion, and the fact that he cannot control it is evidence of his sickness.

AA again fulfills a real need by confronting the alcoholic bluntly with the nature of his problem. The members brush aside his explanations of why he drinks and tell him that he is drinking because he is an alcoholic and cannot help himself. They tell him that, until he accepts this fact about himself, he is powerless over alcohol—that his life has become unmanageable and he will be unable to recover. Here again is an enormously important step in the therapeutic process which AA has discovered: that without this recognition of the nature of the problem, the person who suffers from it will never be able to come to grips with it.

4. AA also fulfills another need of the alcoholic, which is to accept himself as a human being. Alcoholics are apt to be rather Utopian in their concepts. In their immaturity, they have felt that people could be perfect and, finding that neither they nor others have been perfect, have become cynical and disillusioned. Without consciously doing so, AA shows the new members what it means to be a human being; what it means to have strengths and weaknesses, virtues and

flaws; to recognize that every day there will be failure and every day perhaps some success.

They show the alcoholic how he can settle for being a human being, accept himself and live with himself and, being able to do so, learn how to live with other human beings. AA's talk a great deal of the virtue of tolerance; they learn by association with each other how to tolerate themselves and, being able to tolerate themselves, are then able to get along much better with others.

SPIRITUAL HELP

While all these processes are going on—they do not occur, of course, in the chronologic order presented here—the AA novice is also being introduced to the basic source of AA strength: the relationship with God as the members understand Him. It was noted in quoting from the Preamble that AA is not related to any religious sect, and this is true. On the other hand, virtually any member of Alcoholics Anonymous to whom the social worker talks will state that the basis for recovery depends on the ability to relate to a "Higher Power" which is described by the Alcoholics Anonymous group as "God as we understand Him."

This concept is important for the social worker to grasp. It is not a creed to which the members are asked to adhere; there is no theologic description of the Deity. Rather there is the admonition to the new member that if he would remain sober he must develop some concept of God which will be good enough for him to rely on to enable him to break the grip of the alcoholic obsession that is destroying his life.

The concepts of God with which members work are sometimes very crude and slightly shocking. They are very disturbing, sometimes, to ministers and representatives of organized religion; but as the members mature in AA, their concepts tend to become more conventional, and many relate themselves firmly to a church.

The needs outlined above are largely met as the members struggle to live by what they call the program of "Twelve Suggested Steps" to recovery. Social workers will be interested in reading these steps which are printed at the end of this article, to detect the spiritual and psychologic principles upon which they rest. At this point a word of warning may be helpful for the worker. If he cannot accept the validity of a belief in a higher power as a source of strength for an individual's life, he must not try to work with Alcoholics Anonymous. It is not necessary for him to be a believer himself, but he must be willing to recognize that those who believe do find this strength and direction for their lives.

This acceptance of God is not easy for the average alcoholic, but what is amazing is that so many who have been fearful of Him or hostile to Him all their lives, come to a strong and close relationship with Him. They find that in this process they gain release from the grip of the obsession that has chained them so long.

So real is this relationship that for many members Alcoholics Anonymous is in itself a religion. This is perhaps not fortunate and has dangers implicit in it, which many of the older members recognize. But with the absolute freedom given to each member to interpret the program as he sees fit, members who would recognize that AA is not, cannot be, and should not be a religion accept this as valid for those to whom it has meaning.

It is true, as noted before, that generally the Alcoholics Anonymous groups would describe their program as resting on a spiritual base and are free to give the credit where they think it belongs. On any one day, at any given moment, in thousands of groups around the world people are standing up and saying, "I am sober, thanks to AA and the grace of God." In countless AA meeting halls and clubrooms, banners, placards, and illuminated manuscripts hang on the wall, displaying the words "But for the Grace of God."

WORKING WITH AN AA GROUP

No one can really understand the AA program by merely reading about it. The social worker who is interested should inquire as to the location of an AA group and learn when it will have an open meeting he can attend. It is likely that he, as all others that come in contact with the group, will be stimulated, excited, and deeply moved by what he sees going on in the group.

The groups vary in their methods. As a general rule, a number of speakers at each AA meeting describe their alcoholic experiences. The closing speaker will, perhaps, attempt to sum up what the others have said, and frequently will discuss the twelve steps of which the recovery program is composed. There is always an offering—passing the hat, as it is called—and the money is used to pay for the coffee and doughnuts and perhaps a modest rental on the meeting place; for literature to give to new members and outsiders who may be interested; and for support of the national headquarters in New York.

Any social worker who wants to get in touch with AA can consult the phone book. Alcoholics Anonymous is listed under this name in most of the larger communities in the country and many smaller ones. If it is not in the book, the local policeman may know where the groups meet; sometimes the judges know. If the worker cannot find out in his own community, he can write to Alcoholics Anonymous, PO Box 459, Grand Central Station Annex, New York 17, New York, for the location of the nearest group.

It would be wise for the worker to acquaint himself with the working of AA groups near him before attempting to enlist their help in behalf of a specific client. If he could go to one or two groups, introduce himself to the members, search out the secretary and ask for a telephone reference which he could use, explaining his own work and desire to enlist AA's support, he would undoubtedly meet with a universally ready response.

As noted above, AA has only two purposes: to help its members stay sober and to help others achieve sobriety. In pursuit of the second purpose (normally called "carrying the message"), AA members are eager to be called on for what they speak of as "twelfth-step work"—so-called because the twelfth step of the program describes this obligation to help others.

Once the contact has been established and a working arrangement developed, the social worker should always make sure that the client is willing to discuss his problem with a member of AA before asking AA to come in. Invariably the AA member, when approached for help, will ask if the other person wants to see him. It does not have to be any passionate desire or any great interest; a passive willingness to talk to a member of AA will be adequate. If it is possible, the social worker should arrange to introduce the AA member to the client, either bringing the member to the client's home or taking the client to the AA meeting or the AA person's home.

Referral is not good enough and should be avoided wherever possible—referral, that is, in the sense of merely sending somebody somewhere else. The alcoholic has had a long experience of being passed along from person to person, with each one apparently eager to be rid of him. Referral in this way will merely convince the alcoholic that the social worker is like all the rest. If, however, the worker says, "I want to take you to the AA meeting," or "I'd like to bring a member of AA with me when I come to call on you tomorrow night," the situation is completely reversed and the alcoholic is assured at least of an interest deep enough to account for the social worker's trouble in providing the introduction.

The worker must make sure the alcoholic understands that he is not just being abandoned to AA, but that he (the worker) hopes to keep in touch with him and his family to help in any way possible. But he will tell the client that he believes that if he can utilize the services of AA, this will be the best possible thing for him in the months to come. The worker should avoid the impression of dropping his responsibility because AA has been brought into the picture.

The social worker may find that, while AA attracts the client, the latter falls away again. He must be prepared for this and be willing to try some other AA group. AA groups are not all alike. In some parts of the city they are so specialized that they do not have the general appeal that is necessary. A business or professional man, for example, will do better in a group composed of people of similar background than in a group made up solidly of workingmen. By the same token, a woman may feel terribly lonely in an AA group where she is the only woman, but will be happier in a group with other woman members. AA groups themselves will be helpful in matching up their people with the client.

Occasionally, the social worker may get a refusal from AA. When the name of the client is mentioned, the AA spokesman may say that this man is well known to them and they do not believe that he has much interest. The social worker must not be disturbed by this, but may say that he was not aware of it and will talk to his client further. Perhaps the client will admit that he has been exposed to AA before and that it has not seemed to work. If he is willing to try again, AA is usually willing to take another chance with him.

FAMILY AND TEEN-AGE GROUPS

Finally, if the social worker is not able to help the alcoholic, he does have an obligation to his family. There is a fellowship related to Alcoholics Anonymous called the Al-Anon Family Groups, composed of sober relatives of alcoholics. These are predominantly wives, but also husbands of alcoholics; mothers and fathers, sisters and brothers, and even children do belong to Al-Anon groups in certain parts of the country. This movement is growing rapidly, with between 700 and 800 groups in all parts of the United States. The contact with the local Alcoholics Anonymous group will usually produce the name and address of the responsible person for the Al-Anon group in a given community. If none is known in the immediate area, there may be one nearby and its address can be ascertained by writing to the Al-Anon Family Group Headquarters, 125 East 23 Street, New York, New York.

The members of Al-Anon meet not, as one might suspect, to discuss the frightful behavior of the alcoholic husband or wife or son or father, but rather to learn how they, the sober ones, have been contributing to the problem—to discover how they can live with alcoholism and still maintain the home—how they can become better persons themselves. The Al-Anon groups use the same twelve steps and apply the same kind of group sharing of their "experience, strength and hope."

Most wives think their alcoholic husbands are unique. They imagine that no woman has ever known such sorrow and wallow in self-pity. Al-Anon provides a strong corrective to this exaggerated view and brings the problem down to a size where it can be grappled with. Family members learn the techniques of living with an alcoholic and frequently become the medium through which the alcoholic is guided to AA and recovery.

This group also sponsors a third organization called the Alateen group, composed of the adolescent children of alcoholic parents. There are not so many of these, but in some communities they, too, are quite effective in enabling the youngsters to work out their own problems through a group. Children suffer the torments of the damned living in a home with one or both parents alcoholic, until they learn what the situation is. But they, like members of Al-Anon, can be guided to acceptance of alcoholism as a sickness, enabling them to maintain their love and respect for the alcoholic parent even while the drinking goes on. Adolescents advise each other at Alateen about the problem of inviting a date to the house where the father may come home drunk; they learn how to cope with the cruel comments other children make about their parents; they discover how to "handle" mother or father when drunk.

For all social workers who wish to help alcoholics, the fellowship of Alcoholics Anonymous provides one of the most effective sources of assistance. All that is necessary is acceptance of the concept of alcoholics as sick people and a recognition that they can be helped, that none of them is hopeless, that each is a unique individual whose alcoholism has roots which may never be apparent, but whose drinking must be stopped if his life is to be saved; that Alcoholics Anonymous, while not necessarily able to help every person, is able to help a great majority of alcoholics, and that its members stand ready and willing to assist if called upon and enabled to function in their own ways.

Social workers must be prepared to see members of AA violate many techniques and procedures that seem to them almost sacred. If they are wise, however, they will let the AA men and women work at their own tempo and in their own ways, for while they are not very strong on theory, they have worked out excellent pragmatic methods of helping alcoholics. The writer can assure any social worker who avails himself of the support and help of Alcoholics Anonymous of a fascinating experience and a deeply rewarding one. If he has a faith, he will find it deepened. If he has none, he will find his curiosity aroused.

3.   Poison Control

Public Health Aspects of Poisoning*

EDWARD PRESS, M.D.

OUR MODERN ENVIRONMENT is becoming packed with poisons. In primitive societies and in the industrially undeveloped countries, the conditions and agents harmful to human life are primarily those that exist in nature. Formerly, they consisted chiefly of extreme variations in temperature; of predatory animals that ranged from elephants and tigers to rats, lice, bacteria, and viruses; and of vagaries and fluctuations of plant and animal sources of food, with resultant malnutrition or famine. With the advances made in the scientific and sociologic spheres, man has overcome to a considerable extent many of the major hazards to life. Air may be warmed and humidified in the winter and cooled and dehumidified in the summer. Predatory animals may be controlled so well that the macroscopic ones, like elephants and tigers, are museum or zoo specimens and many of the microscopic ones, like typhoid and diphtheria bacteria and smallpox and yellow-fever viruses, are now scarce enough to elicit surprise and concern over their rare or unusual occurence and to arouse the writing instinct of the "printophilic" physician who encounters them.

HAZARDS TO HEALTH DUE TO
MODERN ADVANCES

These advances in modern science and technology have brought mixed blessings. The same advances that have increased the yield of an acre of land by the use of mechanized farming, crop spraying with insecticides, and synthetic fertilizers and that have stretched this yield by the use of preservatives, canning, freezing, rapid transportation, and low-cost, mass-marketing procedures have introduced new hazards to the health of the public. The insecticides that so efficiently poison the insects trying to feed on the crops may be just as efficient poisoning agents if they are accidentally or in-

* Reprinted, with omission of two tables, by permission, from the April 13, 1957, issue of the *Journal of the American Medical Association*, Vol. 163, pp. 1330–1332. This paper was read in the Symposium on Childhood Poisons before the Joint Meeting of the Section on Pediatrics and the Section on Preventive and Industrial Medicine and Public Health at the 105th Annual Meeting of the American Medical Association, Chicago, June 12, 1956. The author is Public Health Director, Department of Health, City of Evanston, Evanston, Illinois.

tentionally used on humans. Indeed, a few drops of some of the insecticides containing organic phosphorus compounds applied to the unbroken skin of a child or adult may cause serious or even fatal results. When this situation is magnified by the large number of insecticides, rodenticides, herbicides, and insect repellents that are now available in so many households for beneficial, proper use or, perhaps, for dangerous misuse, the potential perils of poisoning become apparent. The manufacture and use of fertilizers, if not properly regulated and safeguarded, may also constitute some danger of poisoning, and even the use of artificial preservatives must be continuously scrutinized to make sure that no substances are included that may have harmful cumulative effects. Moreover, the plentitude of food in itself is a hazard. If the temptation against slight, but repeated, overindulgence is not avoided, it may convert the perils of famine and undernutrition to the hazards of obesity and overnutrition.

The threat to the public of poisoning is not limited to these agents alone, as the wide variety of agents, such as drugs; do-it-yourself and home hobby supplies; hair-waving, dyeing, and bleaching solutions; and cleaning, polishing, and disinfecting substances, present in the average household affords a multiplicity of objects available to the inquisitive toddler and child and greatly increases the hazard of poisoning over that existing one or two generations ago. Thus, the modern environment in the United States abounds with readily available poisons in the solid, liquid, and gaseous states. In 1953 there were 5,883 deaths from poisoning.

ESTABLISHMENT OF POISON CONTROL CENTERS

Infants and children, whose main method of learning is by exploration, questioning, sampling, and trial and error, are particularly susceptible to the accidental ingestion of any one of this wide variety of potentially toxic substances that may be found in the average home. Because of the special vulnerability of this age group, the American Academy of Pediatrics pioneered in the establishment of poison control centers in various cities throughout the United States.

Program in Chicago Poison Control Center

With the aid of several local and national agencies, a poison control center was established in Chicago in the fall of 1953. Although there had been other agencies serving as sources of information on the treatment of poisoning in different parts of the United States, this was the first citywide integrated and organized center. It combined the efforts of the departments of pediatrics of all five medical colleges in Chicago, the Chicago Board of Health, the state toxicology laboratories, the Division of Services for Crippled Children of the University of Illinois, and six major teaching hospitals in Chicago into a coordinated effort for the treatment and prevention of poisoning. An advisory committee that included representatives of the American Medical Association, the National Safety Council, and the federal Food and Drug Administration in addition to those of the participating local groups helped in the over-all program.

A summary of references to the basic toxic constituents in the thousands of materials in the average household that could be swallowed and an outline of the best current knowledge of treatment for ingestion of these materials were compiled and placed in each of the participating hospitals. In each of these major hospitals, an attending pediatrician was designated as poisoning control officer or a liaison person to the central committee and was made responsible for seeing that the necessary equipment and supplies were readily available in the emergency rooms, for orienting the hospital staff to the problem of poisoning, and for seeing that the treatment and response of all patients were reported to the Chicago Board of Health.

The board followed up the cases of accidental poisoning in children in an effort to prevent the occurrence of poisoning in siblings of the patients or the recurrence in the patient. The reports were then mechanically tabulated, and the resulting information on the types of poisons, on how the cases of poisoning occurred, and on the treatments and results obtained was made available to the participating hospitals through the central committee. The details of this program have been previously described.[1]

Programs in Other Poison Control Centers

Similar poison control centers, differing in many details of administration but preserving the general principle of the sharing of centralized sources of information on the treatment and prevention of poisoning, have since developed in many other cities. As of April, 1956, there were 18 metropolitan areas with centers in operation. As of October, 1956, there were poison control centers in the following cities and towns:

Albany, N.Y., Atlantic City, N.J., Baltimore, Boston, Buffalo, Chicago, Denver, Durham, N.C., Grand Rapids, Mich., Harrisburg, Pa., Indianapolis, Kansas City, Mo., Lancaster, Pa., Louisville, Ky., Memphis, Tenn., Milwaukee, Montclair, N.J., Newark, N.J., New Bedford, Mass., New York, Nutley, N.J., Oklahoma City, Phoenix, Ariz., Rochester, N.Y., Seattle, Springfield, Ill., Syracuse, N.Y., Washington, D.C., and Worcester, Mass.

There is also a network of poison control centers in 15 cities in Florida, which makes a total of 44 centers in the United States. The manner of organization of each center varies with the community and its medical and related facilities. The core agency around which the program operates may be a health department, a hospital, a medical college, a local medical society, or a combination of these. The number of agencies and institutions participating in these centers may vary from one to over a hundred different ones. The general purpose of the centers is to minimize the damage from potentially toxic substances by improving and extending efforts for the prevention and treatment of poisoning.

The specific objectives of the program in the area of treatment may include improvement and dissemination of knowledge regarding potentially toxic substances and the various measures of general and specific treatment required in the hospital, the physician's office, and the patient's home, as well as efforts to make resources for treatment more readily and widely available and to stimulate research for improved methods of treatment for poisoning by the more common and dangerous chemicals. This would also include methods for making the initial treatment, primarily the proper first-aid measures, more prompt and effective.

PREVENTION

In the area of prevention, the specific objectives may include the development of fuller information regarding the distribution, type, and toxicity of the various poisons, as well as regarding the circumstances in which the poisons are most likely to exert their deleterious effects. Measures for disseminating information and evaluating the most effective, preventive measures, with the aid of professional and lay persons and groups throughout the community, should be an integral part of the activities of poison control centers.

Depending on the size and on the medical, educational, toxicologic, and related facilities of the community, any or all of the following agencies or institutions may participate in various aspects of the program of the center: hospitals, local health departments, State health departments, medical or related professional societies or associations (both general and specialized if the concern is with the problem of poisoning), medical, pharmacy, and veterinary colleges, medical examiners' or coroners' offices, laboratories, and lay groups, such as safety councils, parent-teacher associations, service clubs, welfare councils, and others.

The provision of 24-hour service has posed a problem for some of the centers, but most of them have met this challenge successfully. They have generally utilized the emergency room services already established in many of the hospitals, with slight modification. The information on the medical treatment of poisoning relayed over the telephone consists primarily of comments on the type and effect of the toxic substance contained in the chemicals swallowed and of suggestions for therapeutic procedures. The information on medical treatment is given to the physician treating the patient, and it is made clear that this information is advisory or consultative in nature. The final responsibility for accepting, modifying, or rejecting the advice given over the telephone remains with the physician treating the patient. Telephone inquiries from parents are answered with first-aid instructions and advice to contact their family physician at once or, if this is not possible or feasible, to bring the patient to the poison control center for immediate treatment there—treatment being available on a 24-hour-a-day basis through emergency-room and hospital facilities.

Various types of records, ranging from a simple postcard report form for physicians to fill out to a four-page mimeographed follow-up form for health department personnel, are used in the various centers. Provisions for tabulating, summarizing, and analyzing these reports are generally made. This information would then be available for the education of both lay and professional persons, locally and nationally, to aid in improving methods of prevention and treatment. Several centers issue periodic releases or bulletins warning of new or increased toxic hazards that may have come to their attention, recommending new methods of treatment, or suggesting preventive activities.

A subcommittee on poisoning of the American Academy of Pediatrics maintains a loose, centralized affiliation with all of the poison control centers, and the subcommittee chairman has interlocking membership on the Committee on Toxicology of the American Medical Association and is the staff associate of the subcommittee on chemical poisons of the American Public Health Association, so that an informal framework for correlating the activities of the centers exists. Thus, there may be opportunities for using the experience of several or all of the centers on specific research problems. One such project, the evaluation of the most effective method of treating poisoning due to kerosene ingestion, is already in early phases of operation.

1. Press, E., and Mellins, R. B.: Poisoning Control Program, *Am.J. Pub.Health.* 44:1515–1525 (Dec.) 1954. Mellins, R. B.; Christian, J. R.; and Bundesen, H. N.: Natural History of Poisoning in Childhood, *Pediatrics* 17:314–325 (March) 1956.

4. Epidemiologic Investigations

The Epidemiology of Atherosclerotic Coronary Heart Disease*

JEREMIAH STAMLER, M.D.

MEDICAL RESEARCH has three basic methods for attacking a disease of unknown or obscure etiology. The first, and oldest, is the clinical-pathologic method. It involves the study of sick people while living (clinical investigation) and after death (pathologic investigation).

The second method is animal experimentation. Its prerequisite is the successful reproduction of the particular disease in experimental animals.

Both these methods have made highly important contributions to the solution of the atherosclerosis problem.[1-9 and 9a]

The third method, under discussion in this writing, is the epidemiologic method. This has had a resurgence recently as a fruitful approach to the so-called degenerative diseases, the major Public Health problems today.

DEFINITION OF THE EPIDEMIOLOGIC METHOD

Epidemiology is the study of disease in populations.[2, 9-11] Thus its focus is distinctly different from that of clinical investigation. The latter is generally not concerned with the population of origin of patients. At most this is a matter of incidental interest to clinical investigation. Its chief concern is to achieve a more detailed and profound description and analysis of disease by making a study of its clinical-pathologic characteristics in a series of patients.

The framework of reference of epidemiology is different. Its concern is not with sick individuals but with populations, patterns of disease in populations, and the factors responsible for those patterns. Its approach, therefore, is complementary to that of clinical investiga-

* Reprinted, with omission of 23 figures, by permission, from the May and June, 1959, issues of *Postgraduate Medicine*, Vol. 25, Nos. 5 and 6, pp. 610–622, 685–701. The work by the author summarized in this review was supported by the Chicago Heart Association and the National Heart Institute, United States Public Health Service (H2984 and H4917). The author is Director, Chronic Disease Control Division, Board of Health, City of Chicago, Chicago, Illinois, and was formerly an Established Investigator of the American Heart Association in the Cardiovascular Department, Medical Research, Michael Reese Hospital (Louis N. Katz, M.D., Director), Chicago, Illinois.

tion. It is based on the premise that important leads to the etiology of disease—the central problem of medicine—may be obtained by getting answers to such questions as: Is there more of a given disease today than there was 50 years ago (disease in time) and, if so, why? Is there more of a given disease among Americans than among British, or Italians, or Guatemalans, or Japanese, or Nigerians (disease in space) and, if so, why? Are there varying patterns of a given disease among different population strata of a given country, e.g., by age, sex, place of residence (North versus South, urban versus rural), racial and ethnic origin, income, occupation, smoking and dietary habits, and so on, and, if there are differences, or similarities, why?

In attempting to obtain answers to these questions on patterns of disease occurrence, epidemiology collects data from a variety of sources and in a variety of ways. These include mortality statistics, medical examiners' and coroners' reports, life insurance findings, hospital and clinic records, autopsy analyses, and data from general and special surveys of disease in various strata of the population (Selective Service System findings, National Health Survey reports, labor and management medical observations, special research studies on prevalence and incidence of disease). As in all other research areas, each of these types of epidemiologic data presents its special problems, with which the investigator must be thoroughly familiar if he is to proceed effectively. The idea that epidemiology is confined to working with vital statistics data on mortality is a gross misconception.

The collection of data on the patterns of occurrence of disease in populations may be designated *descriptive* epidemiology, and the attempt to account for these patterns *analytic* epidemiology. This distinction serves to emphasize that the answers to inquiries concerning patterns of disease occurrence are not ends in themselves. They are not decisive objects of epidemiologic research. Rather they are only means to an end. Since the concern is to solve problems of the etiology of disease, the decisive task is to account for observed patterns of disease. Hence the *why* in the foregoing questions.

The delineation of patterns of disease occurrence leads inexorably to a search for etiologic factors responsible for these patterns. Once epidemiology knows that coronary disease occurs much more frequently in middle-aged American men than in women, as is the case, the decisive question arises, why? Similarly, if it is established (as seems to be the case) that coronary disease is relatively rare in middle-aged Guatemalans, or South African Bantus, or Japanese, and is relatively common in middle-aged North Americans, the problem clearly and critically presents itself, why? What are the causative factors responsible for this? The delineation of patterns of disease in populations serves, therefore, to pose a series of crucial questions for further research.

This further research is pursued by epidemiologic, clinical-patho-logic and animal-experimental means, that is, by all three methodol-ogies. For its part, epidemiology seeks to account for observed patterns of disease occurrence by studying the role of multiple factors that possibly may be operative, for example, income, occupation, place of residence, housing conditions, diet, physical activity, smoking, cli-mate, mores, tensions, stresses, antecedent diseases, race, ethnic origin, heredity, and genetics. In assessing these variables, several of which may play a significant etiologic role, epidemiology seeks to determine which one, if any, is decisive in the process of causation. It also concerns itself with how these factors may operate to produce their morbid effects. Income, for example, may be meaningful as a factor in disease causation by virtue of its relation to occupation, or habitual physical activity of work, or nutritional status. Similarly, race may be significant, not because of inherited genetic factors but be-cause of associated socioeconomic conditions. Clearly these complex questions posed by epidemiology can be successfully clarified only by extensive cross-fertilization among many disciplines—sociology, eco-nomics, anthropology, psychology, genetics—and by close coordina-tion among medical investigators utilizing the clinical-pathologic, animal-experimental, and epidemiologic approaches.

In studying the relationships between possible causative factors and the occurrence of disease, analytic epidemiology seeks to deline-ate positive and negative correlations. Thus specific hypotheses are both formulated and put to an initial test, e.g., concerning the role of diet in the causation of atherosclerotic coronary heart disease. It is essential to emphasize that the delineation of such correlations, posi-tive and negative, between possible etiologic agents and occurrence of disease cannot constitute demonstration of cause-and-effect rela-tionships. Such correlations obtained by descriptive-analytic epidemi-ology can by their cumulative impact become indicative of cause-and-effect relationships but they cannot prove them. Further work is necessary. Among other things the epidemiologic data must be evalu-ated in relation to clinical-pathologic and animal-experimental findings concerning the given disease. The indispensability of this interdigita-tion, this shuttling back and forth among the three basic methodologies, is one of the crucial lessons to be learned from the history of medical advance. It is a basic research principle.

It is an equally valid principle that theories of causation—derived from descriptive-analytic epidemiology, clinical-pathologic studies and animal-experimental findings—must sooner or later be critically tested by deliberate planned intervention in the mode of life of human population groups, that is, by *experimental* epidemiology. This in-volves controlled alteration of a specific variable or set of variables, with evaluation of the resultant effects on occurrence of disease.

The success of experimental epidemiology then creates the basis for *applied* epidemiology, the application of new knowledge throughout the population in order to prevent and eliminate disease. This constitutes the acid test of the validity of theories that are concerned with causation.

With these general remarks about the epidemiologic method as background, consideration can now be given to the epidemiology of atherosclerotic coronary heart disease.

ATHEROSCLEROSIS

First a few words are necessary to assure clarity concerning the entity under discussion, which is atherosclerosis, and the distinction between arteriosclerosis and atherosclerosis.[1] As pathology long ago noted, arteriosclerosis is a generic term which embraces several pathologic processes, almost certainly of different etiologies, it might be wiser to use the plural, arterioscleroses.

Atherosclerosis is a specific entity. It is one among the arterioscleroses but by far the most important in respect to morbidity and mortality, not only because of its frequency of occurrence in severe form (at least among the populations of certain countries) but also because of its morphologic peculiarities which lead frequently to the production of serious illness. It is primarily an intimal lesion which impinges on and narrows the arterial lumen with resultant tissue ischemia. It tends to slough, ulcerate, and become a nidus for thrombus formation with closure of the vessel and tissue infarction. The atherosclerotic plaque also tends to become vascularized by capillaries which may bleed with resultant intimal swelling, closure of the vessel, and tissue infarction. All these pathologic features, together with the frequency of occurrence of this process in severe form among middle-aged and elderly persons in a country like the United States, account for the fact that atherosclerosis is the most important of the arterioscleroses and the major producer of mortality in the United States today.

A few other aspects of the pathology of atherosclerosis merit brief attention. Among populations frequently victimized by severe atherosclerotic disease, the process tends to begin in childhood, decades before it becomes manifest as clinical disease. This cardinal fact concerning the natural history of atherosclerosis has been extensively documented in studies on American autopsy material, white and Negro.[12, 13] Its recognition serves to emphasize the important principle, particularly valid for the so-called chronic degenerative diseases, that departure from health is a continuing process. With the years the process of lesion formation tends to proceed inexorably, so that by age 25 many Americans, especially men, have grossly detectable coronary atherosclerosis. By age 45 or 55 this sclerosis is severe in a high percentage of the male population.[2, 12-14]

PRECLINICAL AND CLINICAL ATHEROSCLEROSIS

Fortunately, extensive morphologic lesions frequently exist without the development of frank clinical manifestations. Hence it is necessary to speak of atherosclerosis and atherosclerotic disease. The well-known iceberg analogy serves to point up the distinction between the two: Clinical atherosclerotic disease is the visible one-tenth of the total iceberg; nine-tenths of the whole entity never reveals itself during life.

What factors are responsible for the qualitative change from the occult, submerged, preclinical process to frank clinical disease? Unquestionably part of the answer is quantity, the extent and degree of atherosclerosis. It has been conclusively demonstrated that any group of persons with clinical atherosclerotic disease (e.g., coronary heart disease) has more severe atherosclerosis than a group without clinical manifestations. But it is moot whether quantity is the whole answer. Thus the transition from preclinical to clinical disease is frequently a resultant of the so-called complications of atherosclerosis, e.g., thrombosis on plaques or hemorrhage into plaques, producing vessel closure and tissue infarction. The etiology of these complications may be different from that of the atherosclerotic plaques per se. The study of this problem is therefore an important aspect of atherosclerosis research. It should be kept in mind, however, that these processes are complications of atherosclerosis, particularly of severe atherosclerosis. Were there no severe atherosclerosis there would rarely be complications. It is essential, therefore, to keep the research focus on the central and primary problem, the etiology of atherosclerosis.

ECONOMICALLY LESS DEVELOPED COUNTRIES VERSUS THE UNITED STATES

This paper is concerned with the epidemiology of atherosclerosis and atherosclerotic disease in the coronary arteries. This focus has a threefold basis. (1) Coronary atherosclerosis is the chief producer of morbidity and mortality. (2) The bulk of the available epidemiologic data deals with coronary atherosclerosis. Information is limited on the epidemiology of atherosclerosis in other arterial beds. (3) The correlation between clinical coronary heart disease and morphologic coronary atherosclerosis is of a high order. At least 90% of all cases of coronary disease have marked atherosclerosis as the underlying pathologic process.[2, 12-17] Therefore, data on the occurrence of clinical coronary disease reflect closely the occurrence of morphologic atherosclerosis of severe degree in a population. This correlation does not necessarily hold to a high degree for disease at other sites. With clinical cerebrovascular disease ("strokes"), for example, it is difficult to differentiate among cerebral embolism, hemorrhage, and thrombosis. These are processes having different etiopathologic bases.[10, 18-20] Recent pathologic studies indicate that cerebral hemorrhage in hypertensive persons may be a complication not chiefly of atherosclerosis, as has been widely believed, but of a hypertensive nonatherosclerotic lesion in the small cerebral vessels. Unlike coronary disease, therefore, it is probably not correct to assume that prevalence and incidence rates for cerebrovascular disease reflect the occurrence of severe cerebral atherosclerosis in a given population. This invalid assumption has tended to obscure understanding concerning epidemiologic trends. For valid comparisons cerebral thrombosis (usually atherosclerotic in its pathologic basis) would have to be separated from the heterogeneous cerebrovascular disease grouping.

Consideration may now be given to the available data on the epidemiology of atherosclerotic coronary heart disease and to the meaning of these facts for the problem of causation. It is best to begin with the data on patterns of atherosclerosis in different countries, particularly countries with marked contrasts in the modes of life of their populations, e.g., the United States versus the economically less developed nations of Africa, Asia, and Latin America. Differences between the economically under-developed countries and the United States are multiple and complex—racial, ethnic, climatic, socioeconomic, nutritional, cultural, Public Health, medical, and so on. It is essential for epidemiologic research to concern itself with all these variables, and to focus on those which from initial observation seem to be more closely correlated with recorded patterns of disease occurrence.

Extensive data are available concerning the observed patterns of disease—data collected a generation or two ago as well as recently. The accumulated data are (with a few exceptions of questionable validity) remarkably consistent in their findings.[1, 2, 4, 5, 10, 13, 21, 22] Marked variations exist in the frequency of occurrence of atherosclerotic coronary heart disease in different countries. In the regions less developed economically, clinical coronary disease and severe morphologic atherosclerosis with myocardial infarction at postmortem examination are rarities at all ages. Data leading to this conclusion are available from China, Ceylon, Costa Rica, East Africa, Egypt, Guatemala, India, Indonesia, Iraq, Israel, Malaya, Mexico, Nigeria, Okinawa, South Africa, and Uganda.

THE ROLE OF DIET

What is responsible for this phenomenon? More than 20 years ago it was suggested that life-span pattern of diet is the decisive causative factor.[23, 24] Recent work amply supports this concept. In these economically less developed countries, habitual diets are much different from ours. The overwhelming mass of the population subsists on cheap, high-energy cereal and root foods.[2, 4, 5, 9, 10, 21-24] The diet is low in calories, empty calories (those derived from processed, refined foods high in energy value and low in essential nutrients, foods such as sugar, white flour breads and pastries, or processed fats[28]), foods of animal origin, total fats and saturated fats, cholesterol, refined carbohydrates, total proteins and animal proteins.[9, 10, 25-27]

In recent years this twofold correlation between diet and disease has been extended to a threefold correlation, among habitual diet, plasma cholesterol-lipid-liporotein levels, and occurrence of coronary disease. These peoples, subsisting chiefly on cereal-root diets, have low levels of serum cholesterol and little atherosclerotic coronary disease, clinical or morphologic. This correlation has been consistently observed in every economically less developed country studied to date. It has also been found to hold for Spain, Italy, and Japan, countries somewhat higher in the scale of economic development whose populations en masse nevertheless subsist on cereal-root diets.[1, 2, 4, 5, 9, 10, 21, 22]

In addition to the foregoing findings, other data are available indicating that such variables as race, geography, and climate cannot account for the international epidemiologic patterns. In several countries different social classes have been studied, including the more prosperous urban upper strata whose patterns of diet and physical activity differ from those of the population en masse of their own countries and resemble those prevailing in the United States. Data from Guatemala, South Africa, Egypt, India, Japan, Italy, and Spain indicate that the higher-income groups exhibit levels of serum cholesterol and occurrence rates of coronary disease considerably higher than the bulk of the population.[2, 4, 5, 10, 21-23]

Data are also available concerning the effects of migration, e.g., on Yemenite Jews migrating from Arabia to Israel, Italians from Italy to the United States, Japanese from Japan to Hawaii or the United States.[2, 10] In all cases the attendant socioeconomic changes, including the change in habitual nutrition toward a diet higher in total calories, total fats, saturated fats, and cholesterol, were associated with a rise in serum cholesterol levels and atherosclerotic disease incidence rates.[2, 10]

All of these data are of great importance because they suggest that racial and ethnic origin, geography, and climate are not significantly responsible for patterns of coronary disease occurrence in large population groups. They suggest that socioeconomic factors are critically important. They lend further support to the concept that habitual diet is a decisive influence.

DATA ON 22 COUNTRIES

In addition to the foregoing international epidemiologic findings, an over-all analysis of 1950 data for 22 countries demonstrated statistically significant correlations between death rates and intakes of total calories, total fats, and animal fats.[29] A negative correlation was noted between intake of vegetable lipid and death rates attributed to arteriosclerotic plus degenerative heart disease. This finding is particularly intriguing in view of recent data demonstrating low serum cholesterol levels in American vegetarians and in Yugoslavs subsisting on diets high in vegetable oils.[30, 31] It is also of interest in connection with observation on the reduction of cholesteremia by substitution of unsaturated vegetable oils for saturated fats in American-type diets.[32-36] All these findings emphasize the need for further work on the relationship of high intakes of unsaturated vegetable and marine oils in some countries to the observed patterns of serum cholesterol and coronary disease occurrence.

The cited study also noted a positive correlation between protein intake and arteriosclerotic heart disease death rates.[29] This fact offers a concrete example of the previously mentioned principle concerning evaluation of the cause-and-effect significance of statistical correlations and the need to go beyond the given data in making such an assessment. This particular positive correlation was to be expected once positive correlations were recorded between death rates and total calorie, total fat, and animal fat ingestion. For these intercorrelations among a number of nutritional factors reflect shifts with improved socioeconomic conditions from grain-root to meat-dairy product dietetics. From the nature of the ingested foodstuffs, levels of intake of total calories, total fat, animal fat, cholesterol, total protein, and animal protein would almost inevitably be intercorrelated.

The question therefore becomes: Does the statistical correlation between death rates and levels of total protein and animal protein consumption reflect a cause-and-effect relationship between protein intake and atherosclerotic disease? These data pose this question but cannot answer it. The answer must be sought from other available evidence. Extensive experimental data indicate that this is not the case. On the contrary, they suggest that high protein intake may afford a partial protection against the hypercholesteremic and atherogenic effects of high-fat, high-cholesterol diets.[1, 2, 37-39] On the other hand, extensive clinical-pathologic and animal-experimental data indicate that the correlation between death rates and intakes of total calories, total fats and animal fats is significant in respect to cause and effect.

In this cited study on diets and death rates in 22 countries in 1950 a considerable spread was noted in the data.[29] For several economically developed countries with total fat intakes in the range of 30 to 40% of total calories, age-specific death rates varied from 300 to 600 or more per 100,000 population (Austria, West Germany, Sweden, Norway, Denmark, the Netherlands, Australia, Canada, Finland); the figure for the United States was 739 per 100,000. The populations of some of these countries, for example, Sweden and Finland, exhibited levels of fat intake and coronary disease occurrence rates approximating those observed in the United States. On the other hand a few of these countries manifested middle-aged death rates considerably lower than those for the United States.

Based on such findings, several reports recently challenged the validity of the correlation between intake of lipids (total and saturated) and occurrence of atherosclerotic coronary disease.[29, 40] In evaluating these critiques,[41] it is appropriate to note that the broad statistical data, despite their recognized limitations, verified significant over-all correlations between death rates and intakes of total calories, total fats and saturated fats. These findings, therefore, do not refute the validity of the correlation indicated by a vast array of international epidemiologic data. They merely suggest that the correlation among diet, serum cholesterol, and coronary disease is not a simple one-to-one correlation (see below).

Further, a number of the countries, particularly Scandinavia and the Low Countries, were in 1950 only a few years away from the privations of World War II with its significant restrictions in diet and concomitant declines in arteriosclerotic heart disease death rates.[1, 2] It is highly possible, aside from other considerations, that these effects of World War II still found expression in 1950, particularly since atherosclerosis is a disease which develops over many years.

Moreover, the observed patterns of mortality for these European countries and the United States all range on the high side of a distribution curve for middle-aged population groups, particularly in comparison with the economically under-developed countries. Irrespective of the observed differences in rates, therefore, coronary heart disease is unquestionably a major Public Health problem in these European countries, in contrast to the under-developed nations.

Finally, these differences indicate the need for further detailed field studies, going beyond the over-all national vital statistics and dietary data, studies of the hospital-clinical-pathologic survey type on diet, serum cholesterol, and coronary disease. The several such investigations accomplished in recent years have in fact yielded impressive data supporting the theory of the key—but not exclusive—role of diet.

The findings contained in recent reports from Finland are particularly noteworthy.[42-44] It was found that coronary disease incidence was high in Finland, higher than in any other European country. Further, data suggested that cardiovascular disease was more prevalent in eastern than in western Finland. Serum cholesterol levels were also found to be unusually high, particularly in eastern Finland.

Dietary surveys revealed similar intakes of total fat in western and eastern Finland during summer and winter—in the range of 99 to 105 gm. per person per day (34 to 35% of total calories), with a high intake of saturated fats. Although significant differences in fat intake were not noted between east and west Finland, it was found that intakes of iodine, ascorbic acid, and vitamin E were significantly greater in the west. The low iodine content of the diets in east Finland was associated with a high incidence of endemic goiter with hyperthyroidism, and with high serum cholesterol levels. It was suggested that these dietary patterns, both because of the high content of total fats-saturated fats and because of the low content of iodine, might be a key factor responsible for high serum cholesterol levels and high coronary mortality in Finland in general and in the eastern part of Finland in particular.[42-44]

These findings offer pointed examples of the results to be obtained from a multifaceted epidemiologic approach to the etiology of atherosclerotic coronary heart disease, an approach based on a recognition of the interplay between exogenous (nutritional et al.) and endogenous (hormonal et al.) factors in the etiology and pathogenesis of this disease. It is within the context of this approach that the thesis is advanced of the key—but not exclusive—role of diet in the causation of this disease.

EFFECTS OF WORLD WAR II

As already suggested, this conclusion is amply supported by the findings of time-trends of diet and disease in Scandinavia and the Low Countries during World War II. The marked reduction in intake of total calories, total fats, saturated fats, and cholesterol imposed by German occupation was associated with a gross decline in arteriosclerotic heart disease mortality rates. Similar findings were reported from Leningrad during the World War II siege and from Central Europe during the famine years following World War I.

UNITED STATES TRENDS, 1910 TO 1955

This whole problem of the trend of atherosclerotic disease over the years and its relationship, if any, to evolving dietary patterns has recently received the attention of several investigators.

American and British data suggest a marked increase in middle-age mortality rates in these two countries in recent decades.[2, 4, 10, 11, 40, 45-47] Here it is necessary to emphasize that the evaluation of these trends is complicated by a host of statistical and methodologic problems, some of them permanently beyond precise quantitation because of the nature of the data. Hence it is not surprising that disagreements arise concerning the actual degree and extent of the apparent increases in coronary disease mortality.

In any attempt to arrive at a tentative judgment in this matter the following facts stand out. Cardiovascular-renal death rates (because of problems inherent in the available statistics for arteriosclerotic heart disease per se, the broad term, cardiovascular-renal diseases, is used), for middle-aged white men in the United States have been high throughout the last 30 to 40 years. During these decades the rates for middle-aged white men rose to even higher levels. In contrast those for middle-aged white women declined markedly.[47] The question therefore arises: If the increase in rates for white men is chiefly an apparent one, due merely to changes over the years in diagnostic acumen and death certificate procedures, as some have suggested, why have these changes produced a rising trend for men only? Is there a differential in diagnostic acumen and certification procedures for men versus women, leading to a rise in rates for the former and a decline for the latter? This hardly seems tenable.

As is well known, arteriosclerotic coronary heart disease is common in middle-aged American men, whereas it is remarkably rare in premenopausal women. This sex differential in susceptibility is in the order of from 5 to 25:1 for middle-aged white persons.[1, 2, 10, 48-51]

Given this well-known fact it is not difficult to deduce that the 1920 to 1955 trend of cardiovascular-renal deaths of middle-aged white men versus middle-aged white women in the United States reflects the following: for men, a sizable rise in coronary disease rates, leading to a net increase in cardiovascular-renal disease mortality despite declining death rates for infectious diseases involving the cardiovascular-renal system; for women, continued low coronary disease rates, with little or no rise, and a marked decline in death rates due to the puerperal and infectious diseases of the cardiovascular-renal system, resulting in a gross decrease in over-all cardiovascular-renal death rates.

This tentative conclusion, that coronary disease death rates for middle-aged white men increased sizably, is borne out by other data. While life expectancy at birth for Americans has risen by about 20 years since 1900, life expectancy of white men at age 50 has increased only 2.2 years. In view of the great advances during these decades in the prevention of death in middle age due to pneumonia, tuberculosis, syphilitic and rheumatic heart diseases, and subacute bacterial endocarditis, a greater increase in life expectancy at age 50 might have been anticipated. Almost certainly this absence of a marked improvement is attributable chiefly to an increasing mortality from coronary heart disease in middle-aged white men.[51]

If the foregoing analysis is sound, the qualitative judgment must be accepted that a true increase actually has occurred in mortality among middle-aged white American men due to atherosclerotic coronary heart disease.

What are the factors possibly responsible for this trend? Certainly many changes have occurred in the United States during this period. There has been steadily increasing urbanization, mechanization, sedentary living, use of tobacco, etc. Less and less human energy is expended in work. Muscle power is more and more replaced by non-human energy, from coal, oil, water, or atomic power sources. This, of course, is different from the economically under-developed countries, which as yet have relatively little nonhuman energy and must produce the necessities of life in the old way, by the sweat of the brow. Undoubtedly some people still do heavy work in the United States, but smaller and smaller percentages, compared with previous decades. Many employees, e.g., factory operatives, may have work patterns that are exacting, intense, concentrated, and fatiguing, but the fact remains that diversified large-muscle activity is no longer widespread in our country.

Those are some of the changes. Many observers also believe that life has become more hectic, complex, competitive, insecure, and stressful in the 20th century, particularly since World War I. If this is true, what relationship does this have, if any, to the apparent increase in coronary disease in middle-aged white American men during this 40-year period?

What about evolving dietary patterns? Here again, serious methodologic limitations exist, due not only to a relative paucity of data but to the particular scarcity of information concerning diets in different regions of the country and among different racial, ethnic, and socioeconomic strata at different times (during peace and war, prosperity and depression). With these shortcomings in mind it is possible to delineate the following broad trends. Meat consumption has generally tended to be relatively high in the United States and has remained so, much higher even than in most other economically developed countries.[2, 9, 10, 52-54] Another long-standing, unique American dietary characteristic has been the large intake of butter, lard, and other predominantly saturated fats. This has apparently been further accentuated. In recent decades the composition of ingested saturated fat has tended to change as a result of the introduction in 1910 of the catalytic hydrogenation process for converting vegetable oils into plastic shortenings and margarines. As a consequence of this process, which saturates double bonds, these fats have a high percentage of trans fatty acid isomers (23 to 42%) and a low content of essential fatty acids (2 to 8%).[2, 9, 10, 55, 56] Unless enriched, they are practically devoid of other essential nutrients, e.g., fat-soluble vitamins; hence they are an "excellent" source of empty calories.

Intakes of milk, dairy products, and eggs have also exhibited significant increases. A marked rise in ingestion of refined sugars (100% empty calories) is another important long-term development in the American diet—from 8 lb. per person per year in 1820, to 30 in 1860, 66 in 1900, and 95 today. All these upward trends have been associated with a steady decline in grain consumption of such marked proportions that for tens of millions of Americans today bread can hardly be designated the "staff of life."

A qualitative metamorphosis in flour also has occurred over the decades, that is, a decline in percentage utilization of whole meal. The resultant nutritional losses have been only partially compensated by the limited bread-enrichment measures of recent years. The increased consumption of highly processed, refined foods has also involved a decline in the intake of bulk that is only partially compensated by the increased ingestion of fruits and vegetables. Little work has been done on the possible implications of this trend for health and disease.

Viewed over all, these trends are, within the limitations noted, highly suggestive of a definite increase (relative and absolute) in consumption of total fats, saturated fats, cholesterol and empty calories. This is the path our country has apparently taken nutritionally in evolving its unique pattern of dietary imbalance.

This conclusion, it should be noted, is not shared by all investigators.[2, 57, 58] Some workers emphasize that little information is available on food actually consumed, as distinct from data on food available for consumption. They further stress the difficulty of estimating waste of fats in cooking. Based on these and other considerations they suggest that there has been little or no increase in fat consumption in 20th-century America. These writers are also skeptical about the data indicating an increase in coronary disease incidence in middle-aged men over these years. Thus these authors imply that both fat intake and coronary disease incidence have been high since the turn of the century. If these are actually the facts, and the two phenomena are so correlated, this certainly is not inconsistent with the nutritional-metabolic theory.

In this connection one other problem merits attention. Even if fat intake has increased since the turn of the century, it was, as already noted, high even then. If coronary disease incidence in middle-aged men was much lower then, as some data suggest, why this lack of correlation? This question highlights the need, in evaluating the trends over the last 40 to 60 years, to focus attention not only on evolving dietary patterns but also on the interplay between diet and psychologic stress, and even diet and large-muscle activity.

Thus the apparent changes with time in patterns of diet and disease may or may not be significantly interrelated as to cause and effect. As already suggested, these decades witnessed manifold changes in urbanization, automobile transportation, cigarette consumption, sedentary work, and so on, phenomena emphasizing the need for multifactorial analysis of atherosclerotic disease causation. Because of these complexities and the limitations of both the mortality and the nutritional data, plus the insurmountable obstacles to their further delineation, extreme caution is essential in interpreting them; the danger of "reading" cause and effect into the statistical correlation is particularly acute. With these reservations it is not inappropriate to note both the suggestive positive correlations and their consistency with extensive findings from other sources. Again it is valid to conclude that the concepts of the nutritional-metabolic theory are certainly not contradicted by these data.

THE UNITED STATES AN EPIDEMIOLOGIC "LABORATORY"

Recent years have also witnessed a definite quickening of epidemiologic research of a different type in the United States. It has come to be widely recognized that this country, with its large population stratified by region, occupation, income, ethnic, and racial background, and so on, constitutes an excellent epidemiologic "laboratory." Based on this approach, our group late in 1954 initiated a long-term investigation on the epidemiology of the major cardiovascular-renal diseases in the city of Chicago, in the State of Illinois, and in the United States.

The first phase of this study involved analyses of 1951 and 1953 mortality data for specific groups in the population stratified by age, sex, race, nationality, occupation, and place of residence (including urban-rural), with a particular focus on the middle decades of life.[9, 10, 47, 59-62] For present purposes the following findings assume particular significance. The death rates for arteriosclerotic heart disease were several-fold higher for middle-aged men than for middle-aged women, an observation fully in accord with extensive data from multiple sources.[1, 2, 9, 10, 48, 59] This is the most striking, unquestionably valid epidemiologic fact about coronary disease in the United States. The question forcefully presents itself, why? What is responsible for this gross sex differential?

SEX AND RACE DIFFERENTIALS

Before proceeding to touch briefly on this problem, two further facts, rarely alluded to, are worthy of note. This sex differential, so clearly apparent in the middle-aged white population of the

United States and other economically developed countries, is either absent or much less marked in economically less developed countries. This reduction in the ratio of coronary disease, male to female, comes about principally because of the lower rates which exist for males.[9, 10, 61]

Compare the findings in the middle-aged American Negro population. For the cardiovascular-renal diseases as a whole, virtually no sex differential is demonstrable for Negroes at any time from 1920 to 1955.[10, 47] Also, cardiovascular-renal death rates for Negroes are much higher than those for white persons. Further, arteriosclerotic heart disease death rates for middle-aged Negro men are about the same as or moderately lower than those for white men.[10, 59-61] Finally, arteriosclerotic heart disease death rates for middle-aged Negro women are considerably higher than those for white women. Consequently the sex differential in arteriosclerotic heart disease mortality rates for Negroes is less marked than for white persons. This lower sex ratio, it may be emphasized, is not the same qualitatively as that recorded for the economically less developed countries. In American Negroes it reflects chiefly higher rates in the denominator, i.e., higher rates for Negro women. In the economically less developed countries it reflects mainly lower rates in the numerator, i.e., lower rates for men. The end result in both cases is a similar ratio, but on a different basis.

What is the meaning of all these diverse findings in terms of the problem of causation of coronary disease? Based on present knowledge the following approaches and interpretations may be suggested. It is not likely that nutrition is a decisive factor responsible for the marked sex differential in coronary disease in middle-aged Americans, particularly white persons, since from the limited data available there do not appear to be marked differences in the dietary habits of American men and women. Obesity is, however, less prevalent in white women than in white men. Therefore the matter of dietary patterns in men and women merits further investigation, particularly in view of the paucity of reliable data.

Considerable evidence has accumulated indicating that gonadal function, specifically estrogenic secretion, is a key factor responsible for the high resistance of premenopausal women to atherosclerotic coronary heart disease. Detailed discussion of this aspect of the problem is beyond the scope of this paper, and the reader is referred to other published reports.[1, 2, 48-50]

Does diet enter the picture at all? Data from economically less developed countries indicate that diet is definitely involved. They suggest that a certain nutritional pattern, a habitual diet high in total calories, total fats, saturated fats and cholesterol, is essential to effectuate the metabolic prerequisites for atherogenesis in sizable sectors of a population. Without that dietary prerequisite, atherosclerotic disease rarely develops in middle-aged persons of either sex and the sex differential is absent or slight. With the dietary pre-requisite operating, the susceptible male sex is frequently victimized. The female sex, by virtue of the protection afforded through estro-genic secretion, tends to be particularly resistant in the pre-meno-pausal years. Thus the American woman, particularly the white woman, exhibits a relatively low coronary disease rate in middle age, although this rate is somewhat higher than that of her counterparts in economically less developed countries, where the potential for athero-genesis based on diet is generally low.

This interpretation of the data on the sex differential again em-phasizes the concept of an interplay between dietary (exogenous) and endocrine (endogenous) factors in the etiology and pathogenesis of atherosclerotic disease. It views diet as a key, but not exclusive, causative factor. It is in contradistinction to trends of thinking which demand an either-or, yes-no answer to the problem of the relationship between diet and atherosclerosis.

It is essential to add that the foregoing interpretation of the sex differential is in itself not adequate to account for the apparent find-ings on American Negroes. In this connection it must first be em-phasized that the data on coronary disease in American Negroes, particularly the findings indicating a relatively high arteriosclerotic heart disease rate in middle-aged Negro women, are as yet limited. Further studies on groups of varying geographic and socioeconomic backgrounds are needed to check validity of the data which are extant.

Suppose the validity of this observation that coronary disease rates are higher in middle-aged Negro women than in white women is tentatively accepted. What can be said about possible causes of this phenomenon? Is it related to differences in estrogenic secretion? This should be investigated, but it would appear to be an unlikely possi-bility. Is it related to other endocrine functions—thyroidal, pancre-atic? Is it related to differences in diet and different prevalences of obesity? Is it related to the greater prevalence of hypertension in Negro women? Is it related to a higher incidence in Negro women of genitourinary tract infections and complications of pregnancy (pre-eclampsia, eclampsia, and so on) with consequent renal damage and hypertension? Is it related to socioeconomic and sociocultural differences between the races, in income, employment status, psycho-logic stresses, strains and frustrations (e.g., those relating to dis-crimination and segregation)? All these questions can and should be explored by epidemiologic research in the years ahead.

Further studies are particularly essential in view of the confused, contradictory picture emerging from many papers on coronary disease in Negro men compared with white American men.[2, 10, 59-61] Some reports present data indicating that coronary disease has been occurring much less frequently in Negro men than in white men, an impression receiving some support from recent over-all national mortality data, particularly for men in age groups 55 and over. Other publications contain findings indicating no substantial difference between Negro and white men in age-specific coronary disease rates, particularly in middle age, an impression supported by recent mortality data from large northern cities. These findings are not necessarily mutually exclusive. Rather they may reflect real differences in disease patterns within the Negro population based on socioeconomic differences prevailing during particular decades, in North versus South, in urban versus rural areas, in different income-occupation groups. Additional research, especially in representative samples of the living population, is needed in order to clarify this set of problems.

HYPERTENSIVE DISEASE IN
AMERICAN NEGROES

While this lack of clarity exists concerning coronary disease in Negroes in the United States compared with white persons, it is an unquestioned fact that a gross differential exists between the two racial groups in morbidity and mortality due to hypertensive disease and its sequela, cerebral hemorrhage. The rate of occurrence of hypertensive disease is several-fold greater in Negroes than in white persons. This is the unassailable, outstanding, solid fact of our present knowledge concerning the epidemiology of hypertensive disease in the United States.[1, 2, 10, 18, 47, 59-63]

The highest death rates for cerebrovascular diseases are in Negro women. Also, in contrast to arteriosclerotic heart disease findings, there is an absence of any tendency in either white persons or Negroes for women to exhibit lower mortality rates from these causes. That is, for hypertensive disease there is no sex differential in favor of women. Thus, the data on the epidemiology of hypertensive and atherosclerotic diseases present markedly different patterns. This fact emphasizes the validity of the conclusion that there are two different disease processes etiologically.

It is this high rate of hypertensive disease and its complications (particularly cerebral hemorrhage) in Negroes that largely accounts for the fact that over-all cardiovascular-renal death rates have consistently been higher in Negroes than in white persons during the period 1920 to 1955.

The factors etiologically responsible for this phenomenon remain largely unknown, although it is not difficult to formulate meaningful hypotheses concerning possible variables (nutritional, infectious, psychologic, and so on) to be investigated epidemiologically.

In evaluating the foregoing data on the epidemiology of the

cardiovascular-renal diseases in the United States, it is important to ponder the apparently paradoxic nature of some of the findings. On the one hand, hypertensive disease is several times more prevalent in Negro than white men; on the other hand, the occurrence of atherosclerotic coronary disease is no greater, and may even be less, in Negro than white men. But it has been repeatedly shown experimentally and clinically that hypertension increases the risk of coronary disease. Why then do not Negro men, with so much more hypertension, have more coronary disease? This fascinating and important problem of the coexistence and interdigitation of these two diseases in various age-sex-race-socioeconomic groups certainly merits further investigation in various parts of the country.

URBAN AND RURAL AMERICANS

Several other intriguing sets of data emerged from the analyses of cardiovascular-renal disease mortality in Chicago and Illinois. Urban-rural comparisons revealed high arteriosclerotic heart disease death rates for the city of Chicago, for other Illinois municipalities, and for rural Illinois. However, a considerable differential was noted, namely, relatively high rates for Chicago and lower rates for other municipalities and rural areas.[2, 9, 10, 60] These observations are in accord with mortality data from other States.[64-67] They are also in agreement with the findings of a recent prospective living population study in North Dakota, indicating lower incidence rates of coronary heart disease in farmers compared with nonfarmers.[68] Here and elsewhere (see below), close correspondence obtains in the epidemiologic findings from mortality and living population studies—a point worthy of emphasis in view of the skeptical attitude assumed by some workers toward mortality data.

The question arises of the possible bearing of these urban-rural findings for problems of etiology. Available data indicate that dietary patterns are not different in urban and rural areas of the northern United States.[2, 9, 10, 68-73] In both areas the habitual diet apparently tends to be high in total calories, empty calories, total fats, saturated fats, refined carbohydrates, and cholesterol. If this is the case, it again becomes essential to delineate the interplay between diet and other factors—sedentary living habits, smoking, fatigue, psychologic stress, strain, tension, frustration, etc.—in the etiology of atherosclerotic disease.

In calling attention to this consideration, however, it is also essential to observe that both rural and urban rates are high, particularly when the distribution curve includes the countries of Europe, Asia, Africa, and Latin America. This fact suggests that the high calorie-lipid-cholesterol diet of most Americans, urban and rural, does in fact result in extensive atherosclerotic disease, irrespective of other factors possibly operating to produce moderate differential effects in urban versus rural areas.

NORTHERN URBAN AMERICANS OF DIFFERENT SOCIOECONOMIC STRATIFICATION

The epidemiologic analyses of Chicago mortality data also revealed that coronary heart disease death rates were high for middle-aged men (both Negro and white) of all occupation-income groups.[10, 59, 60] The toll from atherosclerotic disease was at least as great in lower-income strata as in more well-to-do strata, in blue-collar as in white-collar workers, in nonsedentary as in sedentary workers, in people with presumably less responsibility on the job as in persons with presumably more responsibility. Vital statistics data from other cities are essentially similar.[2, 10, 74, 75] In addition, studies of life insurance company mortality experience reveal similar results.[2, 9, 10, 65] Contrary to widely held opinion, lay and professional, coronary disease in the United States is not chiefly an affliction of the more educated, higher-income, more sedentary professional-executive-managerial-proprietary strata. Rather, it occurs with epidemic frequency among all strata of the urban middle-aged male population.

These findings of mortality-analyses have received substantial confirmation in several recent prospective studies on large living population groups.[2, 10, 76-81] A recently completed study by our group[80, 81] dealt with 756 men (737 white, 19 nonwhite) aged 50 to 59 employed by a Chicago utility corporation—virtually the entire labor force (96 per cent) of the company in this sex-age group. Of this base population, 601 (79 per cent) had been in the company's employ for 20 years or longer, 312 (41 per cent) for 30 years or longer.

This population was stratified by several socioeconomic variables —place of residence, education, income, veteran versus nonveteran, indoor versus outdoor work, sedentary verus nonsedentary work, white-collar versus blue-collar work, salaried versus wage work, specific major occupation categories. These subgroups all exhibited high prevalence rates for obesity and hypertension, with no significant differences being noted among them. Preliminary data indicate that they also had uniformly high prevalence rates for hypercholesteremia. They also manifested high incidence rates for coronary heart disease. With the exception of the difference between native-born and foreign-born workers, no significant differences were observed among these subgroups in incidence of coronary heart disease. Other long-term prospective epidemiologic studies of northern urban middle-aged white American men are recording similar findings on socioeconomic subgroups.[2, 10, 76-79]

These observations, particularly the high rates of obesity, hypertension, hypercholesteremia, and coronary disease among all these socioeconomic subgroups, suggest that these subgroups may possess in common certain factors of key significance for the etiology of coronary disease. These presumed common factors are apparently more decisive, in relation to disease causation, than the differences among these subgroups, differences related largely to varying modes of earning a living.

In any attempt to seek out these common factors, the investigative inquiry must inevitably be directed toward five possible areas: improper diet; physical inactivity (inadequate energy expenditure, large muscle activity, physical fitness, etc.); stress (tension, pace and complexity of modern life, frustration, fatigue, etc.); smoking; familial hereditary factors. The question arises: Are these factors—of possible etiologic significance in the genesis of atherosclerotic coronary heart disease—operative to a similar degree among subgroups of the northern urban white American middle-aged male population, subgroups of the kind already discussed?

Before considering this question it is appropriate to relate the aforementioned findings on disease incidence in these subgroups to international data. As already noted, in countries like Egypt, Guatemala, India, Italy, Japan, Spain and Great Britain, different socioeconomic strata of the population exhibit definite differences in coronary heart disease incidence. The more educated, higher-income, more sedentary executives-officials-administrators-professionals-proprietors tend to have higher rates. In contrast, no such differences are apparent among the different socioeconomic strata in the United States (at least insofar as this concerns strata among northern urban middle-aged white men).

What do these seemingly contradictory and paradoxic findings mean in relation to the possible role of the aforementioned factors in the etiology of atherosclerotic coronary heart disease? Let us consider first the possible role of diet, and assess whether these observations are inconsistent with the nutritional-metabolic theory of a key relationship between diet and atherosclerotic disease.

Nutritional patterns among the various socioeconomic strata are different in the United States compared with the aforementioned countries. Correspondingly, important differences exist in the dietary patterns of lower-income Americans and the poorer classes of all these countries (with the possible partial exception of Great Britain). Thus, in contrast to the populations en masse of most of these other countries, the economically less privileged in the United States have been consuming large amounts of meat, milk, eggs, fats and oils, white flour products, refined sugar and salt.[2, 9, 10, 52-54, 69-73] This seems to be generally true with limited possible exceptions (e.g., rural southern Negroes), at least since the end of the depression in about 1940. In contrast to the patterns prevailing in most of the other countries, the intakes of total calories and empty calories, saturated fats (animal and vegetable) and cholesterol among most lower-income Americans are not different from those of their upper-income compatriots. Among the many facts emerging from the latest 1955 comprehensive household surveys of the United States Department of Agriculture, the following may be cited briefly. For urban families in the income ranges of $2000 to $2,999 and $6000 to $7,999, only 18 per cent and 14 per cent respectively had food available for consumption totaling less than 3000 calories per person per day. Only 8 per cent and 3 per cent respectively had less than 36 per cent of total calories from fats; 72 per cent and 80 per cent respectively had more than 40 per cent of calories from fats (predominantly saturated fats).[10, 70]

Moreover, while lower-income Americans consume diets virtually as "rich" in the foregoing constitutents as those of their upper-income fellow citizens, a larger percentage of them tend to ingest suboptimal amounts of certain essential nutrients (vitamins, minerals, proteins, essential amino acids).[2, 9, 10, 69, 70, 82] Rather than eating "too well," as has been alleged, they tend to consume diets that are markedly unbalanced, unique combinations of overnutrition and undernutrition (literally, malnutrition).[83]

Such a unique dietary aberration may be especially pernicious in its potential for provoking the so-called degenerative cardiovascular-renal diseases, particularly atherosclerotic coronary heart disease. The widespread prevalence of this nutritional derangement among lower-income Americans may be a key factor making for extensive coronary heart disease morbidity and mortality among them.

The validity of this imbalance hypothesis needs to be tested in future investigations. Irrespective of the outcome of such studies, however, the evidence is substantial that most social strata in our country, regardless of socioeconomic rank, ingest a habitual diet that is potentially atherogenic. Therefore the finding that coronary heart disease is prevalent among most sections of the American middle-aged population does not contradict but rather lends additional strong support to the theory of a decisive interrelationship between life-span pattern of diet and atherogenesis.

SERUM CHOLESTEROL LEVELS IN
THE UNITED STATES

This concept is further reinforced by abundant data indicating that serum cholesterol levels tend to be high, compared with values observed in the peoples of many other countries, in virtually all strata of the middle-aged United States population.[2, 9, 10, 80, 81, 84]

These international epidemiologic findings are of great importance for another reason. They cast serious doubt on the validity of the standards commonly accepted in the United States for normal serum cholesterol concentration. They pose the questions: Is the life-span pattern of diet inducing a chronic low-grade hypercholesteremia in millions of Americans and thereby creating the metabolic preconditions for widespread atherogenesis? What is an optimal serum cholesterol level for maximal freedom from atherosclerotic disease over a maximal life span?

In this connection it is essential to appreciate that two approaches are identifiable to standards of normalcy for a biologic variable like serum cholesterol. The first, and hitherto predominant, approach in dealing with serum cholesterol concentration involves measurement of the variable in a sample of persons who at that moment are clinically well. The values obtained are then accepted as the mean and range of normal. The second—and, it would seem, more valid—approach to establishment of norms involves consideration of the long-term medical significance of a given value. In arriving at estimates for normal serum cholesterol, this approach requires posing of the question: What values (mean and range) are associated with maximal freedom from atherosclerotic disease during a maximal life span? The recent research data, epidemiologic, clinical-pathologic and animal-experimental, would seem to indicate the need for redefining the standards of normalcy for serum cholesterol, based on the latter approach.

Based on the extensive international epidemiologic data indicating a threefold correlation among habitual dietary patterns, serum cholesterol levels, and occurrence rates of coronary heart disease, the data demonstrating high mean values for serum cholesterol and high prevalence rates for hypercholesteremia in different socioeconomic strata of the United States population are certainly the expected ones. It was to be anticipated that most groups of middle-aged American men, since they ingest life-span diets high in total calories, total fats, saturated fats, and cholesterol, would exhibit high mean values for serum cholesterol concentration, high prevalence rates for hypercholesteremia, and high incidence rates for coronary heart disease.

It is essential that research in this field clearly confront the theoretic problem posed by these data. What is responsible for the distribution of serum cholesterol levels in the middle-aged American male population, and particularly the high mean values, compared with those of other peoples? Extensive data support the concept that this phenomenon is critically a by-product of habitual, life-span dietary patterns. Virtually no evidence to the contrary, convincing or otherwise, has been presented. Nor have any significant data been advanced to support other hypotheses accounting for these patterns of cholesteremia and the associated patterns of coronary disease incidence.

NATIVE-BORN AND FOREIGN-BORN AMERICANS

Available data on coronary heart disease incidence and mortality rates in native-born and foreign-born Americans are also consistent with the foregoing concepts. Death rates for foreign-born Chicago men tend to be high—considerably higher than those for the given nationalities in their countries of origin, but slightly lower than those for native-born Americans.[10, 61] Among the several nationality groups making up the foreign-born, Scandinavian-American, German-American, and Italian-American men tend to have lower mortality rates for coronary heart disease compared with all Chicago white American men.[10, 61]

As already indicated, the living population study in a Chicago utility company recently completed by our group permitted an analysis of coronary heart disease incidence in native-born and foreign-born and employees. Prevalence rates of obesity and hypertension in these two groups were essentially similar.[81] The marked difference in coronary heart disease incidence rates between native-born and foreign-born, and particularly the foreign-born Irish (the only sizable specific nationality group of foreign-born in this company), was statistically significant. This difference between native-born and foreign-born held for the limited group of cases of myocardial infarction and sudden death within the coronary heart disease incidence group as a whole. The incidence rates for myocardial infarction plus sudden death in native-born and foreign-born were 38 per thousand per four years, and 16 per thousand per four years respectively.

While these differences between native-born and foreign-born Americans were significant and noteworthy, it is essential to make the further observation that the rates in the foreign-born were by no means low, in an absolute sense. The foreign-born rate of 34 per thousand per four years represents a risk of about one in six of developing clinical coronary disease during the 20 years of middle age from 45 to 64. This is a substantial risk, particularly compared with that for men of the same age in many other countries.

Since the prevalence rates of obesity and hypertension were similar in the native-born and the foreign-born, the lower coronary heart disease incidence rates in the foreign-born apparently cannot be accounted for on the basis of these variables. However, the prevalence of the combination, hypertension plus obesity, was somewhat lower in the foreign-born than in the native-born (83 per thousand and 138 per thousand respectively). Available preliminary data on mean serum cholesterol levels, obtained during 1958, were as follows: native-born 241 mg. %, foreign-born Irish 222 mg. %, all foreign-born 234 mg. %. Further analysis is pending.

The bulk of the foreign-born, 145 of 267, were skilled workers or foremen. It was therefore possible to compare coronary heart disease incidence rates in native-born skilled workers and foremen (130 men) with those in foreign-born skilled workers and foremen. The coronary heart disease incidence rates were 93 per thousand per four years in the former, and 30 per thousand per four years in the latter. Hence the difference in coronary heart disease incidence rates between native-born and foreign-born does not appear related to their respective occupational backgrounds. It does not appear possible to implicate physical activity of work as a decisive etiologic factor accounting for this sizable differential. Studies on dietary patterns of the two groups remain to be accomplished.

The differences in incidence and mortality rates for coronary heart disease—between native-born and foreign-born Americans on the one hand and between foreign-born Americans and nationals of corresponding countries of origin on the other hand—would appear to merit further follow-up. It is essential first to accumulate further data to validate these observations. In this regard it is to be noted that a recent report from the Framingham study indicated no significant differences in coronary heart disease incidence rates between native-born and foreign-born.[85] The bulk of the foreign-born in Framingham were of Italian origin.

With respect to this whole problem of the effects of migration on disease, it would be invaluable to have data not only on the foreign-born but also on first-generation and second-generation native-born Americans of known foreign descent. One recent investigation presents illuminating data along these lines.[86] This study involved 189 healthy Boston men, aged 20 to 50, whose parents had been born near Naples, Italy, and who themselves had lived all their adult life in the United States. They were found to have dietary fat intakes, mean serum total cholesterol levels, and apparent risks of developing coronary heart disease similar to those of other Americans and significantly higher than those of native Neapolitans.

Assuming for the present that additional data will verify the trends suggested by the foregoing findings, it would appear valid to suggest, as a hypothesis for further testing, that the foreign-born groups bear the stamp of their tenure both in their countries of birth and in the United States—principally the latter. This appears to be true, for example, for their nutritional patterns, which seem to be an amalgam of old-country and American dietetics, resulting frequently in diets of a composition similar to diets of native-born Americans. While other factors of possible significance also need investigation, it would appear reasonable to suggest that the findings on the foreign-born are consistent with the concept that diet plays a key—although not exclusive—role in the causation of atherosclerotic disease.

DIET—A KEY, BUT NOT EXCLUSIVE, ETIOLOGIC FACTOR

In making these observations it is essential to re-emphasize that this concept attributes a key, but not exclusive, role to diet. It in no way implies that atherosclerosis is purely and simply a dietary disease. Such a viewpoint is definitely at variance with well-established facts and therefore untenable. Thus the fact that many persons, eating a typical American diet for decades, reach old age without clinical evidence of atherosclerotic disease—this fact alone refutes any attempt to imply a one-to-one, cause-and-effect relationship between diet and disease. Further, the marked sex differential, the high incidence of coronary disease in middle-aged American men in contrast to women, almost certainly contravenes any pure and simple dietary concept. Similarly the greater incidence of atherosclerotic disease in persons with hypothyroidism, diabetes, nephrosis, xanthomatosis, and hypertension contradicts any exclusive dietary concept. Actually, no serious scientist is making any such futile attempt to "fit" all the phenomena of atherosclerotic disease into the Procrustean bed of a pure and simple dietary "explanation."

As several studies indicate, a remarkable similarity prevails with respect to dietary patterns among large sections of the American population.[68-73] Yet within any sizable groups exhibiting fairly similar nutritional habits, marked differences are to be observed in levels of serum cholesterol and—correlating therewith—in rates of coronary heart disease.

Obviously, as extensive clinical and experimental data also demonstrate, the nature of the organism plays an important role in determining the effects of life-span ingestion of a potentially atherogenic diet. Hence, different persons ingesting similar habitual diets exhibit different levels of cholesteremia and different patterns of atherogenesis. The validity of this interrelationship for individuals in no way negates the important role of diet for populations and for certain susceptible persons.

In individuals, many factors may interact significantly with diet— genetics and heredity, metabolism and endocrinology, clotting and fibrinolytic mechanisms, previous medical history, psychologic make-up and physical condition (fatigue, stress, tension, frustration, etc.), environmental factors. Considerable evidence is now available indicating that smoking significantly increases the risk of coronary heart disease in middle-aged men consuming usual American diets.[2, 10, 68, 85] Antecedent allergic or infectious disease, for example, possibly by damaging vessels and setting up sites of predilection for atherogenesis, may be of great importance in some cases. Hypertension, hypothyroidism, renal dysfunction, diabetes, and xanthomatosis certainly tend to potentiate atherogenesis. The evidence is considerable that estrogenic secretion in women has an opposite effect.

PSYCHOLOGIC INFLUENCES

In recent years, great interest has been aroused concerning the possible influences of psychologic stress and physical activity on the development of atherosclerotic disease, particularly coronary heart disease. Until recently, virtually no reliable evidence was available concerning the first of these, which is understandable in view of the complex and difficult problems of objective mensuration. Within the last year or two, reports were presented on the effects of various types of stress on cholesteremia in subjects ingesting usual American diets. Some findings indicated that periods of marked tension were associated with sizable rises in serum cholesterol levels.[87-89] Limited data were also presented to support the thesis that "high pressure," "high-tension," "time-stressed" persons have a higher incidence of coronary heart disease.[90-92] However, data that may be construed as contradicting this thesis have also been reported.[93] Further information may be anticipated in the years immediately ahead.

EFFECTS OF PHYSICAL INACTIVITY

Epidemiologic data have been reported from Great Britain concerning the influence of physical activity.[2, 11, 45] Comparisons of subgroups within relatively homogeneous socioeconomic strata of the British population indicated that the incidence of coronary heart disease tended to be lower in the subgroups habitually engaged in greater physical activity of work. Data along these lines were obtained in comparisons of sedentary bus drivers versus conductors, sedentary telephone operators versus active postmen, and so forth. However, the differences were not marked; occurrence rates of coronary disease were substantial in physically active men of various social classes. Further, studies in the United States fail to reveal any correlation between habitual physical activity of work and occurrence rates of coronary heart disease.[2, 10, 59, 65, 76, 78, 80] Moreover, all strata of the population in Great Britain, as in the United States and Norway, irrespective of socioeconomic status and habitual physical activity of work, apparently manifest high coronary heart disease incidence rates.

Correspondingly, most recent observations indicate that epidemiologic patterns of cholesteremia and atherosclerotic disease were more decisively influenced by diet than by level of physical activity at work. In South African Bantu with a habitual diet low in total fats, saturated fats, and cholesterol the level of cholesteremia and the incidence of coronary disease were found to be low in both sedentary and active workers.[94] Similar observations were also reported from Japan and Italy.[95] Contrariwise, in Norway and Finland, with habitual diets high in total calories, total fats, saturated fats, and cholesterol, the level of cholesteremia and the incidence of coronary disease were observed to be high in both sedentary and active workers.[43, 44, 96] Similarly, as already noted, recent studies in the United States consistently revealed high levels of cholesteremia and a high prevalence and incidence of coronary disease in virtually all sectors of the middle-aged male labor force, irrespective of nationality, socioeconomic status, income, occupation, physical activity of work, and urban or rural residence.

INTERPLAY OF DIET AND OTHER ETIOLOGIC FACTORS

These data impressively support the concept that diet is a decisive variable determining the pattern of atherosclerotic disease in a population. Nonetheless, research on the interrelationships among nutrition, physical activity, atherosclerosis, and atherosclerotic disease, particularly in countries where large segments of the population ingest diets high in calories, fat, and cholesterol, and lead a relatively sedentary life, remains limited. Recent reports indicate that physical activity may prevent an increase in serum cholesterol, under circumstances when increased fat is ingested to meet greater caloric need. It has also been suggested that continued physical activity through middle age may be a factor in the prevention of atherosclerotic disease, perhaps by influencing the "richness" of coronary collateral vasculature or by other possible mechanisms.[2, 10] Further work is certainly indicated on the effects of energy expenditure and large muscle activity in persons and groups ingesting potentially atherogenic diets.

With respect to the individual, therefore, the relationship between diet and other factors may be formulated as follows, based on our present knowledge. In the individual members of a population group habitually ingesting a potentially atherogenic diet, the development of morphologic atherosclerosis and atherosclerotic disease is influenced by multiple factors. There is a complex interplay between diet and other factors which operate to accelerate or retard atherogenesis. Thus it is not a matter of one factor to the exclusion of others; it is not a matter of either-or. But among these multiple factors interacting to influence atherogenesis, diet is a decisive factor. Thus it would seem valid to designate a certain type of habitual diet as virtually a *sine qua non* for atherosclerosis and atherosclerotic disease, even as the tubercle bacillus is a *sine qua non* for tuberculosis although patently a multiplicity of host and environmental factors enter into complex interrelationship with the decisive causative factor to influence the developmental patterns of the disease. For, without the habitual ingestion of a potentially atherogenic diet, clinical atherosclerotic disease would be rare among the middle-aged members of any population, irrespective of the operation of other factors that were potentially offensive.

SUSCEPTIBILITY TO CORONARY HEART
DISEASE—FACTORS ASSOCIATED
WITH HIGH RISK

These basic conclusions have been designated the nutritional-metabolic cholesterol-lipid-lipoprotein theory of atherogenesis.[2, 9] They have received a significant further verification in recently published findings of prospective epidemiologic studies. In general the results of all these investigations point in the same direction. When sizable groups of middle-aged American men, originally free of clinical coronary heart disease, are followed prospectively, the risk of developing this disease is definitely proportional to levels of body weight, blood pressure, and cholesteremia.[76-78, 80, 81, 85] Thus, from the Framingham report, in the population-at-risk normal with respect to all three of these variables (originally free of clinical coronary heart disease) the four year incidence rate was only 10 per thousand. This is one-sixth the rate of American middle-aged men in general (58 per thousand per four years). In contrast, in the population-at-risk with two or three of these variables abnormally elevated, the four year incidence rate was 143 per thousand, a more than tenfold increase in risk compared with the Framingham normals.

These data re-emphasize the important role of hypertensive disease as a factor in the development of clinical coronary disease during middle age, particularly in populations with the prerequisite cholesterol-lipid-lipoprotein metabolic derangements. Once again, therefore, the conclusion must be reached that a multiplicity of factors (exogenous and endogenous) operate to produce coronary disease and that the critically important nutritional factor has no simple one-to-one interrelationship with atherosclerosis and atherosclerotic disease. At the same time it is also essential to recognize that the incidence of coronary disease was by no means insignificant in the nonhypertensive middle-aged American men followed in these prospective studies. The etiology of coronary disease in normotensive persons therefore remains a key problem.

Similarly, with respect to obesity, while the overweight groups in the Framingham and Chicago studies had coronary disease rates approximately twice those of the normal-weight groups, the rates in the latter were high. In this regard, available data on obesity and cholesteremia are worthy of attention. In at least two studies a positive correlation has been demonstrated between serum cholesterol levels and body weight, but this is a low-order correlation.[84] Put somewhat differently, the middle-aged American population ingesting its habitual diet tends generally to be at least slightly obese and to have high values for serum cholesterol, with or without concomitant gross obesity.

When this high fat, high cholesterol diet is ingested in excess, with resultant gross obesity, serum cholesterol levels tend to be slightly but definitely higher. Given this nutritional-metabolic situation, it is to be expected that incidence of coronary disease would be substantial in middle-aged American men who are not grossly overweight, and that it would be even greater, but not several-fold greater, in the obese. Life insurance data indicate that healthy thin persons have a significantly lower risk of coronary disease.[97] No systematic serum lipid data are available on such persons. In brief, the nonhypertensive, nonoverweight middle-aged American men, better off though they may be, nonetheless still have a significant incidence of elevated serum cholesterol levels and coronary disease. The relationship of life-span diet to these phenomena cannot be gainsaid.

PRACTICAL APPLICATIONS

These data are not only of great theoretic and research significance. They also have profound implications which apply to the practice of medicine.

They pose critical questions concerning the approach of medicine to the prophylaxis of coronary disease. In particular, they pose the question: What can and should the medical profession do for the many middle-aged men who, while not yet victimized by clinical coronary heart disease, run an inordinately high risk of developing it? These are the individuals with two or more derangements—obesity, hypercholesteremia, hypertension, renal damage, diabetes, hypothyroidism, heavy smoking, a poor family history.

Before proceeding to discuss this problem it is advisable to clarify a possible misconception. It has been stated that predictions concerning the development of clinical coronary heart disease in individuals cannot be made based on determinations of their serum cholesterol, weight, blood pressure, etc. This must be clearly and precisely understood.

It is perfectly correct that no one can definitely predict whether a given person will develop clinical coronary heart disease in the next year or two. However, long-term prognostic predictions of the actuarial type, predictions of risk, can be made. Inevitably, a small percentage of these actuarial predictions of risk will be false positives or false negatives. However, these "errors" are of minor importance, reckoned against the achievement, i.e., the ability to identify high-risk individuals with the consequent possibility of successful prophylactic intervention.

Based on recent investigations, it is becoming possible to estimate the scope of this problem of high-risk individuals in specific quantitative terms. It can be roughly estimated that a low-risk middle-aged man, normal in weight, blood pressure, and serum cholesterol, has one chance in 20 of developing clinical coronary heart disease during the age period from 45 to 64. In contrast, a middle-aged man with two or three abnormalities (obesity, hypercholesteremia, hypertension) stands almost one chance in two. These are markedly different risks.

About 10 to 15% of middle-aged American men fall into this high-risk category.[76, 80] When it is further recognized that 20 to 30% of first attacks of myocardial infarction are fatal, the serious nature of the high-risk situation is even more starkly apparent. Is it not extremely valuable for both patients and physicians to be able to identify these high-risk individuals, in order to attempt to do something for them prophylactically?

From the foregoing the critical question emerges with utmost clarity: In high-risk subjects, can risk be prophylactically reduced severalfold by correcting defects? This is perhaps the most compelling practical problem posed as a result of the research achievements of the last 10 years.

It is known that these defects are amenable to correction, in whole or in part, by relatively simple medical-hygienic means, the decisive one among them being dietotherapy. It is not yet known definitively whether coronary heart disease risk can be significantly lowered thereby, although the findings of the life insurance companies on the positive results of correcting obesity are highly suggestive in this regard.[97] Five or 10 years of work still lie ahead before an unequivocal answer will be reached.

Until such definitive data are collected, disagreements among scientists are bound to persist concerning the precise role of diet in the causation of atherosclerotic disease. This situation is virtually unavoidable for the present. Such a phase has occurred with practically every significant new advance in medicine. The important problem is to avoid disorientation amidst the discussion. On the one hand, the disagreements are a product of indubitable important advances in knowledge concerning atherosclerotic disease—advances significant enough to suggest practical conclusions for medical prophylaxis and therapy. On the other hand, the work is as yet unfinished. Definitive evidence from experimental and applied epidemiology is not yet available. The incidence and mortality rates from coronary disease have not yet been decisively reduced by deliberate controlled scientific intervention. This decisive effort is being launched, but its results are several years in the offing. In the interim, irrespective of significant further research advances, *final* judgment concerning theories on the etiology of atherosclerotic coronary heart disease have to be kept in abeyance.

For this interim period, there is widespread agreement among investigators on the individualized prescription of reasonable, moderate, safe, palatable dietary correction in high-risk patients, particularly those with obesity, hypercholesteremia, hypertension, renal damage, diabetes, hypothyroidism, poor family history, etc.[2, 5, 9, 51, 58]

It is, of course, obvious that, particularly during this transition phase of our knowledge, recommendations for prophylaxis should be virtually without danger of any type—biologic, sociologic, or psychologic. For this reason and because the accumulated evidence strongly suggests that the best results are likely to be achieved with dietary prophylaxis (coupled with a good general hygienic regimen, including regular exercise), our general recommendations are focused on this approach.[2, 9]

Finally, it is worth emphasizing that this review on the epidemiology of atherosclerotic coronary heart disease has concluded with a discussion of the status of *applied* epidemiology in this field. For that is precisely what the foregoing discussion of prophylaxis is, a discussion of the implications of recent investigative findings for the day-to-day practice of modern medicine. This is as it should be, particularly since the last decade has witnessed highly significant research advances—epidemiologic, clinical-pathologic and animal-experimental—toward a practical solution, based on scientific knowledge.

It is a pleasure to acknowledge the encouragment, aid, and support for these studies from Herman N. Bundesen, M.D., President, Chicago Board of Health. The vital advisory contribution of the Planning Committe for Epidemiologic Investigation of Cardiovascular Disease in the Chicago Living Population, and of the official Advisory Committee to the Heart Disease Control Program, Chicago Board of Health (Gene Stollerman, M.D., Committee Chairman), is also gratefully acknowledged.

Grateful acknowledgment is extended for the excellent contribution made by the staff of the Heart Disease Control Program and other sections of the Chicago Board of Health, including Frank Bauer, Yolanda Hall, Marcus Kjelsberg, Carl Kolometz, Arthur McCoo, Jr., Wilda Miller, Marilyn Paganin, Barbara Smith, and Marvin Templeton.

1. Katz, L. N. and Stamler, J.: *Experimental Atherosclerosis*. Springfield, Illinois, Charles C Thomas, 1953.

2. Katz, L. N., Stamler, J. and Pick, R.: *Nutrition and Atherosclerosis*. Philadelphia, Lea & Febiger, 1958.

3. *Symposium on Atherosclerosis*, National Academy of Sciences-National Research Council, Washington, D.C., 1954. N.A.S.-N.R.C. Publication No. 338, 1954.

4. Keys, A. (ed.) : *Symposium on Arteriosclerosis*. Minneapolis, Minnesota Heart Association and University of Minnesota, 1956.

5. Symposium: Fats in human nutrition. *J.A.M.A.* 164:1890, 1957.

6. Page, I. H. (ed.) : *Chemistry of Lipids as Related to Atherosclerosis*. Springfield, Illinois, Charles C Thomas, 1958.

7. Pincus, G. (ed.): *Hormones and Atherosclerosis, Proceedings of a Conference*. New York, Academic Press, 1959.

8. Symposium on atherosclerosis. *Am. J. Med.* 23:120, 269, 463, 769, 898, 928, 1957.

9. Stamler, J.: Diet and atherosclerotic disease. Recent pathologic, clinical, animal-experimental and epidemiologic findings. *J. Am. Dietet. A.* 34:701, 814, 929, 1053, 1060, 1958.

9a. Since extensive bibliographies are included in other recent reports,[1, 2, 9, 10] only a limited number of references are cited here. For additional documentation, reference is made to the aforementioned publications with their bibliographies.

10. ———: Epidemiology as an investigative method for the study of human atherosclerosis. *J. Nat. M. A.* 50:161, 1958.

11. Morris, J. N.: *Uses of Epidemiology*. Baltimore, The Williams and Wilkins Company, 1957.

12. White, N. K., Edwards, J. E. and Dry, T. J.: The relationship of the degree of coronary atherosclerosis with age, in men. *Circulation* 1:645, 1950.

13. Holman, R. L., McGill, H. C., Jr., Strong, J. P., Griffin, O. R. and Geer, J. C.: The natural history of atherosclerosis. *Proceedings, sixty-fifth annual meeting, Association of Life Insurance Medical Directors of America, October 1956*.

14. Enos, W. F., Jr., Holmes, R. H. and Beyer, J.: Coronary disease among United States soldiers killed in action in Korea. *J.A.M.A.* 152:1090, 1953.

15. Blumgart, H. L.: Coronary disease: Clinical-pathological correlations and physiology. *Bull. New York Acad. Med.* 27:693, 1951.

16. Spain, D. M., Bradess, V. A. and Huss, G.: Observations on atherosclerosis of coronary arteries in males under age of 46: Necropsy study with special reference to somatotypes. *Ann. Int. Med.* 38:254, 1953.

17. Yater, W. M., Traum, A. H., Brown, W. G., Fitzgerald, R. P., Geisler, M. A. and Wilcox, B. B.: Coronary artery disease in men eighteen to thirty-nine years of age. *Am. Heart J.* 36:334, 481, 683, 1948.

18. Wright, I. S. and Millikan, C. H. (ed.) : *Cerebral Vascular Diseases. Transactions of the Second Conference*. New York, Grune & Stratton, 1958.

19. Adams, R. D.: *Ibid.*[18]

20. Stamler, J.: *Ibid.*[18]

21. Keys, A.: The diet and the development of coronary heart disease. *J. Chron. Dis.* 4:364, 1956.

22. Keys, A. and White, P. D. (ed.) : World Trends in Cardiology: I. Cardiovascular Epidemiology. *Selected Papers From Second World Congress and Twenty-seventh Annual Scientific Sessions of the American Heart Association*. New York, Paul B. Hoeber, 1956.

23. Rosenthal, S. R.: Atherosclerosis: Chemical, experimental and morphologic. *Arch. Path.* 18:473, 660, 827, 1934.

24. Raab, W.: *Diet, Hormones and Arteriosclerosis*. Data and References From the Older European and Oriental Literature. Assembled and published by the author.

25. *Demographic Yearbook*. New York, Statistical Office of the United Nations, Department of Economic Affairs, 1953.

26. *Statistical Yearbook*. New York, Statistical Office of the United Nations, Department of Economic Affairs, 1953.

27. *The State of Food and Agriculture, 1954: Review and Outlook*, Rome, Italy, Food and Agriculture Organization of the United Nations, 1954.

28. Jolliffe, N.: Recent advances in nutrition of public health significance. *Metabolism* 4:191, 1955.

29. Yerushalmy, J. and Hilleboe, H. E.: Fat in the diet and mortality from heart disease: a methodological note. *New York J. Med.* 57:2343, 1957.

30. Hardinge, M. G. and Stare, F. J.: Nutritional studies of vegetarians. II. Dietary and serum levels of cholesterol. *J. Clin. Nutrition* 2:83, 1954.

31. Brozek, J., Buzina, R. and Mikic, F.: Population studies on serum cholesterol and dietary fat in Yugoslavia. *Am. J. Clin. Nutrition* 5:279, 1957.

32. Kinsell, L. W., Partridge, J., Boline, L., Margen, S. and Michaels, G.: Dietary modification of serum cholesterol and phospholipid levels. *J. Clin. Endocrinol.* 12:909, 1952.

33. Beveridge, J. M. R., Connell, W. F. and Mayer, G. A.: Dietary factors affecting the level of plasma cholesterol in humans: The role of fat. *Canad. J. Biochem. & Physiol.* 34:441, 1956.

34. Ahrens, E. H., Jr., Insull, W., Blomstrand, R., Hirsch, J., Tsaltas, T. T. and Peterson, M. L.: The influence of dietary fats on serum-lipid levels in man. *Lancet* 1:943, 1957.

35. Malmros, H. and Wigand, G.: The effect on serum cholesterol of diets containing different fats. *Lancet* 2:1, 1957.

36. Bronte-Stewart, B., Antonis, A., Eales, L. and Brock, J. F.: Effect of feeding different fats on serum cholesterol level. *Lancet* 1:521, 1956.

37. Antischkow, N.: Experimental arteriosclerosis in animals. In Cowdry, E. V. (ed.): *Arteriosclerosis.* New York, The Macmillan Company, 1933.

38. Stamler, J., Pick, R. and Katz, L. N.: Effects of dietary proteins, methionine and vitamins on plasma lipids and atherogenesis in cholesterol-fed cockerels. *Circulation Res.* 6:442, 1958.

39. ———: Effects of dietary protein and carbohydrate level on cholesterolemia and atherogenesis in cockerels on a high-fat, high-cholesterol mash. *Circulation Res.* 6:447, 1958.

40. Yudkin, J.: The epidemiology of coronary disease. *Prog. Cardiovas. Dis.* 1:116, 1958.

41. Keys, A.: Epidemiologic aspects of coronary artery disease. *J. Chron. Dis.* 6:552, 1957.

42. Uotila, U., Raekallio, J. and Ehrmooth, W.: Goitre and arteriosclerosis. *Lancet* 2:171, 1958.

43. Roine, P., Pekkarinen, M., Karvonen, M. J. and Kihlberg, J.: Diet and cardiovascular disease in Finland. *Lancet* 2:173, 1958.

44. Keys, A., Karvonen, M. and Fidanza, F.: Serum cholesterol studies in Finland. *Lancet* 2:175, 1958.

45. Morris, J. N. and Dale, R. A.: Epidemiology of coronary atherosclerosis. *Proc. Roy. Soc. Med.* 48: 667, 1955.

46. Logan, W. P. D.: Social class variations in mortality. *Pub. Health Rep.* 69:1217, 1954.

47. Moriyama, I., Woolsey, T. and Stamler, J.: Observations on possible causative factors responsible for the sex and race trends in cardiovascular-renal disease mortality in the United States. *J. Chron. Dis.* 7:401, 1958.

48. Stamler, J., Pick, R. and Katz, L. N.: Experiences in assessing estrogen anti-atherogenesis in the chick, the rabbit and man. *Ann. New York Acad. Sc.* 64:596, 1956.

49. Pick, R., Stamler, J. and Katz, L. N.: Influence of estrogens on lipids and atherosclerosis in experimental animals. In *Hormones and Atherosclerosis.* New York, Academic Press, 1959.

50. Stamler, J., Pick, R., Katz, L. N., Pick, A. and Kaplan, B.: Interim report on clinical experiences with long term estrogen administration to middle-aged men with coronary heart disease. *Ibid.*[49]

51. Jolliffe, N.: Fats, cholesterol and coronary heart disease. *New York J. Med.* 57:2684, 1957.

52. Cummings, R. O.: *The American and His Food.* Chicago, University of Chicago Press, 1940.

53. Martin, E. W.: *The Standard of Living in 1860.* Chicago, University of Chicago Press, 1942.

54. *Consumption of Food in the United States—1909–52.* Agriculture Handbook No. 62. Washington, D.C., United States Department of Agriculture, Bureau of Agriculture Economics, 1953.

55. Mabrouk, A. F. and Brown, J.

B.: The trans fatty acids of margarines and shortenings. *J. Am. Oil Chemists' Soc.* 33:98, 1956.

56. Sreenivasan, B. and Brown, J. B.: Octadecadienoic acids of shortenings and margarines. *J. Am. Oil Chemists' Soc.* 33:341, 1956.

57. Stare, F. J.: Dietary aspects. *Fed. Proc.* 15:900, 1956.

58. Page, I. H., Stare, F. J., Corcoran, A. C., Pollack, H. and Wilkinson, C. F., Jr.: Atherosclerosis and the fat content of the diet. *Circulation* 16:163, 1957.

59. Stamler, J., Kjelsberg, M. and Hall, Y.: Epidemiological studies on cardiovascular-renal diseases in Chicago and Illinois. I. Analysis of mortality trends by age-race-sex-occupation. (In preparation.)

60. Kjelsberg, M. and Stamler, J.: Epidemiological studies on cardiovascular-renal diseases in Chicago and Illinois. II. Analysis of mortality by age-race-sex-place of residence, including urban-rural comparisons. (In preparation.)

61. Stamler, J., Kjelsberg, M., Hall, Y. and Scotch, N.: Epidemiological studies on cardiovascular-renal diseases. III. Analysis of mortality by age-sex-nationality. (In preparation.)

62. Stamler, J.: Problems of the research utilization of vital statistics on the cardiovascular-renal diseases. Draft report submitted to the Chicago Heart Association Committee on Morbidity and Mortality Classification of Cardiovascular Disorders, 1957.

63. Hoobler, S. W. (ed.): Proceedings of the Conference on Basic Mechanisms of Arterial Hypertension. *Circulation* 17:641, 1958.

64. Gover, M.: Statistical studies of heart disease. IV. Mortality from heart disease (all forms) related to geographic section and size of city. *Pub. Health Rep.* 64:439, 1949.

65. Lew, E. A.: Some implications of mortality statistics relating to coronary artery disease. *J. Chron. Dis.* 6:192, 1957.

66. Parkhurst, E.: Differential mortality in New York state, exclusive of New York City, by sex, age, and cause of death according to degree of urbanization. *Am. J. Pub. Health* 46:959, 1956.

67. Enterline, P. E. and Stewart, W. H.: Geographic patterns in deaths from coronary heart disease. *Pub. Health Rep.* 71:849, 1956.

68. Zukel, W. J., Lewis, R. H., Enterline, P. E., Painter, R. C., Ralston, L. S., Fawcett, R. M., Meredith, A. P. and Peterson, B.: A short-term community study of the epidemiology of coronary heart disease; a preliminary report on the North Dakota study. Presented at the annual meeting of the American Public Health Association, October 30, 1958.

69. Clark, F., Murray, J., Weiss, G. S. and Grossman, E.: *Food Consumption of Urban Families in the United States, With an Appraisal of Methods of Analysis.* Agriculture Information Bulletin No. 132. Washington, D.C., United States Department of Agriculture, 1954.

70. Clark, F., Murray, J. and others: *Household Food Consumption Survey 1955; reports 1 to 10.* Washington, D.C., United States Department of Agriculture, 1957.

71. Adelson, S. F. and Blake, E. C.: *Diets of Families in the Open Country, a Georgia and Ohio County, Summer 1945.* Misc. Publication No. 704. Washington, D.C., United States Department of Agriculture, April 1950.

72. *Family Food Consumption in Three Types of Farming Areas of the South. II. An Analysis of Weekly Food Records, Late Winter and Early Spring, 1948.* Clemson, South Carolina, Southern Cooperative Series Bulletin 20, 1951.

73. Babcock, M. J., Church, H. N. and Gates, L. O.: *Nutritional status of industrial workers.* I. Dietary, blood and physical findings. Milbank Mem. Fund Quart. 32:323, 1954.

74. Lilienfeld, A. M.: Variation in mortality from heart disease; race, sex and socioeconomic status. *Pub. Health Rep.* 71:545, 1956.

75. Kent, A. P., McCarroll, J. R., Schweitzer, M. D. and Willard, H. N.: Coronary artery disease (arteriosclerotic heart disease) death in Manhattan, New York City. (Prepublication report.)

76. Dawber, T. R., Moore, F. E. and Mann, G. V.: Coronary heart disease in the Framingham study. *Am. J. Pub. Health* 47:4, 1957.

77. Doyle, J. T., Heslin, A. S., Hilleboe, H. E., Formel, P. F. and

Korns, R. F.: A prospective study of degenerative cardiovascular disease in Albany: Report of three years' experience. I. Ischemic heart disease. *Am. J. Pub. Health* 47:25, 1957.

78. Chapman, J. M., Goerke, L. S., Dixon, W., Loveland, D. B. and Phillips, E.: The clinical status of a population group in Los Angeles under observation for two to three years. *Am. J. Pub. Health* 47:33, 1957.

79. Pell, S. and D'Alonzo, C. A.: Myocardial infarction in a one-year industrial study. *J.A.M.A.* 166:332, 1958.

80. Stamler, J., Lindberg, H. A., Berkson, D. M., Shaffer, A., Miller, W. and Poindexter, A.: Epidemiological analysis of hypertension and hypertensive disease in the labor force of a Chicago utility company. *Am. J. Pub. Health*. (In press.)

81. ———: *Proceedings, Council for High Blood Pressure Research,* American Heart Association, 1958. (In press.)

82. Coons, C. M.: Family food consumption studies. *Pub. Health Rep.* 67:788, 1952.

83. Stamler, J.: Basic research on atherosclerosis. *J. Am. Pharm. Mfg. A.*, 1955, p. 34.

84. Lewis, L. A., Olmsted, F., Page, I. H., Lawry, E. Y., Mann, G. V., Stare, F. J., Hanig, M., Lauffer, M. A., Gordon, T. and Moore, F. E.: Serum lipid levels in normal persons; findings of a cooperative study of lipoproteins and atherosclerosis. *Circulation* 16:227, 1957.

85. Dawber, T. R., Kannell, W. B., Revotskie, N., Stokes, J., Kagan, A. and Gordon, T.: Some factors associated with the development of coronary heart disease: Six-year follow-up experience in the Framingham study. Presented at the annual meeting of the American Public Health Association, October 30, 1958.

86. Miller, D. C., Trulson, M. F., McCann, M. B., White, P. D. and Stare, F. J.: Diet, blood lipids and health of Italian men in Boston. *Ann. Int. Med.* 49:1178, 1958.

87. Rosenman, R. H. and Friedman, M.: Change in the serum cholesterol and blood clotting time in men subjected to cyclic variations of emotional stress. *Circulation* 16:931, 1957.

88. Thomas, C. B. and Murphy, E. A.: Further studies on cholesterol levels in the Johns Hopkins medical students: The effect of stress at examinations. *J. Chron. Dis.* 6:661, 1958.

89. Wertlake, P. T., Wilcox, A. A., Haley, M. I. and Peterson, J. E.: Relationship of mental and emotional stress to serum cholesterol levels. *Proc. Soc. Exper. Biol. & Med.* 97:163, 1958.

90. Friedman, M. and Rosenman, R.: Association of a specific behavior pattern with increases in blood cholesterol, blood clotting time and incidence of clinical coronary disease. Presented at the annual meeting of the American Heart Association, October 26, 1958.

91. Russek, H. I.: Panel on emotional factors in atherosclerosis, presented at the annual meeting of the American Heart Association, October 25, 1958.

92. Wolf, S. G., Jr.: Panel on emotional factors in atherosclerosis, presented at the annual meeting of the American Heart Association, October 25, 1958.

93. Gertler, M. M. and White, P. D.: *Coronary Heart Disease in Young Adults; a Multidisciplinary Study.* Cambridge, Massachusetts, Commonwealth Fund, Harvard University Press, 1954.

94. Brock, J. F. and Bronte-Stewart, B.: Arteriosclerosis in African populations. In *A Symposium on Arteriosclerosis*. Minneapolis, Minnesota Heart Association and University of Minnesota, 1956.

95. Keys, A., Anderson, J. T., Aresu, M., Biörck, G., Brock, J. F., Bronte-Stewart, B., Fidanza, F., Keys, M. H., Malmros, H., Poppi, A., Posteli, T., Swahn, B. and Del Vecchio, A.: Physical activity and the diet in populations differing in serum cholesterol. *J. Clin. Invest.* 34:1173, 1956.

96. Muller, C., Ustvedt, H. J. and others: Myocardial infarction; an epidemiologic and prognostic study of patients from five departments of internal medicine in Oslo, 1935–1949. *Acta. med. scandinav.* 154 (supp. 315), 1956.

97. Shepard, W. P. and Marks, H. H.: Life insurance looks at the arteriosclerosis problem. In *A Symposium on Arteriosclerosis*. Minneapolis, Minnesota Heart Association and University of Minnesota, 1956, p. 6.

Relationship of Amount of Cigarette Smoking to Coronary Heart Disease Mortality Rates in Men*

ROBERT W. BUECHLEY, M.A., ROBERT M. DRAKE, M.D.,

AND LESTER BRESLOW, M.D.

BERKSON, among others, has pointed out that lung cancer is not the only cause of death, for which increased mortality is observed among heavy cigarette smokers.[1] While mortality from lung cancer is many times higher among heavy smokers than it is among nonsmokers, this increased risk pertains to a still relatively infrequent cause of death. The proportional excess of mortality associated with cigarette smoking is less in the case of coronary heart disease, but this increased risk pertains to the most common cause of death, especially of males in the middle years. The Hammond and Horn data indicate four times as many excess deaths, associated with cigarette smoking,[2] from coronary heart disease as from lung cancer.

The purpose of this paper is to present, for comparison, the several studies that provide mortality rates by smoking class for coronary heart disease; and the several case-control studies that show coronary cases and controls by smoking class, including one study of each type, based on California data.

We consider that these findings, especially their consistency, raise the question whether cigarette smoking may carry greater risk for coronary heart disease than for lung cancer.

In the following pages the reported studies are summarized. As far as the varied reporting systems allow, these have been reduced to comparability. Comparisons may thus be made, and implications drawn, by each reader for himself.

---

* Reprinted with omission of two tables by permission of the American Heart Association, Inc. from the December, 1958, issue of *Circulation*, Vol. 18, pp. 1085–1090. Published by the American Heart Association, Inc., New York, New York. The authors are, respectively, Associate Specialist, Division of Biostatistics, School of Public Health, University of California, Los Angeles, formerly Associate Social Research Technician, Division of Preventive Medical Services, California State Department of Public Health, Berkeley, California; Commander (M.C., USN), Assistant Pathologist, U.S. Naval Hospital, Philadelphia, Pennsylvania, formerly Medical Officer, Bureau of Chronic Diseases, California State Department of Public Health, Berkeley, California; Chief of the Division of Preventive Medical Services, California State Department of Public Health, Berkeley, California, formerly Chief of the Bureau of Chronic Diseases, Division of Preventive Medical Services, California State Department of Public Health, Berkeley, California. This study was supported in part by funds from the Heart Disease Control Program, Division of Special Health Services, and in part by a grant from the National Institutes of Health, United States Public Health Service.

PREVIOUS REPORTS

The positive relationship of smoking to coronary heart disease in men was first reported for Mayo Clinic patients by English, Willius, and Berkson in 1940,[3] following Pearl's 1938 report of an increase in total mortality with amount of cigarette smoking.[4] Mills reported an excess of smokers,[5] and greater amounts of smoking[6] in cases of death from coronary heart disease. Gertler and White[7] found more smokers among cases than among controls. Hegglin and Keiser in Switzerland[8] found more and heavier smokers among male coronary cases. Hammond and Horn[2, 9] and Doll and Hill[10] reported significantly higher mortality rates from coronary heart disease in heavier smokers. The Framingham study, reporting incidence of coronary disease by smoking class, had nonconfirmatory results.[11]

The Study Group on Smoking and Health, sponsored by the American Cancer Society, the American Heart Association, the National Cancer Institute, and the National Heart Institute, recommended ". . . a research program of wide scope that would clarify the relationship and association between smoking and cardiovascular disease." Of particular importance, they considered, were "epidemiologic studies with appropriate consideration of the roles of other factors such as diet, physical activity, and blood lipids."[12]

CALIFORNIA FINDINGS

Information on cigarette smoking and data concerning coronary heart disease are available for two California populations.

The first is a population of 3,994 longshoremen who received a multiphasic screening examination in 1951 and for whom five years of follow-up have recently been completed.[13, 14] The examined men were volunteers from a population of about 6,000 longshoremen, and selection bias occurred—the unexamined men showing higher mortality. The abbreviated question on current (1951) amount of cigarette smoking asked at this examination allows a division of the examined men into two classes: light or nonsmokers (less than a pack of cigarettes per day) and heavy smokers (a pack or more per day, or sometimes two packs). In the first five years of follow-up, 78 deaths from coronary heart disease (International Statistical Classification codes 420.0, 420.1, and 420.2) occurred among men in the examined group. California coronary age-sex-specific death rates applied to the examined population indicate 119 expected deaths. It is thus evident that the mortality rate of coronary heart disease was lower among the examined longshoremen than in a comparable age-sex population of California, and this finding has been discussed elsewhere.[14] Of the observed deaths, 42 occurred among light or nonsmokers, compared with an expected 84, and 36 occurred among heavy smokers, compared with an expected 35. Similar proportions of observed to expected were not found for deaths from any heart disease other than coronary.

A retrospective case-control study, by questionnaire and interview, has been made of Californians reporting coronary disease to the California Health Survey; matched controls came from the same survey, which was based upon a representative sample of the State's population.[15] The persons selected for restudy reported their coronary heart disease, and having survived at least the first coronary attack, they also are in this sense a selected group. The 116 males with coronary disease reported a much higher mean amount of smoking, averaging about 16 cigarettes per day, than the 121 controls, who averaged about 10 cigarettes per day. Twenty-three male coronary patients were nonsmokers, compared with 51 matched controls. Contrary to the trend in the prospective studies of mortality, the differences in amount of smoking are larger at the older ages for this case-control study of coronary heart disease morbidity.

MORTALITY STUDY COMPARISONS

Substantial agreement in results is shown by four prospective studies.[2, 10, 6, and 14] These investigations, including our own study of longshoremen, generally show higher mortality rates from coronary heart disease in each successively higher smoking class. As a simple measure of over-all increase, the difference in mortality rate between the nonsmokers and the heavy smokers in each study at each age has been noted. Similar differences can, of course, be computed for the rates in the other smoking classes.

The four reported studies cannot be exactly reduced to any common denominator, as was done by Edwards for lung cancer,[16] although the rates we have determined are a first step in so doing. Our study of longshoremen did not distinguish smoking categories in sufficient detail. Mill's study did not distinguish the various cardiovascular conditions. Doll and Hill lumped all types of smoking—cigar, pipe, and cigarettes—and reported on grams of tobacco smoked. Hammond and Horn avoided these difficulties, and their reporting as made in 1958 could well be taken as a model. They have adopted Doll and Hill's method of reporting person-years of exposure, which is necessary for computing commensurable rates.

Case-Control Ratios and Incidence Rate Comparisons

The case-control studies are even more heterogeneous. The California study and the Framingham study[11] both utilize cases identified in a representative sample of a specified population. Most of the others report on patients drawn from unknown population bases and compared with controls from the same or other bases. The Framingham study reports an incidence rate, while the other studies report numbers of cases and controls. Despite this heterogeneity, higher case-control ratios for coronary heart disease generally appear in successively higher smoking classes. Gertler and White discount the importance of this increase, although the difference they report is significant by the x^2 test. The Framingham investigators did not consider that the data in their original report demonstrated an association with amount of smoking, but they are continuing to accumulate more data. All other investigators note the relationship, Sigler to the extent of saying ". . . tobacco merely may have some influence in expediting the development of coronary heart disease in a small proportion of the population . . ."[17] and Hegglin and Keiser to the extent of saying ". . . smoking is now the most dangerous drug addiction."[8]

CONCLUSIONS

The heterogeneity of populations, differing approaches and manner of reporting make impossible a good estimation of the magnitude of the relationship between cigarette smoking and coronary heart disease. We have abandoned our attempts to make such an estimate from a combination of studies by various authors. However, the extent of the relationship is generally indicated by the difference in death rate between nonsmokers and heavy smokers. These differences show a strong and consistent relationship between cigarette smoking and coronary heart disease mortality, at least in men 40 to 70 years of age. The difference in mortality between cigarette smokers and nonsmokers at different ages varies from 1 to 7 excess deaths from coronary heart disease per 1,000 men per year.

Smoking rates in the United States are high,[18] and coronary death rates are also high, in comparison with many other countries.[19] Further studies of their relationship are needed.

1. Berkson, J.: Smoking and lung cancer. Some observations on two recent reports. *J. Am. Statistical Assoc.* 53:28, 1958.

2. Hammond, E. C., and Horn, D.: Smoking and death rates—reports on forty-four months of follow-up of 187,783 men. *J.A.M.A.* 166:1159 and 1295, 1958.

3. English, J. P., Willius, F. A., and Berkson, J.: Tobacco and coronary disease. *J.A.M.A.* 115:1327, 1940.

4. Pearl, R.: Tobacco smoking and longevity. *Science* 87:216, 1938.

5. Mills, C. A.: Tobacco smoking: Some hints of its biologic hazard. *Ohio M. J.* 46:1165, 1950.

6. ———, and Porter, M. M.: Tobacco smoking and automobile-driving stress in relation to deaths from cardiac and vascular causes. *Am. J. M. Sc.* 234:35, 1957.

7. Gertler, M. M., White, P. D., and others: *Coronary Heart Disease in Young Adults*. Cambridge, Mass., Harvard University Press, 1954.

8. Hegglin, R., and Keiser, G.: Über Rauchen und Coranererkrankungen. *Schweiz. med. Wchnschr.* 85:53, 1955.

9. Hammond, E. C., and Horn, D.: The relationship between human smoking habits and death rates. *J.A.M.A.* 155:1316, 1954.

10. Doll, R., and Hill, A. B.: Lung cancer and other causes of death in relation to smoking: A second report on the mortality of British doctors. *Brit. M. J.* 2:1071, 1956.

11. Dawber, T. S., Moore, F. E., and Mann, G. V.: Coronary heart disease in the Framingham study. *Am. J. Pub. Health* 47:4, 1957.

12. Strong, F. M., and others: Smoking and health. Joint report of the study group on smoking and health. *Science* 125:1129, 1957.

13. Weinerman, R., Breslow, L., Belloc, N., Waybur, A., and Milmore, B. K.: Multiphasic screening of longshoremen with organized medical follow-up. *Am. J. Pub. Health* 42:1552, 1952.

14. Buechley, R. W., Drake, R. M., and Breslow, L.: Height, weight and mortality in a population of longshoremen. *J. Chron. Dis.* 7:363, 1958.

15. Drake, R. M., Buechley, R. W., and Breslow, L.: An epidemiological investigation of coronary heart disease in the California health survey population. *Am. J. Pub. Health* 47:43, 1957.

16. Edwards, J. H.: Contribution of cigarette smoking to respiratory disease. *Brit. J. Prev. & Social Med.* 11:10, 1957.

17. Sigler, L. H.: Tobacco as a contributing cause of degenerative coronary disease. *New York J. Med.* 55:3107, 1955.

18. Haenszel, W., Shimkin, M. B., and Miller, M. P.: *Tobacco Smoking Patterns in the United States.* Public Health Monograph No. 45, U.S. Department of Health, Education and Welfare, Washington, D.C., 1956.

19. Yerushalmy, J., and Hilleboe, H. E.: Fat in the diet and mortality from heart disease. *New York J. Med.* 57:2343, 1957.

5. Nutritional Health

Malnutrition and the Health of Children*

NEVIN S. SCRIMSHAW

THE HIGH infant mortality rates in technically underdeveloped areas
are widely known, and the plight of children under one year of age in
these countries is often cited as their major health problem. It is true
that infant mortality rates range from three to six times higher in
these countries than in the United States and Western Europe. Of
each 1,000 children born live in 1958 over 100 died during their first
year of life in Colombia, Ecuador, and Guatemala, and over 80 in
Mexico and El Salvador, in contrast to 27 in the United States, and 30
to 31 for other Western countries. While the exact figures vary from
year to year and are beginning to decrease in some of these countries,
they are distressingly high.

Infant deaths result from a wide variety of causes including congenital malformations, birth injuries, postnatal asphyxia and atelectasis, and respiratory infections such as influenza, pneumonia and
bronchitis.[1] As the figures for the United States indicate, not all of
these infant deaths are preventable by good nutrition or by improved
hygiene and medical care.

In technically-underdeveloped countries malnutrition is an important factor in the death of children under one year of age, since
many receive insufficient breast milk. When weaning occurs earlier
than one year of age, a child is often given either milk in dilute form
or a milk-substitute such as sugar water, rice water, or cornstarch
solution, all of which are extremely deficient in both protein and
calories. The result is usually marasmus, a form of partial starvation.
Occasionally, if calories are relatively less deficient, the child under
one year will develop kwashiorkor. This is particularly true of some
urban centers in Africa and Trinidad where early weaning is practiced
so that the mothers can return to paid jobs.

While the high infant death rates, common to most technically-
underdeveloped areas point to a serious problem and should stimulate

* Reprinted, with omission of two tables and some content, by permission,
from Proceedings of the World Health Conference, Los Angeles, California, October 6–7, 1961, published in Los Angeles, UCLA School of
Public Health, 1962. This article was also published in the March, 1963,
issue of the Journal of the American Dietetic Association, Vol. 42, No. 3,
pp. 203–208. The author is Professor and Chairman of the Department of
Nutrition, Food Science, and Technology, Massachusetts Institute of
Technology, Cambridge, Massachusetts.

strong Public Health measures directed at their prevention, they do not begin to indicate either the full magnitude of the problem of high mortality rates among young children in technically-underdeveloped areas or to reveal the consequences of malnutrition among children in such areas. These are best shown by examining not only the mortality rates for children under one year but also those for children one to four years of age. When data from technically-underdeveloped countries are compared with those from the United States, Canada, and Western Europe, the tabulation shows mortality rates not three to six times higher but many which are 30 to 60 times higher.[2, 3, 4] For example, the specific mortality rates, per 1,000 population of children one to four years of age in Sweden, the United States, and the Netherlands, countries where kwashiorkor is unknown, are 1.0, 1.1, and 1.2, respectively, in contrast to rates of 42.7, 55.4, and 60.7, in Guatemala, Guinea, and Egypt, where the disease is common. Malnutrition is directly or indirectly involved in almost all of the excess mortality in the one- to four-year age group. Unfortunately, for general understanding of the nature of the problem, this fact is not revealed in the usual breakdown of causes of death. A major reason is that deaths in technically-underdeveloped areas are largely reported to lay registrars by parents or relatives who, in turn, attribute the death to worms, dysentery, and other infectious diseases, even when they are classical cases of kwashiorkor or marasmus.

Guatemala is a country in which the Pan American Health Organization, Regional Office of the Americas for the World Health Organization, in co-operation with the six countries of Central America and Panama, has established the Institute of Nutrition of Central America and Panama, INCAP, which is studying nutrition problems, training personnel, and conducting educational and applied programs to prevent malnutrition. The mortality rate among children one to four years of age in Guatemala is over 40 times that of the United States. While this figure is lower than Egypt's, it is still one of the highest in the world. Personnel of INCAP selected four villages with an average mortality for children one to four years, of 50 per 1,000, a figure over 50 times higher than in the United States, and investigated the cause of each death by visiting the household.[5]

When the causes of death as reported to the National Department of Vital Statistics were compared with causes assigned by the INCAP workers, only one case attributed to malnutrition was found in the official figures. This was a child who died soon after being brought to the regional hospital and whose death was the only one medically certified. The INCAP workers, on the other hand, found that 38%, or over one-third, of all of the deaths occurred in children with full-blown symptoms of severe protein deficiency or kwashiorkor.

Kwashiorkor is characterized by edema, pigmented skin lesions, changes in the color and texture of the hair, apathy, anorexia, growth failure, serious biochemical imbalances, and pathologic tissue changes.[6] The syndrome is the result of inadequate protein relative to calories and is fatal unless the quantity and quality of protein in the diet are improved. It is important to note that kwashiorkor is nearly always precipitated in an already chronically malnourished child by an infectious episode, which is most commonly either dysentery or a childhood disease such as measles or chickenpox.

Infection exerts its adverse influence on nutritional status in several different ways. Inevitably, a decrease in food consumption due to anorexia, and even actual intolerance of food, results. Even more importantly, in technically-underdeveloped areas, the quality of food offered to the child is changed because mothers and often physicians, too, believe that solid food should be taken away from the sick child, especially from a child ill with diarrhea, and liquids which are generally low in protein are substituted. Similarly, infections result in an increased loss of cellular protein which is manifest by extra nitrogen excreted in the urine and frequently by a significant nitrogen imbalance.

One-quarter of the deaths in the four communities investigated appeared to be a direct result of infectious diarrhea. Few well-nourished children ever die of this cause and almost none within 24 to 48 hours after onset, as occurs frequently in malnourished populations. Most of the remaining deaths, 37%, seemed to result from other infections secondary to childhood disease, but which again would rarely be fatal in a well-nourished child. Thus, even the deaths attributed to infection were really due to the combined effects of infection and malnutrition—a synergism, so to speak, in which the consequences of the combination were far worse than would be predicted for either one alone.

For example, in 1956 the death rate from measles in Mexico was 164 times higher per 100,000 population than in the United States. In Guatemala, it was 228 times higher and in Ecuador, 368 times higher. This was not because the measles virus was more virulent or prevalent in these countries, or even because of the differences in medical care, but because the resistance of the host (the child) was lower in the Latin American countries. We believe that this lower resistance is due primarily to malnutrition. Measles is a good example because it occurs almost universally in children, regardless of social and economic status, and even without medical care is not usually a fatal disease in well-nourished populations.

It should be emphasized that the synergism works both ways. As mentioned previously, most of the deaths attributable to severe protein malnutrition were really attributable to a combination of dietary deficiency and infectious stress. Of course, the relative proportion of deaths due to the synergism between malnutrition and infection varies from one technically-underdeveloped country to another; nevertheless, the principle remains the same. Nearly all of the great excess of mortality among children one to four years of age in technically-underdeveloped countries, as compared with developed countries, is associated directly or indirectly with malnutrition acting synergistically with infection. *In some technically-underdeveloped areas half of the children born alive are dead before age five, as a result of both a high infant mortality and a high mortality in the one- to four-year age group.*

RELATION OF MORTALITY TO MORBIDITY

These mortality statistics are striking, but they tell only a small part of the sad story. For every child in the one- to four-year age group who dies, many more suffer seriously from malnutrition during this age period. In fact, growth and maturation studies among the preschool children in the lower income groups in many technically-underdeveloped countries reveal the fact that nearly all of the children pass through a period of several years following weaning in which growth and development are almost at a standstill. The evidence indicates that this is due primarily to protein malnutrition. The death of so many children during this preschool age period, which is characterized by delayed growth and development, is due to either a lowering of resistance to infection by malnutrition or exaggeration of malnutrition by infection and its sequelae. These consequences include not only loss of appetite and a tendency to withdraw solid food because of the illness, but also the loss of protein from damaged or destroyed cells.

Instead of relying on mortality statistics, the severity of protein malnutrition among preschool children in a community can be judged by the frequency of clinical cases of kwashiorkor, but this requires a house-to-house canvass. Some idea can be obtained, however, by visiting hospital and out-patient clinics. By this means, kwashiorkor has been shown to be a Public Health problem in 19 of the 21 countries of the Americas, all of the countries and territories of Africa south of the Sahara, in India, and in most countries of the Middle and Far East.[7] Clinical cases, whether estimated from mortality figures or surveys of hospital and clinic patients, represent only part of the problem. As has been suggested already, clinical cases of kwashiorkor are more like the tip of an undersea mountain, protruding above the ocean surface but with its hidden vast bulk corresponding to the concealed cases of underlying protein malnutrition.

If the almost universal occurrence of underlying protein malnutrition among children of lower-income groups in technically-underdeveloped areas meant only increased mortality due to a synergism of nutrition and infection, this would be bad enough. If the children who survived suffered nothing more than permanent stunting of their growth and development, this might conceivably be looked upon as a useful adaptation. Unfortunately, recent studies from Mexico suggest that intelligence is impaired as well. Ramos Galvan and co-workers are finding a significant correlation between retardation in height and weight and the score of children reaching school age on the standard Goodenough "Draw-a-Man" test and on the standard Gesell tests.[8, 9] Retardation in weight for age may reflect to some extent current nutritional status, but it is largely a reflection of impaired nutritional status during several of the formative years. Retardation in height is more clearly due to previous malnutrition. If malnutrition during preschool years affects the intellectual performance of children, it is essential to prevent malnutrition in preschool children if educational measures are to have a fair chance of contributing to the improvement of the productivity, prosperity, and democracy of a country. In other words, malnutrition during the preschool years is serious for the children who survive as well as for the many who die as a direct or indirect consequence of it.

OTHER NUTRITIONAL DEFICIENCIES
IMPORTANT IN THE HEALTH OF CHILDREN

While protein malnutrition is the most universal nutritional deficiency among children in the world today, and is a problem likely to become worse in many areas as population growth continues to match or even outstrip increases in food supply, there are other nutritional deficiencies that also seriously affect many of the world's children. One example is infantile beriberi. This condition is characterized clinically by pallor, insomnia, restlessness, anorexia, vomiting, and terminally by cyanosis, dyspnea, tachycardia, and sudden death a few hours after onset.[10] The disease is actually increasing in some parts of Southeast Asia, notably Thailand, because the introduction of gasoline-driven rice mills into small villages has displaced home-pounding which left a greater proportion of hull and thiamine-containing germ. As a consequence, the mothers receive less thiamine in their diet and secrete less thiamine in their milk. If this vitamin is sufficiently inadequate, the child is suddenly likely to develop symptoms at two or three months of age.

In Yugoslavia, Egypt, Basutoland, and a number of other countries, pellagra is still a problem in those portions of the population consuming a predominantly corn diet.[11] Corn is deficient in both niacin and in tryptophan, the amino acid precursor of niacin. Pellagra, due to niacin deficiency, affects children and adults alike and is exacerbated by exposure to strong sunlight. Its occurrence tends to be seasonable because the time of poorest diet coincides with the greatest exposure to sunlight during work in the fields.

Even more widespread is vitamin A deficiency. In mild form, at least, this deficiency almost parallels the occurrence of kwashiorkoı and is responsible for occasional cases of xerophthalmia and keratomalacia superimposed on kwashiorkor and marasmus. In Indonesia, it is responsible annually for many thousands of cases of keratomalacia and much preventable blindness. Like kwashiorkor, it is often precipitated by measles or some other infection in a child whose diet is borderline in vitamin A. A recent WHO report estimates that 5% of all children in Indonesia have impaired vision or are blind as a consequence of vitamin A deficiency.[12]

One indication of the extent to which the child population of Indonesia subsists on a borderline status with respect to vitamin A is indicated by the experience with free distribution of a large quantity of skim milk a few years ago. The augmented protein intake increased the frequency of xerophthalmia and keratomalacia sharply by increasing the requirement for vitamin A, and importation of the skim milk had to be prohibited until arrangements could be made for distribution of supplemental vitamin A capsules.[12] If whole milk with its natural vitamin A content had been used, the incident would not have occurred. Economic factors, however, make it convenient to use skim milk for the prevention of protein malnutrition in many parts of the world.

Another common nutritional deficiency in which children are seriously involved is endemic goiter. Unless the diet includes iodine-containing foods or iodized salt, this condition appears wherever the soil lacks iodine, thus rendering water supplies and locally grown vegetables deficient in this element. The requirements for iodine may be increased by a variety of goitrogenic factors including a chemical substance found in plants of the family *Brassica* to which Brussels sprouts and the common cabbage belong,[13] and also possibly by vitamin A deficiency,[14, 15] and by water supplies rich in lime.[16] Adequate iodine intake will always prevent the condition.

Some idea of the widespread occurrence of endemic goiter may be gained from the realization that it is, (or was until control measures were introduced) a Public Health problem in every one of the countries and territories on the mainland of the Western Hemisphere, in much of Africa, in the mountainous areas of Europe, in parts of India and some countries of the Far East.[17] It is readily surveyed by examining school children whose soft diffuse goiters reflect the current status of iodine nutriture of the population. Administration of iodine causes the majority of goiters in school children to disappear in as short a period as 12 weeks, even in areas where over 50% of the children have goiter.[18] When the goiter persists, it gradually enlarges, becomes fibrous, and turns into the irreversible large visible goiters so common in adults in goitrous areas.

Usually, the hypertrophy of the gland is a successful compensatory mechanism for more efficient extraction of iodine from the bloodstream and is not associated with metabolic changes in children. When goiter occurs in pregnant women, it appears responsible for cases of endemic cretinism and may be associated with an increase in still-births, deaf-mutes, and congenital abnormalities.

Rickets, once a scourge of northern countries because of the wintertime shortage of sunlight necessary for the conversion of ergosterol in the skin to active vitamin D, has all but disappeared in these countries because of the use of vitamin D concentrates. Rickets still occur in children in the tropics who, for special reasons, are not exposed to the sunlight. In the slums of tropic cities children are sometimes deprived of sunlight because they are ill, live in tenements with little opportunity for exposure to the sun, or stay with the working mother whose occupation keeps her within a building during the daylight hours.

1. World Health Organization. *Epidemiological and Vital Statistics Report.* Volume 13, 1960, p. 527.

2. *Summary of Four-Year Reports on Health Conditions in the Americas.* Pan American Sanitary Bureau Regional Office of the World Health Organization, Scientific Publication No. 40. Washington, D.C., 1958.

3. *Demographic Year Book 1957.* United Nations, New York, 1957.

4. *Enquete demographique 1954–1955.* Haut Commissariat de la Republique Francaise.

5. Behar, M., Ascoli, W. and Scrimshaw, N. S. "An investigation into the causes of death in children in four rural communities in Guatemala." *Bull. World Health Organization* 19:1093, 1958.

6. Scrimshaw, N. S., Behar, M., Arroyave, G., Tejada, C. and Viteri, F. "Kwashiorkor in children and its response to protein therapy." *J. Am. Med. Assoc.* 164:555, 1957.

7. Scrimshaw, N. S. and Behar, M. "World-wide occurrence of protein malnutrition." *Fed. Proc.* 18 (Supple. 3):82, 1959.

8. Robles, B., Ramos-Galvan, R. and Cravioto, J. M. "Valoracion de la conducta del nino con desnutricion avanzada y de sus modificaciones durante la recuperacion." *Bol. med. hosp. infantil* (Mex.) 16:317, 1959.

9. Ramos-Galvan, R., Navarrete, J. L., Perez and Cravioto, J. M. "Algunas aspectos de crecimiento y desarrollo en el nino Mexicano." *Bol. med. hosp. infantil* (Mex.) 17:455, 1960.

10. Burgess, R. C. "Infantile beri-beri." *Fed. Proc.* 17 (Supple. 2, Pt. II):39, 1958.

11. Joint FAO/WHO Expert Committee on Nutrition. Report of Fourth Session. *FAO Meetings Report Series* No. 9, Rome. *WHO Technical Report Series* No. 97, Geneva. 1955.

12. Oomen, H. A. P. C. "Clinical experience on hypovitaminosis A." *Fed. Proc.* 17 (Supple. 2, Pt. II):162, 1958.

13. Astwood, E. B., Greer, M. A. and Ettlinger, M. G. "L-5-vinyl-2-thiooxazolidine, an antithyroid compound from yellow turnip and from Brassica seeds." *J. Biol. Chem.* 181:121, 1949.

14. Greer, M. A. "Nutrition and goiter." *Physiol. Rev.* 30:513, 1950.

15. Haubold, H. "Der einfluss des carotinoidmangels auf die nachkriegs-strumen der erwashsenen." *Verhandl. deutsch. Ges. inn. Med.* 57:112, 1951.

16. Murray, M. M. Ryle, J. A., Simpson, B. W. and Wilson, D. C. "Thyroid Enlargement and Other Changes Related to the Mineral Content of Drinking Water (With a Note on Goitre Prophylaxis)." *Great Britain Privy Council, Medical Research Council* (London) *Memorandum* No. 18, 1948.

17. Kelly, F. C. and Snedden, W. W. "Prevalence and geographical distribution of endemic goiter." *Bull. World Health Organization* 18:5, 1958.

18. Scrimshaw, N. S., Cabezas, A., Castillo, F. F. and Mendez, J. "Effect of potassium iodate on endemic goiter and protein-bound iodine levels in school children." *Lancet* 2:166, 1953.

Newer Concepts in The Management of Obesity*

ROBERT W. HILLMAN, M.D.

IN THESE research-structured nineteen-sixties, perhaps more than in any decade since Lavoisier, there is something presumptuous even pretentious about a discussion of "newer concepts" in the management of obesity. From the viewpoint of today's almost frenetic laboratory and clinical pursuit of a solution to this problem, some significant innovation surely would seem implied—if not some scientific breakthrough elucidating its pathogenesis, at least some empirical formula for the effective correction of obesity. Since neither of these hoped for events appears at hand, justification for a review of present thinking must be found principally in the degree to which obesity has become a matter of personal, professional, and public concern.

The importance of obesity derives from three considerations: 1. Its prevalence; 2. Its association with increased morbidity and mortality rates, notably in respect to cardiovascular-renal and metabolic disorders, as well as surgical and obstetric complications; and 3. Its amenability to treatment, as one practical device for the control of these conditions. Although probably an authoritative consensus, each of these categoric assertions requires critical examination and, on the basis of existing evidence, only qualified acceptance. However, since "management" is the designated subject, other aspects of obesity will be considered only as they bear directly on this principal concern.

The reduction of general morbidity and mortality through the correction of obesity presupposes two assumptions: first, that weight reduction can and does lower the risk of disability and death; and, second, that weight reduction can be achieved and maintained.

THE RISKS OF OBESITY

Clinical impressions support the concept of greater risks for obese subjects in respect to most of the major disorders besetting our population. Experimental animal studies seem generally consistent with this belief. Statistical reports, notably from life insurance sources, provide the principal documentation of the increased hazards associated with overweight. Although overweight and obesity are not synonymous, the great majority of overweight persons are obese, i.e., have an excess of body fat. Moreover, although association does not, per se, establish a cause and effect relationship, and although avail-

* Reprinted by permission, with the omission of nine illustrations, from the December, 1962, issue of Health News, Vol. 39, pp. 4–17. The author is Professor, Environmental Medicine and Community Health, College of Medicine at New York City, State University of New York, N.Y.

able information is as yet insufficient to prove beneficial effects attributable to weight reduction, i.e., lowered mortality rates among unselected subjects who reduced, the presumptive evidence for generally adverse effects of obesity seems too massive and too consistent to be ignored. While more conclusive information still must be sought, it seems that the health professions cannot properly wait on the medical millennium before recommending patterns of life for the host of seemingly vulnerable persons in this and similar "well" nourished nations. Unless, and until, unequivocal evidence is forthcoming to the contrary, there appears no reasonable alternative to advising ostensibly well and afflicted individuals alike, in the words of the late, eminent authority, Dr. Norman Jolliffe, "to avoid overweight, and, if overweight, to reduce and stay reduced."

The second assumption, that obesity is amenable to treatment, also must be qualified. Although a negative caloric balance seems within the theoretic capability of almost every correctly advised person, present reported results suggest rather that, beyond relative simplicity of prescription, this frequently sought therapeutic experience is more typically characterized by difficulty of adherence and improbability of achievement. Irrespective of source and of circumstances, reliable, objective, and sufficiently long-term observations continue to indicate poor over-all success for most patients. The term, patients, is employed intentionally not so much to equate obesity with illness or potential illness as to identify those seeking medical advice—a possible nonrepresentative minority of all obese persons, excluding many self-regulating individuals who, once adequately motivated, successfully attain and sustain, if not ideal nutriture, at least desired weight levels.

That obesity is not always amenable to treatment, and that correction of obesity does not insure elimination of the added risks associated with this condition must, therefore, be acknowledged. So, too, must it be acknowledged that the substantial evidence that obesity is generally undesirable is still subject to contradiction; that efforts toward its control seem justifiably predicated on the relative health advantages currently identified with normal weight status.

Since no critical physiologic or pharmacologic advance has been forthcoming or appears imminent in this area, perhaps the chief new contribution to the management of obesity should be depicted as the belated, understandably reluctant realization that obesity is not an entity except in the gross physical sense, and that a single therapeutic solution is unlikely to prove effective in all, or even most, persons manifesting this sometimes only common attribute of adiposity. Although treatment remains as much as ever on an empiric trial and error basis, individualization of patient management has become a necessary and, to some extent, feasible requirement—the initial step towards ultimate identification of the specific metabolic and psychologic aberrations that someday will call for equally specific measures.

CAUSATIVE FACTORS

Existing classifications of obesity now lend themselves to improved understanding of this condition but, beyond the generic, nosologic problems of reconciling etiologic, functional and structural characteristics, there remain the basic difficulties of extrapolating animal experience to man and of interpreting innumerable yet still inadequate and conflicting observations on the human species. With due awareness of the limitations inherent in any current, necessarily tentative classification, students of the subject have implicated: 1. Familial (both hereditable and environmental); 2. Metabolic (endocrine); 3. Regulatory; and 4. Psychologic factors in the complex causation of obesity. Varying with circumstances, including different stages as represented by "active" and "static" obesity, these are presumed usually to be indivisible and, from the practical standpoint, coexistent. Most important in relation to the positive calorie balance that constitutes the basic mechanism in all types of obesity, each of these factors affects the output as well as the intake of energy. Much new evidence suggests that variations in the expenditure rather than in the consumption of calories represent the critical factor for perhaps most obese members of our highly mechanized society.

In part, as a concession to these etiologic concepts but principally for pragmatic reasons, the management of obesity may be divided arbitrarily into four interdependent and overlapping aspects: psychologic, pharmaceutic, physical, and dietary. Collectively, during both the period of active therapy and the long-term follow up, they comprise the general management of this condition directed toward the establishment of optimum energy balance in an individual with the "right kind as well as the right amount of body weight." Proper management necessarily presupposes a correct diagnosis of the obese state *per se* as well as an attempt to assess the "specific" pathogenesis in each instance.

PSYCHOLOGIC CONSIDERATIONS

Psychologic factors are operative in every obese person just as in every nonobese individual. Seemingly, there is neither a single psychologic problem peculiar to the obese state nor one common to all patients with this condition. Although a current consensus indicates no excess of these psychologic problems among the obese, probably just a different expressivity, they nevertheless must be identified correctly and accorded appropriate attention. Whether symbolic meanings are attached to food, to oral mechanisms or to the over-sized body, it is difficult to distinguish the causes from the effects of obesity. Associated psychologic components may be predisposing, pre-cipitating and/or perpetuating—the frequently emphasized "second-ary gain" factor.

The role of conditioning processes must be assessed especially in those instances where anxiety is a conspicuous feature, and the con-sumption of excess calories is not mediated through hunger. Beyond detection of specific neuroses and especially the psychoses, it may be helpful to distinguish between so-called developmental and reactive types of obesity; the latter, with their relatively later onset seem more responsive to treatment. Apparently, too, the juvenile obese patient with a strong psychologic component is relatively unresponsive to treatment, whereas the presence of strong psychologic factors in the adult obese patient is associated with a relatively favorable prognosis. Since it is now realized that attempts at weight reduction may have adverse effects in some individuals with more serious psychologic problems, it is important to preclude or at least to postpone definitive treatment in those comparatively few situations where it actually may be contraindicated.

Psychiatric consultation and/or therapy, as such, is required for only a small proportion of obese patients. The generalist, the internist, or the pediatrician usually can, and for practical reasons also must, provide suitable guidance and support as part of total patient man-agement. The indispensable element of motivation is most readily induced by that physician with the most complete knowledge of the patient, his family, and his unique micro-environment, especially if he assumes responsibility for the patient's integrated over-all care above and beyond the weight reducing regimen *per se*. Rather than the management of the condition, obesity, this therapeutic undertaking now is more appropriately thought of as the management of the patient who is obese—of the whole person.

PHARMACEUTIC PREPARATIONS

The expectation that pharmaceutic preparations comprise most of the definitive new developments in the management of obesity in redundant in the enterprise and vigor with which pharmaceutic research is directed to the solution of major health problems. Al-though it is beyond this immediate province to list, much less to discuss, the many and varied products recently introduced to further weight reduction, these and earlier preparations may be classified into broad generic groups, notably: anorexiants, euphoriants, tran-quilizers, sedatives, metabolic activators, bulk producers, antiabsorb-ents, cathartics, and diuretics. A broad range exists with respect to both effectiveness and tolerance; considerable variation is noted within as well as between these groups. Preparations still to be formulated are certain to include improvements combining enhanced and sustained activity with fewer adverse reactions. At present, however, widely used pharmaceutic and related adjuncts appear to have only limited and temporary value and, in some instances, actually may be detrimental. Predominantly dehydrating devices, for example, seem hardly consonant with the objective of long-term correction of adiposity, as such, and lend themselves too readily to exploitation. Agents that reduce food intake sometimes are advocated initially or, in stubborn cases, as short-term adjuncts to dietary treatment provided they do not compromise consumption of essential nutrients. Beyond their specific actions, these pharmaceuticals admittedly meet the frequent need for a "gimmick," the element of magic for which the wavering will power inevitably reaches out. Since, however, they also serve as a crutch, detracting and diverting from essential emphasis on dietary regulation and, at best, appear to afford only initial temporary help, present disposition is not thus merely to postpone the day of necessary self-confrontation but, preferably, to avoid pharmaceutic agents in the management of obesity at all stages and in almost all cases.

PHYSICAL FACTORS

Among the current though scarcely new developments in the management of obesity is the revised emphasis on the role of exercise. Once regarded as a major factor in the treatment of overweight, physical activity later was accorded less importance in the wake of revelations that considerable effort was required to shed even one pound of adipose tissue. Energy equivalents such as a 36-mile walk, a six-hour swim, discouraged a majority of would-be reducers who were too readily convinced that they lacked the resources to work off even this small part of their surplus. Moreover, they found spiritual as well as bodily comfort in some expert opinion that calories expended through exercise would be immediately replaced as a result of an automatic increase in appetite. The only exercise that mattered, they were persuaded, was the thrice daily practice of pushing away from the table "soon enough and far enough."

At present, fortunately for fitness as well as for fatness, exercise has been restored to grace, enjoying not only physiologic but also psychologic and even social respectability. In contrast to the sedentary interlude when the pursuit of vigorous activity was reviewed with the skepticism and amused tolerance now reserved for the food faddists, exercise is once more acceptable in the smart set. The reactivated heel-and-toe fraternity is even now eschewing the pointed and spiked footwear that discourages walking. The tandem bike, a tougher triumph for togetherness, is coming back and may yet supplant the sports car as a status symbol. If they hearken to Drs. Paul D. White, Irvine Page and other advocates of the active life, the self-propelled squares of today will become the literally not too big wheelmen of tomorrow.

Exercise is advocated for at least three reasons: First, it promotes caloric expenditure.* Moreover, within the usual range of activity, as Dr. Mayer has shown, exercise need not provoke a commensurate increase in appetite to, as inevitably, negate the energy deficit. It is also emphasized that while the energy equivalent of a pound of adipose tissue remains approximately 3500 calories, weight loss obviously need not be effected in decrements of precisely this amount. Fractions rather than multiples of this standard, but nonetheless arbitrary unit of surplus, represent a more practical realistic daily objective compatible with the usual personal resources of time and physical condition. Instead of the exhausting, often impossible 36-mile hike within the span of hours, a walk of just one extra mile per day for 36 days is a simple, even pleasant device for shedding an extra pound of fat. The total loss of 10 pounds thus readily achieved in a period of a single year represents a rate of loss which, with few exceptions, is greatly in excess of that at which corpulence is acquired by the average individual who typically accumulates his 10 to 30 per cent surplus over a span of as many years. Obviously, while extremes of physical exertion are not called for and may even be contraindicated, regular exercise consistent with reason and tolerance can contribute significantly to a negative energy balance. Although much more evidence must be gathered in this area, regular physical activity in the process of burning excess calories probably also enhances general metabolic efficiency, resulting in reduced hormone needs and improved utilization of energy sources.

Exercise manifestly furthers physical, mental, psychologic and social fitness. It provides an outlet for emotional tensions, promotes self-confidence, and enhances the real, albeit intangible, sense of general well-being that lends strength of purpose as well as will power to confront and to master personal challenges, including a reducing regimen.

Of more than parenthetic importance to patients concerned about the topical arrangement as well as the amount of their excess fat, present evidence indicates that while body contours may be favorably

---

* Although the energy cost of specific activities can now be measured with fair precision under experimental conditions, it is difficult to estimate the time actually devoted to these activities in usual, everyday situations. Marked differences in intensity as well as duration of participation— during work, recreation, and as recently emphasized, even sleep hours— probably account for greater variations in caloric expenditure than has hitherto generally been appreciated.

altered by muscle development, physical activity—general or local, active or passive—does not *per se* modify the constitutionally determined distribution of adipose tissue.

DIETARY ASPECTS

Newer developments have significantly failed to bring rejection of the predictably durable axiom: a proper diet remains the *sine qua non* for the successful, long-term management of obesity. Although there is now an, if possible, even wider divergence of opinion concerning both the components and the scheduling of food intake, the consensus is that there is no substitute for this fundamental aspect of weight and, hopefully, of over-all health regulation. It is generally agreed that given adequate motivation, weight loss can be achieved on virtually any dietary regimen, good or bad, that insures a negative energy balance. It is equally apparent that many diets are only temporarily effective and do not further the fundamental objective of permanent weight loss, not to mention good eating habits.

The cardinal principles of the good reducing diet continue to be essentially these:

1. The diet should be individualized in accordance with economic, ethnic, and personal circumstances, literally a personalized prescription.

2. The diet should be practical, consistent with work patterns and other everyday obligations and responsibilities. It should keep the individual functioning at optimum levels, at his usual job and not conduce to invalidism, real or imagined. Inappropriate or excessive devotion to diet above and beyond actual need can be still another form of iatrogenic disability.

3. The diet should be flexible, employing a system of exchanges (specific foods, not merely caloric equivalents) with provision for individual preferences and idiosyncrasies. Elasticity of prescription should be combined with reasonable rigidity of adherence. Deviations, if any, should be planned, deliberate and by design rather than by default. For instance, special temptations such as ice cream may be prescribed, not just permitted, once or twice weekly.

4. The diet should utilize readily available commonly preferred foods as distinct from unusual or "dietetic" foods which all members of the family can be encouraged to enjoy.

5. The diet should be consistent with established or accepted health practices and compatible with regimens prescribed for concurrent medical conditions such as hepatic, renal, and cardiac disorders.

6. The diet should be balanced and complete in conformity with the Recommended Dietary Allowances of the National Research Coun-

cil. These, it must be stressed, afford a margin of sufficiency above minimum "requirements."

7. The diet, basically, should be a pattern for life not only for the period of weight reduction but also for the long-term maintenance of "normal" weight and optimum health.

Specific aspects of the dietary regimen may be divided into the so-called academics and mechanics of food consumption. The former, relating to the essential components of the diet, still presuppose the fundamental importance of calories (they really *do* count) while taking cognizance of newer concepts concerning the respective roles of individual macro- and micro-nutrients. The latter, embracing the size, timing, and specific food items of meals, necessarily also consider recent observations on the effects of frequent feedings as well as of short-term starvation.

In respect to each of these aspects, there is the over-all basic requirement to recognize that by reason of inherited as well as acquired attributes, patients differ metabolically as well as psychologically and, pending an improved ability to distinguish between biotypes, dietary recommendations remain largely general and empirical.

ADJUSTING CALORIC LEVELS

The total caloric prescription remains a function of the weight level and of the desired rate of loss—a decision based on the physician's estimate of the optimum rate for the individual patient and consonant with psychologic and physiologic requirements, including the patient's personal priorities and values. Excessive rates of loss not only fail to provide an adequate period for adjustment to a revised living pattern but, particularly in grossly overweight adults, appear to increase the risks of serious cardiovascular mishap. The usual goal of one or two pounds' loss per week is achieved by a daily deficit of 500 or 1000 calories, respectively from the estimated caloric intake needed to maintain prereduction weight. However, prescriptions range widely and commonly are set at some arbitrary level between 1000 calories and the energy level sufficient to maintain the estimated desirable body weight. The nomogram may be used for this purpose. However, satisfactory working estimates may be computed as readily through such simple formulas as 15 calories per pound of desired weight with no reckoning for physical activity, or 25 calories per kilo of desired weight with, in this instance, an additional 25 per cent to 50 per cent depending on physical activity. This factor often is the crucial element. Obviously the calorie level can and should be adjusted in accordance with response. There is no substitute for the therapeutic trial. It is also currently emphasized that 1000 calories represent the smallest, practical energy vehicle that can provide the recommended daily allowances of essential micro-nutrients through usual food sources. For children, notably during puberty and adolescence, the minimum figure for a satisfactory balanced pattern is closer to 1600 calories, with 1800 often recommended to insure a margin of safety as well as to encourage adherence.

The protein component of the diet usually is calculated at one gram per kilo of ideal body weight, of which at least two-thirds should be of animal origin, i.e., of high biologic value. Although this represents 12 per cent to 20 per cent of the total calories, higher proportions still are advocated by some, more in the interest of lowered fat and carbohydrate content than of nitrogen balance.

Fat should contribute 25 per cent to 30 per cent of the total energy supply; however, 45–50 grams seem a minimum for practical purposes considering its satiety and energy values as well as its usual sources.

The carbohydrate remainder, some 40 per cent to 60 per cent of the total calories, should include a minimum of simple sugars and a maximum of polysaccharides. It should also provide suitable bulk with sufficient fiber content for optimum bowel function and, it is now thought, to sustain generally beneficial intestinal flora.

These represent tentative, average and admittedly arbitrary proportions of the principal aliments. Enthusiasms for more extreme prescriptions, e.g., high fat, high carbohydrate, are revived periodically by experimental and clinical observations which suggest something more promising than the present generally ineffective regimens. Although these programs commonly are without adequate scientific foundation, applicable to only a relatively small proportion of obese patients, inconsistent with good long-term dietary practices, and operate through psychologic even more than metabolic mechanisms, they have the partial virtue of emphasizing both current therapeutic limitations and the need to investigate these aspects more thoroughly if the management of obesity is to become more effective.

Notwithstanding emphasis in some quarters on a large number of so-called trace elements, the diet prescription for uncomplicated obesity usually gives special attention only to calcium, phosphorus and iron needs. Adult calcium requirements generally are met through one pint of skimmed milk or cottage cheese equivalent daily. Phosphorus needs are readily supplied through usual milk, meat and fat (phospholipid) sources. Ordinary iron needs are satisfied by inclusion of liver once or preferably twice weekly. Potassium requirements, less commonly a cause of concern, are readily met through meat, milk, and, particularly vegetable sources.

Salt intake, although ordinarily in excess of needs, should not be restricted on reducing regimens except where dictated by specific individual complications. In all likelihood, interdiction of salt has contributed indirectly to weight reduction, at least until adaption through decreased food appeal as well as water loss.

Vitamin requirements, while theoretically met through the diet, are probably best insured by prescribing one supplemental multi-vitamin capsule daily, particularly during the early phases of weight loss wherein endogeneous fat sources contribute significantly to the high energy output. The purely supplementary role of the vitamin preparation must be emphasized notably where patients may be disposed to substitute this for preferred food sources.

Fluids should be consumed ad lib, preferably in sufficient quantities to permit a daily urine output of at least one liter, while combating the tendency to constipation that sometimes troubles patients in the initial stages of a reducing program. Although newer evidence concerning the physiologic as well as anatomic relationships between the "aquastat" and the "appestat" suggest that fluid restriction may conduce to food restriction, there is at present insufficient information to recommend routine limitation of fluid intake as a means of long-term caloric control.

Liquid formula diets unquestionably have helped many persons to lose weight. Although some of these preparations combine the merits of economy, acceptability, and nutritional balance, these too lend themselves chiefly to short-term intensive weight loss, postponing the day of reckoning when practical considerations inevitably oblige the patient to return to more usual and probably more complete foodstuffs. Without the essential conditioning and educational components of the reducing regimen, the prospects for effective maintenance of desired weight seem little better than in those instances where other pharmaceutic products are utilized.

DIETARY OBJECTIVES

Together with the academics, the primary objectives of the mechanics of the diet are: 1. Attainment of optimum nutriture in terms of function as well as structure; and 2. Education of the patient not only as an immediate device for weight reduction but, more important, as a means of inducing a permanent, satisfactory, nutritional way of life, i.e., "loss of weight without physiologic or psychologic derangement."

Since eating patterns from the outset should be directed towards the patient's future as well as present nutritional objectives, meal schedules generally should conform to conventional practices, avoiding any aura of ritualism that tends to segregate patients into special food-phobia fellowships.

The total day's prescription may perhaps for some individuals be distributed among three meals with calories represented equally or, perhaps more realistically, in a two-fifths, one-fifth, two-fifths pattern, 40 per cent breakfast, 20 per cent lunch, 40 per cent dinner. Each meal should contain all the aliments, especially complete proteins in the light of current evidence, and essential nutrients in suitable proportions, that is, balanced and complete in itself.

Recent reports indicate that smaller, more frequent feedings may be more conducive to weight loss than the more usual three meal regimen. As observed by Dr. Cohen and his colleagues, smaller segmented, isocaloric diets also may be more protective against metabolic derangements and diseases. Somewhat in contrast, short periods of fasting are advocated by other competent clinicians whose patients have achieved impressive weight loss on surprisingly well-accepted regimens involving periodic complete abstinence without apparent adverse effects. Hospitalization is sometimes recommended, at least initially, in these and other instances where close supervision is essential.

TIMING OF MEALS

Of great importance, but commonly ignored, is the timing of meals; these, whatever their number, should be consumed at regular, though not necessarily equal, intervals. Meal schedules should be set and followed consistently seven days a week. Only in this manner can the rhymthic pattern be developed that is essential for long-term adherence to a reducing and especially a maintenance regimen. Also emphasized, meals should be leisurely, stress-free, preferably family occasions wherein adverse emotional elements do not interfere with the consumption, retention or utilization of essential nutrients. Here too the sound general nutrition practices embodied in the reducing regimen hopefully will be emulated by other nonobese and especially younger members of the family circle. In the event of discrepancy, it is they rather than the patient who must be urged to conform.

The successful management of the patient with obesity requires continuous supervision and evaluation. This is almost always required, particularly in the interest of avoiding the too commonly observed oscillating up-and-down weight pattern which, according to current belief, may have serious physiologic as well as psychologic effects. It may be preferable to remain obese than to alternate rapidly between obesity and a normal weight pattern.

Results unquestionably are a function of the frequency with which the patient is seen, notably in the early stages of the regimen when weekly visits are all but essential. The desired permanent state commonly is achieved in practical stipulated stages through a succession of short-term goals. Although planned plateaus reportedly are desirable in some instances, therapeutic weight loss seems generally best implemented without interruption. Weight objectives may be set for periods of four to 12 weeks; progress may be checked by means of such devices as the "performance index," a ratio between the actual and the predicted weight loss. Irrespective of the criteria adopted, the patient should be given support throughout the period of weight loss. This support should continue to the point where his maintenance program hopefully will become an all but automatic way of life, free from the thrice or more daily deliberations that jeopardize adherence to the permanent program of weight control and compatible with his total physical, psychologic, and social well-being. Weight reduction, the patient must be convinced, is never an objective in itself. It is part of the physician's total program for helping the obese person to become a generally well-nourished, adjusted, and productive member of the community.

Just as a consensus concedes that the symptom, obesity, must be managed in different ways in different individuals at different times and under different circumstances, so it is generally agreed that the treatment of obesity is for the most part unsatisfactory, at least in terms of weight loss effected and sustained. It is also true, however, that while obesity *per se* is too infrequently corrected, many overweight persons nevertheless do profit from the nutritional advice. Improved eating habits often result even though desired weight levels, possibly the most acceptable term if not criterion, may not be achieved. Current emphasis rightly seems on qualitative as well as quantitative change, the kind as well as the amount of tissue. The patient may become in part a "better" person without necessarily becoming a smaller one through improved over-all tissue status. While not unmindful of the distinction between obesity and overweight, some physicians now are less concerned about a slightly or even moderately obese person who eats a well-balanced diet than about a nonobese subject with a qualitatively poor intake.

THE ROLE OF GOOD NUTRITION

Also, it must be emphasized, good nutritional therapy directed to an obese person irrespective of the effect on the weight of the patient *per se* may favorably influence the eating pattern of other members of the family notably in the case of the young mother who plans, purchases, and prepares the meals for her spouse and children. The resulting general improvement in dietary habits should help to prevent all types of malnutrition including hyperalimentation.

Patently, since there is nothing really new in the management of obesity, emphasis must be on this and other preventive aspects especially in the younger age groups among whom so many are otherwise destined to join the hard core of relatively refractory obese adults. Family physicians and pediatricians from their tactical vantage point can do much here to control this serious threat to the physical and psychologic well-being of a significant segment of our society. The serious, sustained cooperation of parents unquestionably is essential but a coordinated school program is equally important. Emphasis should be on the positive, dynamic ("thou shalt" rather than "thou shalt not") approach to weight control as an integral part of physical and total fitness. Example must be provided as well as encouragement; the need at all levels and in all areas of health education is for exponents rather than mere proponents. The educational potential of the school lunch program surely can be exploited to greater advantage and school athletic facilities can be utilized more fully within as well as beyond scheduled class hours.

Finally, as long as the natural countryside continues to be sacrificed to urban expansion, adequate and accessible open spaces also must be assured. At a time when the health professions are concerned with other serious aspects of the "metronoses," it would be ironic, not to say inconsistent, if we were to contemplate with equanimity the ominous disappearance of our outdoor recreation areas, retreats in spirit as well as in substance, until our conspicuous consumption of these and other vital resources invoked a less rational and certainly less happy "solution" to the problem of obesity.

6. Home Care

Home Care Programs*

CECIL G. SHEPS, M.D., AND JACK KASTEN, M.P.H.

HISTORY AND DEVELOPMENT

HOME CARE has been with us as long as medicine has been practiced. In recent years, however, these two words have taken on a special significance and have come to represent a new modality of patient care. It is generally agreed that the first organized home care program in the United States was started at Boston Dispensary in 1796. It should be pointed out that there were somewhat different reasons for the development of the Boston Dispensary program from those that brought forth our modern home care programs. At the time of the inception of the Boston Dispensary program, virtually all medical care for self-supporting people was provided in the home. For the indigent, some medical care was available in dispensaries and hospitals. Thus, the objectives of the Boston Dispensary program were described as:

1) The sick, without being pained by separation from their families, may be attended and relieved in their own houses.
2. The sick can, in this way, be assisted at a less expense to the public than in any hospital.
3. Those who have seen better days, may be comforted without being humiliated; and all the poor receive the benefits of charity, the more refined as it is the more secret.[1]

Throughout the 19th century the circumstances governing the delivery of medical care remained about the same. Medical care was given by the general practitioner, who made home visits using a bicycle or a horse and buggy and who had one or two diagnostic instruments as the only supplements to his physical senses.

Changes in the first half of the 20th century affected society's attitude toward many aspects of medical care. During this period, the hospital evolved as the center for the care and treatment of major illness. With the increased use of aseptic technics, hospitals became safe. Scientific discoveries provided the physician with a wide array

* Reprinted, by permission, from the May, 1962, issue of *Rehabilitation Literature*, Vol. 23, pp. 130–135, 144. The authors are, respectively, Professor of Medical and Hospital Administration, Graduate School of Public Health, University of Pittsburgh, Pittsburgh, Pennsylvania; and Research Associate, Medical and Hospital Administration at the Graduate School of Public Health, University of Pittsburgh, Pittsburgh, Pennsylvania.

of tools for diagnostic use and an increasing number of therapeutic measures to aid him in his practice. These developments led to a sharp growth in the number of new professions represented in the hospital. Social workers, psychologists, therapists, and others came onto the scene with their skills and technics for helping the sick. Nursing personnel grew in number and scope of responsibility and subdivided into various levels of ability and training. Technicians were needed to operate new equipment and laboratory facilities. As new avenues were explored and developed by medical science, new areas of service were added to the hospital program.

The expansion and change in medical service have been accompanied by an increase in costs of care. New methods of payment have developed a variety of organization. Organizations for payment have an effect on the public's view of how medical care should be provided and on how medical care actually is provided.

The predominant trend in medical care practice in this country has been the emphasis on hospital care. There has been a consistent tendency on the part of the physician to use the hospital as a center for his activities. It has come to be considered as the best way of treating patients, and it is also the most convenient. All health workers have encouraged the community to think of the hospital as the place to get well rather than the place to die. This attitude was eventually accepted and by the early 1940's we find communities generally considering the hospital as the center for the care of major illness and an essential to the delivery of high-quality medical care.

Now that the image of the hospital as the best place for treatment of illness has been accepted, there is some difficulty in reversing attitudes. The doctor, as well as the patient, has a great sense of security in the hospital. When a doctor visits a home he gives advice. When he goes to the hospital he gives orders. In many ways this might be a more comfortable situation for the doctor and, perhaps, even on occasion for the patient.

In the last 25 years, there has been a sharp decline in the number of doctor-patient contacts within the home. In 1928–1931, 40 per cent of out-of-hospital doctor-patient contacts were in the home, but by 1957, this had decreased to 8 per cent.[2] (p. 5)

Along with the changes in the place of care, a variety of changes has occurred in the pattern of medical care needs. In the last half century, the nature of the population has changed from predominantly rural to an urban-centered metropolitan type of life. Greatly improved transportation facilities have lessened the problem of travel and distance. There has been a decline in the number of generations of a family living under one roof, or even in the same community. Today we are faced with a large and ever-growing number of persons of advanced age. The bulk of chronic illness is found in this same group. Often these patients have more than one disease condition. The increasing number of patients with chronic disease in the community presents a particular problem for the general hospital. There have been studies that point to the malutilization of hospitals and to the extent to which hospitals are being used as a substitute for other services less complicated but otherwise not available. The best known of these is the study conducted in four general hospitals in Boston.[3] (p. 145) It was found that about one-third of the patient days of care was given to persons who remained in the hospitals 30 days or longer, and that one-half of those patients did not require the full range of hospital care. This represents almost 15 per cent of the total days' care rendered in these four institutions.

In 1944, Jensen, Weiskotten, and Thomas published a report of an imaginative and decisive experiment in medical care through which the services of the medical staff of a hospital were extended beyond the walls of the institution.[4] This study was based upon a philosophy developed by the faculty members of Syracuse University College of Medicine. Since they believed medical education was becoming too institutionalized, a program was introduced into the undergraduate curriculum giving each student the responsibility of making a complete study of at least one patient, including a personal investigation of the home and living and working conditions. A senior medical resident was assigned to the program to bear the ultimate responsibility for follow-up of discharged patients. This pilot study began on July 1, 1940, and involved all patients discharged from the medical wards of the University Hospital up to February 1, 1942.

Some of the most significant findings in this study were:

1) 84.1% of the patients admitted to the medical wards were suffering from chronic diseases.

2) Only 59.3% of the patients discharged to private physicians and 23.2% of those discharged to the free dispensary reported to them without follow-up action by the medical resident. The activities of this resident increased these percentages to 78.8% and 84.2% respectively.

3) The organization and administration of the experiment revealed that the lack of integration of sources of medical supervision in the community makes continuous care for the medically needy difficult unless a plan is made for their co-ordination.

The final paragraph in the summary of this report states:

The information revealed by this experiment tends to reemphasize the fact that the hospital is the pivot around which should revolve the various services, inpatient care, outpatient clinics, and public welfare programs, which maintain the health of the people. The provision of home care for discharged medically needy patients is one further step toward a more economical and beneficial use of the hospital in the care of the indigent. Unless we are prepared to furnish a qualified physician to pilot the medically needy patient suffering from chronic disease on his course after leaving the hospital, we shall continue to waste time, effort, and many thousands of dollars by hauling him back to port for repairs each time he goes on the rocks.[4] (p. 79-80)

A few years later, in 1948, Montefiore Hospital in New York City developed its organized home care program.[5] This program extended the service of the hospital into the home by providing medical, social, nursing, rehabilitative, and related services to patients through a department of home care. The announcement of Montefiore Hospital's success evoked widespread interest in this modality of care. Many papers were published. Speeches were made both to community groups and in professional associations. Similar programs were launched in other communities. In light of this widespread interest it is surprising and disappointing to find that, after over 10 years, there are only some 50 home care programs operating in the entire country.

DETAILED PROGRAM DESCRIPTION

As an example of the more highly organized programs, comparable to the Montefiore program and one which the authors know best, the home care program of the Beth Israel Hospital in Boston will be described in some detail. There the following principles were agreed upon before the program was started in 1954:

1) This would be the extramural arm of the hospital for patients with long-term illness.

2) A service program would be designed to meet the needs of patients, teaching and research being second and subservient objectives.

3) It would serve patients not able to afford private medical care.

4) Duplication of existing services would be avoided through cooperation with existing community resources.

5) We considered that the program would not be an entity in itself but a bridge in the continuity of care.

6) Immediate readmission to the hospital when needed was guaranteed.

7) In accepting a patient for the program there would be three primary considerations:

   a) The patient must be medically suited for home care.

   b) The social situation in the home must be suitable, with a responsible member of the patient's family available to provide certain elements of care and support.

   c) The patient must be unable to afford private medical care.

In addition, the patient must be within a 30-minute driving radius of the hospital so that there can be prompt response of a doctor in an emergency as well as regular calls. Also, this would speed readmission to the hospital if this should become necessary.

Referrals to the home care department are accepted from the ward service and outpatient department, from other community health and welfare agencies, and from members of the hospital staff. Staffing is provided by full-time or part-time paid professional staff. Nursing care in the home is provided through contractual arrangements with the visiting nurse services in various communities in metropolitan Boston.

Services provided by the visiting nurse associations generally consist of the evaluation of the physical facilities in the home for the suitability of nursing, physical therapy, competent and skilled diet therapy, and instruction of the family in simple nursing procedures.

Homemaker services are arranged as needed through various community agencies or directly by the home care department.

The three foundation stones for the program are: comprehensive care, co-ordinated services, and continuity of responsibility. These are suggested as three *minimum* criteria by which to determine the effectiveness of a home care program.

Here then is a hospital that opens its doors and reaches out into the community. Its services are provided on a co-ordinated basis. In addition to services of the physicians on the program and consultants when needed, care includes nursing, social service, laboratory and x-ray work, physical and occupational therapy, homemaker services, with medications and equipment of various kinds provided.

Whenever necessary, all the consulting services of the hospital are brought to bear on the needs of the patient. Studies that can be made available in the home, including blood tests, x-ray studies, and electro-cardiographs, are so arranged. Otherwise, the patient is brought to the hospital. This applies also to special forms of treatment, such as blood transfusions, abdominal paracentesis, and the application of casts. Patients are given round-the-clock coverage. They are instructed that if they telephone to the hospital, day or night, their needs will be immediately referred to the covering physician, who will take care of them.

Upon acceptance into the program all the patients and their families are informed that, if hospitalization seems indicated, they will be admitted immediately. Of course, this is of tremendous importance in terms of assurance to both the patient and the family when he is leaving the protective atmosphere of the hospital ward.

The cornerstone of this program in terms of its quality and effectiveness is the *team approach*, which involves, among other things, two types of formal meetings that are held each week. One is for the evaluation of cases referred; the other is held to evaluate the progress of patients already under care. The conference brings into play various skills of diverse professional people who may have a contribution to make to the understanding of the needs of the patient. Of 273 patients referred to the program in the first 5 years of operation, two-thirds were found suitable for home care. At this point in the development of this particular program at Beth Israel Hospital, the average number of patients being cared for was 45. Most are in the older age group, 72 per cent being at least 60 years of age.

An examination of the first 25 patients treated in this program provides interesting information about diseases represented and what kind of care they received. The 25 patients had 38 major conditions. Eleven had heart disease, 9 cancer, 7 diabetes, and 6 peripheral vascular disease. These are the major medical conditions one finds in patients who are referred and found acceptable for home care.

An analysis of the volume of and types of visits for these first 25 patients shows that in this period there were 816 physician visits, 783 visits by the visiting nurse, 153 visits by a social worker, 81 visits of patients to the outpatient department, and one visit to the emergency department.

The breakdown of the length of time that the first 25 patients were followed on home care shows that 12 were followed for less than 3 months, 19 for less than a year, 3 for 2 years or more, and one for 4 years or more. In this period of 59 months, just a month short of five years, there were 19½ patient years of continuous care given these 25 patients, 91.4 per cent in the home, 7.1 per cent in the hospital, and 1.5 per cent in a convalescent home.

Now what happened to these patients in terms of basic issues such as life and death? Seventeen of them died during this span of time. Five of them were discharged from the program as being able to carry on simply as outpatients. Two of them transferred to a long-term hospital and one patient still is on home care.

Many of us who view these matters have a tendency to think in terms of statistics only. It is important to remember that statistics are "human beings with the tears wiped off." Therefore, it is helpful sometimes to think of home care in human terms. This point can be illustrated best by telling of the effects of home care on one patient.

Mrs. B. is a woman of 68, whose husband receives public assistance. Total income for both from all sources is $126.00 a month. The patient suffers from a group of chronic disabling diseases, including heart failure, bronchial asthma, postoperative ventral hernia, and bilateral pyelonephritis, to name only a few. In the 25 years from 1930 to 1955, she was admitted to the Beth Israel Hospital 29 times. In the five-year period before she was accepted on home care, she was admitted to the hospital 6 times for a total of 331 days of care.

After almost four years of receiving continuous, coordinated, comprehensive care from the home care department, Mrs. B. has recently said, "I never wanted to be an invalid; home care came along and now I no longer am an invalid." Since she has been on home care she has been admitted to the hospital only twice, for a total of only 20 days. Each admission was for diagnostic purposes only.

Thus, a dramatic change in the lives of this couple is seen. They maintain their home and Mrs. B. receives a high quality of care with a minimum of cost and a maximum of effect.

One-third of the patients in this particular program are receiving public assistance. The welfare department pays the cost of their care on a per diem, not a per visit, basis. The balance of the cost of the home care program is borne by private voluntary community philanthropy.

A somewhat different type of program worthy of attention is the one operated by the New York City Department of Hospitals. Although much of the over-all structure is the same as the program previously described, there are certain unique features. Size alone is a distinguishing feature of this program. There are 16 home care units with a total average census last year of 2,207 patients. Each of the 16 units has a capacity of 100 patients or more.[6] All the units operate within one general policy laid down by the department of hospitals. There is, however, some variation in individual programs. Social work services are available in most of the units in the same manner as in the previously described program, but, in at least one of the City hospitals, the ward social worker follows the inpatient into the home care program, thereby performing the functions of a home care social worker.[7] Another way in which this program is different is in the availability of physicians for emergency service. Calls for emergency visits after 5 p.m. are referred to the emergency ward of the hospital.[7] (p. 376) Thus patients are brought to the hospital rather than medical service being sent to the patient in his home.

The home care physician in the City hospital program does not take part in the evaluation process for admitting patients to the program. There are some programs in which an effort is made to assign groups of patients to particular physicians. However, in most of the operating units a different physician may make each home visit.[7] (p. 376) Thus, the opportunity for a continuous relationship is lost. Referrals in all the units are from the hospital's own inpatient wards with a few instances of referral from another City hospital or from the outpatient department of the hospital operating the program.[7] (p. 370)

Another type of program that should be differentiated from the typical program described is the community-based home care program.

A good example of such a community-based program is the one in Detroit operated by the Visiting Nurse Association in association with the Michigan Hospital Service (Blue Cross).[8] This program does not provide physician services. Instead, a condition of acceptance to its home care program is that the patient have a private physician in attendance at home. There is an evaluation of each applicant, but the service to patients is more a co-ordination of services that are rendered in the home than a controlling function in establishing and carrying out a program of continuous care for the patient at home. Since this program is predicated on shortening the hospital stay, it functions for discharged patients only.

This home care program as an entity does not guarantee the patient a hospital bed, since it has none formally at its disposal. The over-all supervision and management of the patient and rehospitalization, if necessary, is left to the private physician in attendance. In programs such as this one, the personal physician's participation in establishing a long-term program of care and in periodic conferences on patient progress has been less than would seem desirable. Also the volume of referrals to home care has depended on the amount of work done by a liaison person from the home care agency with the medical staffs of the hospitals in the program.[9 (p. 1684)]

The descriptions given above cover most features in typical home care programs. The authors feel, however, that optimum home care service can be rendered only if the following essential elements are part of the program.

1) The home care program *as an entity* must accept the total responsibility for care of the patient.

2) Physician services must be available 24 hours a day, 7 days a week.

3) Immediate hospital admission for patients on home care must be guaranteed without the necessity for the patient to meet any criterion other than referral by the home care physician.

4) There must be a formally structured group comprised of at least a physician, a Public Health nurse, and a social case worker responsible for the operation of the home care program.

5) Patients must be formally referred and there must be an initial evaluation, a review of the patient's record at least monthly, and a final discharge conference. The physicians who give actual service in the home must be present at conferences involving their patients.

6) Patients must be selected for participation on the basis of need for the organized approach of the home care program, rather than any single home health service. The home must be physically and socially suitable.

REHABILITATION AND HOME CARE PROGRAMS

Physical restoration and rehabilitation have played a major role in organized home care programs. By the very nature of the population group treated by those programs, there is great need for rehabilitation services. A number of programs, however, have had some difficulty in staffing their units with qualified rehabilitation personnel. A study of organized home care in New York City (1956) showed that 10 of the 19 programs in the study had neither a physical therapist nor an occupational therapist. Six had one, but not both, and three had both. This report also showed that, in the programs in the study, only 10% of the patients on home care received rehabilitative services.[7] (p. 108)

Goldmann and Fraenkel, in their study of patients on home care programs, showed that 56.6% of the patients received some service from a physical therapist, occupational therapist, or speech therapist during the one month in which a detailed breakdown was made.[10] (p. 83)

The *Inventory of Coordinated Home Care Programs in the United States,* now in the process of publication, received reports from 48 administrative units (16 of these are in the New York City Department of Hospitals Program) on services available for patients.[6] Forty-six have arrangements for the provision of physical therapy service, 32 provide occupational therapy, and 33 make provision for speech therapy.

One of the major problems in any rehabilitation program is re-employment. Home care programs have been looking into the possibility of jobs for the homebound. A pilot project was developed at Montefiore Hospital, New York, at its home care unit. At the conclusion of the pilot program, jobs for the homebound project became a regular home care service. Their experience indicated that appropriate work can be found for homebound, chronically ill patients and that this work activity can be included in a medical home care program at a reasonable cost.[11]

In addition to the great interest in rehabilitation services in organized home care programs, there has been a new development in recent years. Rehabilitation programs per se have developed home care services for their patients. There are at least three programs (Delaware County, Pennsylvania Stroke Program; Jewish Chronic Disease Hospital of Brooklyn Cerebral Vascular Accident Program; Continuation Care Program, Hospital Center at Orange Rehabilitation Service, Orange, N.J.) in which either demand for inpatient beds or a desire to extend the rehabilitation program into the community has stimulated the establishment of a home care program by a rehabilitation agency. Although these programs are limited to the particular kind of patient in which the rehabilitation agency is interested, it is possible, and in at least one case probable, that these programs meet all the criteria set up for the essentials of organized home care.

Although there is an attempt to provide rehabilitation services within the framework of home care, and home care services within a rehabilitation agency framework, intensive rehabilitation service should be rendered only in the hospital. Also in the light of the shortage of rehabilitation personnel, home care might be used as an additional method by which the training experience of physical therapists, occupational therapists, and students of other rehabilitation disciplines might be broadened.

ACHIEVEMENTS AND CURRENT INTEREST

The benefits of organized home care programs are of two major types. The community gains by more efficient utilization of its resources. The patient gains by the focusing of medical services on individual needs. The achievements of such programs are:

1) By providing care in the hospital only for those in need of total hospital care, more effective use has been made of community facilities.

2) Continuous care of the patient upon leaving the hospital has greatly facilitated rehabilitation to maximum functional capacity in the patient's normal environment.

3) It has been possible to provide a high standard of total medical care in terms of the services needed by patients rather than in terms of services available in a particular institution that would be less flexible and more restricted than the home care plan.

4) Patients have made better progress in the normal home environment, where they receive the devoted and affectionate care of their families. This helps to preserve family unity, which is so often disrupted by long illness.

Patients are therefore happier. When properly selected, they progress as well, often better than in the hospital. There is no reduction of quality or effectiveness of service and there is reduced cost. A home care program through its operation gives the hospital or community the equivalent of an extra ward. The great difference is that the patients are scattered throughout the city with the hospital as the focal point instead of the patients being retained within the walls of the hospital itself.

There is now more interest than ever in home care. It has progressed to the point where national organizations are beginning to work *together* to bring the story of home care to the people who can operate such programs. In April, 1960, the American Hospital Association, American Medical Association, Blue Cross Association, Blue

Shield Medical Care Plans, and the U.S. Public Health Service joined together to sponsor a national workshop on home care services. After this national meeting, these same organizations sponsored regional workshops. They are now also co-operating in the publication of an *Inventory of Coordinated Home Care Programs in the United States.*

Governmental agencies are vitally interested in the promotion of home health services. In the implementation of the Kerr-Mills Medical Aid for the Aged program, at least one state (Pennsylvania) specifically designated home care as a service that will be paid for under the plan. The federal government in its administration of this program has encouraged this by stipulating that at least 10% of the services paid for be "out-of-hospital" services. The U.S. Public Health Service's Long-Term Illness Program is encouraging the establishment of educational institutes on home care. Two were held in Pittsburgh and in St. Louis and more are in the offing. Thus, more and more information is being disseminated about the operation of home care programs, and professional health workers are taking this information to their communities in an effort to introduce this modality of care into the spectrum of health services.

This type of medical care is not second best and it is not "cutrate." It provides the best of modern medical care, makes it possible for the chronically sick to be looked after in their own homes, and provides them with the wide range of professional services that is not easily secured through a single physician. Organized home care has proved its worth and it can be recommended to the communities of the nation as a valuable and essential addition to the totality of medical resources for long-term patients.

There is a tremendous unfilled need for home care. The unavailability of home care for those patients for whom it is best constitutes a denial to them and to their communities comparable to the denial of any other essential service such as a hospital bed or a new and effective antibiotic. All persons and organizations who have responsibility for any aspect of patient care have a stake in the provision of organized home care services to meet the needs across the nation because this provides a segment of care that clearly satisfies the twin criteria of effectiveness and economy.

1. *150 Years of the Good Samaritan.* Boston: Boston Dispensary, n.d.

2. The Increased Use of Medical Care. *Progress in Health Services,* Health Information Foundation. Oct., 1958. 7:8:1–6.

3. Rosenfeld, L. S., Goldmann, F., Kaprio, L. A., Reasons for Prolonged Hospital Stay. *J. Chronic Diseases.* Aug., 1957. 6:2:141–152.

4. Jensen, F., Weiskotten, H. G., and Thomas, M. A., *Medical Care of the Discharged Hospital Patient.* New York: The Commonwealth Fund, 1944.

Cherkasky, M., Hospital Service Goes Home. *Modern Hosp.* May, 1947. 64:5:47–48.

6. *Inventory of Home Care Programs in the United States.* In process of publication.

7. Hospital Council of Greater New York, *Organized Home Medical*

Care in New York City: a Study of Nineteen Programs. Cambridge, Mass.: Commonwealth Fund (Harvard University Pr.), 1956.

8. Michigan Hospital Service and Detroit Visiting Nurse Association, *Home Care Project, a Report of the First Year of Operation, July, 1961.* Detroit: The Service, 1961.

9. Peabody, S., The Home Care Program of the Detroit Visiting Nurse

Association. *Am. J. Public Health,* Nov., 1961. 51:11:1681–1687.

10. Goldmann, F., and Fraenkel, M., Patients on Home Care: Their Characteristics and Experience. *J. Chronic Diseases.* Jan., 1960. 11:1:77–87.

11. Clarke, M., Developing Useful Work Opportunities for the Homebound Patient. *Am. J. Public Health.* Jan., 1962. 52:1:47–54.

PART SIX

Some Technics: Innovations and Adaptations

1. Multiphasic Screening	749
2. Periodic Health Examinations	759
3. Immunizations	783
4. Crash Teams	792
5. Community Self-Study	799

THE STRATEGIES and emphases of Public Health programs are in constant change as new knowledge and technics make it possible to move from one level of prevention, cure, or rehabilitation to another. To devise the best possible program at any time, and to help define where future changes might be sought, Public Health constantly experiments with new technics that demonstrate the practicality of aiming new approaches at particular targets. When tested, these innovations may become part of the foundation of long-range "master plans" for control of a particular disease or social problem.

This section reviews a few such innovative technics or demonstrations: case-finding for disease detection in large populations; community organization for mass immunization; mobilization of an international team to cope with a health crisis transcending local resources; and considers the implication of power relationships for community organization.

1. Multiphasic Screening

Multiple Screening in the
Baltimore Study of Chronic Illness*

DEAN W. ROBERTS, M.D., AND CHARLES M. WYLIE, M.B., CH.B.

MUCH OF THE current need for custodial care of persons with advanced chronic illness stems from the fact that much illness reaches an irreversible point before diagnosis is made and definitive treatment undertaken. An effective approach to this problem must include consideration of procedures for earlier detection and diagnosis. When progress is made in this area, more people can receive treatment early in the course of disease when a better therapeutic response can be achieved.

In its deliberations, the Commission on Chronic Illness concluded that case-finding of asymptomatic disease should employ all of the available technics, the usefulness of which has been demonstrated. The commission recommended that:

All persons should have a careful health examination including selected laboratory tests at appropriate intervals. The medical and dental professions must specify the desirable scope and frequency of this examination, taking into account age, sex and other biosocial factors. Such examinations must then be made practical and realistic, and be incorporated in the day by day practice of modern medicine and dentistry.

Screening tests for early case-finding are an essential device in prevention. Used discriminately, these tests should be undertaken in physicians' offices, hospitals, industrial health services, schools and health centers. Local health departments especially should foster efficient screening programs for large groups of the population.

* Reprinted by permission, with the omission of three tables, from the August 11, 1956, issue of the *Journal of the American Medical Association*, Vol 161, pp. 1442–1446. This study was from the Commission on Chronic Illness. The authors are, respectively, Executive Director, National Commission on Community Health Services, Inc., Bethesda, Maryland, formerly Executive Director of the National Society for Crippled Children and Adults, Chicago, Illinois; Associate Professor of Public Health Administration, The Johns Hopkins University, School of Hygiene and Public Health, Baltimore, Maryland, formerly Research Associate, Public Health Administration, School of Hygiene and Public Health, Johns Hopkins University.

The editors would like to point out that an evaluation of multiple screening has been reported at a later date by Dr. Wylie in his article "Use of Death Rates in Evaluating Multiple Screening" in *Public Health Reports*, Vol. 76, pp. 1111–1116 (Dec.), 1961.

The commission also recognized that present technics for early diagnosis leave much to be desired and that research is needed to develop valid and feasible tests that can be widely and inexpensively applied. In considering screening programs the commission concluded that:

> The successful operation of programs for making screening tests available to large groups of the population cannot be accomplished until a number of problems are solved. Administrative research is needed to seek solutions to such questions as: the appropriate relationship of mass screening programs to the practice of medicine, the creation of a demand for services after screening which cannot be fulfilled with existing resources, a standard of reasonable cost for screening. There are other similar questions stemming from present-day traditions and attitudes about which administrative research should be undertaken.

Published opinions on the value of multiple screening vary from enthusiastic endorsement[1] to complete condemnation.[2] Although multiple screening programs have tested some two and one-half million persons in the United States in the past decade,[3] relatively little has been learned about their efficacy. Perhaps the programs have yielded so little information because their organizers have concentrated on persuading the public to take the tests, without conducting a corresponding study of what happens to persons with abnormal screening tests who are asked to visit their physicians for further examination.

In considering multiple screening as a device for early detection of chronic disease, the commission conducted studies in Hunterdon County, New Jersey, and in Baltimore. Both studies included operation of experimental screening clinics for specified samples of the populations. This article presents some of the findings of the screening phase of the Baltimore study, with particular emphasis on the follow-up of individuals for whom test results were positive in the more important screening tests.

WHAT IS MULTIPLE SCREENING?

Screening tests are procedures that sort out persons who probably have abnormalities from those who probably do not.[4] Well-known examples are the miniature chest roentgenograms for pulmonary tuberculosis and blood and urine sugar tests for diabetes mellitus. Multiple screening is the use at one time of two or more screening tests to identify persons who probably have abnormal conditions and to refer them for diagnosis and, if indicated, for further medical care. If conclusively proved to be of value, multiple screening may develop as an adjunct to the periodic physical examination procedure. Thus it would enable the physician to concentrate his efforts on persons (with abnormal screening tests) who are more likely to have disease or abnormalities.

WHO ATTENDED THE CLINIC?

The study, of which the Baltimore Multiple Screening Clinic was a part, has been described elsewhere.[5] The total project had the approval of the local and State medical societies. Invitations to attend the clinic were mailed to 7,000 persons, aged 17 years and over. If the mailed invitation produced no response, it was followed by a phone call or home visit if necessary. These 7,000 persons were the less disabled members of a sample chosen by the census bureau as being representative of the Baltimore population. Most of these individuals, when previously interviewed at home, reported that they were healthy or that they had only minor ailments. A small number reported more serious conditions, for some of which they were under the care of their personal physicians.

During the 10 weeks that the clinic was active, 2,024 (29%) of the 7,000 persons took the screening tests. The age, sex, and racial characteristics of the screenees were studied. It was found that a greater proportion of white than nonwhite individuals attended, and that a higher percentage of those between 25 and 54 years responded than in the younger and older age groups. There was no consistent difference between the two sexes.

SCREENING TESTS

A committee composed primarily of practicing physicians advised the commission in selecting the tests. A detailed description of the tests is given later in this report. Briefly they consisted of (1) height and weight, for obesity; (2) self-screening questionnaire for heart disease; (3) six-lead electrocardiogram; (4) blood pressure determination; (5) visual acuity test; (6) hearing acuity test; (7) miniature chest roentgenogram for tuberculosis, heart disease, and other chest conditions; (8) test for urine albumin; (9) test for urine sugar; (10) test for blood sugar; (11) determination of hemoglobin level; and (12) serologic test for syphilis. The tests were usually completed in one hour. A dental examination, not used as a basis for referral, was also carried out in this period.

PROCEDURE AFTER TESTS WERE COMPLETED

Before leaving the clinic, each individual was interviewed by a Public Health nurse who explained the method of sending the results to the physician and to the screenee. The nurse also emphasized that tests were not done for conditions that could be found only on physical examination.

Four weeks later, a complete copy of all the test results, including a copy of the electrocardiographic tracings, was mailed to the screenee's physician. Two days later, one of several letters was sent to the screenee. If the tests were completely negative or if only a minor abnormality was present, the letter said so and did not urge a visit to the physician at the time but did recommend regular medical examinations at least once a year. If a serious abnormality appeared to be present, the letter said that the person appeared to have a condition for which he should consult his family physician. All letters emphasized that screening procedures do not replace the periodic physical examination.

Screenees were classified as having a major abnormality when positive results were obtained in any of the following tests: self-screening questionnaire for heart disease, electrocardiogram, determination of blood pressure, chest roentgenogram, test for urine albumin, blood and urine sugar tests, determination of hemoglobin level, and serologic test for syphilis. Follow-up figures were sought on all persons with major abnormalities, unless they had marked on the questionnaire that they were already aware they had conditions that would produce the positive tests.

To obtain the follow-up results, the staff got in touch with the screenee by mail, or by phone or home visit when necessary, to find out if he had visited his physician. Of the 607 individuals who were referred on the basis of the above tests, 393 reported that they had consulted their physicians about the results. In turn, the physicians of these 393 individuals were contacted. The necessary information was obtained, by mail or by phone, from the physicians of 351 of the persons referred. In comparing the results of the screening and follow-up steps, one must remember that 42 per cent of the persons referred were lost to the study, either because they did not visit their physicians or because no report was obtained on the diagnostic examination.

GENERAL SCREENING RESULTS

Thirty-seven per cent of all screenees had no abnormal test results. An additional 31 per cent were regarded as having minor abnormalities only. These persons had positive results only in the tests for obesity, hearing, vision, or glycosuria (without hyperglycemia). Thirty-two per cent of the screenees failed in one or more of the remaining tests. Of these latter 652 persons, 45 had answered in the questionnaire that they were already aware of the condition at which the positive test was aimed. The remaining 607 individuals were asked to visit their family physicians for further advice.

INDIVIDUAL TEST RESULTS

The number of persons taking each test was not constant, since one of the tests was sometimes not done on an individual or the result was unsatisfactory for various reasons. Although each person referred to his physician did not indicate on his questionnaire that he already knew of the condition at which the positive test was aimed, a considerable proportion of the confirmed cases were stated subsequently by the physicians to be previously known to them.

The people who benefit from the screening procedure, the yield of the tests, are the screenees in whom positive test results were confirmed for conditions previously unknown to their physicians. In reality, the benefit is theoretic for persons who may have conditions for which no specific treatment is available. On the other hand, this loss in yield is probably counterbalanced by screenees whose positive test was not confirmed by diagnostic examination but who were found in the examination to have some other condition that would respond to medical treatment.

BLOOD PRESSURE. Blood pressure was taken with mercurial sphygmomanometers after the screenee had been reclining for five or six minutes. The criteria for referral were as follows: (*a*) above 150 mm. Hg systolic and 90 mm. Hg diastolic, if below 35 years of age; (*b*) above 160 mm. Hg systolic and 96 mm. Hg diastolic, if 35 to 50 years of age; and (*c*) above 170 mm. Hg systolic and 100 mm. Hg diastolic, if more than 50 years of age.

In 31 of the 67 persons referred, presence of hypertension was confirmed. Twenty of the confirmed cases were already known to the physicians, however. This situation is readily understandable, since many physicians will not mention the presence of this condition to their patients. Thus the patient may be wrongly referred by the screening clinic on the assumption that the doctor does not know of the condition. The measurement of blood pressure, using higher levels for older age groups, appears to be a fairly satisfactory method of screening for hypertension. Most screening programs have had similar satisfactory results.[6]

ELECTROCARDIOGRAM. The three bipolar and three unipolar limb leads were taken while each screenee was reclining. The cardiologist reading the tracings used the Framingham criteria of abnormality as a guide in classifying the result.[7] If the result was doubtful, the screenee was invited to return for a 12-lead electrocardiogram. The

179 screenees with abnormal readings, and 15 with doubtful results who failed to return for their chest leads, were referred to their physicians for further examination. In 43 of the persons referred, presence of heart disease was confirmed. As with the blood pressure test, two-thirds of the confirmed cases were already known to the physicians. The yield of new cases was almost entirely confined to those of persons over 45 years of age.

As used in Baltimore, the electrocardiogram discovered more previously unknown cases of heart disease than did the chest roentgenogram and questionnaire. The bipolar and unipolar limb leads, when taken on persons in the older age groups, appear to be a screening test of some promise in detecting previously unknown heart disease. Other studies[8] suggest that the use of the lead 1 tracing alone, while greatly simplifying the test and reducing its cost, results in a too-high proportion of false-positive results.

CHEST ROENTGENOGRAM (FOR HEART DISEASE). A chest physician read the 70 mm. chest films for heart abnormalities. Because of suspect or abnormal readings, 155 individuals were referred to their family physicians. In 29, presence of heart disease was confirmed, confined mainly to those over 45 years of age. Only eight patients had conditions previously unknown to their physicians. As used in the Baltimore clinic, the chest roentgenogram detected fewer cases of heart disease than the six-lead electrocardiogram. One reason was the higher proportion of follow-up results completed with the electrocardiographic test. However, other programs[9] confirm the low sensitivity of the chest roentgenogram as a screening test for heart disease.

SELF-SCREENING QUESTIONNAIRE. The self-screening questionnaire contained seven brief questions designed to obtain information on conditions that were already known to the screenee and to obtain the name and address of the family physician. Two questions, found elsewhere[10] to have some degree of specificity in testing for cardiac disabilities, were used for referral when positive answers were given for both. These questions were as follows: 1. Do you ever have distress, pain, or an uncomfortable feeling in the chest while walking on the street or up inclines or steps? 2. While walking, are you forced to stop in order to rest? These questions were much less effective than the electrocardiogram in screening for heart disease. The test result was more frequently positive in women, and all five confirmed new cases were in women. The use of questionnaires in other screening programs has usually given poor results.[11] Only one study reports a more optimistic conclusion, and this does not appear justified by the findings of the study.

CHEST ROENTGENOGRAM (FOR TUBERCULOSIS). The chest physician read each film for tuberculosis and other chest conditions, as well as for other heart abnormalities. A full-size film was taken at a later date when recommended. When the large film confirmed the suspect finding or when the screenee failed to have the large film taken, the individual was referred to his family physician. The yield of new active cases was low and the proportion of false-positive results high, as much more extensive chest x-ray surveys have already shown. However, the importance of early detection of tuberculosis justifies the widespread use of this screening test. The effectiveness of the chest roentgenogram in screening for other chest conditions in the Baltimore clinic was poor.

URINE ALBUMIN TEST. A sulfosalicylic acid test (with use of Bumintest reagent tablets) was used to determine presence of albumin in the urine. A result of 1+ or more was used to indicate the need for referral. Of 37 screenees who consulted their physicians, in only two instances was presence of proteinuria confirmed. This low yield of new cases and high proportion of false-positive results has been obtained in other screening programs.[12] A urine albumin test does not appear worthy of inclusion in a multiple screening program.

URINE SUGAR TEST. The test for urine sugar (with use of Clinitest reagent tablets) was carried out about 45 minutes after the screenee had taken an orange-flavored carbonated drink containing 50 gm. of glucose. In 54 screenees, the test gave a positive result of 1+ or more. However, only 15 of these persons had tests with positive blood sugar results, and these persons were referred to their physicians as possible diabetics. Other screening programs confirm the low specificity of the urine sugar test in screening for diabetes mellitus.[13] Indeed, the urine sugar test appears to be unnecessary when a blood sugar test is carried out after the administration of glucose.

BLOOD SUGAR TEST. A venous blood specimen was taken for the blood sugar test about 50 to 70 minutes after the glucose drink, and the true-glucose values were obtained by the Wilkerson-Heftmann method. When the one-hour value was above 160 mg. per 100 cc., the screenee was again tested at the end of the second hour. In 33 persons, the tests were positive at one hour, and results were either confirmed above 130 mg. per 100 cc. or the persons were not retested at two hours. Fifteen of these screenees had positive urine sugar tests and were regarded as probable diabetics. Of the nine who were known to have consulted their physician, in five presence of diabetes mellitus was confirmed. The yield of previously unknown diabetics was smaller than that obtained in other screening programs. It seems likely that a number of diabetics with a high renal threshold were missed because referral was carried out only when the urine sugar test was positive.

HEMOGLOBIN LEVEL. The hemoglobin level of the venous blood was determined by use of the copper sulfate specific gravity method. Men were referred when the hemoglobin level was below 12.3 gm. per 100 cc., women when below 11.0 gm. per 100 cc. The eight previously unknown cases of anemia were all in women. Other screening programs[14] confirm that the screening of men for anemia is a relatively nonproductive procedure.

SEROLOGIC TEST FOR SYPHILIS. A serologic test for syphilis was carried out on each blood specimen. A positive test usually resulted in referral for further examination, especially when the Treponema pallidum immobilization test, done in a proportion of screenees, was also positive. Of the 53 persons referred, 45 were Negroes. Fourteen consulted their physicians, who confirmed three previously known and one new case of syphilis. This low yield is partly due to the small proportion of persons referred who consulted their physicians. The results of selective programs, testing much larger numbers of persons, suggest that the serologic test for syphilis is a useful screening test for groups in which the prevalence of syphilis is high.[13c]

HEIGHT AND WEIGHT. Because they were 30% or more above the central weight for persons of medium frame of the Metropolitan Life Insurance tables, 106 individuals were referred to their physicians. Those between 20 and 29% above this weight were merely informed that they were moderately overweight. No follow-up was carried out for this test, nor for the vision and hearing tests.

VISUAL ACUITY. The American Optical Company Sight Screener was used to determine visual acuity. The results obtained while the screenee was wearing glasses (if any) determined the need for referral. When vision in each eye was 20/40 or less, or vision in one eye was 20/50 or less, the individual was advised to obtain a more thorough examination to determine the need for glasses. Using these criteria, 530 persons, slightly over one-fourth of those tested, were abnormal.

HEARING ACUITY. The test for hearing acuity was deliberately made more thorough than usual to obtain exact information on the prevalence of hearing difficulties in the population. In brief, the screenee was advised to seek medical advice when the better ear had a hearing threshold averaging 30 db. or more at frequencies of 500, 1,000, and 2,000 cps.

LIMITING FACTORS

A screening procedure may fail at any one of four points. First, the screening test may perform so poorly that for considerable numbers of screenees the tests are wrongly classified as positive or negative. This study can give no estimate of the false-negative results, i.e., in individuals who have the disease but for whom tests are classified as negative. Second, a large proportion of the screenees for whom the tests are positive may fail to go on for the diagnostic examination by their family physician. In this study, no follow-up results were obtained on 42% of the persons referred. Therefore, the proportion of wrong referrals tends to appear larger than it really is.

Third, the diagnostic examination may be inadequate, so that the condition is not confirmed although it actually is present. Other studies, particularly after diabetes detection drives,[15] suggest that, in a proportion of persons for whom the tests are truly positive, presence of the condition is not confirmed because of inadequate diagnostic examination. This study can give no estimate of the diagnostic error. Fourth, presence of the condition may be confirmed on diagnostic examination, but the person may fail to return for treatment or may have a condition for which there is no specific treatment. These persons do not really benefit from the screening procedure, and they reduce the yield of the test. Neither this nor other published studies have investigated this phase of the screening procedure.

SUMMARY AND CONCLUSIONS

The results of the Screening Clinic of the Baltimore Study of Chronic Illness have shown that multiple screening is a procedure of promise, although some tests will require further development and study before they come into widespread use. Multiple screening has other aspects, briefly mentioned here, that require further study to clarify the usefulness of the procedure.

1. Getting, V. A., and Lombard, H. L.: Symposium: Multiphasic Screening Programs: Cost and Evaluation of Multiple Screening Procedures, *New York J. Med.* 52:2605–2609 (Nov. 1) 1952.

2. Smillie, W. G.: Multiple Screening, *Am. J. Pub. Health* 42:255–258 (March) 1952.

3. Study of Multiple Screening: A Bibliography with Abstracts, Chicago, Council on Medical Service, American Medical Association, 1955, p. 13.

4. Breslow, L., and Roberts, D. W.: Symposium: Screening for Asymptomatic Disease, *J. Chron. Dis.* 2:363–366 (Oct.) 1955.

5. Roberts, D. W.: Baltimore Study of Chronic Illness, *Maryland M. J.* 2:297–299 (June) 1953. Roberts, D. W., and Wylie, C. M.: Multiple Screening: Its Place in Baltimore Chronic Illness Study, *ibid.* 3:557–562 (Oct.) 1954.

6. (*a*) Hilleboe, H. E.; James, G., and Doyle, J. T.: Cardiovascular Health Center: I. Project Design for Public Health Research, *Am. J. Pub. Health* 44:851–863 (July) 1954. (*b*) Kurlander, A. B.; Hill, E. H., and

Enterline, P. E.: Evaluation of Some Commonly Used Screening Tests for Heart Disease and Hypertension, *J. Chron. Dis.* 2:427–439 (Oct.) 1955.

7. Footnote 6*b*. Dawber, T. R.; Kannel, W. B.; Love, D. E., and Streeper, R. B.: Electrocardiogram in Heart Disease Detection: Comparison of Multiple and Single Lead Procedures, *Circulation* 5:559–566 (April) 1952.

8. Footnote 7. Weintraub, H. J.: Evaluation of Lead 1 as Screening Technique for Heart Disease, *J.A.M.A.* 158:178–179 (May 21) 1955.

9. (*a*) Footnote 6*b*. (*b*) Phillips, E.; Chapman, J. M., and Goerke, L. S.: Relative Values of Techniques Used in Detection of Heart Disease, *Am. Heart J.* 45:319–330 (March) 1953.

10. (*a*) Footnote 9*b*. (*b*) Phillips, E.: Cardiac Screening Procedures, *California Med.* 82:118–120 (Feb.) 1955.

11. (*a*) Footnotes 9 and 10*b*. (*b*) Breslow, L.: Multiphasic Screening in California, *J. Chron. Dis.* 2:375–383 (Oct.) 1955 (*c*) Weinerman, E. R., and others: Multiphasic Screening of Longshoremen with Organized Medical Follow-Up, *Am. J. Pub. Health* 42:1552–1567 (Dec.) 1952.

12. (*a*) Footnote 11*b* and *c*. (*b*) Getting, V. A., cited in footnote 3, p. 60. (*c*) Kurlander, A. B., cited in footnote 3, p. 62.

13. (*a*) Footnote 11*b*. (*b*) Derryberry, O. M., cited in footnote 3, p. 33. (*c*) Smith, C. A.; Donohue, J. F., and Stuart, J.: Blood Test Screening in Syphilis Control, *J. Chron. Dis.* 2: 480–486 (Oct.) 1955.

14. Footnotes 11*c* and 13*b*.

15. McLoughlin, C. J.; Petrie, L. M., and Hodgins, T. E.: Diagnostic Significance of Blood Sugar Findings, *J.A.M.A.* 153:182–184 (Sept. 19) 1953. Loube, S. D., and Alpert, L. K.: Evaluation of Screening Procedures in Diabetes Detection Drive: Follow-Up Survey of Individuals Found to Have Positive Urine Tests, *Diabetes* 3:274–278 (July–Aug.) 1954.

2.   Periodic Health Examinations

The Values and Limitations of Periodic
Health Examinations*

NORBERT J. ROBERTS, M.D.

PERIODIC HEALTH EXAMINATIONS are being increasingly advocated and performed, especially within industry.[1] Is this desirable? Review of some of the background of such examinations and of evidence and opinions concerning their value and limitations may clarify our thinking on the subject.

Periodic health examinations or evaluations are, as the terms imply, examinations of individuals performed at periodic intervals to determine the status of their health even if they are symptom free and seem to be well.

Such examinations are usually done with the goal of helping those examined retain or even improve their health. When carried out as part of a company's occupational medical program, this may be their goal, or they may be done exclusively or additionally (1) to help assure the continuing fitness of those examined for the duties which they perform, especially when their own safety or that of others depends upon their fitness, and/or (2) to help assure that the health of those examined is not being adversely affected by any potential hazards of their working environment.

There is no purpose in our debating the value of examinations performed when indicated for either of the latter two reasons, assuming that those performing and interpreting them have the skill and judgment required. Whatever may be the limitations of periodic health examinations, it is unlikely that any physician would suggest that the periodic evaluation of the health of airplane pilots or workers exposed to known carcinogens would be without value. Organized medicine has extended its endorsement to such examinations.[2] Let us, therefore, confine our critical discussion of periodic health examinations to those which are performed purely for the purpose of health maintenance or improvement, recognizing that many of the values and limitations we mention would be equally applicable to such examinations no matter what their purpose.

* Reprinted by permission, with the omission of one table, from the February, 1959, issue of the *Journal of Chronic Diseases*, Vol. 9, pp. 95–116. The author is Associate Medical Director, Standard Oil Company of New Jersey, New York, N.Y.

In 1861, Dr. Horace Dobell[3] proposed ". . . that there should be instituted, as a custom, a system of periodical examination, to which all persons should submit themselves, and to which they should submit their children." In the interval between then and now, this proposal has been endorsed by many others.

Barès,[4] writing in France in 1902 on the possible necessity for periodic examinations, was enthusiastic about the wealth of knowledge that could be expected to result from analysis of the observations made in the performance of such examinations.

In the interval between 45 and 30 years ago, physicians in Public Health, in the insurance industry, in industry generally, and in the military services, together with others in private practice, attempted to stimulate the widespread performance of periodic examinations for the purpose of health maintenance.

In 1914, S. S. Goldwater,[5] referring to data collected at the Massachusetts General Hospital and at Cornell and to the finding that 62 per cent of 800 New York garment workers examined were in need of medical treatment, wrote: "I, for one, am not willing to cease short of a radical change in the manner of applying medical knowledge. Preventive medicine cannot do its utmost good until physicians are regularly employed by the entire population, not merely for the treatment of acute and advanced disease, but as medical advisers in health." He concluded that: "The next great task of preventive medicine is, therefore, the inauguration of universal periodic medical examinations."

In 1919, Mock[6] summarzied his writings of preceding years, and the reports of others, concerning the desirability of such examinations in industry, advocating that: "Every employee, male and female, from the head of the concern down, should be examined."

In 1922, the House of Delegates of the American Medical Association adopted this resolution: "Whereas, the need and value of periodic medical examinations of persons supposedly in health are increasingly appreciated by the public, it is recommended . . . that the county medical societies be encouraged to make public declaration that their members are prepared and ready to conduct such examinations. . . ."[7]

In 1923, Roger Lee[8] spoke and wrote impressively about the importance, limitations, and opportunities of periodic health examinations. In 1924, physicians were told that they "must recognize a rising movement among the laity demanding that physicians prepare themselves to make intelligent reports on the physical state of adults who are apparently healthy" and that the time had come for the medical profession to "take up the subject of periodic examinations as one of its major activities."[9]

The next year, the American Medical Association published a manual on the conduct of such examinations.[10] In 1927, Eugene Lyman Fisk, after more than 20 years of experience, study, speaking, and writing on the subject, published, with Crawford, a book on the method of performing periodic examinations.[11] Already at that time—over 30 years ago—his list of references on this subject required 8 pages of print.

Since then, a number of people in our country have sought, and most of them have obtained, periodic examinations from their personal physicians or at clinics or from medical groups that have been more active in their performance. Pediatricians and our dental colleagues especially, and to some extent ophthalmologists, obstetricians, and gynecologists—among others—have for a number of years allotted varying but appreciable portions of their time and efforts to periodic examinations of patients not known to require treatment.

Nevertheless, even today, only a relatively small portion of our people, and of physicians themselves, are being examined periodically.[12] Many who champion such examinations would endorse the continuing accuracy of Edie's[13] statement, made in 1925, to the effect that: "The proposal that healthy people be examined at regular intervals . . . is notable for the logic of its theory and the slowness of its adoption" and describing those proposing such examinations as "voices in the wilderness."

We ought, therefore, to review critically the evidence for and against such examinations and to consider the factors influencing their value and the performance of them. In doing so, let us first present some of the most frequently expressed criticisms of such examinations and then examine these and some of the evidence and other opinions pertinent to them.

COMMON CRITICISMS OF PERIODIC EXAMINATIONS

Perhaps the most common basis for criticism of periodic health examinations is an attitude summarized succinctly by Christ almost 2,000 years ago: "It is not the healthy who need a physician, but they who are sick" (Matthew 9:12).

The physician often points out that he studied medicine to help the sick and that his interest is in sick people and their diseases. He may add, accurately, that he is already entirely busy caring for people who are ill and need his help. He may even summarize his attitude toward such examinations by saying: "I can't think of anything duller than doing a bunch of routine physicals." He often wonders sincerely if any physician doing many such examinations can keep from losing his clinical skill or if these examinations are not usually being done by physicians who already feel themselves inadequate for more dramatic clinical work.

Many physicians feel that examinations of this sort are not worth their while when their total yield is weighed against the time, skill, energy, facilities, and money involved. They believe that a large proportion of the diseases or defects discovered during such examinations are not important. Many, they feel, do not need treatment or even observation, and many others cannot be helped. They express the opinion that most of the diseases or defects found that are of real importance would bring the patients to the doctor eventually anyway and doubt that much is gained by the time "saved."

A great many physicians emphasize the limitations in our ability to measure health with accuracy, often quoting an instance where an individual has died soon after being reassured about his health on the basis of a periodic examination. They take exception to the false sense of security that they feel patients obtain from these examinations. They caution about the frequency with which we may do harm by making those we examine over-anxious concerning their health.

Many physicians are convinced that even if we wished to do such examinations widely at present, we do not have the doctors, nurses, technicians, and facilities needed to do them. They doubt that patients would be willing or able to spend the money that would have to be charged for a thorough health evaluation. Further, they ask how we could ever convince patients that examinations of this sort are desirable if we cannot even persuade doctors themselves to have them.

Some physicians, observing the performance of periodic health maintenance examinations as part of occupational medical programs, ask why the American businessman, whom they recognize as the champion of free enterprise and fair competition, gives employees these examinations without cost. They point out that in their opinion this is hardly fair competition for the physician who is practicing medicine privately as a free enterprise.

To what extent are these criticisms justified?

DISCUSSION

First, it is generally true, of course, that the sick man needs a physician more than the healthy. The ill cannot go unattended while physicians tend the healthy. But in considering this concept, we must be reasonable. Would we condemn physicians immunizing the still-healthy in the midst of an epidemic as behaving undesirably in failing to devote their attention exclusively to the unfortunates already ill?

Christ, in speaking of the sick man's need for a physician, was likening that need to the sinner's need for His help, and theologians would not interpret His quoted words as meaning that Christ's help would not be available as well to the good man or that the latter were independent of it.

How does a physician know whether an individual is healthy without examining him if, to beg a question momentarily, asymptomatic disease is as common as it is claimed to be? Let us admit that the completely healthy individual does not need a physician. Evidence exists, however, to indicate that it requires thorough medical examination to separate those who are in good health from those who believe themselves to be in good health but in fact are not. Reports indicate, at least with respect to the adult male, that thorough examination will usually reveal that actually only 10 to 25% of those who seem healthy are quite entirely healthy and that from 25 to 35% of those being examined for the first time will be found to have some significant disease which was not previously known to exist.[14-22]

With reference to why most physicians seem to lack interest in the performance of periodic health maintenance examinations, one of the most commonly expressed reasons is the doubt that the examinations require sufficient skill to be challenging or offer sufficient opportunity to earn the satisfactions sought by physicians in the practice of medicine. Of course, such doubts alone could not justifiably dissuade a physician from performing these examinations if, his goal being the patients' welfare, it could be demonstrated to him that the examinations can contribute appreciably to the maintenance or improvement of his patients' health.

If evidence exists that a patient's prognosis is better if his malignancy is diagnosed early, it becomes difficult, of course, to try to weigh the accomplishment of a physician who examines many people to find a single early asymptomatic malignancy against the accomplishment of his professional colleague who, dealing with sick people over the same time interval, diagnoses and treats 2 or 3 well-along symptomatic malignancies.

Physicians, daily reaping the satisfaction that results from the immediate and obvious expressions of gratitude by patients and their families for efforts in their behalf at a time of rather dramatic need, might not find appealing the prospect of trading this for satisfactions that must often be derived interiorly and can be enjoyed only in smaller doses at less frequent intervals. Here again, however, if it could be demonstrated to them that their patients' prognoses would be better, perhaps they could be convinced that their eventual net income, in satisfaction would be great indeed.

Does it require less skill to do periodic health examinations than to handle sick patients? Need the performance of "routine physicals" be boring?* Ought they to be relegated to physicians who, with or

---

* The word "physical," if used to refer to an attempt at measuring an individual's health, is an unsatisfactory designation in many ways, and physicians should cease to use it in this fashion. The physical examination is but one step in the evaluation of a person's health, and to exclude from any examination the obtaining of any information or the making of any observations about elements of health that are not physical is unrealistic. Examinations should be referred to as medical or health examinations, except when we refer specifically to that part of an examination which deals as exclusively as it can with the patient's physical status.

without justification, lack confidence in themselves? These questions do not lend themselves to exact measurements. However, some opinions pertinent to them merit attention.

Although any physician who approaches and performs periodic examinations "routinely" in the unsavory connotation of that adverb will undoubtedly be bored, some might be challenged would they but contemplate seriously the possibility that it may require more skill and more knowledge of health and normalcy as well as of disease to recognize an early stage of a disorder than it does to recognize a later stage of the same disorder. Although less skill might be needed for the effective treatment of early disease, this still could be sufficiently challenging to be satisfying, and the patient and his family would not be disappointed if his illness could be treated successfully with less than maximum skill.

In 1861, Dobell[3] wrote ". . . the manner in which man is to exercise his instrumentality for the prevention of disease, the prevention of the vestiges of disease, and the prevention of fatality in disease, is to search out those earliest evasive periods of defect in the physiological state, and to adopt measures for their remedy. *This appears to me to be highest, the most enobled duty of the physician, calling for the most abstruse knowledge of the science of life, the deepest experience in disease, the keenest exercise of the perceptive faculties, the calmest, most far-sighted reasoning, and the wisest judgment—a duty as much above the management of acute disease as to rule an empire is above fighting a pitched battle.*"

In 1942, an outstanding clinician serving as Professor of Medicine in one of America's finest medical schools wrote ". . . the public must be taught not only that *a periodic health examination* is a valuable investment for better health, but that it *is perhaps of all tasks the doctor is asked to perform, the one that calls for the greatest skill and wisdom.*"[23]

But in 1958 several keen young medical students, soon to graduate with an impressive amount of knowledge from this same medical school, told me that their interest is in clinical medicine and that they hope to be real clinicians and cannot possibly imagine themselves being interested in examining people who seem to be well.

It is evident that both undergraduate and postgraduate medical education today are oriented so heavily toward the ill patient and his disease that those attempting to focus the attention of future physicians on health and well people have little success. They do, of course, interest some students, but relatively few in a deep and lasting fashion. We must, therefore, add to the criticisms of periodic examinations already listed the doubt that most of us, as physicians, are adequately prepared, either in orientation or by training, to do such examinations. Further, we must also face the fact that we do not seem to be adequately preparing medical students to do them in spite of the efforts of many teachers who are sincerely convinced of the desirability of this goal. Illustrative of the limited progress being made is the likelihood that relatively few of the students graduating as physicians this year have ever had a really thorough evaluation of their own health.

Many physicians whose only clinical work is the periodic examination of supposedly well people have concluded that, as has been suggested, it is truly difficult to maintain clinical skill if such work is one's exclusive clinical activity. The clinician who has accumulated and can retain easily a splendid fundamental knowledge of health and disease, who is possessed of an inquiring and analytic mind, and who uses it might thrive and progress through many years of doing such examinations alone. But, unfortunately, most of us do not have this capacity, and we need the assistance of continuing contacts and study to maintain our knowledge and acuity about things infrequently encountered. Rigler,[24] in a fine discussion of one type of periodic examination, cautions about "the psychology of the negative," the negative-mindedness that is risked. This is a matter to which doctors doing health maintenance examinations exclusively must consistently and regularly give attention, and which will in most cases require adherence to a program of planned medical reading, study, and periodic contacts with professional colleagues, medical teaching environments, and broader clinical horizons.

To discuss the relationship of the yield of periodic health maintenance examinations to their "cost" in terms of the time, energy, and patience of those examined, and the money, and the technical and professional time, energy, skill, facilities, equipment, and material involved, we must ask what the yield has generally been from the performance of such examinations.

As has been pointed out, and it seems to be true, such yields would be expected to vary in the sexes, with age, race, location, socioeconomic, and other factors, with the caliber and thoroughness of the examinations and examiners, the cooperation of the examinees, and the effectiveness of follow-up observation and treatment.[25] In spite of this, when we review what various physicians over the past 45 years have reported as their findings when they examine groups of supposedly well individuals, most of whom have been adult males, there is an impressive consistency with which at least 15% and up to 40% of those examined are found to have a significant disease or defect of which they are unaware. In as many as one-half to two-thirds of the cases, these disorders are still asymptomatic when so discovered. Further, in a like number of those examined (15 to 40%) there is usually found some known disease or defect for which only about half are obtaining indicated treatment or medical observation.[5, 10, 14-22, 25] Most who report on this subject classify as "significant" any disease or defect able or likely to shorten life or result in some incapacity or disability.

MOST COMMON FINDINGS

The disorders most frequently diagnosed in adults at the time of initial or subsequent periodic examinations and the percentage incidence among those examined[14-22, 16-30] were: obesity 10–30 per cent; arthritis 10–20 per cent; hypertensive disease 5–20 per cent; arteriosclerotic heart disease 5–20 per cent; hemorrhoids 5–20 per cent; anxiety state 5–20 per cent; rectal or sigmoid polyp or adenoma 5–15 per cent; vasomotor rhinitis 5–10 per cent; peptic ulceration 5–10 per cent; and inguinal hernia 5–10 per cent. The variations in frequency are results of differences in the scope of examinations performed, the interests and training of the physicians performing them, the age distribution in the groups examined, and the diagnostic criteria used.

Observing the occasionally great variations in the reported incidence of a specific disease in different groups examined, we may either be tempted to doubt the accuracy of the observations or be understandably confused about factors that could explain such variance. For example, while Densen, D'Alonzo, and Munn[31] report no diabetes mellitus whatsoever among the employees in 10 different plants with a total population of at least 3,000 individuals, Tupper and Beckett[29] report 37 definite cases and 31 suspected cases of diabetes among 294 University of Michigan faculty members. Unless patients with diabetes are excluded from employment in the plants studied by the former authors and preferentially are selected for employment, or inbred, at Michigan, it is difficult to understand the difference in incidence of this disease in these two groups and the difference between its incidence in each group and that usually reported in the general population. No practically imaginable divergence of diagnostic criteria could explain differences of this degree.

Reviewing the reported findings on periodic examinations, any of us would be tempted to challenge the justification for labeling certain of them as significant, especially in view of the infrequency with which they are demonstrated to produce disability or shorten life. Admittedly, too, with respect to many findings that obviously are significant, we would have to acknowledge our complete or relative ineffectiveness at the present time in altering the course of the patient's disease.

We must face frankly the areas in which we are thus far completely frustrated. We are entitled to be disappointed, but we are not, of course, entitled to be discouraged. Although, for example, we must admit that the majority of patients with primary carcinoma of the lung may not be saved by present-day treatment received even before their initial symptoms appear, it does seem, as will be illustrated, that at least a few extra patients in each hundred treated while still asymptomatic do survive in spite of the limitations in our effectiveness.

MacDonald and Kotin[32] have pointed out that their studies caused them to conclude that "the concept that the early diagnosis of carcinoma of the stomach may improve the end results is not only fallacious but is in fact the reverse of the truth." Although in support of their conclusion they could point to higher survival rates in patients with carcinoma of the stomach whose symptoms were of longer duration and to lower survival rates in those whose symptoms were of shorter duration, the conclusion itself would appear unjustified. The important point that these two workers emphasize—the extent to which a specific tumor's nature predetermines significantly the patient's possibilities of survival—worked, it would seem likely, to select into the groups with symptoms of short duration those patients with highly anaplastic, fast-growing, and early-metastasizing tumors and into the other groups those with more differentiated, slowly-growing, and late-metastasizing carcinomas. They do not present, and we do not know of, any real evidence that patients whose carcinomas of the stomach are diagnosed and treated early fare less well than those with comparably anaplastic or differentiated carcinomas diagnosed and treated later in the course of the disease.

While some may be awed, and we must all be impressed, by the extent to which in many malignancies the patient's destiny seems so much predetermined by the nature of his tumor and by his own susceptibility to it, we must continue to attempt the earliest practical recognition and treatment of such lesions.

Happily, there are relatively bright areas. Even those who feel that the threat of carcinoma in situ is being exaggerated can hardly fail to be impressed by the limited but accumulating evidence of more favorable survival rates in those who receive treatment for certain types of carcinoma in the earlier states of their disease, especially while still asymptomatic. Survival rates in patients with carcinoma of the stomach, colon, rectum, larynx, breast, and uterus, and even in patients with carcinoma of the lung, as pointed out before, do seem better when the disease is treated early, in spite of some of the skepticism that has been voiced.

Robbins and Bross[33] have pointed out the significance of delay with respect to patients having carcinoma of the breast. Boucot and Sokoloff[34] report 20 per cent of their patients with asymptomatic carcinoma of the lung surviving 3 years or longer, as opposed to the rate of 9 per cent among those with symptoms. Overholt, Bougas, and Woods[35] report 3-year survival rates of 30 per cent as opposed to 12 per cent, and Davis, Peabody, and Katz[36] report the survival for 2 years or longer of 52 per cent of patients without symptoms as opposed to 14 per cent of those having symptoms. The latter authors point out that, of 14 patients with small, solitary, circumscribed, asymptomatic bronchial carcinomas operated upon 5 or more years ago, 11 (78 per cent) are still alive and well.

Hufford and Burns[37] report that 5-year follow-up studies revealed only 2 of 22 patients with asymptomatic carcinoma of the uterus had died of carcinoma, whereas 22 of 41 patients with symptomatic carcinoma had died over the same interval. Hitchcock and Aust[38] report 17 of 18 patients with asymptomatic carcinoma of the colon and rectum well up to 5 years after the time of diagnosis, whereas only 3 of 8 patients with symptoms still survive. Six out of 9 of their patients with asymptomatic carcinoma of the stomach were alive up to 5½ years after diagnosis, whereas only 1 of 5 patients with symptomatic gastric carcinoma survived.

While these quoted experiences deal in some instances with small or relatively small numbers of cases and in others with too-short (even though comparable) periods of observation, the same general trend in the large amount of data available to the American Cancer Society and the National Cancer Institute has caused the Joint Committee on Cancer Statistics of these two groups to concur in some interesting pertinent estimates shown in Table I. If we grant that localized carcinoma should be "earlier" carcinoma, the extent that it is "earlier" admittedly varying widely with the nature of the tumor and other factors, these estimates give us some clue to possible benefits that might be derived from the combination of earlier diagnosis and good treatment.

Lest it be felt that too much emphasis is being placed upon the possibility of the earlier diagnosis of malignancy influencing survival rates, we need only consider the fact that present data indicate that in our country 1 out of 4 persons develops a malignancy some time during his life.[1]

With respect to diseases other than malignancies, we know beyond doubt that treatment can help at least a portion of the patients with some of the diseases encountered relatively commonly, such as hypertension or diabetes. It may seem prematurely optimistic to suggest that patients in whom coronary atherosclerosis is recognized early will be in a position to be helped appreciably, but nonetheless this is the impression of many.

Unfortunately, although we have many reports telling us what asymptomatic disorders can be found by periodic examinations, we have few that include follow-up studies that enable us to compare the ease or success of treating patients whose disease is so discovered with that of treating comparable patients in whom the disease is

Table I. Present and Potential 5-Year Survival Rates for Patients With Malignancies[39]

Site of Malignancy	Per Cent of Patients Presently Surviving 5 Years*	Per Cent of Patients That Could Possibly Survive 5 Years or More Were Tumor Discovered and Treated In Localized Stage†
Tongue	17	68
Esophagus	2	3
Stomach	6	48
Colon	29	50
Rectum	25	77
Larynx	37	64
Lung	4	34
Breast	46	81
Cervix	53	69
Body of uterus	62	78
Ovary	24	48
Prostate	21	32

* Based on Connecticut experience; cases diagnosed 1947–1951.
† Based on experience of specialists reporting at the Third National Cancer Conference; cases diagnosed 1946–1950.
Adapted from tabular material contained in Minutes of the July 26, 1956, meeting of the Joint Committee on Cancer Statistics of the American Cancer Society and the National Cancer Institute.

discovered after, and because, it becomes symptomatic. We have little evidence of the frequency with which patients seek and obtain the care or observation advised and with what results.

Whalen and Woodward,[40] studying what happened in the cases of 100 patients in whom a significant new diagnosis was made at the time of periodic examination, found that 68 per cent promptly sought and obtained the care or observation needed. Fifteen per cent delayed from one to several months but eventually sought and obtained it; 11 per cent promptly sought it but obtained it only after delay. Six per cent of the patients could never be persuaded to seek or accept treatment, including one with a carcinoma.

Prickman and his associates[22] studied the extent to which 231 executives having at least two periodic health maintenance examinations at the Mayo Clinic complied with medical and surgical advice. They found that 65 per cent complied fully, 18 per cent not at all, and the balance partially, for example, accepting care for a medical problem but declining recommended surgery. They noted a slightly greater tendency for patients to comply with advice given after a second or third examination than with that given after an initial visit.

Mitchell,[26] reporting in 1943 on 1,580 individuals examined two or more times, indicated the frequency with which defects discovered at initial examination had been eliminated by the time of follow-up examination. For example, he noted that only 9.7 per cent of those obese at the time of their first examination were no longer obese when re-examined. Only 19 per cent of those having inguinal hernias had

had them corrected by the time of subsequent examination. Thus we note that the discovery of such disorders is very often not followed by successful treatment, even if good treatment is available.

Baker and his associates,[41] re-examining 106 people found to be obese at the time of previous examination, found that 15 per cent were no longer so when re-examined, 34 per cent had improved, 40 per cent were unchanged, and 11 per cent were worse. The same workers reported cure or improvement of 83 per cent of the patients in whom anemias were diagnosed, cure or improvement in 31 per cent of those with hypertensive vascular disease, and improvement in 20 per cent of those with hypertensive cardiovascular disease.

Franco[17] reported that follow-up studies of the diseases found in 707 patients over a 7-year interval revealed 20 per cent of his patients had been cured, 33 per cent were improved, 31 per cent were unchanged, and the balance were worse (8 per cent), retired as disabled (3 per cent), or dead (5 per cent). He indicates, however, that only 35 per cent of the patients with asymptomatic disease were cured or improved, whereas 68 per cent of patients with symptomatic disease were cured or improved. Such results would seem truly disappointing to the advocates of the early detection of disease. However, the different results in these groups may well have been far more influenced by differences in the nature of findings in the two groups than by whether the patients had symptoms or not.

It is true, of course, that even in the best of hands periodic health evaluation may fail to detect life-threatening disease, as, for example, the reported failure of one group to detect 9.4 per cent of the malignancies occurring in the patients studied by them, about half of these being frankly missed and the other half undiagnosed because of a lack of patient cooperation.[38] Guiss[42] reports the death of 27 individuals from carcinoma of the lung within a year of the time that 70 mm. screening films of their chests failed to reveal evidence of such a tumor, although it should be noted that, on the positive side, the same screening program resulted in the finding of 213 other cases.

Most physicians have had the sad experience of seeing a patient die soon after an examination which revealed no threat to his life. Most commonly, such episodes have been related to our inability to demonstrate coronary atherosclerosis with consistency. But as long as we face such limitations, and work to eliminate them as completely as we are able to practically, this need not be discouraging when weighed against what can be accomplished.

Care must be taken, of course, that patients do not obtain an unjustified sense of security on the basis of an essentially negative health examination. It is true that those examined are sometimes unqualifiedly assured of the excellence of their health after grossly inadequate examinations. In view of the recognized inadequacies in even the best of examinations, we advise that patients always be told something of the limitations in our ability to measure and predict health and that they be cautioned to seek assistance promptly for any new, recurring, or persistent symptoms that trouble them between scheduled periodic examinations. The necessity of doing this, if it is done properly, need not deprive patients of the satisfaction of being reassured in general concerning the status of their health, if such reassurance is justified, nor need it cause them to become overanxious or hypochondriac. My associates and I, who believe ourselves sensitive to these possible complications, seldom indeed encounter evidence of a patient's having suffered any ill effects traceable to an unjustified sense of security resulting from such an examination. Nor do we often see a patient become overanxious about his health upon the basis of one. Both hazards do admittedly exist, and probably the fact that we consistently and conscientiously guard against them explains the infrequency with which we see them. From the positive viewpoint, it is worth noting that we are often able to allay a patient's anxiety about his health following an examination which reveals no justification for such anxiety.

With reference to the concept that at present we do not have sufficient physicians, nurses, technicians, and facilities to examine everyone periodically, it can only be admitted that this is unfortunately true. Some feel, however, that quantities of these *"sine qua nons"* might be freed for such work if the ill, who now require so much of their energy and time and space, could be treated much earlier in the course of their disease so that their treatment could be, at least in some instances, more simply and promptly accomplished.

Admittedly, if all the general practitioners and internists in our country were sufficiently free and interested now to examine 3 or 4 people thoroughly each of their working days, this still would not suffice for annual health evaluation for all of our adults. But if each such physician examined only 1 to 2 patients daily, each could be offering 500 patients annual or biennial health maintenance evaluations. This itself might diminish the need of this segment of their patient population for more time-demanding care and might permit a gradual shifting of the emphasis in their practice toward more preventive health maintenance and earlier therapy.

Basically it seems evident, however, that, for thorough health maintenance service to be widely available at the same time that patients needing therapy can obtain the optimum amount and quality of care, and for necessary medical research, teaching, and Public Health work to be accomplished, we do need more doctors, especially good general practitioners and internists whose services are available to the public.

When we come to the question of the willingness and ability of people to pay the necessary cost of thorough health maintenance services, we can only point out that many have already evidenced their willingness to do so and express our conviction that many others, even if not all, can be educated to be willing.

Rutherford and Banks[43] reported recently that when they offered their patients, without particular enthusiasm, the opportunity to revisit them periodically for examination even in the absence of symptoms, the number of visits made by patients for this purpose soon became so large that they were forced to restrict them in order to continue their regular practice. Fremont-Smith[44] says that on the basis of 40 years' experience he has learned well that people will pay for a thorough examination and will return for others year after year.

That education can stimulate people to accept such examinations and respect their value is evidenced by the continuing and growing percentage of employed individuals who voluntarily have them periodically when they are offered. Under these circumstances, they are usually without cost to the employee, which is a factor of importance. However, in our experience, almost 60 per cent of those participating in our program continue to seek such examinations from their personal physicians after they retire when they themselves must pay for them out of their reduced retirement income.

In most instances, two basic considerations have undoubtedly encouraged the acceptability of these examinations to employees. First, wherever their own safety or that of others does not depend upon their fitness, the examinations have usually been offered rather than required and participation in the health maintenance program has been on a voluntary basis. In some well-established programs, as many as 90 to 100 per cent of those eligible have participated.[28]

Second, but of singular importance, has been the assurance the employee has had that results of the examination will be treated confidentially and not revealed to anyone except at his request. It is perfectly evident that the value of periodic examinations is distinctly limited whenever the individual being examined cannot be assured that information learned about him in the course of the examination will be kept confidential.

It is clear that both of these factors, the voluntary and the confidential nature of the program, are important in encouraging the complete and frank cooperation of those participating. An additional criticism of periodic examinations performed in industry has been based upon the possibility or likelihood that the patient will not give a frankly honest health history either because he is being examined involuntarily or because he lacks conviction that information learned about him will be treated confidentially and not used against his interests. In our experience, however, even those employees required by the nature of their work to have examinations have usually participated unreservedly upon recognition of the goals of the examination and upon demonstration over the years of the confidential and ethical nature of the patient-physician relationship involved.

It is truly a biting indictment that it has not been possible to persuade most physicians to have health maintenance examinations themselves periodically. This, however, seems primarily a matter of education—a failure in communication. Unfortunately, a great proportion of physicians are not only unacquainted with the facts concerning such examinations but are even more inclined than the laity to dismiss them without interest or with comments more emotional than scientific. Unreasonable as it may seem, fear of what might be discovered is probably as often the reason a physician avoids examination as it is the layman's for doing so. This attitude is compatible with the observation[45] that there is essentially just as much delay in the diagnosis and treatment of malignancies among physicians as there is among the laity.

While the cost of such examinations carefully performed is appreciable, we do not believe ourselves entitled to assume that it is beyond the capacity of a great portion of our population to budget for them. When we weigh the potential importance of these examinations against that of innumerable other expenditures regularly made without great resistance, we cannot doubt that education on the matter and good judgment might inspire many people to provide such examinations for themselves and their families, especially if we are imaginative enough to design and offer practical and ethical plans to prepay for their cost. Further, with the efficiencies and economies that can be realized, the cost of these examinations need not be so high as many are publicized to be. Some groups in private practice already include them in services offered on a prepayment basis at a cost that a good number of people of modest socioeconomic level are paying.

Why should these examinations be offered employees by their employer without cost? The reason seems to be that the employer has been persuaded that they help assure him of an effective, productive work force and hence help assure the success of his business. Were his employees seeking and obtaining health maintenance services from their personal physicians, the employer might have little incentive to do more than assure his employees' fitness for their work and freedom from undesirable effects of their work environment. These latter assurances must often be obtained from a physician who is a specialist in occupational medicine because they require a familiarity with the worker's duties and with the often-complex physical and psychologic aspects of his working environment. Inasmuch as the private practitioner cannot be expected to gain and retain the specialized knowledge and competence required for this and some other work in this field, we shall continue to have occupational medicine as a specialty.

It does seem, however, that most employers who are providing their employees with periodic health evaluations solely for the purpose of helping them maintain or improve their health are doing so only because they feel the examinations are desirable and will not often be done, or done with interest and thoroughness, unless they provide them.

Where these examinations are performed as part of a company's occupational medical service, they are not, and in our opinion should not be, offered to an employee as a fringe benefit or as a form of compensation in lieu of cash. They are but one of many steps taken and one of many investments made to help assure a company's success. Fortunately, the employee's welfare and the company's welfare are both best served by his remaining healthy, and his welfare is quite obviously even more immediately served than is the company's by steps taken to help him preserve his health.

Where services that include periodic examinations are paid for entirely from union funds, the situation is different, of course, in that under these circumstances the employee is spending for such an examination money which he has earned but which has been set aside for this purpose under a program arranged for him by his union.

SCOPE OF THE PERIODIC EXAMINATION

What should be included in a good examination designed to evaluate an individual's health? Wade[46] defines health as the optimal adjustment of the total person—physical, mental, social, and spiritual—to his total environment—microbes, automobiles, ideas, etc. Accepting this definition, we would desire a good health evaluation to include a measurement or determination of these adjustments. It would require, to be complete, the taking of a good health history, the making of a good physical examination, and the performing of certain supplementary laboratory and x-ray studies, all planned with attention to the adjustments listed, and would require as well the satisfactory recording, analysis, and communication of the results of the examination to the patient and usually to one or more physicians unless the examination has been done by the patient's personal physician. Although Fisk[47] pointed out over 30 years ago that it is idle to set up standards for these examinations which are beyond what the general practitioner can attain, it would seem best to describe what appears to be desirable regardless of the practical obstacles which might necessitate compromise under some circumstances.

The health history should, of course, be a complete one, although in health maintenance examinations it does not so often contribute to the discovery of a disease or defect as do the physical examination or supplementary studies.[14, 18, 27] For those accustomed to handling ill

patients in contradistinction to the supposedly well, it comes as somewhat of a shock to realize that the history they prize so much seems
less productive than the other elements of the examination. However,
when we pause to consider the frequency with which diseases discovered during such examinations are still asymptomatic, this is
exactly what we should expect. There remain, however, many diagnoses and important observations that can be made only on the basis
of a thorough and carefully taken history.

While there is no satisfactory substitute for a careful interview of
the patient to develop needed details concerning a complaint or illness, we find that a thorough health questionnaire completed by the
patient in advance of a health maintenance examination contributes
greatly to the effective use of the time he and the physician can spend
together for a history interview and assures a thoroughness, as
demonstrated by the Cornell group,[48] that is not achieved without it.
The use of such a questionnaire to shorten the amount of time that
the physician must allot to the examination is one evident manner in
which the cost of such examinations might be reduced.

My associates and I, who prided ourselves on our ability to take
good and complete medical histories, find that in up to 15% of
the patients we see the complete health questionnaire which we use at
present elicits potentially significant health history information that
we doubt we would have elicited by the interview techniques in which
we had so much confidence before designing and using our health
questionnaire.

After the patient has completed the questionnaire, it is our procedure, before going on with the physical examination, to interview
him in the indicated degree of detail concerning all of his responses
that are not negative, and to discuss with him a number of health-
related matters not adequately covered by the questionnaire.

In addition to eliciting current and past information concerning
the patient's organic health, family history, and occupational history,
we interrogate him tactfully but in detail concerning his relationships
with others, the strains and satisfactions in his work life and family
life, his sense of values and his goals, his anxieties, his reactions to
frustrations, and his health-related interests, activities, and habits. We
also attempt to assess his maturity, his sense of responsibility, and his
acceptance of reality.

The physical examination must, of course, be done carefully and
completely. We hear occasionally of so-called examinations for which
the patient is not asked to undress. We see the frequent omission of
such a relatively simple step as the testing of visual acuity. Distressingly, we note the infrequency with which a digital examination of
the rectum is included. Such examinations are not adequate ones. As a
matter of fact, there is no excuse for short-cutting in health mainte-

nance physical examinations. The ocular fundi should be as carefully explored, the thyroid as carefully palpated, the spleen, lymph nodes, and peripheral arterial pulsations as carefully felt for as they would be in any obviously ill person. A basic neurologic survey should be included.

Although it is not usually described as part of the physical examination, we feel that a proctosigmoidoscopic examination should be included. With good preparation of the patient made so simple today by the use of the disposable enema, with the examination itself so simple that any physician can learn to do it (perhaps with some of the less adept or courageous limiting themselves to the 7-inch instrument), and with the positive findings upon such examinations so consistently high, it seems evident that an examination of this sort ought to be included in a physical survey far more consistently than it is. Time-consuming, yes. Awkward and undignified, yes. Initial reluctance on the part of the patient, yes. But under many circumstances, all of these problems can be surmounted. It need not be pointed out that a health maintenance examination of a woman remains sadly incomplete until a pelvic examination has been performed.

With respect to the laboratory and x-ray studies that should be included regularly, a urinalysis, hematocrit or hemoglobin determination and a scanning of a stained blood smear, and an x-ray examination of the chest would seem quite consistently indicated. In some groups, or in some locations, or at varying intervals, other tests might always or occasionally be done. Any tests indicated by any symptom or sign should be obtained.

In women, especially those over 35, a cervical smear for cytologic study ought to become routine. In men over 35 or 40 and women over 45 or 50, electrocardiography might well be done regularly, whereas in younger patients only a base line tracing and relatively infrequent repeat studies might be deemed required in the patient whose initial tracing is normal.

In some areas, the stool should regularly be examined for ova and parasites. In certain groups or areas, regular serologic testing for syphilis would be indicated, whereas under other circumstances this might be done less frequently with little risk. Some examinations might be done once, and seldom, if ever, repeated without indication —for example, an x-ray examination of the gall bladder at the age of 45 or 50. Other studies, such as a complete blood count or determination of the serum cholesterol level or of blood glucose following the ingestion of a test amount of sugar, might be done intermittently. Some might desire to use the erythrocyte sedimentation rate regularly.

In those middle-aged or over, intermittently ascertaining the presence or absence of free hydrochloric acid in the stomach by a "tubeless" gastric analysis, and at each examination testing the stool for occult blood with an agent of appropriate sensitivity or insensitivity would allow the recognition of some patients in whom gastrointestinal x-ray studies would be justified. We hesitate to advocate x-ray studies without some justification but would feel, for example, that the potential yield in so examining an older man with achlorhydria or definite occult blood in the stool would outweigh the undesirable effects of the radiation involved. We do not, of course, advocate x-ray examination of the abdomen of the fertile woman or of the male genital area without some indication for it. Indicated but elective x-rays of the abdomen are postponed in women until the cessation of a menstrual period in order that we might have this degree of assurance that the patient is not pregnant.

An obvious consideration with reference to these supplementary studies is the accuracy of the laboratory and x-ray services available, as illustrated by Bolt, Mallery, and Tupper,[49] and Hitchcock and Aust,[38] among others.

The frequency with which a few commonly performed supplementary laboratory and x-ray studies may be "positive" in the supposedly healthy is illustrated in Table II.

The basic examination described will require from 45 to 90 minutes of the physician's time, the amount being influenced by the patient's health problems or freedom from them and by the physician's thoroughness, pace, and working habits. The patient would have to invest from 90 to 150 minutes, including the time required for the completion of the health questionnaire in advance.

After the examination, what? It is impressive to read how much can be found on periodic health maintenance examination, but the findings are relatively meaningless unless the follow-up procedures assure that diseases and defects that are found receive the medical care or observation required. We feel that the best way to communicate the results of an examination to a patient is to schedule him for a 15 to 30-minute revisit with the physician, usually several days later, following completion and interpretation of laboratory and x-ray studies. (And we should have a better designation for the supposedly healthy examinee than "patient.") During this visit, an attempt is made to tell the patient in terms he will understand what has been found in the course of his examination and its meaning to him. We not only encourage him to ask but attempt to extract from him any questions that might come to his mind. As indicated earlier, through all of this we guard as religiously as possible against precipitating anxiety in the patient.

If the patient has any disease or defect requiring treatment or observation and has been examined by someone other than his personal physician, he should be referred at once to the latter, to whom a copy

Table II. Results of "Routine" Use of Certain Examinations

Examination	Per Cent "Abnormal"
Urine for sugar	2.6
Urine for protein	2.2
Blood for hemoglobin	6.7
Blood for sugar	4.1
Blood for syphilis	5.6
Stool for occult blood	15.7
Electrocardiogram	11.9
Cytologic study of cervical smear	0.49 (asymptomatic carcinoma)
Proctosigmoidoscopy	0.3 (asymptomatic carcinoma)
Proctosigmoidoscopy	8.2 (asymptomatic polyps or adenomata)
Chest x-ray	2.88 (abnormality of some type)
Chest x-ray	0.16 (active pulmonary tuberculosis)
Chest x-ray	0.72 (abnormal cardiovascular silhouette)
Chest x-ray	0.01 (primary pulmonary malignancy)

These figures are derived from reports of screening and periodic-type examinations summarized in *The Early Detection and Prevention of Disease*, edited by John P. Hubbard, New York, 1957, McGraw-Hill Book Company, Inc.

of the record of the examination should be forwarded—but not carried by the patient. As pointed out earlier, all patients do not seek or obtain promptly the treatment or observation needed, so that some provision should be made to remind or reurge those patients that require such to obtain it. Unfortunately, some patients who visit their physicians promptly to seek indicated treatment or observation do not succeed in obtaining it, sometimes because the physician they consult is unimpressed with their still early and mild disease and suggests to them that they ignore it unless or until it becomes more of a problem.

To realize the full potential benefits of periodic health examinations performed in industry, it is necessary that a formula be found and followed to assure cooperation and understanding between occupational health service physicians and the private physicians of employees examined.

FREQUENCY OF PERIODIC EXAMINATIONS

How often should periodic examinations be performed? Reports indicate that examinations subsequent to the initial one yield enough to justify their regular performance, for example, at annual intervals. As would be expected, the more frequent the examinations, the lower will be the yield in new findings. However, in the experience of some, the yield on annual examinations seems sufficient to justify their repetition that often. Bolt, Tupper, and Mallery[15] discovered new significant disease in from 13 to 20 per cent of those having examinations subsequent to an initial one; Elsom, Spoont, and Potter[18] found the same in 22 per cent of 150 patients re-examined one to two years after their first examination. Hitchcock and Aust[38] report that 45 per cent of 147 malignancies discovered by their group over a 6½ year period in 6,754 individuals were found at the time of re-examination rather than at the time of initial examination.

Specific findings or circumstances in the case of an individual may sometimes indicate examination even more frequently than once yearly. On the other hand, while in our experience the yield at the time of initial examination of younger individuals is quantitatively (although not qualitatively) roughly the same as that in older individuals, there does seem to be a lower yield when younger people are examined each year. For this reason, many have adopted the practice of examining younger patients less frequently—for example, those under 30 years old only every third year, those between 30 and 40 every second year, and only those 40 or over every year.

Rather than permit younger people to go as long as 3 or more years without examination of any sort, it would seem to us preferable to examine them annually but to perform briefer examinations, perhaps largely of a screening sort, in the intervals between more thorough examinations every second or third year.

The limitations of multiphasic screening types of examinations are well recognized, but they can be of distinct and measurable usefulness if they are understood and interpreted properly. Profiting by what has been demonstrated with respect to such examinations, it might be suggested that in interval years between thorough examinations the patient could complete a health questionnaire, have certain basic observations about his health recorded by a nurse, such as his height, weight, temperature, pulse rate, blood pressure, and general appearance, have a few basic laboratory tests including chest x-ray performed, and be seen only very briefly by the physician, or, if necessary, not at all unless something in his responses to the questionnaire, the nurse's observations, the x-ray examination, or other tests reveals the desirability of a physician's attention. Used between more thorough ones, an examination such as this, preferably with at least a brief interview and examination by the physician after completion of the "screening" and without a revisit unless indicated, might at least for the present serve as a practical adjustment to the shortage of medical, nursing, and technical personnel previously discussed and to the expense of annual thorough examinations.

With further respect to the frequency of health maintenance examinations, it seems to have been well demonstrated that the incidence of most diseases is no greater in executives than in other employees, so there does not seem to be need for more frequent examination of the executive group.[21, 30, 50, 51]

Last, with reference to the frequency of periodic examinations, it is self-evident that the physician should be guided in the individual case by his findings upon examination of the patient concerned, especially with respect to indications for more-frequent-than-usual examinations and with respect to special problems created by the patient's environment at work or otherwise.

SUMMARY AND CONCLUSIONS

Attempting to view periodic health maintenance examinations in proper perspective, the following conclusions would seem justified:

With Respect to Their Limitations

Periodic examinations are not the keystone of preventive medicine, as they were identified to be in the title of a recent round-table discussion on the subject. There are many other activities that come under the heading of preventive medicine, such as Public Health services, that more consistently and very importantly contribute to our health. As Sir Adolphe Abrahams[52] has pointed out, many things that we do every day or could be doing are more capable of influencing our health favorably than are periodic examinations.

Many of the criticisms of such examinations, as listed and discussed, are justified to varying degrees and in varying circumstances and frequency.

We have enjoyed relatively little success in "selling" them thus far to the public or our own profession.

But With Respect to What They Can or Could Accomplish

Their yield is measurable in the discovery of previously unrecognized disease, an appreciable portion of which is still asymptomatic. Evidence exists that the early diagnosis and treatment of some diseases increase the likelihood that their treatment will be successful.

They allow us an opportunity to stimulate patients to obtain care or observation needed for known but neglected disease as well as for newly diagnosed disease.

They provide us with base line data which often prove useful later in making the correct diagnosis of an acute or chronic illness when this depends upon the recognition of *changes*.

While they do not *prevent* disease, of course, they do, as a result of its early detection, frequently offer the possibility of preventing some of the complications or disabilities of disease and occasionally offer the possibility of stimulating action that *will* prevent disease.

Thorough analysis of the observations made during great numbers of such examinations, for which purpose the keeping of good records which lend themselves to such study is an obvious necessity, would probably contribute greatly to the store of our knowledge concerning both health and disease.

Finally, although this defies actual measurement, one of their greatest yields—possibly the greatest—is their educational value. They offer an opportunity to teach a patient in a highly personalized fashion something about the maintenance and improvement of his health. They direct his attention, at least intermittently, to an asset of untold value that he may otherwise tend to neglect and ignore. They help him develop the degree of respect for his health and the awareness of it necessary to stimulate him to have complaints or problems referable to health investigated promptly.

1. 1959 *Cancer Facts and Figures*, New York, 1958, American Cancer Society.

2. American Medical Association, Council on Industrial Health: Scope, Objectives, and Functions of Occupational Health Programs, *J.A.M.A.* 164:1104, 1957.

3. Dobell, H.: *Lectures on the Germs and Vestiges of Disease and the Prevention of the Invasion and Fatality of Disease by Periodical Examination*, London, 1861, J. & A. Churchill, Ltd.

4. Barès: Sur l'utilité d'un examen periodique des individus sains ou paraissant tels, *Congrès français de médecine*, 6th, Toulouse, Paris, 1902, Compt.-Rend, p. 130.

5. Goldwater, S. S.: *The Next Step in Preventive Medicine*, New York, 1914. (In Dept. of Health, City of New York, Reprint series, no. 18, June, 1914.)

6. Mock, H. E.: *Industrial Medicine and Surgery*, Philadelphia, 1919, W. B. Saunders Company.

7. Dodson, J. M.: The American Medical Association and Periodic Health Examinations, *Am. J. Pub. Health* 15:599, 1925.

8. Lee, R. I.: The Physical Examination of Apparently Healthy Individuals: Its Importance, Limitations, and Opportunities, *Boston Med. & Surg. J.* 188:929, 1923.

9. Periodic Medical Examinations, *A.M.A. Bull.* 19:120, 1924.

10. American Medical Association: *A Manual of Suggestions for the Conduct of Periodic Examinations of Apparently Healthy Persons*, Chicago, 1925, A.M.A.

11. Fisk, E. L., and Crawford, J. R.: *How to Make the Periodic Health Examination*, New York, 1927, The Macmillan Company.

12. Wells, R. L.: Medical Examinations in Industry, *A.M.A. Arch. Indust. Health* 14:503, 1956.

13. Edie, E. B.: Health Examinations Past and Present and Their Promotion in Pennsylvania, *Am. J. Pub. Health* 15:602, 1925.

14. Huth, E., and others: *Periodic Health Status Examination Program*, 1954. Unpublished report.

15. Bolt, R. J., Tupper, C. J., and Mallery, O. T., Jr.: An Appraisal of Periodic Health Examinations, *A.M.A. Arch. Indust. Health* 12:420, 1955.

16. Baker, J. P., and others: The Effectiveness of Periodical Medical Evaluation, *Indust. M. & S.* 25:248, 1956.

17. Franco, S. C.: The Early Detection of Disease by Periodic Examination, *Indust. M. & S.* 25:251, 1956.

18. Elsom, K. A., Spoont, S., and Potter, H. P.: An Appraisal of the Periodic Health Examination, *Indust. M. & S.* 25:367, 1956.

19. Carryer, H. M.: The Health of an Executive, *A.M.A. Arch. Indust. Health* 16:267, 1957.

20. Guidotti, F. P.: Periodic Health Examinations in the Hotel Industry, *Indust. M. & S.* 26:506, 1957.

21. Wade, L.: Physical Examinations for Executives, *A.M.A. Arch. Indust. Health* 17:175, 1958.

22. Prickman, L. E., and others: Does the Executive Health Program Meet Its Objective? *J.A.M.A.* 167:1451, 1958.

23. Pepper, O. H. P.: Preclinical Medicine and the Periodic Health Examination, *in* New York Academy of Medicine: *Preventive Medicine in Modern Practice*, New York, 1942, Paul B. Hoeber, Inc. p. 57.

24. Rigler, L. G.: Periodic Roentgen Examination—Drudgery or Challenge? *J.A.M.A.* 163:530, 1957.

25. Roberts, N. J.: The Periodic Evaluation of Health, *Indust. M. & S.* 27:153, 1958; *Med. Bull.* 17:1, 1957.

26. Mitchell, T. H.: Observation on Periodic Examinations, *Med. Bull.* 5:374, 1943.

27. McCombs, R. P., and Finn, J. J., Jr.: Group Health Surveys in Diagnostic Center, *New England J. Med.* 248:165, 1953.

28. Saunders, G. M.: Executive Health Programs, *A.M.A. Arch. Indust. Hyg.* 9:133, 1954.

29. Tupper, C. J., and Beckett, M. B.: Faculty Health Appraisal, University of Michigan, *Indust. M. & S.* 27: 328, 1958.

30. Martin, C. E., and Hanley, M. J.: Do Periodic Health Appraisals Pay Dividends? *Indust. M. & S.* 27:461, 1958.

31. Densen, P. H., D'Alonzo, C. A., and Munn, M. G.: Opportunities and Problems in the Study of Chronic Disease in Industry, *J. Chron. Dis.* 1: 231, 1955.

32. MacDonald, I., and Kotin, P.: Biologic Predeterminism in Gastric Carcinoma as the Limiting Factor of Curability, *Surg., Gynec. & Obst.* 98: 148, 1954.

33. Robbins, G. F., and Bross, I.: The Significance of Delay in Relation to Prognosis of Patients With Primary Operable Breast Cancer, *Cancer* 10: 338, 1957.

34. Boucot, K. R., and Sokoloff, M. J.: Is Survey Cancer of Lung Curable? *Dis. Chest* 27:369, 1955.

35. Overholt, R. H., Bougas, J. A., and Woods, F. M.: Surgical Treatment of Lung Cancer Found on X-ray Survey, *New England J. Med.* 252: 429, 1955.

36. Davis, E., Peabody, J., and Katz, S.: Solitary Pulmonary Nodule: Ten-Year Survey, *J. Thoracic Surg.* 32:728, 1956.

37. Hufford, C. E., and Burns, E. L.: Papanicolaou Test in the Early Diagnosis of Uterine Cancer, *Ohio M. J.* 44:900, 1948.

38. Hitchcock, C. R., and Aust, J. B.: Diagnosis of Asymptomatic Malignant Disease, *Postgrad. Med.* 17:145, 1955.

39. Joint Committee on Cancer Statistics of the American Cancer Society and The National Cancer Institute, Minutes of Meeting, July 26, 1956. (Unpublished.)

40. Whalen, E. J., and Woodward, W. M.: A Follow-up Study of 100 Cases in Which Significant New Diagnoses Were Made During Health Maintenance Examinations, Exhibit at the Annual Meeting of Industrial Hygiene Foundation, Pittsburgh, Pa., Nov., 1954.

41. Baker, J. P., and others: Executive Health Examinations, *South M. J.* 46:984, 1953.

42. Guiss, L. W.: Mass Roentgenographic Screening as a Lung-Cancer-Control Measure, *Cancer* 8:219, 1955.

43. Rutherford, R. N., and Banks, A. L.: Value of Yearly Physical Survey in the Adult Female, *J.A.M.A.* 160:1289, 1956.

44. Fremont-Smith, M.: as quoted by B. S. Miller: Cancer Detection in Daily Practice, *Merck Rep.* May, 1956, p. 5.

45. Robbins, G. F., McDonald, M. C., and Pack, G. T.: Delay in the Diagnosis and Treatment of Physicians With Cancer, *Cancer* 6:624, 1953.

46. Wade, L.: What is Executive Health and How Should it be Maintained? *Med. Bull.* 18:154, 1958.

47. Fisk, E. L.: The Value of Complete Routine Examination in Supposedly Healthy People, *Boston Med. & Surg. J.* 195:740, 1926.

48. Brodman, K., and others: The Cornell Medical Index-Health Questionnaire, II, As a Diagnostic Instrument, *J.A.M.A.* 145:152, 1951.

49. Bolt, R. J., Mallery, O. T., Jr., and Tupper, C. J.: An Appraisal of Laboratory Procedures in Periodic Health Examinations, *A.M.A. Arch. Indust. Health* 12:253, 1956.

50. D'Alonzo, C. A., and others: Prevalence of Certain Diseases Among Executives in Comparison With Other Employees, *Indust. M. & S.* 23:357, 1954.

51. Lee, R. E., and Schneider, R. F.: Hypertension and Arteriosclerosis in Executive and Nonexecutive Personnel, *J.A.M.A.* 167:1447, 1958.

52. Abrahams, A.: Periodic Medical Overhaul, *Lancet* 2:670, 1953.

3. Immunizations

Two Voluntary Mass Immunization Programs Using Sabin Oral Vaccine*

RICHARD B. JOHNS, M.D., STANFORD FARNSWORTH, M.D.,

HUGH THOMPSON, M.D., AND FREDERICK BRADY, M.D.

IN SEPTEMBER OF 1961, a group of pediatricians, concerned about the low level of polio immunization in Maricopa County, Arizona, considered the possibility of a mass immunization program. Previous programs in the county, using the Salk vaccine, had failed to bring polio immunization to a satisfactory level. Consequently, an intensive campaign using Sabin oral vaccine was considered, though only type 1 and type 2 were licensed. The proposal to conduct a county-wide program was presented to the local pediatric society in September and was approved by that group. In October, the idea was presented to the total membership of the Maricopa County Medical Society. This society not only approved the plan but decided to sponsor the effort.

Thus began the largest voluntary mass immunization program in the nation to date.

This paper will describe the planning and actual conduct of the polio immunization programs in two Arizona counties, Maricopa and Pima. These two counties contain the two largest cities of the State, Phoenix and Tucson. Their population is approximately 700,000 and 300,000, respectively. The early planning was done by Maricopa County, then Pima followed Maricopa's lead, beginning in December, 1961. Consequently, the first part of the paper will deal primarily with Maricopa's experience. Though each program was conducted separately, basically they followed the same pattern. Variations will be noted when these occurred.

Once the medical society had decided to sponsor the program, a steering committee, under the chairmanship of a Phoenix pediatrician, was appointed to guide the over-all planning. The committee consisted of representatives of the medical society, the Maricopa County

* Reprinted, by permission, with the omission of one illustration, from the January 19, 1963, issue of the *Journal of the American Medical Association*, Vol. 183, pp. 171–175. The authors are, respectively, a Pediatrician (Children's Medical Center), and Chairman of the Maricopa County Medical Society Polio Committee, Phoenix, Arizona; Director, Maricopa County Health Department, Phoenix, Arizona; Pediatrician (The Tucson Clinic), and Chairman of the Pima County Medical Society Polio Committee, Tucson, Arizona; and Director, Pima County Health Department, Tucson, Arizona.

Health Department, the county pharmaceutical association, the National Foundation, a wholesale druggist, a reporter from one of the daily papers, and a representative of the pharmaceutical house that manufactured the vaccine.

Early in the program a full-time coordinator was appointed to work with all committee members in planning and following through with details. The associate executive secretary of the medical society was chosen for this key post.

One of the problems that had to be faced was that of clinic sites. Maricopa County is large, covering an area of 9,228 sq. mi. All population groups had to be considered. At first it was thought that physicians' offices should be used as clinics. However, this was impractical from several standpoints: (1) space in the physicians' offices was inadequate to meet the needs of such a mass program, (2) parking space was usually inadequate, and (3) physicians' offices were not always conveniently located for the population of an area. It was decided that schools would provide the most ideal places for the clinics. The county school superintendent was consulted, and his approval was obtained. Each district school superintendent was then contacted, in addition to school principals. Before the final selection of schools that would serve as clinic sites, the health department made a statistical breakdown of the county population, and the schools were selected by geographic location to cover all areas of the county. Sixty schools were then chosen to serve as clinic sites.

In early planning meetings, several important decisions had to be made. The dates for the program had to be set. Two successive Sundays in January of 1962 were selected—Jan. 14 and Jan. 21—for administration of the type 1 polio vaccine. These dates were selected because it was the earliest possible time to allow for complete organization of the program, yet still allow time to complete the type 2 immunizations and type 3, if authorized, before the coming polio season. Sundays were selected as clinic days because it was felt that this was the day when families were more likely to be together than at any other time. This was cleared with church groups in the area, and the decision was made to open the clinics at 11 A.M. and to continue until 7 P.M.

Several methods of administering the vaccine were considered, and the "sugar cube" method was selected. Droppers would be provided to give the vaccine directly into the mouths of babies too young to eat a sugar cube.

Financing the program also had to be considered. The medical society agreed to underwrite the vaccine purchases, and arrangements were made with the Maricopa County Health Department for the use of any excess vaccine in the six days following the clinics. The county health department also agreed to use and to pay for any unthawed vaccine, since this was nonreturnable vaccine. The vaccine was given at cost—25¢ for those who could pay, free to those who could not. With higher voluntary contributions in many cases, the money collected at the clinics completely covered the cost of the vaccine in both the type 1 and type 2 programs.

In the Pima County program, full advantage was taken of the Maricopa experience. Modifications were of a minor nature because the methods of staffing, financing, and selection of time and places of administration had already proved their worth. The steering committee in Pima County included officers of the PTA and women's auxiliary of the medical society and representatives of the clergy, as well as of the groups active in Maricopa County.

Pima County, with an area of 9,241 sq. mi., is sparsely settled except for the Tucson area and the city of Ajo, 120 mi. away. Of the 38 sites selected, 33 were in the Tucson metropolitan area and 5 were in small rural schools. The hours of administration were from noon to 6 P.M.

PUBLICITY

Getting the information to the people of Maricopa County presented a unique problem because of the vast area involved and the various language and cultural groups. Because of this, a public relations consultant was hired to handle the entire publicity campaign. It should be noted here that this was the only paid person in the entire SOS program. SOS (Sabin Oral Sundays) was chosen as the name of the campaign since the initials SOS usually attract attention as the old Morse code signal for help.

The first public announcement of the program appeared in one of the daily papers on Nov. 9, 1961. It told of a program whose goal was the eradication of polio as a Public Health problem in Maricopa County. From that time on, the progress of the committees was reported in newspaper stories almost daily. An intensive publicity campaign was started during the period between Christmas and New Year. Every available means of publicity was utilized, including news releases to all media; preparation and release of spot announcements to radio and television; posters displayed in doctors' offices, drug stores, health department clinics, schools, and other prominent places throughout the county; displays in shopping centers and in store and bank windows; marquee displays; bumper stickers; and more flamboyant methods such as "flying billboards." The flying billboards used here were flashing neon signs attached to the underside of the wings of a small plane. The plane flew over population centers of the county from dusk until 10:00 P.M. on the two evenings immediately preceding each clinic day.

Coverage by newspapers, radio, and television was outstanding. In addition to printing daily stories, the newspapers printed the registration forms on the days before the clinics and urged their readers to have these forms filled out and ready when they arrived at the clinic. They also publicized the clinic sites and time of the clinic openings and closings.

During the week before the first clinics, Phoenix mayor, Sam Mardian, Jr., issued a proclamation making the clinic dates "Sabin Oral Sundays." This proved to be excellent publicity for the program.

The publicity committee of the over-all steering committee checked all news releases and assisted the public relations consultant throughout the campaign. At the request of the consultant and with the full approval of the medical societies, attempts at anonymity were abandoned for the physicians on the steering committee. Direct quotes and photographs were used freely.

As a part of publicity, the health department mimeographed notices, including registration forms, for distribution through the county schools.

Another publicity device was the small notice, signed "Your doctor," which was included with the physicians' mailing of monthly statements.

In Pima County, the initials "PPS," for Polio Prevention Sundays, were used. Because of the hope that all three types could be administered, with appropriate intervals between, before schools closed in June, only three weeks were allotted for publicity before administration of type 1. The response of public media following a press conference was almost phenomenal.

STAFFING

The medical societies assumed responsibility for physicians' staffing. At least one physician was assigned to each clinic. The physician assumed complete charge of his clinic.

Nurses' staffing was done as a joint effort of the health department and the district nurses organization.

The Maricopa County Chapter of the National Foundation assumed the task of a lay volunteer staff which was used primarily for record-keeping, age count, and lines direction.

The county pharmaceutical association recruited pharmacists for mixing vaccine at distribution headquarters and one pharmacist for each clinic site to supervise dropping the vaccine on the sugar cubes.

In Pima County, the PTA's recruited the volunteer staff. For the most part these volunteers were members of the school's own PTA.

A Boy Scout council was responsible for staffing each clinic with

Boy Scouts and with at least one scoutmaster per clinic to direct traffic and to collect money.

The complete staff of each clinic numbered from 12 to 20 at a time. The physicians and a few other personnel worked the entire day; other volunteers worked only half the day.

DISTRIBUTION AND PURCHASING

The steering committee had the responsibility of purchasing all supplies for all clinics. This included ordering vaccine, sugar cubes, paper cups, droppers, record forms, bottles, and all other supplies. It also arranged for the distribution of supplies to the clinics.

In Pima County, purchase and distribution were arranged by representatives of the retail and wholesale druggists.

Method of Distribution of Vaccine and Supplies to Clinic Sites

In both Phoenix and Tucson, a large wholesale drug house served as distribution headquarters. There the vaccine was thawed, diluted, and bottled by pharmacists the morning of the clinic. Sugar cubes, paper cups, and other necessary supplies were packaged with the vaccine for delivery to the clinics. A variety of methods of delivery was used: Some physicians picked up supplies for their clinics directly from the wholesale house; the county sheriff's department, the city police, and State highway patrol delivered them to others. Retail and wholesale druggists' trucks were also used. All supplies reached the clinics well in advance of the opening hour. The amount of vaccine sent to each clinic originally was determined by the estimated total population in that clinic area. (The population estimates were based on the 1960 census tract data, projected to the present, using current school enrollment figures.) Also taken into consideration were the distance of the clinic from headquarters and the relative difficulty of restocking. On the second Sunday of each series, one more factor had to be considered: the percentage of the population served by each clinic that had been immunized on the first Sunday. A general guide to recommended amounts of vaccine for initial dilution and distribution was as follows: first Sunday, vaccine for 34 per cent of the population kept on hand at the vaccination sites, and on the second Sunday, 25 per cent; first Sunday vaccine for 10 per cent of the population kept in cars with radio equipment, and on the second Sunday, 5 per cent; and on the first Sunday, vaccine for 3 per cent of the population held at headquarters, and on the second Sunday, 3 per cent. The total for the first Sunday was for 47 per cent of the population, and for the second Sunday, 33 per cent.

At the headquarters on each polio Sunday were the chairman and several other physician-members of the steering committee. One of these assumed the responsibility of determining if and when additional vaccine was to be thawed and diluted; others answered telephone inquiries and kept in touch with the clinic sites. Several of these acted as "trouble shooters." Each visited a group of clinics early in the day to discover and correct existing problems.

Redistribution was extremely important. Each clinic director had been supplied with the telephone number of distribution headquarters so that he could reorder supplies if needed. Five telephones were staffed to receive incoming calls at headquarters. When the reorders were received and filled, they were sent out to the clinic immediately. Volunteer drivers from the health department, the sheriff's posse, and others transported the supplies. In Maricopa County four National Guard helicopters with volunteer reserve pilots speeded reorders to clinics in outlying areas.

On the second Sunday in Maricopa County an additional method of redistribution was introduced. Ham radio operators with mobile equipment were stationed at strategic points throughout the county to pick up supplies and vaccine from nearby clinics and take them to the clinic requesting additional supplies. As a later innovation, these operators in both counties were provided with stocks of vaccine at the beginning of the day and received directions by radio from headquarters so that vaccine could be delivered in a matter of minutes to the schools in their areas. Toward the end of the day they aided in the transferring of stocks between schools. This transferring allowed for great saving in unused vaccines. In Pima County on the second Sunday, only 6,400 doses were left over from all 37 clinics. This represented approximately 5 per cent of the total diluted vaccine!

CLINICS

The clinic layouts were planned well in advance for maximum efficiency and speed in administering the vaccine. Although the initial layout was designed to handle 2,500 persons per 8-hour clinic day, it was found that the exact layout was adequate to handle up to 10,000 persons per clinic day. In several clinics where the population was greater, the same layout was used, but the stations were doubled or tripled, as necessary.

Because of the swift processing, few lines developed, and a few of the larger clinics immunized up to 5,000 persons per hour. Another reason lines moved fast was that approximately 80 per cent of the people had completed their registration forms before coming into the clinic.

Vaccine was not given to patients to take home to a member of the household who failed to appear. On the other hand, those in cars but not able to stand in line were given the vaccine by a nurse who walked out to the car. Special parking places near the door were provided for cars bringing the handicapped.

HEADQUARTERS ORGANIZATION

The headquarters organization was geared to supply adequate doses of vaccine without diluting a large excess. To accomplish this purpose, responsibility was given to a single individual to determine if and when additional doses were to be thawed and diluted. His decision, in turn, was dependent upon good intelligence from the sites.

A large tote-board was set up showing the sites and number of doses originally given out, followed by recorded data showing time and size of additional orders received and time of their dispatch. In addition, clinic directors were asked to report on their supplies periodically so that excess stocks would be known to headquarters.

One group of headquarters personnel was chosen to answer inquiries and another group to "troubleshoot" sites while the clinics were in operation. The headquarters also served as a central clearing house for press information. In one instance, a radio station was informed that preschool children were not appearing in adequate numbers at several school sites. This announcement was put on the air, and a response was noted in about 10 minutes.

Runners between the various areas were found to be more useful than telephonic intercommunication.

USE OF VACCINE DILUTED BUT
NOT USED ON SUNDAY

In both counties, thousands of doses of vaccine were available as unused supplies from the various sites. These doses were distributed to hospitals and institutions (including jails), made available at small clinics run by the health department and county hospitals, and were given distribution to the home-bound by a civic organization assisted by pharmacy students. By these devices many thousands of additional persons were immunized.

RECORDS

Record forms were kept as simple as possible. In fact, the major record used was the registration form which was filled out by all persons who were immunized. This form contained the name and age of each person, and, in the case of minors the signature of the parent or guardian was added. Maricopa statistics were taken from this form.

"Tick-off" tally sheets were used which were broken down into five age groups. These tallies could at any time be used to estimate the approximate number of doses dispensed and, after each was rechecked, served as the basis of the total count.

The physician in charge of the clinic was responsible for collecting all records, money, and leftover supplies and for returning them to headquarters. Here tabulations were made immediately of money collected and of the number of persons immunized. Further evaluation was completed later by the statistician and his staff at the county health department. Armored car service was used at this point to collect the money and take it to a local bank for recounting and deposit.

Estimates of population were based on calculated growth since the 1960 census. However, a number of factors affected their accuracy, such as visitors in the area and the population on Indian reservations and on military posts. It was also recognized that the tallies were not always accurate in recording all takes of the vaccine. Recognizing that these factors could not be determined, the following data, developed from tallies, are presented in Table 1 without any correction factors.

The reasons for the differing age percentages in the two counties are not known but may be related to the publicity presentations. For example, the possible role of the elderly as "carriers" was stressed in Pima County, which may account for the higher turnout of this age group. The better elementary school response in Maricopa County may have been due to classroom discussions before the campaign started. These and other factors will be the subject of future studies.

Table 1.—Percentage of Proportion of Population Taking Oral Vaccine by Age Groups*

| | Maricopa County | | | | Pima County | | | |
| | PER CENT TAKING | | | | PER CENT TAKING | | | |
Age	Population Estimate	Type 1	Type 2	Type 3	Population Estimate	Type 1	Type 2	Type 3
Under 3 mo	4,500	—	—	—	1,900	—	—	—
3–11 mo	13,500	78.1	77.5	79.8	5,600	84.8	77.1	77.8
1–5 yr	86,000	85.2	84.0	83.1	35,500	84.1	82.0	83.5
6–14 yr	138,000	98.5	96.4	94.6	55,400	93.4	92.7	96.3
15–39 yr	242,000	74.3	72.7	70.5	104,100	77.7	77.8	80.0
40 yr and over	222,000	57.2	59.5	56.8	97,100	71.6	65.9	70.5
TOTALS	706,000	74.6	74.2	72.1	299,600	79.1	76.1	79.2

* At the time this paper was prepared, Maricopa County had not completed the type 3 immunizations, and Pima County had not completed either types 2 or 3. Percentages for these programs were added to this table by the authors just prior to publication.

REPOSITORIES OF DILUTED VACCINE

Because of the perishable nature of the vaccine, the thawed and diluted vaccine can be used for only seven days. If an excess was prepared, it had to be discarded; and if too little was prepared, the sites could not be supplied fast enough to immunize waiting people. With the use of stocks in cars with radio equipment, the diluted vaccine was held in three locations: headquarters, clinics, and radio cars. As a result of the experience of Maricopa and Pima counties, information on recommended repositories was included for the initial distribution of supplies.

RESULTS

The high percentage of people responding will give Maricopa and Pima counties good protection against the wild spread of poliomyelitis viruses in these communities. Probably of even more importance are other less tangible values of the campaign. One of the first obvious results of this program was the improved relations between the organizations which worked together to provide this program for the counties. The other important result is the improved image of the Medical Society in the eyes of the public.

4. Crash Teams

Rehabilitation Operation for
10,000 Moroccan Paralysis Victims*

G. GINGRAS, M.D., AND M. H. L. DESMARAIS, M.D.

THE WORLD WAS SHOCKED to read in mid-November, 1959, that human greed was the underlying cause of an outbreak of over 10,000 cases of paralysis in Morocco.

The first cases appeared between August 31 and September 2, 1959, in the city of Meknes and rapidly spread throughout various parts of the country; by the third week of September, 200 to 300 new cases were being reported daily. Because opinion was divided as to whether the disease was due to an infection or to a toxic factor, and because it was unable to trace the cause of the mysterious "epidemic" to a common etiology, the alarmed Moroccan Government finally appealed to the World Health Organization (WHO) for urgent assistance.

WHO DETECTION

In response, Doctors H. Smith and J. M. K. Spalding of Oxford visited Morocco from September 25 to October 2, 1959, as WHO temporary consultants to investigate the cause of the paralyzing disease. Study of the epidemiologic and statistical information already collected by the Moroccan health authorities, and made available to the WHO experts, revealed that the incidence was still rising rapidly, the outbreak was centered on Meknes and the nearby towns of Sidi Slimane and Khemisset and that only the Moslem Moroccans of the

* Reprinted, by permission, from the December, 1960, issue of the *Archives of Physical Medicine and Rehabilitation*, Vol. 41, pp. 559–563. This paper was presented at the 3rd International Congress of Physical Medicine, Session on Neuromuscular Diseases, Washington, D.C., on August 24, 1960. The authors are, respectively, Professor and Director, School of Rehabilitation, Faculty of Medicine, University of Montreal, and from December 1959, to February 12, 1960, Senior League Delegate and Medical Liaison Officer of the League of Red Cross Societies' International Relief Action for Moroccan Paralysis Victims; Director of the Departments of Physical Medicine of the Municipal Hospitals, St. Boniface Hospital and Misericordia Hospital of Winnipec, Manitoba, and from February 12, 1960 to May 15, 1960 served in the same capacity as Dr. Gingras in Morocco.

artisan class were affected. After investigating both the infective and toxic theory, the cause of the paralysis was proved to be due to intoxication by tri-ortho-cresyl-phosphate found in a dark-colored cooking oil which recently had appeared on the local markets under a well-known trade name. The source of the toxic substance was traced to a lubricating oil used to flush aviation engines and sold as surplus material by the soon departing United States Air Force to a Moroccan dealer. The lubricating oil was eventually purchased by unscrupulous Moroccan merchants who, to realize greater profit, mixed this cheaply bought lubricant with edible oil in proportions from 5 to 80% and put the contaminated mixture on the market as a cooking oil. This accounted for the sparing of other ethnic and religious groups. Jews have their own supervised markets; pilgrims ordinarily bring their own food; Europeans and wealthier Moroccans could afford a better quality of cooking oil while the poor could hardly afford to purchase any oil at all.

CLINICAL PICTURE

Examinations conducted shortly after the appearance of symptoms showed areflexia and a flaccid paralysis mainly of the distal parts of the upper and lower extremities. Symptoms were symmetric in the majority of cases. Paresthesia and loss of superficial sensitivity with a glove-like or sock-like distribution were noted by a number of examiners, but rarely confirmed on more intensive investigation or during regular followup. Patients complained that the affected limbs felt cold, and this was confirmed on palpation. However, interestingly enough, if the temperature of the limbs was elevated somewhat by immersion in warm water prior to testing or treatment, the sensitivity phenomena disappeared in almost all cases. Muscle atrophy became particularly evident in the upper extremities especially involving the flexors and opponens of the thumb. In the lower extremities, drop foot was the common denominator and victims were easily identified at a distance by their "steppage gait." There were no urinary or intestinal symptoms. In conclusion, the clinical picture and evolution were essentially that of acute peripheral neuritis.

Later statistics revealed that 50% of the victims were children and adolescents from five to 18 years of age, and that adult women were affected in greater proportion than men. This is explained by the fact that women ingested more of the contaminated oil through the tasting of the food during preparation and eating all their meals at home, whereas many of the men work outside and have their mid-day meal away from their homes. There have been no reported deaths directly attributable to the intoxication.

PREVIOUS T.O.C.P. INTOXICATIONS

This form of poisoning has been reported in the past in several countries, but never on such a large scale. Tri-ortho-cresyl-phosphate is highly toxic to the peripheral nervous system; it was held responsible for the great outbreak of paralysis in the United States in the early 1930's and in Germany and Switzerland during World War II. In the United States it was known as "Jake Paralysis" because the toxin was present in a soft drink called Ginger Jake or Jamaica Ginger. In Switzerland, 80 soldiers suffered severe poly-neuritis in 1940 and, although prompt and adequate measures were available and applied immediately, the Swiss victims show sequelae of the toxic paralysis even 20 years after the ingestion of a single mas-sive dose of the toxicant. Thirty-three % of these victims are still totally disabled.

REHABILITATION PLAN

An outbreak of 10,000 cases of paralysis in a population of 10 million is a staggering situation in any part of the world. It is disastrous when it occurs in a country like Morocco, a four-year old nation, completely lacking in rehabilitation personnel and equipment. Because of this lack, a French professor Denis Leroy, was sent to Morocco by WHO as a temporary consultant from October 23 to November 6, 1959, to study the incidence and evolution and to make recommendations with reference to the possibilities of organizing re-habilitation centers.

INTERNATIONAL RELIEF ACTION

As it was realized by the Moroccan Government that its national resources could not cope with the situation, an appeal was made to the League of Red Cross Societies for assistance with urgent rehabilitation measures. After a meeting on November 18 at Geneva between representatives of WHO, the Moroccan Government, the League of Red Cross Societies and other international agencies, the League launched an emergency appeal to its national member societies to cover a certain proportion of the medical and material needs while WHO, the Moroccan Government and other United Nations organi-zations endeavored to provide the remainder.

The response was immediate and heartwarming. More than 200 tons of material and equipment were delivered mainly by air from 14 countries, funds from eight countries, and 55 professional rehabili-tation personnel (14 physicians, most of whom are specialists in physical medicine and rehabilitation, 31 physical therapists and 10 nurses), arrived within six weeks from 15 countries. WHO provided an Administrator Delegate, two physical therapists, and two units of electromyograph apparatus. The United Nations Childrens Fund (UNICEF) provided equipment for child patients.

MOROCCAN PROGRAM

The Moroccan Government's program to provide facilities and welfare payments is well under way. A special division was created within the Ministry of Health to operate the Paralysis Program. This division is headed by Doctor A. Faraj, one of the pioneers in the field of health in Morocco.

Establishment of Indoor and Outdoor Rehabilitation Centers

In the program's special division are integrated WHO and League personnel to staff:

Four rehabilitation centers for treatment on an outdoor basis in Sidi Slimane, Sidi Kacem, Khemisset, and Meknes;
One hospital rehabilitation service (indoor) established in a reconverted former military hospital in Alhucemas; and
One hospital rehabilitation center (indoor) being established in Fez.

Because of the geographic distribution of the toxic paralysis cases the possibility of opening other treatment centers is being studied. This would enable the treatment of patients nearer to their homes instead of having to transport them hundreds of kilometers from their communities.

The rehabilitation centers are all improvised and established in large depots, hangars, and abandoned barracks, and each is equipped for simple and uniform mechanotherapy and hydrotherapy according to the plans outlined by Professor Leroy. Each center is designed and equipped as a unit to treat 400 patients excepting Sidi Kacem, where double facilities lend themselves to two units, permitting the treatment of 800 patients daily.

Staffing

The Senior Delegate of the League of Red Cross Society is in charge of directing, from Headquarters in Rabat, all medical and technical aspects of the program. All staff members from all sources operate under him. Each center is provided with a chief physical therapist and nurses. The government provides, through provincial health offices, supporting personnel and social workers. Adhering to initial policy, staffs are of mixed nationalities, thus permitting the maximum utilization of individual experience and knowledge of languages. The Canadian personnel is particularly useful in this respect as they are proficient not only in English but also in French, the latter being the second language of Morocco.

Medical Testing and Treatment

Although the international personnel arrived at their postings in the field while renovation and alterations were still in progress, they nevertheless proceeded with the first step, testing and evaluating patients. A standard and precise record and identification system was developed which also is used by social workers since welfare payments are graduated according to the degree of paralysis and the patient's role in the family unit.

Treatment now is being given in all the centers. The majority of patients are treated as out-patients, reporting to the centers by their own means or transported by government vehicles (which were scarcely available at first). As the usual practice of individual treatment is impossible with such a mass of patients, and since symptoms are similar, patients are divided and treated in groups of approximately 10 each, and the therapy classes are led by the nurses and physical therapy aides under the general supervision of qualified therapists. However, individual treatments and intricate or special therapeutic measures that may be prescribed by the physiatrists are applied only by the qualified physical therapists.

The plan for the care of the approximately 600 quadriplegics and 1,000 children is to accommodate them in the former military establishment which is being transformed into an indoor treatment center in Fez, where the children will have the benefit of combined treatment and schooling. Plans are being drawn up to bring these children from all provinces into Fez, thus relieving somewhat the load on the outdoor centers.

Statistics provided by the Ministry of Health at the end of January, 1960, listed a total of 9,991 victims, of whom 6,242 were examined and tested by the international teams by mid-February. These preliminary statistics would indicate the following prognosis: 6% will remain quadriplegics, confined to bed or wheelchair; 15 to 20% will need short term or no treatment; and the balance will require treatment for extended periods of time. By mid-April, a total of 9,081 patients had been examined and tested.

As muscle activity is subject to variation during the clinical course and subsequently, electromyographic studies were carried out in a number of selected cases, not only for statistical information but also to note the variations, permitting immediate appropriate measures such as intensification or reinstitution of treatment. This study was carried out by Dr. Erland Svennilson of Stockholm, who soon will publish his findings.

Referring to the past experiences of others in similar outbreaks, it is too early to forecast a definite prognosis. All that is clear at the moment is that provision must be made for long-term treatment.

Training of Moroccan Personnel

Special introductory 10-day short courses have been started to train Moroccan male and female nurses aides to send into the field as physical therapy aides. The goal is to provide 250 physical therapy aides; more than 100 had been trained by April, and it is reported that their services are proving useful. After postings to the centers, they receive additional instruction and practical training on the job.

With the approval of the government, WHO has developed a special 12-month physical therapy training course for selected Moroccan nurses. This will be the first School of Rehabilitation in North Africa, and the Moroccan graduates will enable the foreign staff to be released. The plan is the basis for the League's agreement to ask the National Societies to continue professional aid through 1960. This course will be established in line with the recommendations of the World Confederation for Physical Therapy, Second Congress, held in New York on June 20, 1956, pertaining to the initiation and development of programs of Physical Therapy Education and Service in under-developed countries. This type of program already has proved satisfactory in Venezuela and Guatemala.

NEW PROBLEM

Upon discovery of the tri-ortho-cresyl-phosphate as the toxic agent there was confiscation and destruction of all suspicious edible oil in retail establishments as well as impounding of all stocks in refineries until tested; but in spite of warnings to the public, small quantities of the toxic oil seeped into isolated communities and cases have continued to appear at widely separated points. This occurred because the rural population makes infrequent visits to markets for provisions which they purchase in quantity, because they have little contact with the exterior, and also because the criminal merchants deliberately dispatched the contaminated cooking oil to remote areas hundreds of kilometers from Meknes after the public warnings were issued. In order to examine and evaluate these isolated cases, the Senior League Delegate built two mobile teams consisting of a doctor and physical therapists to visit patients in the remote areas. By mid-April, 1,517 of these patients had been tested and evaluated, and recommendations were made for the transfer of the patients requiring treatment to appropriate rehabilitation centers.

INTERNATIONAL COOPERATION AND LIAISON

The headquarters staff makes regular field trips to the centers to maintain close contact and to make on-the-spot decisions jointly to solve problems.

This is one of the largest and most tragic peace-time operations in which physical medicine and rehabilitation have been called upon, and we must continue to assist and help prepare the burdened Moroccan collaborators who will have to carry on the rehabilitation task.

We share a common interest and responsibility, as well as a tremendous opportunity—the welfare of the people. The speed and volume of international aid that has come to the help of a stricken nation is a shining example of international sharing of knowledge and skill and illustrates the fact, as stated by Doctor Howard A. Rusk, when informed of the action, "that medicine and human compassion know no international boundaries."

5. Community Self-Study

What Makes Communities Tick?*

PETER H. ROSSI, PH.D.*

THE TITLE of this paper is in two senses misleading. First, it implies that there is some sort of standard mechanism in all communities which produces the ticking noises we hear when we examine their bodies politic. We are aware of the striking differences among communities; the social forces which they share in common can scarcely be reduced to a machinelike model.

The second sense in which the title is misleading is its overly ambitious scope. I plan to atone for this deception by discussing some generalizations concerning the forms of decision-making in American local communities and indicating what these generalizations imply for techniques of community organization.

These ideas are based on the published literature in this field and data collected by colleagues and me in half a dozen studies of communities scattered over the northeastern third of the country.[1,2,3,4] These communities vary considerably in size and in economic and social composition, ranging from a neighborhood in Chicago at one extreme to a middle-sized southern Ohio city at the other. They do not constitute any sort of fair sample of U.S. communities.

COMMUNITY SOCIAL STRUCTURE

When compared with the U.S. community of the 19th century, the most striking characteristic of contemporary cities is the relative drop in the importance accorded local government, not only in comparison with State and Federal governments, but also in relation to the importance accorded local voluntary associations. To understand what is happening within a contemporary community an investigator cannot confine himself to the official table of organization for municipal government but must also consider a host of voluntary associations which act on behalf of the community and which, with the formal structure of local government, form the basic organizational framework of the local community.

There is no doubt that this is the age of the "community project."

* Reprinted by permission from the February, 1962, issue of *Public Health Reports*, Volume 77, pages 117–124. The author is Director of the National Opinion Research Center, University of Chicago, Chicago, Illinois.

Significant community enterprises are often initiated outside the framework of local government, aided and abetted by a proliferation of civic associations and citizen committees.

In many communities the mayor and city council often appear to be dragging their heels while organized prominent citizens exhort the community to push toward progress. The voluntary associations, ranging from the more permanent varieties—the community chest, chambers of commerce, and service clubs—to the *ad hoc* citizens' committees, have taken over many of the functions of initiating social change and marshaling community support for such changes that are formally allocated to local government and to political parties. While in many cases these voluntary associations eventually must move local political authorities, the initial spark and much of the task of mobilizing public opinion have been performed in advance by the non-political groups.

This is a peculiarly American pattern, not to be encountered in England or in other Western nations. In England particularly, local government agencies well staffed with experts are the prime movers of social change in the community.

Another striking characteristic of the American community in comparison with the past is the status gap between the personnel of local government and the local elites of wealth, intellect, and status.[5] The local echelons of the party organizations and the elective offices of municipal, county, and even State governments are manned by persons whose social positions are often several or even many levels below the denizens of the country club, Rotary Club, and the chamber of commerce. The city fathers and the county commissioners are often recruited from among local lawyers of somewhat uncertain income and miscellaneous clientele or from among small proprietors or professional politicians. Money, status, and intellect seem to cluster in one place and political control in another. Such anomalies lead to the hypothesis that things are really not what they seem and that somewhere there are strings by which local government is guided from without.

How things get done has therefore become more and more problematic as the lack of articulation grows between the political elite and the industrial, commercial, and professional elites. It is hard to believe that the corner grocer elected mayor can govern in his own right in a community with branch factories of several national firms, a local elite of some wealth, and several large commercial establishments.

This apparent mushiness to the local community gives rise to problems common to both the community sociologist and the community organizer. It is hard to understand what makes a community tick and it is hard to grasp how to operate the machinery. It is difficult to understand why one community is run with admirable attention to modernization while another, apparently similar, stagnates.

POWER STRUCTURES

There is a great temptation to resort to the explanation that the ultimate source of innovation and social change in the local community is in either a single individual or in a small group of men. I do not deny that there is evidence that this explanation is warranted in some communities or that some data on all communities tend to support this viewpoint. However, I deny that this is always the case or even that it is the case more often than not.

The existence of power phenomena on the local scene cannot be denied. Citizens are not equally interested and involved in local affairs, and decision makers are not equally sensitive to the opinions of every citizen. It is this inequality of status, wealth, leadership, and involvement which is at the base of community power.

Tied to this inequality are two important issues: first, what accounts for the differentials in effectiveness, and second, over what kinds of decision makers is power particularly effective.

In each of the several communities which we have studied, the wishes and desires of the same types of persons carried particular weight with decision makers. The set of effective power wielders varied somewhat according to the decision maker and the issue. But, in each community it was possible to discern for that particular issue some overall ranking of effectiveness along which prominent citizens could be ordered unidimensionally.

The way in which the content of an issue determined who would be effective in moving a decision suggests that it would be difficult to define a single overall pyramidal power structure. Yet, there is an overall pyramidal structure of power, not of exercised power, but of power potential. In other words, men and social positions could be ranked unidimensionally according to how much weight they could possibly carry, but not according to how much weight they actually throw around. This implies two things: first, the exercise of power is voluntary and some persons of considerable potential elect not to employ it. Second, power rarely is used in all the spheres of community life where it might be employed. In part, this is because partisans seem to specialize in some areas of community life, and in part, some areas of community life are more immune to power.

What are the social positions or the attributes of people who can wield effective influence? Following is a partial catalog of bases of power.

Control over Wealth and Other Resources

This alone is rarely sufficient. Wealth needs to be turned into control over resources or institutions such as banks, land, or mass media that can be used to exercise sanctions or it needs to be accompanied by a tradition of community activity and concern. Thus, in "Bay City," Mass., one wealthy family was powerful because in the past as well as in the present it had contributed heavily to the community by endowing hospitals, playgrounds, and the like, and was recognized as having a claim to be heard. Another family, equally wealthy but without such a history, would have been resented if it had tried to exercise such claims on the community.

Control over Mass Media

Any newspaper publisher is ipso facto powerful whether or not his newspaper wields a great deal of influence with the public. Thus, in a southern Ohio town the newspaper has a poor reputation in the eyes of the public, yet the publisher plays an important role in the community decisions. The controllers of the mass media are in a strategic position because they can either give or withhold attention and approval. These powers are exercised within limits, since a newspaper still must publish some news.

Control over Solidary Groups

Persons who head cohesive organized groups or who are reputed to have influence over large segments of the public can wield power by threatening to withhold support. Even when support by public opinion is not strictly necessary to the carrying out of a decision-maker role, as in a chamber of commerce campaign to get new industry into town, the threat of withholding public support may be an effective sanction.

Control over Values

The social positions of minister, priest, and certain of the professions which are concerned primarily with the interpretation of cultural values wield power by virtue of their right to make value judgments. A minister's moral judgment counts more because this is his specialty.

Control over Prestigious Interaction

Control over entree into desirable social circles is an important sanction over the behavior of decision makers. The transformation of a rough-and-tumble labor leader into a tractable and well-behaved member of the Community Chest board in a large industrial city was accomplished by tempting him into the social circles of high-level management.

In considering this list, it is important to note that it may not be the objective facts which count so much as the reputed facts. For example, the managers of industrial establishments in a southern Ohio city are ranked in power roughly according to the perceived size of each firm. However, size is rarely seen accurately but distorted to fit the rank order of power. Similarly, the Protestant Republican politicians in "Bay City," Mass., saw the Catholic priests as important leaders in the Democratic Party who through control over their flocks prevented the politicians' access to the Democratic masses. In fact, a majority of the priests were Republican in their personal political convictions (Bay City Study by J. Leiper Freeman and co-workers, unpublished).

The manipulation of the appearance of power is, of course, a major technique of the skillful would-be leaders. The source of power which is most easily manipulated in this sense is leadership in organized groups. Few organized groups on the local scene have the power to mobilize public opinion that they are reputed to have.

Who has power over whom? Perhaps the clearest distinction is between the two areas of community life, local government, and the voluntary community associations. For local government officials who are ultimately brought to the bar of public opinion on election day, the leaders of solidary groups normally on their side carry the most weight. Insofar as wealth and the mass media are seen as potential influencers of public opinion, they too are powerful. Within the voluntary community associations which depend largely on the bounty of large contributors, wealth and its control play the major role.

Another distinction must be drawn according to types of issues. An issue which divides the community (or which potentially might divide the community such as integration in public housing or public schools) can be moved to a decision point only by solidary groups. Projects which can be achieved without striking deeply at the gains of one particular group are perhaps best moved by the elite of wealth and status. The best way to get a hospital drive underway is to get together a committee of prominent citizens, but the best way to get a fair employment practices ordinance is to prove that some significant portion of the electorate is for it. This is what is meant by nonpolitical policy issues.

While this diagram of power structures is probably true in a last-analysis, ultimate showdown sense, it should not be taken as the norm for day-to-day activities. The potential for power is only intermittently exercised. By and large, a city council goes its own way, the mayor himself makes the major part of his own decisions, the chamber is guided by its full-time secretary, and so on. Decisions are made with the potential power structure in mind, but few issues are clear in their implications for the powerful.

A tremendous amount of energy is expended in negotiating consent and support for community projects. The urban renewal of Hyde Park-Kenwood in Chicago, for example, required thousands of hours of negotiation between and among politicians, university officials, community leaders, and downtown businessmen. Much of the negotiation at first glance appeared unnecessary and redundant. The explanation for this activity was the profound uncertainty of the decision makers concerning the ability of individuals and groups to veto the plan. In particular, it was necessary to convince the mayor that no significant group opposed the plan and that positive benefits to the mayor's career could be gained by going along with it. Generally this process consists, in part, of showing that persons in opposition represent only themselves, while the supporters represent widespread consensus among large segments of the population.

The practical significance of this view of community power structure is on a general level. The community organizer bent on getting some change introduced into a community has a wider range of alternative tactics from which to choose than would be possible if a single pyramidal model of community power structure fitted all communities. The community organizer's task is to identify which portions of the potential power structure it is possible to enlist and which would be most effective in moving the community toward a decision.

Two specific tactics are also implied in this model. First, in order to enlist the aid of the voluntary association sector of the local community, it is important to define the issue as noncontroversial and the proposed change as a benefit to all groups or at least a detriment to no groups. Second, it is important to appear to recruit mass support through the aid of reputedly solidary organizations if you want to move local government and, as a corollary, it is important to move masses of resources if you want to move the voluntary organization sector.

Perhaps the most important task of the community organizer is the negotiation of consent and support from possible sources of opposition. The most successful community organizers whom I have encountered were extraordinarily skilled at this prime task and spent upward of half their time at it.

ORIGINATION OF CHANGE

In studying the local community, the topic that engages attention more quickly than any other is how social action, the deliberate changes, comes about.

The first question is where do these changes originate? Typically, there are several sources to be encountered within a community. Individuals in professional occupations centrally concerned with community institutions are a major source of innovations. Part of the responsibility in certain occupations is constantly to propose changes in community institutions. Such professional roles as city managers, school superintendents, Public Health officers, and the like carry within themselves the notion of constant improvement in services.

For example, the major source of change within school systems stems from the school administrators. School administration as taught within the three graduate schools of education with which I am acquainted is haunted by the dilemma that a superintendent's worth in the profession depends on how many changes he can introduce into his system, but his tenure in the community often depends on completely different criteria. School superintendents and other community professional persons faced with similar dilemmas react to this conflict by an extraordinary mobility rate.

Another point of origin for social action lies in the competition among community leaders. Often enough, local politics appears to be a wild search for issues, with issue after issue being offered up to the public. While few such attempts succeed in capturing public fancy sufficiently to develop into large-scale controversies, this possibility is another specter that haunts every community leader and public official. This anxiety is the ultimate source of the nonpartisan citizens committee and the desire to take politics out of schools, highways, police protection, and the like.

Finally, one must acknowledge the elusive but fairly important role played by general U.S. value standards. The cult of civic improvement has many devotees in the typical American community. They are found in greatest number within the chamber of commerce and the service clubs. The search for something to do in the way of improvement and amelioration and especially to supply symbols of progress, preferably concrete, provides a constant stream of community projects. Indeed, the demand for community projects is sufficient to support a small industry replete with publications, training sessions, and the like to supply the demand. Certainly the existence of community service organizations like that at Southern Illinois University or at Michigan State University is partially in response to this demand.

Hunter's study of "Regional City,"[6] particularly shows how a group of restless and energetic businessmen spent a significant portion of their time organizing projects to improve their city. In the achievement of an urban renewal project around the University of Chicago, not the least expenditure of effort came from the high-level businessmen closely connected with the university.

It is important not to accept a glib but unsophisticated interest explanation for the participation of high-level businessmen in civic activities in the local community. If it is to the interest of business enterprises to expend funds and permit their managers to spend time on community projects, the interest is far from nonspecific to the business enterprise. Furthermore, among those enterprises with fates most closely linked with the local community, the small commercial establishments, civic participation is weakest.[2]

For an explanation of business participation in community projects, it is more useful to look to the social functions of such participation within the business community. Community projects are so much a part of community life, as lived in the middle and upper echelons of the business world, that these projects provide a measure of the prestige positions of firms and business managers on the local scene. Business peers judge the power and prestige of the businessman and his firm in proportion to the importance of their roles in community projects. While the public relations office of the firm may rationalize the expenditure of resources as an investment in community goodwill, the primary audience in fact turns out to be the rest of the business community; the general public remains virtually unaffected.

In a way, the community chest or the hospital drives are nonwasteful potlatches in which both firms and individuals validate their bids for prestige by the amounts of money they contribute. Conspicuous charity and civic good works in the middle 20th century have replaced the conspicuous consumption and private piety of the late 19th century, aided considerably by the contributions to charity provisions of our income tax laws.

It is characteristic of charities and community projects that those who foot the bill call the tune. These community organizations are not democratic institutions, ultimately responsible to a constituency widely defined. Rather they are ruled by boards and committees who nominate and choose their own successors. Thus a structure of power is more clearly visible in this area of community life than in any other. The boards and committees heavily weighted with large contributors most closely approximate the pyramidal model of a power structure. In this area of community life, wealth and power go hand in hand. Participation in such activities becomes a way of cashing in the resources that one may control, transforming money into prestige. It is this tie-in between prestige and participation in the community affairs which makes it easy to recruit those of high rank in the business and professional worlds to serve on the boards and committees of community organizations.

One latent consequence of this tie-in is that participants in civic activities tend to shy away from the controversial and to stick to things with which no one could possibly disagree. Favorite projects for the chamber of commerce in a southern Ohio community included a clubhouse for youth and rounding up votes for a school bond issue. Nobody in the business community would tackle fair employment laws or even fluoridation for fear that failure of the project would jeopardize the prestige position which participation validates. Similarly, businessmen joined in the fight for urban renewal in Hyde Park-Kenwood only when it was clear that there was no significant opposition to the plan and that the plan would eventually be approved. This pattern is one of the major explanations for the businessman's aversion to politics.

The practical implications of this pattern are considerable. First, it points to a remarkable source of manpower for the citizen committees of community projects. Second, it underscores the necessity for making sure that a project is not going to be controversial if business community support is to be recruited. This gives rise to a new public relations art, that of coopting a sufficient portion of community leadership to take the potential sting out of any proposed community project.

CITIZEN PARTICIPATION

Citizen participation is a social invention which is characteristic of U.S. community life. The idea of ordinary citizens taking part in improving the commonweal is congenial to our conception of democracy in which superior wisdom is imputed to an enlightened citizenry. According to its proponents, much good is credited to this social invention. A minimum claim is that when the ordinary citizens of a community get together, the final outcome is something that has an easier chance of widespread community acceptance. Some claim that better decisions result. Some extreme proponents have claimed all sorts of miracles; one psychiatrist has claimed that better mental health results in the community when participation really works.

Over the past several years, my co-workers and I have studied the effectiveness of citizen participation in the urban renewal planning of Hyde Park-Kenwood, the neighborhood surrounding the University of Chicago.[4] If ever citizen participation was to achieve its claimed effects, this was the neighborhood in which success was most likely. The density of liberal, intellectual homeowners probably exceeds that of any comparable urban area. In fact, this may be the only urban neighborhood in this country in which intellectuals occupy the highest prestige rank, a phenomenon which results from 85% of the faculty residing within one-half mile of the University.

The area can be characterized as hyperorganized. The local citizens organization, the Hyde Park-Kenwood Community Conference, has 4,000 members on its rolls. Block groups affiliated loosely with the conference claim an additional 4,000 persons, excluding overlapping membership. Thus approximately 40% of the families in the area are connected organizationally with the conference. Of the non-members, "fellow travelers" account for an unknown but undoubtedly large proportion.

The expertise within the membership of the conference is nothing short of fabulous; prominent social scientists, city planners, geographers, real estate moguls, lawyers, all of first rank, are active members and participate vigorously in the conference's many committees. Thousands of man-hours and thousands of dollars of foundation funds went into the stimulation and organization of citizen participation in the replanning. Block groups met, considered plans drawn up by professional planners, made recommendations which were carried to the planners, new plans were communicated to the block groups, and so on.

The achievements of the conference must be judged considerable but only in some directions. The plan was changed in numerous minor ways such as which house on a block was to be demolished to provide playground space around a public school. Undoubtedly, the level of anxiety in the neighborhood concerning the meaning of the plan to individual householders was lowered. Intense popular support was mobilized for the final plan. But missing from it were certain points close to the central ideologic goals of the conference, such as provisions for middle income housing and public housing, guarantees surrounding relocations of displaced residents, and the like.

The lesson of Hyde Park-Kenwood for the student of community organization was that citizen participation is a cooptation device which progressively committed the citizens to the plan while their right to dissent was being undercut. This occurred because a large group of citizens, no matter how well trained, working on a part-time basis can only come to a firm consensus on general goals and hence is in an inferior bargaining position vis-a-vis a smaller but full-time group of professionals. (There are, of course, other elements at work in this urban renewal project which complicate the matter and which must be omitted in this short paper.)

The Hyde Park-Kenwood experience raises serious questions in my mind concerning the effectiveness of citizen participation in achieving some of its goals. Grass roots groups like the conference can only react to proposals made by professionals, and, despite the professional competence of members of such an organization, its major function turns out to be that of giving the appearance of consent upward and the appearance of participation downward. While the participation of citizens and their wholehearted involvement made it easier for the plan to be accepted, it can hardly be said to be a plan made by the citizens themselves.

The lesson for the community organizer is plain: the function of citizen participation is to support, not to create. The function of the professional is to create.

CONCLUSIONS

In this paper I have tried to draw upon my research experiences to uncover some of the clockwork mechanisms which make some communities tick. There are many brands of clocks in this market, each operating according to somewhat different principles, but just as in the case of time-measuring machines, there are some underlying uniformities.

First, a community is like an iceberg in that the portion which is visible on the surface is only a small part of the total bulk. There is differential influence, power, and authority.

Second, to move the local community toward change from within procedures must be adapted to the various institutions. Politics is the realm of combat and you had better have troops. The community service voluntary areas are the arena of negotiation and some hard cash on your side is handy.

Third, citizen participation is a good way for a professional to operate to get things done, but there is no superior wisdom in the local masses, merely superior strength.

Fourth, the critical role in social change can often be played by the professional who stirs things up, presents, and then organizes mass support.

1. Rossi, P. H.: Community Decision Making. *Administrative Science Quarterly* 1:415–443 (March) 1957.

2. Rossi, P. H.: *Industry and Community*. Report No. 64. Chicago National Opinion Research Center, (Oct.) 1957, [mimeographed].

3. Rossi, P. H., and Cutright, P.: The Impact of Party Organization in an Industrial Setting, in Janowitz, M., and Enlan, H., eds.: *Community Political Systems*, First International Yearbook in Political Behavior Research. Glencoe, Free Press, 1961, pp. 81–116.

4. Rossi, P. H., and Dentler, R.: *The Politics of Urban Renewal: The Chicago Findings*. Glencoe, Free Press, 1961.

5. Brotz, H. M.: Social Stratification and the Political Order. *American Journal of Sociology* 64:571–578 (May) 1959.

6. Hunter, F.: *Community Power Structure*. Chapel Hill, University of North Carolina Press, 1953.

PART SEVEN

Special Studies: Resolving the Unpredictable

Iatrogenic Disease   812

Iatrogenic Disease

A Study of the German Outbreak of Phocomelia: The Thalidomide Syndrome*

HELEN B. TAUSSIG, M.D.

IN LATE JANUARY, 1962, I heard that a large number of infants had been born in West Germany with severe malformations of the extremities and that a sleeping tablet was suspected as the cause. I immediately went to West Germany to investigate the situation and traveled throughout West Germany with the exception of West Berlin.

It was indeed true that a new clinical syndrome had appeared. The outstanding feature was phocomelia. Phocomelia means "seal extremities"; the word comes from two Greek words *phokos* meaning "seal" and *melos* meaning "extremities." In phocomelia the bones between the hand and the shoulder are defective or absent and the hands or rudimentary fingers arise directly from the end of the affected bone as the flippers of a seal. The first two such cases were presented by Kosenow and Pfeiffer[1] as an exhibit at the German Pediatric Meeting in Kassel in 1960. At this exhibit Kosenow and Pfeiffer reported that no hereditary factor was found, nor was any blood incompatability demonstrable and no chromosomal abnormality was detected. Little attention was paid to the exhibit. Dr. Guido Fanconi, however, studied the cases and stated he had never seen the clinical syndrome. In retrospect, it is surprising that so little attention was paid to this exhibit because during 1960 infants with this syndrome had been brought to almost every pediatric clinic in West Germany.

Phocomelia has long been known as a rare malformation but usually affects only one limb. Dr. Grüber of Göttingen, who is now 86 years old and has devoted his life to malformations in man and animal, told me he had seen as many individuals with two heads as he had with phocomelia.

Suddenly in 1961, the incidence of phocomelia increased rapidly. Almost every clinic in West Germany admitted three times as many such infants in 1961 as in 1960. The incidence which was reported to me in March, 1962, by various university pediatric clinics in West Germany and also in three centers in the British Commonwealth, was

* Reprinted, with omission of three tables and seven illustrations, by permission, from the June 30, 1962, issue of *The Journal of The American Medical Association*, Vol. 180, pp. 1106–1114. The author is Professor of Pediatrics, The Johns Hopkins University, School of Medicine, Baltimore, Maryland.

as follows: 1949–1959, three to four per year at two clinics, including peromelia, amelia, and micromelia; 1959, 17; 1960, 136; 1961, 515; and in the past three years 678. By the time of the 1961 pediatric meeting in Düsseldorf almost all pediatricians were aware of the outbreak of phocomelia.

In September, 1961, Wiedemann[2] reported the first series of 33 such children, and delineated the clinical syndrome. As in most malformations, the severity varies but the pattern is remarkably specific. The essential feature of the abnormality concerns the long bones of the extremities. The prehensile grasp is lost. The hand arises directly from the distal end of the affected bone. The radius is absent or both radius and ulna are defective; in some instances only one short bone remains; in extreme cases the radius, ulna, and humerus are lacking and the hand buds arise from the shoulders. Both sides are affected but not usually with equal severity. The legs may be affected in the same manner; in most instances the deformity of legs is less severe. The tibia fails to form. The fibula also may not form and the femur may be short. The hip girdle is not fully developed and there is a dislocation of the hip with external rotation of the stub of the femur. The feet are externally rotated. Polydactylism and syndactylia of the toes are common. In the extremely severe cases the arms and the legs are missing. In some instances the external ear is missing and the internal auditory canal is abnormally low. Usually hearing is not grossly impaired. Unilateral facial paralysis is relatively common. The vast majority of children are of normal mentality.

Pfeiffer and Kosenow[4] noted that a mid-line facial hemangioma on the forehead which extended over the nose to form a "moustache" on the upper lip was almost pathognomonic of the syndrome. A saddle nose was also common. These features diminish and tend to disappear as the infant grows. In some instances, usually in severe cases the internal organs are affected. Malrotation of the gut occurs with duodenal stenosis and anal atresia. Asplenia may occur and the musculature of the uterus may be so affected as to make a bihorned uterus. A variety of cardiac malformations have also been reported but these did not fall into any specific pattern. Thus hypoplasia of the aorta, defects of the auricular and ventricular septa, all forms of transposition of the great vessels, tetralogy of Fallot, and pulmonary stenosis have all been reported. Pfeiffer and Kosenow[4] reported extensive family studies on 34 children. They found no similar traits among the relatives and no consanguinity among the parents. Chromosomal analysis of 12 patients showed no chromosomal aberration either in the number or form of the chromosomes. Four of six pairs of dizygotic twins had the same type of malformation, but the twins were not equally affected. These investigators thought that the causative factor was exogenous, and acted during the critical phase of development, i.e., between the third and sixth week of pregnancy.

Although the critical time was similar to that of German measles, viral infection was excluded by the steady increase in the number of patients over a two-year period and also by the distribution of the cases. Viruses know no territorial borders. This epidemic remained strikingly centered in West Germany. German pediatricians became aware of the problem. Extensive studies had been instituted in a number of centers. Lenz in Hamburg, Weicker in Bonn, Wiedemann[2] in Kiel, and Pfeiffer and Kosenow[4] in Münster each undertook special studies. Many doctors suspected radioactive fallout. Lengthy questionnaires were sent out inquiring about x-ray exposure, hormones, detergents, foods (and food preservatives), contraceptive measures, and tests for pregnancy. Most of these were retrospective studies. Dr. Lenz's initial studies showed that approximately 20% of his patients had taken Contergan. On Nov. 8 it occurred to him that Contergan was the cause. He requestioned his patients and the incidence promptly rose to about 50%. Many of the patients stated that they had considered that drug too innocent to mention it on the questionnaire.

THE DRUG

Contergan is the West German trade name for thalidomide, a synthetic drug which, as the story is told in West Germany, was first conceived and made by Ciba and found by them to have no effect on animals; therefore, it was discarded. In 1958, Grünenthal developed the drug and tried it on animals; they, too, found it had no effect on animals. Thereupon it occurred to the inventors that it might be useful in epilepsy and was marketed as an anticonvulsant drug. It was soon found to be worthless for epilepsy, but it caused sleep. Thereafter, it was sold as a sleeping tablet, a sedative, and tranquilizer. It had a prompt action, gave a natural deep sleep and no hangover. It appeared innocent and safe. Man could not commit suicide with it. It became West Germany's most popular sleeping tablet and was widely used in hospitals and in mental institutions.

Thalidomide was added as a sedative to other drugs such as algosediv (thalidomide and acetylsalicylic acid), peracon expectorans, grippex, and polygripan; thus it was used for grippe, neuralgia, asthma, and as a cough medicine. A liquid form was made for children. It was used in hospitals to quiet a child for an electroencephalogram. It became West Germany's baby-sitter. It was also found useful as an antiemetic in pregnancy. The drug was manufactured "by the ton" and sold without prescription. Inasmuch as the drug was cheap and an excellent sedative, the sale was tremendous.

The rights to market the drug were sold to pharmaceutical firms in other countries. In the British Commonwealth it was marketed by Distillers (Biochemicals) as Distaval. In Portugal it was sold as Softenon and it was manufactured in the United States as Kevadon (but it was never passed by our Food and Drug Administration). It was sold both as Kevadon and Talimol in Canada. Thalidomide was also added to the English drugs known as Valgis, Tensival, Valgraine, and Asmaval. I do not know whether the drug was added to any Portuguese preparations.

In April, 1961, a new form of polyneuritis appeared: tingling of the hands, sensory disturbance, and later, atrophy of the thumb and motor disturbances. It was soon recognized that the long continued use of Contergan in adults was responsible for polyneuritis; furthermore, unless the drug was promptly discontinued, the polyneuritis was irreversible. Thereafter, the drug was placed upon prescription. Nevertheless, it remained a popular drug and continued to be widely used in hospitals and also in the home.

CAUSAL RELATIONSHIPS

As previously stated, on Nov. 8 it occurred to Dr. Lenz that Contergan was probably responsible for the catastrophic outbreak of phocomelia. On Nov. 15 he warned Grünenthal that he suspected Contergan was the cause of phocomelia and that the drug should be withdrawn. On Nov. 20, 1961, at the Düsseldorf Pediatric Meeting, Lenz[5] reported he suspected a specific drug was the cause of the "Wiedemann syndrome" and that he had warned the company that the drug should be withdrawn. He did not name the drug. That night a physician came up to him and said, "Will you tell me confidentially, is the drug Contergan? I ask because we have such a child and my wife took Contergan." In the next few days he received a half dozen letters asking the same question and saying, "My wife took Contergan and we have such a child." A couple of days later it was generally known among the doctors that Contergan was the drug under suspicion. On Nov. 26 Grünenthal withdrew the drug from the market.

On Nov. 28 the Ministry of Health issued a firm but cautious statement that Contergan was suspected to be a major factor in the production of phocomelia, and stated that the drug had been withdrawn from the market. Women were warned not to take the drug. The announcement was carried on the front page of every newspaper, on the radio, and on television.

Phocomelia not only suddenly appeared in Germany, but the same unusual type of malformation equally suddenly made its appearance in Australia. In April, 1961, Dr. W. G. McBride[6] in a relatively short time saw three babies born with severe phocomelia. He saw no more such infants until the fall of 1961. In October and November, 1961, he saw three more such infants. Thereupon he reviewed the six cases and he found that all six mothers had received Distaval in early pregnancy. Dr. McBride communicated his findings to the Australian Branch of Distillers Limited and they in turn cabled their London office on Nov. 27, 1961. Distaval is the English trade name for Contergan. Thus, within a couple of days the English firm received similar reports from two widely separated countries. The drug was promptly withdrawn from the market. The latest report is that it is available to hospitals in limited sales.

McBride[7] in a brief note in the Dec. 16 *Lancet,* reported a 20% increase in severely malformed babies from the use of Distaval in early pregnancy. The malformation affected the mesenchymal tissue, both the long bones, and the musculature of the gut. Had anyone else seen anything like it? Lenz[8] replied to his letter in the Jan. 12 issue of the *Lancet.*

Spiers[9] in Stirlingshire, Scotland, had seen 10 infants with severe phocomelia during 1961. He immediately set to work to ascertain whether his cases were associated with Distaval. On questioning mothers and doctors he obtained a history of Distaval in two of the patients. Then he went to the office where all prescriptions are filed, and with the names of the patients and the approximate date on which the medicine was given, he asked to have the prescriptions checked. It took three weeks. During this time he interviewed the mothers and in two instances the mothers finally remembered they had taken sleeping tablets and produced the bottles from which the tablets had been taken. The tablets therein were stamped DT/DL. Ultimately, he obtained positive proof that eight out of 10 of these patients had taken Distaval in early pregnancy.

Thus, between Nov. 20, 1961, and January, 1962, the circumstantial evidence rapidly accumulated in different parts of the world which indicated that thalidomide played an important role in the production of phocomelia.

Further studies were instituted everywhere. Many clinics reported a history of the ingestion of Contergan could readily be obtained from the women in one-half of the instances but not in all cases.

A few, but remarkably few, prospective studies were instituted. One obstetrician asked each of 65 patients whether Contergan had been taken in early pregnancy and obtained a positive reply in only a single instance. He said if that woman had an abnormal baby he would believe Lenz. She did!

Professor Von Masselbach made a prospective study of 350 patients in his obstetric clinic. Thirteen women had taken Contergan, six in the second half of pregnancy and seven in the first half, i.e., in the first 4½ months. Among these seven women, two had babies with phocomelia, one had a baby with an anal atresia, and four were normal.

In Düsseldorf, in a group of 300 women who had not taken Contergan, all the babies were healthy, whereas one-half of the women who took Contergan had abnormal children. These investigators also had collected 40 cases over a two-year period. Seventy-five % of these mothers gave a history of Contergan. Since the records were not checked, the history of Contergan was recorded as probable but not proven. Dr. Weicker[10] in Bonn was collecting 100 cases of phocomelia with a history of Contergan. In March, 1962, when I was in Bonn, he had over 90 such cases.

Dr. Lenz[13] undertook a study to ascertain in how many patients who had given birth to infants with phocomelia he could obtain proof that the mother had taken Contergan during early pregnancy. He considered a case as proven only by a photostatic copy of a prescription or by a hospital record showing the date and amount of Contergan given. The difficulty in obtaining such information was great because prior to April, 1961, the drug was sold without prescription. By and large, women in the early months of pregnancy are not cared for in a hospital. Dr. Lenz, however, found that a number of women had been admitted to a hospital for some minor operation before they knew they were pregnant. Many of these patients had received a sleeping tablet while in the hospital and thereby Dr. Lenz could obtain proof that Contergan had been prescribed. In many West German hospitals sleeping tablets are given by the nurses as freely as laxatives are given in the United States.

Few of us can remember what medicine we took a year or more ago. Far less, exactly when and how much we took. In some instances, however, special events enabled the patient to remember the date or the approximate time during which she took a sleeping tablet. Travel was a common event. Many people do not sleep well when traveling. Such persons usually know if and approximately when they took sleeping tablets. One woman knew the date she took a sleeping tablet: it was the night the neighboring farm house had burned down. Another woman recalled she had taken Contergan for three nights after her father-in-law had been murdered. The date was clearly imprinted on her mind. Two other incidents reported by Dr. Lenz illustrate how difficult it may be to obtain accurate information. In one instance in which the mother gave birth to a baby with phocomelia, the doctor swore the mother had not received Contergan. He had prescribed an entirely different sedative. On investigation at the pharmacy where the mother had bought the medicine, Dr. Lenz found the prescription was stamped "drug not in stock, Contergan given instead."

In another instance in which Dr. Lenz talked with the parents for more than one-half hour and both denied the mother had taken

Contergan, three weeks later Dr. Lenz received a letter saying: "I have been told not to write but I can no longer sleep without telling you I did take Contergan but, as my husband was once in a hospital for drug addiction, I had promised I would never take such a drug; I could not tell him I had broken my promise."

By the middle of March, 1962, Dr. Lenz had analyzed 50 cases[13] in which he interviewed parents, reviewed hospital records, and determined the date of the last menstrual period, and in many instances he obtained the date of conception and also had proof of the date on which Contergan had been taken. Forty-five of 50 women had taken the drug between the 30th and 50th day and five had taken it between the 50th and 60th day after the last menstrual period. Among the 21 instances in which the date of conception was known, the mothers had taken Contergan between the 28th and 42nd day (inclusive) after conception. Although the exact time during which the drug has a teratogenic action may be found to vary slightly, the period in which it affects the development of the embryo appears to be relatively brief.

These observations clarify the finding of Dr. W. Hillmich[14] of Göttingen who made a prospective study of 99 patients who had taken Contergan during pregnancy. He found none had taken the drug in the first three weeks; one had taken it in the fourth week, none in the fifth, one in the sixth, none in the seventh, and one in the eighth week. All of the remaining patients had taken the drug after the ninth week of pregnancy. The mother who had Contergan on the 42nd day after the last menstrual period was the only one who had an abnormal baby. The woman who had taken Contergan in the 6th week had taken it on the 51st day after her last menstrual period which is probably safe provided she had a normal ovulation time. All others had taken the drug well after the sensitive period.

OCCURRENCE

The incidence of phocomelia in West Germany is extremely high. Studies from the Institute of Human Genetics in Münster showed that between 1949 and 1959 they saw an average of four children per year, as mentioned, with severe malformation of the extremities. These malformations included peromelia (amputation of a limb), amelia (absence of a limb which may be the extreme either of peromelia or of phocomelia), micromelia (a small limb), and phocomelia. Even the phocomelia of former years differed from the present phocomelia in that it was usually unilateral. Suddenly, in 1959, three cases of bilateral phocomelia were seen in that institute; 26 cases occurred in 1960 and 96 cases in 1961. Furthermore, to date,

13 pairs of twins have been registered; hence they estimated there should be 1,300 cases.

The Minister of Health of Westphalia has set up a name registry for all children with defective hands and arms, i.e., all children who would need orthopedic help. This registry included clubbed hands and polydactylism as well as phocomelia. They estimate that about 80 per cent of these cases will be phocomelia. As of Jan. 1, 1962, they had 800 registered cases and at that time reports had been received from only one-half of Westphalia. I saw the stack of records for January and February, 1962. These had not yet been counted but there must have been approximately 200. This indicates that there will be probably 1,500 to 2,000 such children in Westphalia and the North Rhineland by August, 1962. This estimate agrees with the estimate from Münster. Westphalia is but one section of West Germany. Thus the estimation of 3,500 to 4,000 cases appears to be a minimal figure. Probably the number will be far larger. Two-thirds of the children are expected to live.

We visited Freiburg for it was reported that there were 100 cases there. At the University Clinic, Dr. Keller advised me that they had seen approximately 10 or 20 cases and showed me one infant in the hospital. He kindly offered to look up the exact number. Subsequently, he wrote me that they had seen 37 infants in the clinic and they had received reports of 200 such infants born in the environs of Freiburg.

In contrast to these findings, Dr. Immon at the Headquarters of the United States Army of Occupation in Heidelberg told me on March 6 that he was reasonably confident that there had been no cases of phocomelia among the 16,000 babies born in the U.S. military hospitals in Germany in 1961. He had traveled extensively and had visited all their hospitals. He had been shown the unusual cases, but had seen no infants with phocomelia up to March 12, 1962. Further, they were certain that all such infants would be immediately evacuated to the United States. All evacuations passed through their office, and no case of phocomelia had been reported. As of April 14, no such cases had been received from overseas at the Walter Reed Hospital in Washington, D.C. In a recent letter, Dr. Immon reported one infant born with phocomelia in a U.S. Army hospital. The infant's mother, who was a German, volunteered the information that she had taken Contergan in early pregnancy.

Alas, the incidence in England is also high. Reports are steadily appearing in the *Lancet* of the occurrence of phocomelia in infants born of women who have taken thalidomide in early pregnancy. Dr. Clifford Parsons[15] advised me that at a recent medical meeting almost everyone in the audience had seen at least one such case. The total incidence is expected to be in the hundreds but fortunately not in the thousands.

Reports are still coming in from all over the world which show that phocomelia has occurred where Contergan has been used. As of March 22, seven cases were reported in Sweden in which Contergan had been purchased in Germany; two cases in Belgium and the Contergan was known to have been bought in Germany; four cases in Switzerland with a history of the ingestion of Contergan; seven cases in Lebanon where the Portuguese preparation, Softenon, is available; one case in Israel and the mother took Distaval; one case in Peru and the father had obtained Contergan in Germany. Seven cases have been reported in Canada in women who had taken Kevadon in early pregnancy. One sad instance in the United States is that of a German woman who had married an American, and brought Contergan with her to the United States. She took the drug and has given birth to twins; one has phocomelia and the other duodenal atresia and a rectovaginal fistula. As yet, I have received no information of the incidence of phocomelia in Portugal. Dr. Lenz, however, has written me that he has learned of an outbreak of phocomelia in Brazil associated with thalidomide.

There are, however, still many perplexing problems. One concerns twins. Usually both twins are affected even when they are dizygotic but not always to the same extent, as in the above mentioned case. Another case is known in which one twin died at five months and was delivered at term with the living twin. The living twin had a phocomelia and the bones of the dead twin were normal.

I learned of a physician who had taken Contergan until she developed peripheral neuritis. Thereupon she stopped taking the drug until she was pregnant and then took it again through two successive pregnancies and both children were normal. The question arises as to how early in pregnancy did she take the drug, or is she one of the fortunate women?

Everyone admits that no information is available concerning how many women may have taken the drug in the sensitive period and have had a normal child.

Some doctors in Germany are still doubtful about the exact role of Contergan. Most doctors, however, believe that Contergan plays a major role. Dr. Pfeiffer remarked that most phenomena are more complicated than they seem, and therefore he cannot believe that the cause of phocomelia is as simple as Contergan alone. Nevertheless, he, too, believes that Contergan plays a major role. Many English physicians believe there must be some other substance or factor which also causes phocomelia because a history of Distaval cannot be obtained in every case. No relation has been found between the amount of the drug ingested and the severity of the malformation. A single dose of 100 mg. is thought to be sufficient to cause severe phocomelia, and repeated doses may give only a mild abnormality.

The only other drug with which I am familiar which is similar to Contergan is glutethimide (Doriden). Although in a few instances, a history of glutethimide, not Contergan, has been obtained, glutethimide has been widely used in Switzerland since 1955, and phocomelia was not known until 1961 and then only a few cases were seen and in most instances, a history of Contergan was obtained.

My attention has recently been called to 2 other drugs which contain radicles similar to thalidomide, namely, bemegride (Megimide) and chlorthalidone (Hygroton).

Little is known concerning the metabolism of thalidomide or how it is excreted from the body, nor the length of time the teratogenic factor persists in the body. Virtually all that is known is that it is insoluble in water and in fat. It affects the nervous system of mature people and the mesenchymal tissue of the embryo.

LABORATORY TRIALS

Few animal experiments have been done. As previously mentioned, thalidomide does not induce sleep in the usual laboratory animals. Grünenthal has tried to reproduce phocomelia in rats, mice, and rabbits and has failed. In Keil, the drug was fed to hens, and the chicks were normal.

Grünenthal has shown that the drug passes through the placenta of rabbits but in their experience the offspring were normal. Somers[16] has, however, recently reported the production of abnormalities in rabbits which are remarkably similar to those in infants. Although the offspring were not equally affected, the extremities did appear to be grossly abnormal and radiologic examination of the extremities showed that the long bones were defective. Although Somers believes the ill effects of thalidomide are proved, others disagree. Murphy[17] has recently reported the production of phocomelia in the offspring of a rat by intraperitoneal injection of an enormous dose of thalidomide on the 12th day of pregnancy. Clearly these observations require confirmation. Should the observation not be confirmed, it should be remembered that thalidomide makes a horse sleep. Therefore, the horse might be found to react as man does. Simian experiments would also be of interest.

Once a susceptible animal has been found, a new avenue of approach to malformations will be available. It is quite clear that the drug acts during the period in which the embryo is developing, as is the case with the virus of German measles. It is equally clear that it acts at a different point or in a way different from that of the virus of German measles; the resultant malformations are totally different. Furthermore, thalidomide is a synthetic chemical, and it should be possible to test the action of the separate chemical radicals from which the drug is compounded.

RECOMMENDATIONS

Even though this drug has not been conclusively demonstrated to have the same effect on animal and man, it does indicate that all new drugs which circulate through the blood stream should be screened for their effect on the offspring of pregnant animals. Distillers Limited is already attempting to develop tests by which to screen drugs for this serious untoward effect. It is, however, an extremely difficult problem and it demands extensive study. Our Food and Drug Act, although better than most of the other countries, should be strengthened. Women in the child-bearing age must be educated not to take new drugs. Often the harm is done before they know they are pregnant, and with the best of medical knowledge some other harmful preparation may be incorporated into some drug. We do not know how to eradicate completely such a danger, but let us do what we can.

Thus, the tragic effects of thalidomide have opened up a new avenue of approach to the etiology of malformations. What is the precise factor that causes phocomelia? Where does it act? How does it inhibit growth? Many physicians have also asked how about its effect on cancer? One sad story is, we hope, coming to an end. It should be the dawn of new and better control of drugs. Let us hope that it is also the dawn of new knowledge.

SUMMARY

In 1960 Kosenow and Pfeiffer reported a new clinical syndrome; the essential feature was phocomelia. The incidence of the malformations rapidly increased and by the end of 1961, thousands of children had been born with severe malformations of the extremities. The causative factor appeared to be an exogeneous agent. Many retrospective studies were instituted.

Almost simultaneously Lenz in Hamburg and McBride in Australia suspected that the malformations were caused by taking thalidomide in early pregnancy.

Thalidomide is a synthetic drug developed by Grünenthal and marketed in Germany as Contergan, in England as Distaval, in Portugal as Softenon, as Kevadon in the United States (though not released by our Food and Drug Administration) and as Kevadon and Talimol in Canada. It was an excellent sleeping tablet and tranquilizer, and was added to a number of other compounds which were used for the relief of grippe, migraine, and asthma and also for expectorants.

The circumstantial evidence is overwhelming that this drug does cause severe malformations of the extremities. Grünenthal showed that the drug passed through the placenta of rabbits. Distillers, Ltd., in England, have reproduced the malformations in rabbits by feeding the drug to pregnant animals. Murphy has produced phocomelia in the rat by an enormous dose of thalidomide given intraperitoneally to a pregnant animal.

Certainly new drugs, which are of use to persons of all ages and which enter the blood stream, should be screened for possible teratogenic action. Furthermore, young women must learn that nothing is foolproof and new drugs should not be taken unless absolutely necessary, as the damage often occurs before the woman knows she is pregnant.

This drug shows how serious the side effects of drugs may be and it also opens up a new avenue to the study of the etiology of malformations.

GENERIC AND TRADE NAMES OF DRUGS

Thalidomide—*Contergan* (West Germany), *Distaval* (British Commonwealth), *Softenon* (Portugal), *Kevadon* (United States and Canada), *Talimol* (Canada).

Thalidomide is also a constituent of the following drugs: algosediv, peracon expectorans, grippex, polygripan (West Germany); Valgis, Tensival, Valgraine, Asmaval (British Commonwealth).

Glutethimide—*Doriden.*

Bemegride—*Megimide.*

Chlorthalidone—*Hygroton.*

1. Kosenow, W., and Pfeiffer, R. A.: Micromelia, Haemangioma und Duodenal Stenosis Exhibit, German Pediatric Society, Kassel, 1960; reported by title in Monat, *Kinderheilk* 109:227 (March) 1961.

2. Wiedemann, H. R.: Himweis auf eine dezeitige, Häufung hypo-und aplastischer Fehlbildungen der Gliedmassen, *Med Welt* 37:1863–1866 (Sept. 16) 1961.

3. Wiedemann, H. R., and Aeissen, K.: Zur Frage der derzeitigen Häufung von Gliedmassen-Fehlbildungen, *Med Mschr* 12:816–818, 1962.

4. Pfeiffer, R. A., and Kosenow, W.: Zur Frage einer exogenen Verursachung von schweren Extremitaten-missbildungen, *Muench Med Wschr* 104:68–74, 1962.

5. Lenz, W.: Kindliche Missbildungen nach Medikament während der Gravidität, *Deutsch Med Wschr* 86:2555–2556 (Dec. 29) 1961.

6. McBride, W. G.: Personal communication from Distillers, Ltd., in London.

7. McBride, W. G.: Thalidomide and Congenital Abnormalities, *Lancet* 2:1358 (Dec. 16) 1961.

8. Lenz, W.: Thalidomide and Congenital Anomalies, *Lancet* 1:45 (Jan. 6) 1962.

9. Speirs, A. L.: Thalidomide and Congenital Abnormalities, *Lancet* 1: 303–305 (Feb. 10) 1962.

10. Weicker: Personal communication to the author.

11. Lenz, W.: Thalidomide and Congenital Abnormalities, *Lancet* 1: 271–272 (Feb. 3) 1962.

12. Lenz, W.: Eintstehung von Missbildungen durch Medikamente, *Arzt Mitt* 47:494 (March 3) 1962.

13. Lenz, W.: Personal communi-

cation to the author; full report to be given at International Pediatric Congress, Lisbon, Sept., 1962.

14. Hillmich, W.: Personal communication to the author.

15. Parsons, C.: Personal communication to the author.

16. Somers, G. F.: *Lancet*, April 28, 1962; personal communication, Brown and Somers of Distillers, Ltd., London.

17. Murphy, M. L.: Reported at meeting of American Pediatric Society, Atlantic City, May 10, 1962.

PART EIGHT

Goals and Priorities in a Changing World

1. The Foundations for a Social Epidemiology
   of Health   827

2. The Dynamics of Planned Change   838

3. The Goals of Public Health   852

4. After Civilization What?   866

"All things flow," said Heraclitus, "we do not bathe in the same river twice." The revolutionary pace of scientific advance and social change in our time dissolves old perspectives and new problems, undreamt of a decade before, emerge on the human scene.

Based on the accumulating knowledge from biologic and behavioral science, Public Health is constantly evaluating its day-to-day strategies, while considering whether its long-range goals remain constant or are themselves in flux.

The papers in this final section depict the forces that promote and inhibit technologic and social change and that shape the perspectives of Public Health. They probe deeply, sometimes speculatively, into the future of a field whose policies cannot but be dynamic and change-oriented if it is to realize its prodigious potentialities for human betterment.

1. The Foundations for a Social Epidemiology of Health

Man and His Changing Environment: Health and Disease and the Changing Social and Cultural Environment of Man*

EDWARD STAINBROOK, PH.D., M.D.

IN A SMALL British village the local apothecary shop displays as its sole identifying legend, "Prescriptions dispensed with deadly accuracy." This, I assume, is also an exemplary, if somewhat ambivalent, aspiration for the shaping of far-ranging descriptions of the too-often subtle and ambiguous happenings which constitute the cross-organization of man and his environment. But, as Pascal wrote many years ago, "The nature of man is his whole nature," and wholeness always challenges adequate and accurate comprehension. The mind is strained to perceive in one intellectual grasp the molecular and the molar conceptions of the same living event. Happily, however, in current medical thinking about man and his actions, there is progressively less tendency to avoid the threat of complexity by willfully impoverishing the rich reality of the human situation or by reducing the perception of life to nothing but the metabolic fires in which it burns. In contemporary medicine we have come to a tentative agreement, at least, that a theoretic model of an interpenetrating system-organization of the physical world, biologic processes, actions describable as human behavior, and happenings between persons, determined in part by the social and cultural conditions of the life-space which they inhabit, is a necessary way of talking about human living in the experience of being well or of being ill.

Psychiatry, itself, has frequently and justly been criticized for admonishing the other medical disciplines that the body is also a person while proceeding in its own work as if the person were not also a body. The necessary resolution of this dialectic is not only to put the mind back into the brain conceptually, where it undoubtedly

* Reprinted, by permission, from the July, 1961, issue of the *American Journal of Public Health*, Vol. 51, pp. 1005–1013. Copyright by the American Public Health Association, Inc., 1790 Broadway, New York 19, N.Y. This paper was presented before the Association Symposium of the American Public Health Association, at the Eighty-Eighth Annual Meeting in San Francisco, California on October 31, 1960. The author is Professor and Chairman, Department of Psychiatry, School of Medicine, University of Southern California, Los Angeles, California.

belongs, but also to put the brain back into life and into living, where it inexorably is.

A field theory of human action in a far more complicated sense than that envisioned by the early 20th century Gestalt and topologic psychologists underlies the modern medical and Public Health concerns with the social and cultural environment. For not only is each individual a highly differentiated and organized living system integrated into an organized and differentiated world, but much of the here-and-now behavior of the person is dependent upon the life history of the encounter with his society and culture which has already transformed him.

Many of the treatment attempts of contemporary medicine fail and are irrational because they try to change the effect of history, of the influence on the individual of his prior learning, not by more experience in living, but by direct biochemical or surgical intervention designed to alter immediately biologic states and functions. The burgeoning, exuberant, and highly undisciplined field of psychopharmacology is being greatly overstimulated by the widespread clinical practice of assuming that the behavior an individual brings to the present, as well as the behavior induced in him by his conditions of life, can be changed rationally by influencing pharmacologically, in a relatively nonspecific way, biologic functions which are what they currently are largely because of the human experience they have had and are having.

The laws moderating the selection, differentiation, organizing, and reorganizing of experience into its representations in living systems cannot be ignored so impatiently. In the individual, as in the collectivity, so much of the effect of history can be changed radically only by more history, that is to say, by more human experience and learning. And the new learning and experience as it becomes history must be innovative and not, as is so usual of human behavior, merely repetitive. Originality, as Wallace Stevens observed, is the escape from repetition.

We seek, then, in a discussion of medicine, society, and culture, conceptual models for the physical world, for the body, for the person, and for the human group in its various complexities of social organization. All these theoretic models have in common words and sentences for making a structure-function analysis of their object of study and for describing their action through time. By symbolic association and participation in the social and cultural learning of the person, even the unlearned functions of body and of organs learn how to be human. The body is full not only of life but of living. Each system is differentiated and organized as the result of its history. For the person, and therefore also for his body, much of his history can be self-reported, and a significant determinant of his behavior in the present will be his and his society's forecast of the future.

Since there are concomitant physiologic processes associated with every individual behavioral event, and since probably no act of individual behavior is unrelated to the social space in which it is occurring, body and society are in constant transaction across a total field of reciprocal determination. In many constantly shifting patterns, body and person are the environment of society as society becomes the environment of person and body.

It is in this latter sense that in relation to health and disease social medicine has been concerned for so long about cultural values and behavioral life-styles, as well as about economic conditions, sanitation, housing, and other more tangible definitions of social space. To paraphrase Wystan Auden, even cultural ideas and values modify, and get modified in the guts of living.

Moreover a comprehensive theory of disease, interrelating body, person, human group, and the physical environment, signifies, diagnostically, an insistence upon etiologic patterns or fields even if the major search for structural defect or dysfunction is confined to the body. Hence, every disease, in some balance of etiologic patterning, is a psychosomatic, a psychosocial, and a biosocial ill-at-easeness.

Rational treatment and rational prevention follow from the determination of the causative pattern. What part of the disease causation is in the body, the person, or the human group is the rational cue for intervention with methods appropriate for correction in the biologic, the behavioral, or the interactional social processes sustaining the illness.

All these statements are a theoretic prelude to an insistence that much of what goes on inside bodies is intimately related to what goes on between bodies. The understanding of the structures, functions, and values of social organization is not optional and elective for medicine and the Public Health, but imperative. The sciences of social man and of individual behavior, the behavioral sciences if you will, are an integral part of basic medical science. We shall consider, therefore, some present trends in society and culture with particular reference to medical theory and practice and not merely in relation to the general humanistic concerns overlying our immediate professional roles.

Certain it is that not many of us can even pretend to know what history is up to. At best, we can only try to be aware of what may be happening to us. At the risk of continuing to be perceived as too abstract, I should like, nevertheless, to suggest that one of the basic changes in the culture of modern Western man is a growing awareness of how much of his essential humanity must be self-created and self-sustained. The steadily diffusing and intensifying scientific scrutiny of biologic man, of man's individuality and uniqueness, of man's interaction with other men, of the general nature of human nature, and finally of the character of a centerless universe in which actually or metaphorically man can be lost—this view of ourselves creates either a tragic sense of despair or a sober determined faith in the power of man to manage his own destiny.

But whether most of our population can be engaged in a confident, active, participant engagement with the increasing knowledge of our time, and on the basis of that knowledge make responsible decisions for themselves and for others, depends not only upon the implicit and explicit values with which they identify, but also upon conditions of social organization affecting their access to knowledge and information and their approach to social resources for the implementation of decisions.

Since values are what men live by, it may be well to think for a moment about our immediate cultural heritage with respect to the contemporary images of man. Only a little longer than a half-century ago, an already existing preoccupation with the irrational needs and motives of men was dramatically catalyzed by the application of psychoanalytic theory to the understanding of human behavior in many contexts, within and without medical practice. Out of this reflection on human nature came the now widespread awareness that much of the motivational push of human action is the repetitive seeking in the present for old goals once obtained and never wholly given up, or once desired and still sought. Moreover, it is also evident that these insistent needs which distort the present to fit the perceptual and conceptual organizations of self and of the world learned under the aegis of the childhood past are the sources of much of the irrational in us. And, certainly, we have made an heroic gain by becoming aware of and accepting responsibility for our own irrationality. But let us not be intimidated by the irrational, nor despair about the capacities of the rational man. More things, to somewhat translate Tennyson, are wrought by rationality and consciousness than this world dreams of.

One insistent task of the contemporary culture, therefore, is to restore strength, security, and confidence to the image of the rational man thinking his way constructively through life, but with full acceptance and with no denial or disclaiming of the awful power of the irrational.

Obviously, many other implicit and explicit expectations and value-decisions about ourselves and our society are determining our behavior in medical thought and action. Our necessity is simply to be as aware of what determines our individual and collective behavior as our current knowing will allow. Many of our contemporary ways of seeing ourselves and our world may be including or excluding perceptions and assumptions, outside of our accepted awareness, that may defeat our control over and our effective responses to urgent and significant aspects of our situation. We believe so much of what we see because so much of what we see is what we already believe. Perhaps some of our most significant breakthroughs in creativity and reasoning come not only when, as Nietzsche suggested, we see what nobody else has seen but when we see what everybody else sees but think something new about it.

It is usual to think about society and culture in terms of the trends of change. But all the institutions of a society exist in a natural system of mutual response and adaptation so that countertrends are always being engendered as reactions and resultants to what are described as the major trends. One of the intellectual dangers in the use of a natural system model of society, however, is that the assumption of built-in, spontaneously correcting homeostatic principles may lull the initiative for planned and active countertrends. It is well to remember that the dinosaur became extinct because it had no adequate strategy of countertrending. Hence, an effective and vigilant department of countertrends should be part of the organizational structure of many social institutions.

The family, as the basic social organization in which we all learn not only how to be human but also how to remain that way, has been changing significantly through recent social and cultural time. In American society the basic functions of reproduction, physical, biologic, and psychologic maintenance, socialization, social control, and social class and status ascription are achieved in a relatively small conjugal group, tending to change its abode rather frequently and in many instances living quite apart from other kinship families or persons.

Additionally, every family group, and every individual, if identified adequately in social space, must be given a social class subscript as a general index of probable cultural orientation and probable characteristics of social action and participation. Indeed, many human ecologic and epidemiologic studies are disappointingly uncertain because their "political arithmetick," as Sir William Petty in 1690 referred to social statistics, does not specify the social class stratification of their populations. In an affluent society, where material wealth and economic gains are widely diffused, the relations of individuals to health values, resources, and practices and to the acquisition, communication, and development of disease seem increasingly to focus medical attention upon cultural, social, and psychologic "impoverishment" rather than only upon economic poverty. A basic finding of the Commission on Chronic Illness was that attitudes toward medical care were a major obstacle to the utilization of therapeutic measures which could have prevented secondarily a worsening of disability in one-third to one-half of the persons studied.

With specific relation to the family group and its behavior, social class IV and V families, which comprise the home social space for about 60 per cent of our population, are characterized frequently by less than a completed high school education, by more homes broken by separation, divorce, and death, by a higher infant mortality, by a lower life-expectancy, by a greater incidence of many disease conditions, and by a more rapidly developing mortality for some diseases once the sick role is overtly accepted. The possible relationship between the socialization of illness in the sick role and social class and culture also entail some consideration of the organizational structure and function of hospitals and other medical helping agencies and their response to the detection, acceptance, and treatment of illness. But we must first explore more fully some characteristics of the modern family and their import for medical concern and care.

In the pursuit of this task we must be fully aware of the integrative, need-satisfying, and resourceful aspects of contemporary family living with its high regard for child care and for the health, education, and welfare of its members. Indeed, if medical practice must continue to be office-centered and the physician must maintain his reluctance to visit the family, the entire family, because of its child-centered concerns and its emphasis on the personal well-being of its members, may increasingly be induced to come to the doctor's office or to the clinic as a group. Of course, this will require teaching physicians and other health personnel methods of group interviewing and for therapeutically altering behavior in small groups. The use of group methods, particularly with the family group, has hardly been explored in general medical practice, not only for health education, but for the reduction of intrafamilial tensions that produce dys-ease and for the changing of family-induced countermotivations militating against bodily, psychologic, and social health.

Most American families today, like most individuals, have more time and more affluence to be concerned about themselves. Hence, in many families, whether we see increased strain, mutually hostile dependency, intensification of conflicts, anxiety, lack of affection and intimacy, more demanding and less giving, or, on the contrary, increased companionship, personal ease, and a relatively strainless resolution of conflicts and deprivation depends to a significant extent on the relation of the family and its members to the social context of life beyond the home.

The family as a social system is a means of adaptation by which persons satisfy needs and reduce tensions, many of which may have been evoked in individuals by the conditions of participation in the organizational life of other social systems, such as the school, factory, office, agency, or hospital. As Nathan Ackerman has pointed out, the emotional alienation induced in people toward values and knowledge as well as toward other people by the organizational behavior in various social institutions may lead family members to demand, excessively and urgently, esteem, succor, and reassuring affection beyond the capacity of the family, particularly of the wife and mother, to satisfy.

It may also be important with especial reference to psychologic health and illness that the very structure of the small and kinship-isolated conjugal American family tends in itself to intensify emotional interaction in the family, particularly between the child and his mother. Using the epidemiologic model of infectious disease, the child has thus much more intimate contact with a possibly noxious agent and runs a greater risk of being affected by a possible psychologic illness of the mother.

The American family is also a mobile group, both geographically and somewhat less so sociologically. It is estimated that each year about one person out of five moves to another house. From a general overview, out of the 33 million people or so who move in any one year, about one-third of them move as far as another county and about one-sixth move to another state. All these moves produce a more or less disruptive state of transition and challenge the family to restore adequately and with minimal strain its articulations with a new neighborhood and community, both in terms of knowing about what is happening and existing in the community, as well as in feeling secure about access to the resources of the new environment, especially those of health and medicine.

Perhaps it is important to remark here that the danger of isolation and ineffective reestablishment of neighborhood and community associations may be greater with some social class groups than with others. Some families, whether entirely class-determined or not, suffer much more alienation from work and community. Not only is there greater danger of social pathology occurring in the socially isolated and alienated, but the adaptive attitudes of de-emotionalization, and lack of involvement, participation, and commitment learned in the work organization are generalized to all other social participation. Where, because of various industrial and technologic trends, the factory, shop, or job has created the conditions which have brought about the lack of worker interest in work, society must itself develop resources of recreation, education, and voluntary community associations to make possible a moral equivalent for committed work. Otherwise we shall be developing not only a mass society, but an immoral, indulgent, and irresponsible society.

Other Public Health concerns also relate to the present image of the family. Infant mortality has been reduced by two-thirds within the last few decades and is now at a rate where further reduction may be achieved more by what Sir James Spence calls "maternal capacity" and to which I see no reason for not adding "paternal capacity." In general this means "family capacity" for child rearing. This must be maintained and further potentiated even though 29% of all married women are now in the labor force and about one in four of all children have working mothers.

Since the first year and the last year are the most dangerous medically of one's life, it is also evident that many of our geriatric problems are related to the sociology of the contemporary family and the associated cultural values about aging. An excessively facile equation of aging and illness, the conception that the sick role is necessarily experienced in an institution, isolation from kinship support, downward social mobility which retirement and loss of work-given status may seem to imply, the trajectory model of the life-span rather than a model of continuing development and differentiation— all these factors unduly and perhaps unnecessarily stress the aging person in our society.

Let us look now at the larger social system of the city. Most of us I think will agree that the best things and the worst things happen in cities. In cities we deal almost in pure culture with the man-made environment and with the environment-made man. Indeed, in less than a century, we shall have most of our then 600 million people in the unnatural space of the city. Social pathology and urbanization are highly correlated, but an historic look at the trends in criminal action, for illegitimate births, and other evidence of an inadequately organized society indicates that the greatest amount of deviant behavior, as well as the greatest mortality in cities, coincides with periods of high immigration and rapid population growth. When metropolitan growth rates have been slow, social pathology has declined even in the presence of significantly reduced business and economic activity. In times of concentrated population influx the social organization of the city cannot properly "process" all the humanity which comes to it. Hence, individuals and families may search for or organize a subculture which permits them to act out deviantly and relatively anonymously the hostile, retaliative, or self-seeking motivation induced in them by the failure of social integration. Others may become deviant or sick in other ways. Some will feel powerless and helpless because of a very low expectation of influencing or controlling the events which affect them. Still others may feel meaningless and unrelated.

Studies on psychiatric illness in migrants into cities, whether the move is from one county to another, one state to another, or one nation to another, indicate that the incidence is greatest in the first six months of the transition.

The highly publicized problems of juvenile delinquency and drug addiction are closely related to our ineffective countertrending against the inadequate organizational integration of our cities. At the 1957 rate of delinquency incidence, 12 per cent of all adolescents will soon be involved in at least one court delinquency action, and if boys alone are considered this percentage becomes 20 per cent. To react fully to the import of this in absolute numbers it is necessary to remember that there will be 50 per cent more boys and girls in the 10–17 age group in 1970 than now.

The countertrends initiated by civic action and particularly by public administration seem to suggest rapid and adequate decentralization of Public Health, welfare, recreational and educational services, and for adolescents, especially, attention to organizational and administrative changes in the school system which facilitate meaningful participation and involved commitment in the school society.

It may not be too offensively utopian even to suggest the creation, ultimately, of departments of social behavior in city and county administrations as an aid to public executives in developing information about the collective behavior of the city and in planning the organizational direction necessary to assure maximal community integration.

We must, finally, look at the changing scene in relation to social organizations in general and specifically to the sociology of health organizations and institutions. In his provocative book, "Post-Historic Man," Roderick Seidenberg speaks of social organization, and of organizing, as translating ". . . under the influence of intelligence, the implicit possibilities of life into those explicit patterns of living that distinguish our conscious social processes and social relationships."

The organization, therefore, is not necessarily something which opposes and suppresses individualism, creative uniqueness, or personal leadership and responsibility but, on the contrary, is an adaptive system of resources, functions, and social relationships by which we potentiate constantly the greatest human actualization and fulfillment of the individual. The organization man is intimidated into conformity, unimaginative compliance, and passivity not because of too much concentration upon organization but because of too little.

Progressively we are creating for ourselves an almost totally manmade physical, social, and cultural environment. Diseases and illness —accidents, air-pollution reactions, psychosocial stress responses, suicides, and health problems complicated or engendered by people-deficiency and by meaning-deficiency, faulty sick role experience, and inadequate, reluctant, or tardy access to the social and cultural resources for the prevention of disease and uneasiness and for the prevention or retardation of its worsening—all these illnesses can be encompassed sufficiently within medical awareness and influence only by the intelligent organization of countertrends and by the utmost administrative use of the disease-detection and disease-treating processes to increase and maintain wellness and to reduce both the prevalence and the duration of illness.

For where, indeed, is illness bred? In the heart or in the head? Or in the body politic? Whatever the determining pattern, as soon as the individual can accept himself as ill he may then turn to the medical helping institutions to become legitimately sick and a patient. He may, of course, experience a more or less prolonged struggle within himself before achieving his self-definition of being ill. This is not only a psychodynamic struggle with himself. It is also related to his social class and social space perceptions of the meaning of being ill and of the prospective sick role experience. It is salutory to remember that many patients do not deny their self-perception of being ill. They do avoid entering the sick role experience and becoming patients under the conditions they perceive as associated with the patient role. Hence sick role expectations and the actual social behavior related to the destined patient role of various persons, loosely defined by social class, may be as important in early case-finding and early initiation into treatment as the assessment of the financial and physical adequacy of the health facilities themselves. Potentiation of social and psychologic access to the already existing health resources is, as we all know, a continuing task of all Public Health personnel.

An important health observation here is that the prevalence and the incidence of much disease is greatest in social class IV and V and, generally, for many diseases the mortality seems to be greater during the same amount of overt and formal sick role time for these social classes than for persons in classes I and II.

If the patient role is socialized by participation in a hospital society, then the various ways in which the hospital organization may unwittingly increase the stress of the patient and thus interfere, even physiologically, with the optimal dynamics of healing and repair puts the organizational function of the hospital intimately into the treatment process.

Here, again, the possible apathy, anxiety, resentment, and the low involvement, participation, and commitment of health personnel to the medical tasks of the hospital may be the result not only of the intrinsic organizational and administrative behavior of the hospital but may also be due to the failure of the hospital to countertrend successfully against the adaptations to work which have been learned elsewhere in the society.

What many hospitals need today is a doctor of the hospital—someone who is an expert in both medicine and social science—who can diagnose and treat the organizational uneasiness of the hospital and who understands how to use the sociability of man to engender maximum commitment and excitement in the work of the hospital. The urgent need is for administrators who can treat patients, not with a fragmented, sometimes unrelated and even hostile therapeutic aggregate of individuals, but with the whole integrated social system of the hospital.

The same obligation to achieve awareness of how we are being organized by our society and culture, and of how our effective control of events must be achieved by rationally and consciously taking responsibility for organizing ourselves applies obviously to medical education, medical research, and to all our medical institutions. We must, ourselves, arrange and administer our organizations so that each of us can integrate himself into his organization with the high security of knowing adequately what is happening in the organization and of feeling certain that he has access to and can mobilize the resources of his organization to do his work and to facilitate constantly his own progressive development and his own creative and productive individuation.

In his penetratingly compassionate thinking about the evolution of man, Père Teilhard de Chardin concludes that: "The history of the living world can be summarized as the elaboration of ever more perfect eyes within a Cosmos in which there is always something more to be seen. . . . Man, the center of perspective, is at the same time the center of construction of the universe. And by expediency, no less than by necessity, all science must be referred back to him. If to see more is really to become more, if deeper vision is really fuller being, then we should look closely at man in order to increase our capacity to live." As trustees of the public well-being, we are charged with the wholeness, the health of man. What else can this imply except the most urgent, assertive, and forthright devotion of all the sciences of man, physical, biologic, and behavioral to the increasing actualization of the human condition? The time, all over the world, is noon.

2.   The Dynamics of Planned Change

Psychodynamics of Group Opposition to Health Programs*

JUDD MARMOR, M.D., VIOLA W. BERNARD, M.D.,
AND PERRY OTTENBERG, M.D.

HEALTH PROGRAMS generally derive from scientific progress and scientific recommendations. Despite this fact, it is not unusual for such programs to meet with intense and determined opposition on the part of various groups in our society. It is the purpose of this communication to outline the nature of this group opposition, to attempt to delineate its features, and to identify some of the psychodynamic and sociodynamic factors which are involved in its existence.

There is a not infrequent tendency on the part of the scientifically oriented person to generalize about the people who make up this opposition and to characterize them all as being malevolent, ignorant, or members of the so-called "lunatic fringe." A dispassionate study of the problem, however, reveals that such a generalization is unwarranted and is itself the expression of a prejudice which tends to strengthen the very opposition at which it is aimed. The fact is that most group opposition to scientifically motivated health legislation runs a wide gamut of heterogeneity. There is usually a broad spectrum of opposition, with arguments ranging from highly rational and scientific ones to completely irrational and delusional ones; from genuinely selfless considerations to deliberately power-seeking ones; from unconscious motives to consciously manipulative ones.

RATIONAL AND IRRATIONAL OPPOSITION

Since health legislation ordinarily is introduced only after having been first recommended or endorsed by responsible scientific authorities, it is not surprising to find that, in the opposition which

* Reprinted with the omission of one footnote and four illustrations, by permission, from the April, 1960, issue of *The American Journal of Orthopsychiatry*, Vol. 30, pp. 330–345. This paper was presented at the 1959 Annual Meeting of the American Psychiatric Association. The authors are, respectively, Clinical Professor of Psychiatry, University of California, Los Angeles, California; Associate Clinical Professor of Psychiatry, Columbia University, New York, New York; and Associate, Department of Psychiatry, University of Pennsylvania Medical School, Philadelphia, Pennsylvania.

develops, the part which is based on rational considerations tends to occupy a considerably narrower band on the spectrum than that which is irrational and unconsciously motivated or else deliberately dishonest. Nevertheless, the former group is an extremely important one, not only because it lends prestige and scientific authority to the opposition and so influences large numbers of people whose resistances might otherwise not have been aroused, but also because its arguments often point up realistic flaws or inadequate safeguards in the health program, which might otherwise go unnoticed.

Thus some of the objections raised to the Alaska Mental Health Bill (a bill designed to provide a mental hospital for the territory of Alaska) in its original form dealt with ambiguities in some of its phraseology, which might conceivably have led to misinterpretation or abuse—for example with respect to a patient's right to a jury trial. Similarly, one of the scientific objections raised to water fluoridation has been that, although it indeed protected the enamel, it could lead to pathologic bone changes from disturbances in calcification. This sort of honest disagreement, whether it be right or wrong, stimulates further research and observation, which ultimately serve to clarify the issue further. An example of this kind of clarifying research was the 10-year controlled epidemiologic study of two population groups which checked, among other things, on possible significant bone changes due to ingestion of fluorides in drinking water and found none; published by Nicholas C. Leone, Michael B. Shimkin, *et al.*, under the title Medical Aspects of Excessive Fluoride in a Water Supply, *Public Health Representative*, 69:925–936, 1954.

SCIENTIFIC CONSERVATISM

Rational opposition to health legislation often grows out of a scientific conservatism, which looks askance at all innovations until they have been proved beyond all peradventure. Such conservatism is by no means without value and serves to protect the public against premature exposure to untested procedures at the hands of misguided enthusiasts. Thus, the American Dental Association and the Public Health Service both refused to endorse water fluoridation when it was originally proposed. The British Royal Society rejected Jenner's findings concerning cowpox and vaccination when they first appeared. As a rule this kind of scientific resistance tends to melt away when the proof of the adequacy of the new procedures has been fully established. Unfortunately, the original withholding of endorsement by reputable groups or individuals is often used and quoted by less rational opponents of a measure long after the scientific dissidents have withdrawn their opposition.

CULTURAL PATTERNS

As one examines this problem more deeply, it becomes apparent that one important aspect of it impinges on the broad problem of social reactions to change in general. Mores and beliefs of people of any given community are not accidental or unrelated phenomena. They are integrated elements in a cultural system that has gradually evolved in time, and a basic change in any one of these elements can have important reverberations affecting the entire network of habits and beliefs.

Not all cultural patterns, however, are of equal importance to the system. Some are more central, others more peripheral. Hence some habits or beliefs are easily altered, while others arouse great resistance. In general, whenever an attempted change challenges established beliefs or practices which are fundamental to the stability of the particular social or cultural or psychologic system involved, one may anticipate serious group resistance to change. An example of this is the reaction of a large segment of our Southern white population to desegregation—a social change which threatens cultural patterns, balances of power, and psychologic needs which are at the very core of a long-established way of life in that area. On the other hand, the attitude of our population toward the Japanese people has undergone a considerable reversal in the past 15 years without comparable upset to basic cultural integrations.

Among the Zulus, conceptions about tuberculosis are extremely difficult to change, because the symptoms of this disease have long been assumed to be due to witchcraft, and the entire topic is surcharged with powerful feeling.

Similarly, as John and Elaine Cumming[1] recently demonstrated, ideas about mental illness in some groups within our own culture can be just as deeply irrational as those of the Zulus about tuberculosis, and just as resistant to alteration.

The nature and sources of these unconscious and irrational anxieties are of particular interest to us as psychiatrists, and we shall examine them in detail a little later in this communication. For the moment, however, let us continue to survey briefly some of the more conscious and *external* sources of group opposition to health legislation, which often interact with the unconscious and internal sources of opposition.

EXTERNAL SOURCES

Sometimes a proposed change threatens or seems to threaten the power, prestige, or economic security of certain special segments within a society. This is generally the basis for variations in

response to changes that occur on an ecologic or demographic basis—
such as differences in response between Northern and Southern areas
of our country, or between rural and urban groups. We can expect that
specially threatened groups or individuals will do all in their power to
mobilize public opinion against the change. Thus, the introduction of
vaccination completely displaced the practitioners who favored inoculation by variolation, or the direct transference of smallpox infection.
In the antivaccination campaign which followed Jenner's discovery,
the opposition of these groups was particularly virulent and all kinds
of fantastic charges and slanders were spread by them.

Some of the most powerful opposition to polio vaccination and
water fluoridation has come from groups whose vested interests bring
them into direct conflict with the theories of organized medicine and
dentistry. Prominent among these are naturopaths, chiropractors,
cancer quacks, some Christian Science groups, and small but im-
pressive-sounding organizations like the "American Association of
Medico-Physical Research," founded by Albert Abrams, who achieved
notoriety by the claim that he could diagnose any disease from one
drop of the patient's blood, and could, with his "electronic reaction"
machine, cure any illness.

Similarly, efforts of governmental experts to introduce a model
health, education and welfare project in a Mexican rural community[2]
in 1943 met with intense opposition from local officials and wealthy
farmers, because they feared the project as an ultimate threat to their
power. Such power groups or leaders, whatever their nature, do not
hesitate to play deliberately upon the irrational fears, anxieties, and
prejudices in the population at large to achieve their ends.

Some opponents of the Alaska Mental Health Bill raised the cry
that it was an effort to set up a Siberia for the U.S.A., and darkly
hinted that it concealed a nefarious plot by Communists to hospitalize
and brainwash their opponents. Others were certain it was part of an
international Jewish conspiracy, and one retired general was equally
sure that the Bill had been engineered by the Roman Catholic hierarchy in this country as part of its campaign to "destroy our freedoms
under the Bill of Rights." In the controversy over fluoridation also,
certain groups tied their opposition to the "Communist conspiracy"
theme, claiming it was a Communist plan to "rape" the people,
weaken their minds and make them "moronic, atheistic slaves."

Sometimes the general public is misled when opponents to health
legislation carry the insignia of esteemed authorities. Thus, an M.D.
or a Ph.D. degree is not always a reliable indicator of scientific objectivity when borne by individuals whose personal bias outweighs
their rationality. Similarly, the position of the *Brooklyn Tablet*, a
Catholic weekly, against fluoridation and the Alaska Mental Health
Bill, gave many people the false impression that the Catholic Church

was officially opposed to these projects, and that the undertakings themselves were anti-Catholic—a potent accusation in a city like New York with its large Catholic population.

Another "external" element which plays a partial role in group opposition is the factor of coercion. The word "compulsory" is a negatively loaded semantic concept in societies with a democratic tradition. Occasionally some political liberals may see in compulsory health legislation an invasion of individual freedom. This issue was strongly raised by many in the fight against water fluoridation. It is interesting to note that not infrequently such "liberal" opponents find themselves joined in their opposition to such programs by political conservatives, who see in the same legislation an advance toward the socialistic state. Thus certain opponents of water fluoridation and mental health legislation like the California Community Mental Health Services Act (Short-Doyle Bill) saw, or claimed to see, in these measures dangerous trends toward socialized medicine and governmental infringement upon individual liberty.

Although it is true, therefore, that social changes which are allowed to take place spontaneously, so to speak, are less likely to arouse organized resistance, a governmental agency is faced with the necessity of weighing the pros and cons of such an approach in each specific situation. Where the health or welfare of an entire community is jeopardized, as by a threatened smallpox epidemic, for example, circumstances may not permit the luxury of voluntary gradualism as far as vaccination is concerned.

Related to this factor of coercion is the factor of time. Generally speaking, the more rapid and energetic the attempt at social change, the greater the opposition that is apt to be aroused. When more time is allowed for education and preparation of the group for the proposed change, there is less likely to be misunderstanding or resistance. The historic decision of the Supreme Court on desegregation took cognizance of this temporal factor when it called for its implementation not immediately, but with "deliberate speed" depending on the problems of the local communities. On the other hand, occasionally when an agency allows *too much time* to pass before implementing a proposed change, group resistances to it *may* become more solidly organized and congealed. This was clearly demonstrated in the efforts to introduce water fluoridation and desegregation. In many communities, in which they were introduced with relatively little fanfare, they aroused little anxiety or opposition, while in others, where their adoption was delayed and subjected to prolonged debate, their opponents were able to mobilize sufficient public anxiety and doubt to defeat them. Leonard Duhl[3] has suggested that one of the reasons for popular opposition at such a point may be displaced resentment that some people in modern society feel at being cut off from many areas of governmental decision-making.

This raises the question of the value of education of the public in preparation for proposed health legislation. Since, as we shall see later, some of the most important sources of opposition to such legislation come from unconscious and nonrational sources, it is not surprising that educational appeals to conscious reason often fail to dissipate the opposition. This is not to imply, however, that educational efforts are without value. By no means. Often more important, however, than such specific educational campaigns is the *basic* educational and economic level of the various groups within a society. A number of studies have shown that group resistance to scientifically oriented social change is most apt to come from the less educated and lower economic groups within any given community. There are several reasons for this. For one thing, "scientific thinking" tends to be limited to the more highly educated minority, especially those who have gone to college.

Equally important, however, is the over-all cultural "climate" as regards science and scientists. In the past decade in America we have witnessed an instance of the periodic emergence of a rather widely prevalent anti-scientific and anti-intellectual attitude, epitomized by the opprobrious term "Egghead." This appears to have been part of a broad, defensive reaction to the threat of Communism, a reaction which led to such political extremes as McCarthyism, and which included in it a distrust of scientists in general as tending to be too "liberal," and hence as being actual or potential "subversives." This distrust has been an important factor in causing various organizations, in the name of patriotism, to link certain scientifically based health proposals to the threat of Communist subversion. Situations in which this link was charged include such diverse proposals as the Alaska Mental Health Bill, the California Community Mental Health Services Act, the polio vaccination program, and fluoridation of water.

The insidious pervasiveness of this antiscientific attitude in our country was illustrated by a recent study of the "Image of the Scientist Among High School Students," by Margaret Mead and Rhoda Métraux.[4] Their study of a nationwide sampling revealed the existence of an "overwhelmingly negative" image of the scientist, when students were asked for their reactions to science as a career, or to the scientist as a person.

Another study was conducted by the National Association of Science Writers in conjunction with New York University and the Survey Research Center of the University of Michigan on "The Public's Image of Science and Scientists."[5] This study, based on interviews with 1,919 questionnaire respondents in a representative nationwide sampling, indicated that even though the majority of the respondents held a positive view of science and the scientist, there was a significant minority who viewed science with antagonism and suspicion, and who variously described the scientist as someone "socially inept, introverted, hard-to-know . . . neurotic, queer, crazy . . . mildly eccentric, absent-minded, out of touch . . . ideologically and politically deviant . . . too powerful, able to control lives, with powerful and dangerous things within his control."

There are some evidences, however, that this antiscientific cultural climate in the United States has begun to shift recently, mainly as a reaction to the impact of the realization that the Soviet Union has been overtaking, and in some areas surpassing us scientifically and technologically. Part of this shift, it is true, may merely be the other side of the coin of the image of the scientist as having magical power, power that now is seen as an important ally in the struggle against potential enemies and the frightening mysteries of outer space. Nevertheless, it is possible that with such a change in our society's attitude toward science, there may be some diminution in the distrust encountered by scientifically sponsored health programs.

In any event, this problem of group attitudes tends to highlight the importance of the role of leadership in the fate of such programs. When the leaders of a community are lukewarm or antagonistic to a legislatively ordained change, and consequently make no effort to enforce it legally, it has been found that group resistances become intensified. A dramatic example of contrasting types of leadership and their consequences was afforded in September 1957 in Little Rock, Arkansas, and Nashville, Tennessee. In Little Rock, a plan of gradual desegregation had majority public acceptance and the support of municipal officials. The opposition of the State's governor, however, had the effect of encouraging and legitimizing violence against desegregation. The subsequent chain of events has been such that the desegregation situation in Little Rock is still tense. Around the same time an elementary school was dynamited in Nashville, where a few Negro children were entering a previously all-white school. Police restrained prosegregationist demonstrators, and arrested a score of them. The State's governor promptly made it clear that the law of the land would be upheld in Tennessee, even though he did not personally like integration. By the end of the month the school scene was peaceful in Nashville and has remained so. Apparently under certain conditions, legally enforced behavioral changes may have to precede attitudinal changes. Such a sequence has been observed following enforced desegregation in the Armed Forces.

UNCONSCIOUS SOURCES

The part played by the opposition leaders in the attacks upon health legislation is an extremely important one and impossible to deal fully with here. In general these leaders fall into two main groups, with considerable overlapping: 1) those who are motivated by factors of personal power, prestige or gain; 2) those who are motivated by powerful anxieties or hostilities, the true sources of which are unconscious. They are often individuals of great ability, intelligence, and capacity to arouse intense fervor and passion in others. In extreme forms they assume the role of the godlike crusader, the charismatic leader, who is ready even to endure martyrdom for the sake of the "cause." Their function must be understood not only in terms of their capacity to arouse their followers to what seem to be potential threats; they are also an important factor in trying to hold rigidly to a fundamental conservatism which may provide a sense of security to the groups which they lead. Some aspects of the psychology of such leaders and many of their supporters are discussed in what follows.

Granted the existence of all of the external factors which tend to mobilize opposition to certain health programs, the problem still remains to explain the degree of irrational anxiety which these programs often evoke in significant segments of our population. For it is clear that if only external factors were involved, educational campaigns presenting the scientifically proven facts and demonstrating the general benefits involved in the health program ought to have been more successful than they have been. Obviously the appeal to reason fails so often precisely because the popular anxieties which have been aroused have an *irrational* and *unconscious* source.

It is this fact which explains one of the most interesting features of the phenomenon we are considering, namely, the fact that *we find the same groups of people involved over and over again in opposition to widely diverse and disparate health programs.* Thus, many of the same individuals and organizations that are active in the fight against water fluoridation can be found in the ranks of those opposing mental health programs, compulsory vaccination either of animals or humans, and vivisection. As an extreme example, the American Naturopathic Association is on record as opposing not only fluoridation, but also vaccination, immunization, pasteurization, vivisection, drugs, narcotics, alcohol, tobacco, tea, coffee, cocoa, cola drinks, and compulsory medication!

What is the common denominator behind the opposition to such varied stimuli? To answer this question we must examine the problem of the psychic significance of health and sickness in the life history of the individual. Good health is linked in the unconscious with basic needs for survival, security, and mastery. Ill health is connected with fears of bodily disintegration, dissolution, and death. Even more important are the conditioning factors that are experienced in early development, and related to the experience of health or sickness. For all people, for example, what goes into their mouths, and by extension, into any part of their bodies, is strongly associated with good and evil.

"Eat this—it's good for you," and "Don't put that in your mouth—it will make you sick," are among the earliest aspects of enculturation probably in all cultures. "Good" food is "pure," "clean," "wholesome"; "bad" food is "impure," "dirty," "poisonous." To eat well is to be secure, healthy, and happy. The converse means insecurity, starvation, and death. Little wonder that when psychotics experience a weakening of their ego boundaries, one of their commonest delusions is of being poisoned; or that elderly and sick people, as their ego-integrative capacities become impaired, often become overwhelmingly preoccupied with problems of diet and bodily health, thus regressing to earlier patterns of adaptation in their efforts to achieve a sense of security and ego mastery. (This, in all probability, is why disproportionately large numbers of elderly people are so often found in the ranks of those who feel irrationally threatened by certain health legislation.) But it is not only the sick and elderly who are beset by such anxieties. Any individual whose life experiences have been such as to leave him with deep feelings of vulnerability—either physical or psychologic—in the struggle for existence, is apt to respond with anxiety to anything which he perceives as a threat to his sense of intactness—or which, by virtue of being coercive, arouses in him fears of being overwhelmed or dominated by forces which are endowed by him with mysterious or superhuman power.

Adorno, Frenkel-Brunswik and others have described the developmental backgrounds of some of these people in *The Authoritarian Personality*.[6] Often these people come from homes in which rigid, repressive, and authoritarian patterns have dominated their early developmental years, with consequent patterns of deeply repressed hostile, dependent, libidinal strivings. To protect themselves against the emergence of these impulses, such individuals develop patterns of intense characterologic rigidity, repression, and an ever-ready tendency to discharge their repressed hostility, or project their repressed sexual strivings, whenever a convenient cultural scapegoat is presented to them.

To such individuals purity is equated with security, and health with wholeness. They are equally concerned with pure food, pure morals, and pure races. They are excessively preoccupied with fears of sexual attack, bodily poisoning, or ideational contamination. Safety lies in what is old and familiar. The new and the unfamiliar are threatening. New habits, new foods, new drugs, or new ideas are all viewed with suspicion and apprehension. Fundamentalism is the cornerstone of their philosophy—a determined and rigid adherence to convention and tradition.

This sense of vulnerability is equivalent to what has been symbolically described in psychoanalytic theory as "castration anxiety" and its developmental precursors. To express this in less technical terms, it is our conviction that the basis for most of the irrational anxiety that some health measures arouse in certain individuals is that the measures are perceived as constituting a threat either to their sense of bodily wholeness, or their sense of psychic wholeness, or else to the wholeness of what we might call their "life space." These, of course, are often interrelated and interconnected. This is the common denominator which explains our finding the same individuals passionately defending themselves against the forcible entry of any "foreign body"—whether it be a vaccination, a mental health proposal, interracial contact, or a wave of immigrants from overseas.

Measures which involve introducing something foreign into the human body, such as fluoridation of water, or vaccination, are perceived by such individuals as threatening their bodily integrity. Terms like "rape," "poison," "murder," and "paralysis" figure importantly in their impassioned arguments against these measures. By a simple process of extension or displacement, one generally finds these same people fighting vigorously against similar measures involving animals, such as vivisection, or antirabies inoculation for pets.

On the other hand, the intense fear that mental health proposals arouse in certain people seems to derive from feelings of being threatened psychologically. The reactions of some of these persons seem to reflect a fear that any psychiatric insights may expose their own underlying mental instability, much as a patient who fears that he has cancer of the lung may be terrified of a chest X-ray. Terms like "mental rape," "brainwashing," "hypnotism," and "thought control" are commonly used by such opponents. As one hostile witness put it in the Alaska Mental Health Bill hearings, "What is mental health? By whose standards can we deduce one person is normal and another is not?" It is noteworthy that in recent years a small but exceedingly vocal group has been attacking the entire field of psychiatry as something alien and dangerous. This group, interestingly enough, is equally vociferous against other forms of health legislation—such as water fluoridation and polio vaccination, as well as school desegregation.

John Kasper, who achieved notoriety in Clinton, Tennessee, by organizing White Citizens Councils to fight desegregation, was also active in the fight against fluoridation and the Alaska Mental Health Bill. Here is an excerpt from his testimony on the latter issue: "Psychiatry is a foreign ideology; it is alien to any kind of American thinking . . . its history began with Sigmund Freud who is a Jew . . . almost 100% of all psychiatric therapy . . . and about 80% of the psychiatrists are Jewish . . . one particular race is administering this particular thing." The attack on Freud and psychoanalysis is often linked with the implication that psychiatrists, Jews, and Communists are somehow involved together in a sinister plot to brainwash loyal Americans. (The hostile association of psychoanalysis and Jews with

Communism is particularly ironic when we recall that in the Soviet Union psychoanalysts and Jews have been subjected to the analogous charge that they are tools of Capitalism!) Similar attacks on the mental health movement are being repeatedly made in various extremist publications throughout the country. Regardless of the motives of the publishers of some of these sheets, there is no doubt that many of their readers fall into the group we are describing, and are genuinely frightened by what they are being told.

The concept of the threat to the life-space implies that the individual perceives the threat as going beyond his personal physical and psychic integrity to involve the entire position of himself and his group in the world. It is what he is apt to call a threat to his whole "way of life." The intense panic reactions which many people felt to the news of Russia's Sputnik are an illustration of this kind of response. The reactions of their contemporaries to the discoveries of Galileo, Darwin, and Freud are other examples in point.

EFFECTS ON SUPPORTERS

Up to now, in accordance with our topic, we have concentrated on the psychodynamics of those opposed to health programs, Closely related, however, are the emotional effects of these various kinds of opposition on the programs' supporters. The psychodynamics of the proponents' responses to attack warrant our attention, at least briefly, especially with regard to the deterring effects on scientific progress and the public welfare. Extremist attacks on responsible professional experts and governmental authorities have indeed frequently succeeded, at least temporarily, in blocking various programs such as water fluoridation, desegregation, and mental health legislation. Aside from defeating a specific legislative or administrative proposal, however, such attacks can retard or prevent Public Health programs in ways that are less obvious, harder to assess, and more far-reaching through their psychologic effects on initiators, endorsers and advocates of such measures, present and future.

Once a scientific program is rendered socially and politically risky, no matter how irrationally, the extent to which its adherents can withstand the attack and afford, emotionally and practically, to continue its support depends on many variables for each individual. One set of such variables includes personality attributes, values, convictions, motivations, and the person's degree of insight, as well as commitment to the issue. Another set of variables concerns the extent of the threat to his reputation, tenure of office, or professional job security. Sometimes people in these situations successfully withstand intimidation and slander from the opposition when they feel that their own leadership and associates are standing firmly together, but become embittered and defeatist if these fail them by capitulating to the power of the antiscientific opposition. The importance of enlightened and courageous leadership in withstanding the pressures of such opposition can scarcely be overestimated.

Individuals and organizations often face a dilemma in deciding whether to continue striving for a particular measure which has aroused intensely heated denunciation. A civic group, for instance, might recognize the merits of the measure, the irrationality of the opposition, and the validity of basing its stand solely on the facts and the public welfare. Yet, in deciding on its own course of action, the organization must weigh those considerations which dictate support of the measure against the risk to other valuable parts of its present and future program that may depend on the good will and cooperation of powerful factions or individuals in the community who are currently lined up against the proposal. In such circumstances, a realistic and conscious decision is sometimes made to sacrifice a potentially valuable program which has aroused such vehement antagonism in order to safeguard other social objectives of the individual or organization, such as survival and potential for effectiveness. A realistic decision of this type is to be distinguished from the rationalizations that are also a frequent response to a conflict situation of this kind: where actions really based on unacknowledged expediency and on fears for self which are not ego-acceptable masquerade under cover of this more respectably altruistic reason. Such rationalizations usually engender guilt feelings and self-contempt that reduce people's over-all effectiveness. Contemporary versions of Galileo's famous predicament and recanting of his recanting are still to be found.

Sometimes proponents of scientifically grounded health programs react to unreasonable opposition, not by withdrawal, intimidation, counterattack, or unperturbed determination, but by an intensified advocacy. Apparently the experience of being attacked in these ways can stimulate deep personal anxieties and unconscious patterns of defense. As a result, a person's prior scientific basis for supporting a health measure may shift to a blindly emotional espousal of a cause, with all the concomitant drawbacks that this entails. We have already referred to a spectrum of opposition to health legislation which ranges from rational to irrational. The advocacy of these measures can occupy a similar spectrum, however, for the proponents and the opponents are likely to be the reverse of each other.

The general public loses from the inactivation of scientific workers and public officials when, under the pressure of social penalties and demoralization within their own group, they withdraw, emotionally as well as physically, from further endeavors to raise the community health level. Some of those in the health professions retreat into less controversial areas of work. The laboratory may feel safer than the market place. But the public is deprived of the benefits of the laboratory if research findings that are developed and tested there cannot find their way into general application. For each constructive health program that is halted by extremist opposition, it appears likely that an inestimable number of potentially constructive programs fail of inception because officials and scientists fear the real or fantasied power of antiscientific opposition.

When the social climate renders the risks especially great, as during the height of McCarthyism, not only may the public be deprived of the applications of scientific progress, but that progress itself may be hampered by the extension of the inhibiting forces into certain areas of research. Prejudice, superstition, fear, and ignorance have been mobilized against attempted research projects in the fields of preventive mental health and human relations in the same way as against legislative health proposals. Apparently the spur to such opposition is the possibility that the research investigation may produce findings which might lead to broad-scale legislative and administrative applications that threaten these opponents along the lines discussed above. Research in publicly supported institutions is especially vulnerable to this type of attack, and its defenders relatively weak in the face of it. Indirect pressure has also been exerted, however, on non-public sources of support, as when private foundations are dissuaded from granting funds to projects because they fear these may foment adverse public opinion and threaten their tax-exempt status.

We are aware that many aspects of this complex topic need further study. How do people who feel compelled to do something actively about their convictions differ from the great majority who may hold similar convictions but never feel the need to commit themselves to action? How does unrealistic *complacency* in the face of realistic danger differ psychodynamically from the unrealistic *anxieties* we have been discussing? We recognize also that today's scientific proposal can end up as tomorrow's fad. Many of us can still remember, for instance, the scientific zeal with which tonsils, teeth, and other supposed "foci of infection" were removed in wholesale proportions. How does such "rational" zeal differ from the "irrational" opposition to such measures?

We are aware that not all scientific proposals have been equally validated—witness the differences that exist among reputable scientists as to the degree of harm that is being done by radioactive fallout. Does the degree of validation of a scientific proposal make any difference in the degree of opposition which it arouses? These and many other questions warrant separate communications.

SUMMARY

To summarize briefly then: We have tried to demonstrate that opposition to scientifically motivated health legislation covers a wide range of heterogeneity—from groups whose opposition is based on science and reason, to those whose objections appear to be based on self-aggrandizement or political considerations, and finally to those whose opposition stems from irrational anxieties or ignorance. We have indicated that the problem is part of the broader problem of reactions to social change in general. Opposition to social change derives from factors which are external to the individual as well as internal within his psyche. Some of the external factors involved include threats to the power, prestige or economic security of certain groups, the factor of coercion, problems of timing, the attitudes of leadership, and various educational, socioeconomic and cultural factors. The internal factors involved appear to be centered on feelings of vulnerability in relation to the sense of bodily wholeness, psychic wholeness, or wholeness of the individual's "life-space." An awareness of both external and internal factors, and of the way in which they interact in any given "field" situation, is essential for a fuller understanding of this complex group reaction. Although many questions still remain unanswered, it is hoped that this discussion will stimulate further interest in a problem which has, we believe, significant psychiatric as well as social ramifications.

1. Cumming, John and Elaine: "Mental Health Education in a Canadian Community," in *Health, Culture and Community* (B. D. Paul, Ed.), pp. 43–69. New York: Russell Sage Foundation, 1955.

2. Lewis, Oscar: "Medicine and Politics in a Mexican Village," in *Health, Culture and Community*, ibid., pp. 403–434.

3. Duhl, Leonard: *City Responsibilities in Problems of Mental Health* Presented at 34th Annual Congress of the American Municipal Assoc., San Francisco, Dec. 3, 1957.

4. Mead, Margaret, and Rhoda Métraux: Image of the Scientist among High School Students. *Science,* 126:384–90, 1957.

5. Kreighbaum, Hillier: "The Public's Image of Science and Scientists," in *Science, the News and the Public*, pp. 35–42. New York: New York Univ. Press, 1958.

6. Adorno, T. W., *et al.: The Authoritarian Personality.* New York: Harper, 1950.

3.   The Goals of Public Health

What Sets the Goals of Public Health?*

SIR GEOFFREY VICKERS, V.C.

I AM DEEPLY GRATEFUL to those who have honored me by this invitation; the more so, because I am a layman, unqualified in the sciences of your field. I comfort myself with the reflection that we are all
laymen for most of our time, especially in a field so close as yours is
to problems of decision and action. And further, that it is as laymen,
not as academics, that we make our most daring speculations. The
scientist with a reputation to lose may not speculate too far beyond the
evidence, at least in public, but the layman with a job to do must
make whatever assumptions are needed for decision, and he is content
if he can reduce by even a little the random element in his behavior.
So it is not inappropriate that it should be a layman who invites you
to pursue a speculation that will take us beyond the boundaries of the
known, even beyond the scope of our present conceptual apparatus,
but never beyond the challenges of practical life.

I ask what sets the goals of Public Health. I do not ask how we
choose them, for manifestly our choice is only one element in a manifold process. When we open our eyes to the scene around us, we find
goals already set. Policies are being implemented; institutions are in
action with all the historical momentum of buildings and establishments. Men are in mid-career. Budgets, even budget headings, have
acquired prescriptive rights. This dynamic configuration is resistant
to sudden change. So the most obvious answer to my question springs
to mind at once. History sets the goals of Public Health. We influence
them no more and no less than we influence the course of history.

The process of interaction and mutual adaptation that we call history is an obscure though familiar mystery. Looking into the future
we see a widening vista of possibilities. Tomorrow is almost committed, but next year, 10, 20 years hence, what might not be possible?
Yet, when we look into the past, the vista seems to narrow from past
to present. We see a thin line of actualities detaching itself from all

* This paper was presented at a public health forum at Harvard School
of Public Health, Boston, Massachusetts on November 26, 1957, and is
reprinted, by permission, from the March 20, 1958 issue of the *New
England Journal of Medicine*, Vol. 258, pp. 589–596, and from the March
22, 1958 issue of *The Lancet*, Vol. 1, pp. 599–604 where it was published
simultaneously by special arrangements. The author is Chairman, Research Committee, Mental Health Research Fund, Goring-on-Thames,
England.

that might have been, and those who will someday look back over what is now the uncommitted future will see the same. Of all that competes for realization, only a tiny fraction is realized and in the process excludes a host of alternatives. The eternal enigma of history is: "Why from all these possibilities did these rather than any of the others come to birth?" Somewhere in the answer to that question lies, among many other things, the scope and meaning of human initiative.

HUMAN NEED

Among the forces that make history, one of the most obvious is human need. Some would say that need sets the goals of Public Health. New needs emerge and evoke the measures which will satisfy them. At any moment, with a more or less significant time lag, the goals of Public Health reflect the dominant needs of time and place.

This statement is not so simple as it looks. The needs that evoke response are those which are recognized as needs, and this process of recognition has odd features. Our culture accepts some conditions of living that in other epochs would have moved slaves to rebel, such as going to work on a rush-hour subway, and on the other hand insists on others that other epochs never thought of, such as having its bread wrapped in cellophane. Why this particular selection of needs? Again, we cannot satisfy all the needs we recognize. Our age, with Public Health services more abundant and more active than any before it, is probably more aware than any other of unsatisfied needs. How are they resolved, the conflicts between needs fighting for satisfaction? Are they resolved by human choice? And, if so, by what criteria?

In answering these two questions we discover how significant that time lag may be. In 1946 the British Parliament, with the passing of the National Assistance Act, thought that it had destroyed the last vestiges of the "New Poor Law" that the reformers of 1834 expected to abolish destitution. Yet every page of the new statute reflects attitudes that are not responses to the future but protests against the past. It is not only soldiers who start each war perfectly equipped to win the one before.

Previous ages had neither subways nor cellophane, so they had no occasion to opt for or against them. The thought suggests another. To some extent, at least, technics set the goals of Public Health. For technics not only enlarge our responses; they mold our expectations.

Most obvious is the impact of therapeutic technics. Pasteur set the goals of Public Health for many decades ahead. Every new technic, by opening a possibility, awakens a need—at least in our Western culture, where in matters of health we have a highly developed sense that whatever is possible for any should be available to all.

Industrial technics are no less potent. Apart from the technics of the pharmaceutic industry, on which all chemotherapy depends, the engineering industry is the main executant of sanitation. Equally important are administrative technics. Large-scale public works are only possible in societies that are capable of administering them and of collecting and spending the money they involve, societies, moreover, tolerant of high taxation and of land requisition and accustomed to think in terms of social and geographic areas commensurate with the problems involved.

LIMITATIONS

These factors also limit the goals of Public Health. As we, looking back a few decades ago, see our societies at a stage that not only did not attempt but could not have attempted much that we regard as a matter of course, so a not so distant future age may see us enmeshed in limitations of administrative vision that we cannot yet discern.

These limitations are manifold. Every executive authority concerned with Public Health is limited not only by money and technical skill, but also by the area of space and the span of time over which it is free to plan, and by its own past experience, which goes far to determine how it shall set about its new problems. And apart from these direct limitations, each authority is limited by its own current activity. For our powers of attention are limited, and the habit of placing something at the focus of our attention implies the habit of leaving other things in the periphery.

Technics limit us in yet another way. A technologic age expects to deal with its problems technologically. Consider the growing hazard of noise. To the earlier ages, the natural remedy would have seemed to be to make less noise. That, I fear, would seem regressive and defeatist to us. So many alternatives are open. We might take to wearing helmets that excluded all noise absolutely. Dual, or better triple microphones around the helmet could be so devised that they could distinguish and reject sounds, however loud, which came from remote sources, admitting only those which arose nearby. We could thus converse in comfort, while the roads roared with machinery, and the air screamed with jets. The helmets would be bad for our hair, but we should not want hair if we were always to wear helmets. Medical technology would devise a painless and permanent method of depilitating the scalp, and fashion stylists would have greater scope with our helmets that they could possibly have with our hair. Each new problem would be a new opportunity for technology. Furthermore, we should have achieved a moral advance in at least two directions. By getting rid of our hair, we should have abolished one of the tiresome hereditary differentials that conflict with our ideas of equality. And

we should have enlarged the area of human freedom by giving ourselves new powers of choice in deciding to what we should attend.
Above all, we should have again eluded the regressive, defeatist solution of saying "no." The engineers would no longer be threatened
by the limitation of what our ears would stand. Progress would have
burst another barrier.

To be exact, we should have avoided saying "no" in the one field
where that word is unacceptable to us. Our impoverishment would
fall only in areas of life that are commercially insignificant.

If this forecast of a brave, new world sounds fanciful, does it seem
any more fanciful than the thought of a technologic age deliberately
choosing to be less active in order to be less noisy?

So let us add another to our list of goal setters. Ideology sets the
goals of Public Health.

Needs, technics, ideologies—these are names for aspects, dimly
understood, of the mutually adaptive process called history. But among
the interacting forces is one, unique and clearly identified—our human
selves; no mere pointers recording the resolution of external forces
but pointers dynamically charged, themselves contributing to the
forces they record. We must determine our own role if we are to
complete our analysis of what sets the goals of Public Health.

GOALS AND THREATS

This is perhaps the moment to question whether Public
Health has any goals. Is it not governed rather by avoiding threats?
Let us not confuse ourselves by saying that a threat is only a negative
goal. The psychologists have wrought havoc with our understanding
by popularizing the term "goal-seeking" as if it covered all purposive
behavior. It begins now to be widely recognized that threat-avoiding
differs from goal-seeking in important ways. One of the most important
is this. If I successfully seek a goal, I still ultimately find it, and then
I shall discover whether I really like it. But if I successfully avoid a
threat, I shall never experience it, and so I shall never discover
whether it was worth avoiding.

Threat-avoiding bulks large in individual motivation, and I fancy
that it plays an even larger part in the collective decisions of larger
and less coherent bodies. In individual motivation the psychologists
tell us how much of our behavior is directed to avoiding what we
recognize, often unconsciously and often wrongly, as a threat. The
landmarks of political, economic, and social history are the moments
when some condition passed from the category of the given into the
category of the intolerable. The welfare legislation of my country is
based on a report that identified "five giant evils" as goals for attack
—disease, unemployment, ignorance, squalor, and want. I believe

that the history of Public Health might well be written as a record of successive redefinings of the unacceptable.

It is safer, nonetheless, to assume that Public Health knows goals as well as threats, but it is not safe to assume that these are interchangeable, positive and negative ways of saying the same thing.

In any case, goals and threats are not ultimate governors of behavior; on the contrary, they are the most superficial of all. Much of the confusion that surrounds the discussion of ends and means comes from the fact that a "goal" or "end," if it is attainable once for all, is never more than a "means" to maintaining some relation that must always be sought anew. My dinner is a "goal," something I seek and either find or do not find, but it is only a means to maintaining that rate of metabolic exchange that must be maintained through time as long as I live. The specific goals we pursue—I will call them objectives—are always means to attain or preserve a relation, internal or external, that we need or think we need. The specific threats that we seek to escape are threats to some relation—events that we think might strain it beyond repair. These continuing relations I call norms. We seek to maintain them; when we deviate from them, we seek to return. But they have thresholds beyond which we may not, or think we may not, deviate without disaster, thresholds that in the clearest cases mark points of no return; these I call limits.

Physiologically, our needs for food and drink and air fall readily under these descriptions. They are relations with the environment; they have an optimal position, and they have thresholds beyond which they cannot deviate without disaster. Our psychologic and social needs, so far as we can discern them, seem to be of the same kind. "To be secure," "to be successful," "to be happy," are relations that no one expects to attain once and for all.

Health is clearly a norm, not a goal, according to this terminology, a relation not to be attained once and for all but ever to be renewed. Disease is a deviation from this norm, and includes a series of limits beyond which irreversible change takes place, the most dramatic being death.

This is not the normal meaning of health and disease. The constitution of the World Health Organization does indeed define health as a state of complete physical, mental and social well-being and not the mere absence of disease or infirmity. But who is to define for each person the state of multiple excellence that under this definition would constitute health for him? It is easier to equate the norm with the normal, and to count as disease only what falls below this assumed level of normality. Yet few, I think, would quarrel with the implication of the World Health Organization constitution that health is a form of individual excellence.

It is common today to describe human striving in terms of tension reduction, and this serves well enough to describe the norm-seeking and limit-avoiding that I regard as the basic governors of our activity. But it is not always remembered that our norms and limits are to some extent self-set. The architecture of our expectations determines the operative tensions, whether positive—between what is and what "ought to be"—or negative—between what is and what "ought not to be;" the process of adaptation consists no less in the redesigning of our own expectations than in the manipulation of our environment.

There is an intimate mutual relation between these two processes. The development of the automobile did more than provide us with new means to satisfy our needs. It set new needs, new expectations, new norms of mobility, even new limits of unacceptable immobility. The essential character of industrial expansion and the root of its basic instability is precisely that it creates and continually changes the expectations to which it is supposed to minister. Commercial advertising is socially significant not as a medium for proposing and indirectly defining the specific goals or objectives through which our expectations can be satisfied, but rather as a means of setting and constantly resetting the expectations themselves.

The process by which we set and revise our governing expectations is obscure, largely unconscious, and immensely important. Consider in how short a time your country has developed among a population so large and so diverse the wide conformity of expectation that is understood by the American way of life. I do not seek to explore that astonishing achievement here. It may serve to illustrate the fact that the character and coherence of a society, or of an individual personality, is largely a function of its governing expectations, the norms and limits that describe its setting as a dynamic system, and that the crucial task of adaptation is the adjustment of this inner architecture so as to maintain effective contact with the environment without losing the inner balance of forces whereby the individual or the society hangs together.

The process of history is a process of mutual adaptation. Every organism and every society is a dynamic system, an ever-shifting balance of forces, and it has continually to solve a double problem. It has to regulate the interaction of its inner forces, whereby it hangs together; and it has to regulate the interaction between itself as a whole and its environment. Neither configuration is infinitely plastic; each can be changed only within limits and notable within limits of time. Thus, the creature must learn to find the food it can digest or learn to digest the food it can find. And it survives only so long as it can find a viable compromise between its needs and its opportunities. Its possibilities in either direction are limited; within the limitations that are rooted in its unchanging nature are others that it can learn to transcend only with time.

I invite you, then, to consider our behavior in the field of Public Health as one aspect of that historic process in which we are engaged, a process of adaptation in which, consciously and unconsciously, we continually modify both our external environment and our inner system of expectations, behavior that can be defined at any given moment in terms of the relations that it is set to maintain, and the limits that it is set to avoid, but such behavior is as much and as properly concerned with redesigning its norms and limits as with modifying its external environment. It is within this process, still largely blind, that human initiative plays whatever may be its part and thus takes a hand in setting the goals of Public Health.

I hope I have made it clear that I regard the process by which these goals are set as largely beyond our control—largely but not wholly. Our conscious contribution, though limited, may be crucial. To explore its possibilities, I shall consider the kind of situation in which it seems most operative—that is, in the taking of concrete decisions.

Suppose someone has to decide whether a particular child, at present neglected and ill used, should be given institutional care or left in its ill found home. The decision is taken within a framework of half-conscious value judgments about the relative importance of children's rights and parental rights, the proper limits of official interference, the effect on children of separation from parents at different ages, or the merits and demerits of institutional as against familial care. These judgments reflect the governing expectations of the deciding minds at the time, the norms and limits by which they are regulated, their "setting," if they are regarded as dynamic systems.

But within this framework of norms and limits a set of practical considerations of a different kind operates. Is there a place in a suitable institution? What is the quality of institutional care available here and now? The answer to the particular case may well be given by these practical considerations alone.

But the particular case is by no means all that is being decided. It serves to confront today's expectations with today's possibilities, and thus to release into the stream of policy making the consciousness of a disparity, a maladaptation. The institutions available now were built in response to the felt needs of an earlier decade. Today's revised intuitions of need will not be realized in terms of buildings, budgets, staff, or training for some decades to come. They are already muted by the past, for our inherited institutions have themselves contributed to our current ideas of what institutional care connotes; our revised ideas, on the way to realization, will have to fight for their lives against other equally valid intimations in totally different fields, which compete with them for resources, space, skill, and attention. Yet it seems to be through the deciding of concrete cases today that we crystallize the insights and the discontents that mold the standards and the institutions of tomorrow.

I have taken this cursory look at the historic process in the hope of discerning where human initiative comes in. So far the answer is far from clear. All decisions, it seems, are choices between a limited number of specific alternatives, all sometimes highly unwelcome. They challenge us first to distinguish these alternatives and to evaluate them. They challenge us further to inquire how those choices came to be posed, and to consider through what inner and outer adjustment they may be answered more acceptably in future. The possibilities in this second field are, I think, the wider, and it is chiefly through them, in my view, that we have the power to take a hand in setting the goals of Public Health—and not the power alone but also a duty and a need of unusual intensity today.

CHALLENGES OF PUBLIC HEALTH

For Public Health in our Western culture seems to be at a crossroads. For a hundred years it has been concerned mainly with the age-old threats that beset a species not too firmly established on the earth—the threats of deficiency in basic metabolic needs for enough food and rest, and of competition from the only other genus that still disputes with us for mastery of the planet, the bacteria. In its battle with deficiency and with infection Public Health achieved spectacular success. True, that success does not look so final today as it did 20 or 30 years ago. The world still contains many under-nourished people, and it is not clear that their numbers will be less a hundred years hence. Bacteria and viruses become resistant to our present methods of attack, and continually threaten us anew. The fact remains that Western societies are less preoccupied than ever before with the control of deficiency diseases and infectious diseases.

They are, however, no less concerned with disease. Metabolic disorder, mental disorders, disorders of excess rather than deficiency, have risen in importance as others have declined, and with these we are at present less well equipped to deal. Our hazards from excess range from excessive nuclear radiation, through excessive smoking to the excessive consumption of ice cream—products that have in common the fact that their superabundance is our own doing. Even the still obscure concept of "stress" as a cause of mental ill-health connotes excess, the impact of more challenge than the organism is able to bear.

A technologic age was well equipped to partner Public Health in its attack on the deficiency diseases and the infectious diseases. Even where the new hazards were partly the creation of industrialization, as in the growth of mammoth cities, industrialization had the tools to remedy its own defects. It was as much at home providing a water supply and a sewerage system as in building a hydroelectric power station or an arterial road. It was possible for Lewis Mumford to describe the evils of industrialization as merely features of an eo-technic age.

Today, it is far from clear that a technologic age is as well equipped to partner Public Health in the next stage of its journey. On the contrary, it is likely in my view that the requirements of Public Health will cut ever more sharply across the valuations of an industrial age. What matters most to human well-being in the coming decades may well be conditions that industry cannot provide and is, in fact, chiefly instrumental in denying.

These changes will affect every aspect of Public Health. Public Health, as I see it, has three main concerns: with health services; with health conditions; and with the concept of health itself. In all three fields it faces important tasks of revaluation.

In my country the introduction of a national health service has helped to clarify our understanding of health. At one point it was widely, if half-consciously, held that a health service was a self-limiting service. When the demands of health were fully met, there would be nothing more to do. Indeed, better preventive services might in time reduce the total resources needed to provide optimum health for all. It is clear, I think, that health services are not self-limiting in this sense. The amount of effort that can plausibly be devoted to the health of the individual and the community increases with every scientific development and will, I think, increase indefinitely.

Thus, the services that might be provided may well continue to exceed, perhaps by an ever-increasing margin, the services that can in fact be provided, since the total will be limited by the number of resources available, having regard to conflicting demands. Consciously or unconsciously, we shall still have to decide what is to be the total volume of resources devoted to Public Health and how it is to be distributed among different services, different needs, and different classes of beneficiary—for example, between the young and the old. These decisions will grow harder, not easier, with the passage of time.

Public Health has always been especially concerned with preventive medicine; here, its function has been to establish the conditions of health, primarily in the physical environment, but also in the structure of society and of the individual personality. To change, for example, social attitudes toward mental illness or individual attitudes toward prenatal and postnatal care is to change the conditions of health, no less than to lay a water main. Here, it seems that a much wider field is opening.

Your current culture is sometimes criticized by your social psychologists on the ground that it builds up and sanctions too many expectations that it does not allow to be satisfied, and thus produces more frustration than most people can safely take. However this may be, it is clear that the culture and structure of society, including the many subcultures of which it is composed, set conditions that are potent for good and ill. These conditions are not under the control of Public Health, but they are not beyond its influence and its criticism.

For Public Health has a unique opportunity, as well as a duty, to clarify our understanding of health and disease, and hence our attitude toward it, and this field clamors to be further explored. Even the etiology of the disorders that have hitherto been most prominent is far from fully understood; still more obscure is that of the diseases that claim priority today. The distribution of disease, even within the crude categories of our present statistics, is full of oddities. In my country, though infant mortality has vastly declined over the past 50 years, the relative differential between the rates in different income groups has not been reduced but has, if anything, increased. Why? Schizophrenia is known to have a genetically predisposing cause; yet its reported incidence in the lowest income group is many times that in the highest. Why? Such challenging enigmas could be multiplied, I expect, among your statistics, as among ours.

These thoughts arise only from the indexes that we at present use. But we have no reason to think that our present classifications of people are the most significant. We badly need a more adequate classification of human types, and, perhaps, of human situations also.

This, again, may give us a new idea of the conditions of health. We already know, though it is easy to forget, that a "society" at any moment of time contains people of two sexes and all ages, and that the health of each of these is a condition to be preserved through the span of a lifetime. Add to this that these people consist not merely of an "admired type" and varying degrees of deviation from it, but of a wide variety of types each of which can claim the respect we accord to the normal. To do justice to all these diverse claims may well call for a concept of the conditions of health more penetrating than any we use now.

So let me add another answer to the question that we are asking. I should like to think that, so far as the goals of Public Health are consciously set, they will be set increasingly by practitioners of Public Health and especially by physicians, epidemiologists, and social scientists working together, with the more abundant technics and data now available to us, to disentangle more clearly the nature of the dynamic balance that we should recognize as health, and the conditions that favor or threaten it. And I shall devote the last part of this paper to describing what I think we might expect of such an effort.

ACHIEVEMENT OF GOALS

There are, I suggest, three contributions that Public Health can thus make to the setting of its own goals. It can evaluate health by the criteria that we currently use. It can criticise these criteria, and thus help to deepen and refine them. And it can explore the processes of decision by which Public Health policy is defined and implemented.

The first is a familiar function. Public Health is at present measured largely by statistics of mortality and morbidity. Even these rough indexes, as I have already mentioned, disclose differences between localities and categories of people and changes with time that cannot be explained and challenge us to research. Moreover, this information, at least in my country, is analyzed today under categories that are almost certainly more inadequate and inept than they need be. This is serious, for the categories under which information is gathered are immensely important. They not only influence what we think about; they limit what we can think about.

There is thus much to be done in interpreting our simplest indexes and in refining the tools and the methods whereby we work on them.

Next, there is much scope for refining the criteria of breakdown that we regard as indexes of ill-health, individual or social. Already, we use many beyond the basic figures of mortality and morbidity that not long ago would have seemed an adequate measure of Public Health. Alcoholism and drug addiction, crime and perversion are readily used as indexes of breakdown, but how are we to interpret them? Shall we seek the cause in the nature and history of the individual or in the structure of society? In reaction against the long centuries in which the criminal, the drunkard, the addict, the pervert were regarded as enemies of society, we tend today to assume that they are its victims. Fromm and Kardiner have used such statistics to impugn the health not of the individuals concerned but of the society that destroyed them.

Clearly, these indexes and their interpretation are the concern of Public Health. Clearly, too, their interpretation is more complex than a decision whether they indict the individual or his society, for the interaction between the two is far too subtle and involved to permit any such simple alternative.

And here, I think, we are helped by another important change in our approach to health. It seems to me that Western medicine is at last getting around to the question that patients have always asked, but only witch-doctors have hitherto taken seriously. This is the question, "Why me?"

Smitten by accident or disease, the savage, as I understand, asks,

"Why me?" Granted that boughs fall and snakes bite, why should I be the victim, rather than another? The question would have seemed trivial to the Public Health of only a few decades ago. Suffice it to eliminate, so far as may be, the risks from falling boughs and biting snakes or their equivalent in our day. What matter whether A or B is the unlucky one? It makes no difference to the statistics. Yet medicine has always known that immunity and vulnerability are in some measure characteristics of the individual. In its attack on the infectious and deficiency diseases, medicine is increasingly concerned to build up the inner immunity of the individual, rather than to eliminate the risk from the environment, and the study of individual variations in immunity is an increasing part of medicine's activities.

Vulnerability is the opposite side of the same penny. The study of psychosomatic disease leads medicine to view an increasing field of illness as highly individual behavior, the response of a particular person to a situation to which he is vulnerable. Even having an accident is coming to be regarded as a form of such behavior. The concept of accident proneness plays an important part in industrial medicine, and its exploration provides ever more material to answer the question, "Why me?"

This concept of immunity and vulnerability as a characteristic of the individual applies no less to mental health and mental disorder and may find here its most important developments. We assume that here also there is need of a dual approach, on the one hand, to reduce the hazards of the environment, and on the other to increase the immunity of the individual. But we know much less about the meaning of either term. "Stress" in the psychiatric, as distinct from the physiologic, sense is an imprecise concept; equally unsure is our understanding of the conditions that make the individual relatively vulnerable or immune to it. Even a small enlargement of our understanding here would alter our concept of health.

What is the relation between these two approaches to Public Health—the approach that reduces hazard and the approach that increases immunity? Each has its own undisputed territory. We rely largely on the first to control malaria, and largely on the second to control smallpox. But between the two there is a no-man's-land, in which the two approaches are alternative and even antagonistic. As people eat an ever larger proportion of food prepared by an ever more sterilized food industry, their immunity to the risks of natural foods decreases. We cannot have both protections to the full at the same time. Where should we draw the line? An Englishwoman living in the Near East remarked, "I would rather have Gippy tummy once or twice and get immune to it than give up strawberries and cream." Such choices may confront us in more subtle and important matters.

In the field of mental health it seems unlikely that we shall suffer in the near future from any lack of hazards. It is the more important that we should get a better understanding of the nature of immunity. This, it seems, is a function of the way in which the individual organizes his experience on the one hand and his expectations on the other—if that word "expectations" is allowed to stand for all the norms and limits that define the setting of his system. The two must be so related that the individual can remain internally coherent and externally effective—I should say "adaptive," if that word had not acquired so one-sided a connotation.

Psychiatric literature is full of warnings against allowing our governing expectations to diverge too sharply from the realities of the world in which we live. Socially, it may be even more disastrous if they diverge too little, for it is precisely through our sense of this divergence that we exercise over events whatever initiative we can win. Every adaptive society must have its protestants, for protest is the mainspring of any adaptation that is not purely passive. And since the protester gets more than his share of stress, he needs more than his share of immunity.

We need, then, a concept of health that will take account of the individual's ability both to live in his society without breakdown and to resist its pressures. We are still so far from this that laymen at all events do not distinguish the immune from the well adapted or even from the conformist. Yet, if we had an adequate idea of what adaptation means, we should, I think, recognize the distinction as crucial. Adaptation is a continuous process. Its agents are not those who are commonly called the well adapted, still less the conformist; they are those who can carry within themselves without injury a more than usually large measure of tension—tension between the norms of individual and social experience, between the "is" and the "ought to be," between the present and the future, in a word, those who have a high degree of immunity to the pressures that threaten our mental health. I have no doubt that such a concept of health and its conditions would incidentally give a new clarity to our understanding both of individual freedom and of the process of democracy, for I believe that both freedom and democracy depend on this rare quality.

And, finally, I suggested that it was within the field of Public Health to explore the processes of decision whereby the policy of Public Health is defined and implemented. These processes are important because in them the process of adaptation breaks the surface of consciousness and becomes open to analysis at a new level. If we observed the behavior of officials and politicians, of committees and pressure groups in the making of some policy, might we not get some more precise insight into the way in which the disparate forces I have noticed combine to set the goals of Public Health?

Such a research, if it could be designed and mounted, would, I think, land us in successive areas of doubt, each more recalcitrant but also more fruitful than the one before.

First, we should find, I hope, that the decision that came out of the deciding machine bore some relation to the information that went in, and we should confront the problem of how to make available to policy makers, predominantly lay, the knowledge and attitudes of rapidly expanding sciences.

Secondly, we should find that the decision that emerged was a choice between a few specific alternatives, and we should be led to ask how these alternatives were selected and why others were ignored. We should encounter the enigma of attention.

Thirdly, we should observe that the alternatives between which the policy makers chose were disparate. In the budgeting of resources that underlies all decisions, they have to weigh against each other short-term proposals and long-term proposals, preventive proposals and therapeutic proposals. At one level a pediatric project is competing with a geriatric one. At another level a whole Public Health program is fighting for a place in the national budget with something as disparate as a hydrogen bomb. How in the world do the policy makers weigh against each other alternatives so different in character?

We should observe men in the process of answering that critical and ubiquitous question, "What matters most now?" And we should thus observe valuation in action.

And here we should find that the alternatives that these men were comparing with each other were by no means so simple or so stable as they appeared. No issue ever is or ever ought to be decided "on its merits," if that is taken to mean without reference to its repercussions on other issues which its decision will affect.

The views people take of an issue depend on how they "see" it. It can be seen as part of many different questions; people will see it as part of the questions that most concern them. They cannot be proved wrong; they can all be proved right. So what? Does valuation dissolve in discrimination, and is discrimination simply a matter of what one fancies?

Perhaps research would tell us the answers to these questions. They are important, and they are real. One thing I am sure of: it would tell us. The way we see the question depends on the kind of question we are accustomed to deal with. Our society is run by people who are accustomed and professionally trained to see and answer technologic questions and financial questions and legal questions and administrative questions. Only few people are accustomed and professionally trained to see and answer human questions about people as people. We may be thankful that their number is increasing, for this imbalance cannot fail to distort the goals of Public Health. But this alone, I think, is only a small part of the answer.

I have suggested a few of the ways in which we can hope to build up our knowledge of ourselves and of the processes of which we are part—of all fields of knowledge, the most intractable and the most important. I believe that this knowledge will never equal the other sciences in giving us the power to predict, but that it can nonetheless promise something different and far more important—a greater power to understand. And it is this that will determine how much and how wisely we can contribute to the seeking of our own health in all its implications. Tyrants may shout orders, within us and without, but the voice we obey in the end speaks quietly in the indicative mood.

After Civilization What?*

KENNETH E. BOULDING

WE ARE LIVING in what I call the second great change in the state of man. The first great change was from precivilized to civilized societies. During the first 500,000 years or so of man's existence on earth he puttered along in an astonishingly stationary state. Whatever changes there were were unbelievably slow. About 10,000 years ago, there was an acceleration in the rate of change. This became noticeable 5,000 years ago, with the development of the first civilization with written records.

The details of this first great change are probably beyond our recovery. We do know that it depended on two phenomena: the development of agriculture and the development of exploitation. In a hunting and fishing economy it seems to take the food producer all his time to produce enough food for himself and his family. With agriculture's superior employment of human resources, the food producer can produce more than his family can eat. This in itself is not enough to produce civilization. In some societies in these happy conditions, the food producer has simply relaxed and indulged himself with leisure. As soon, however, as we get politics, that is exploitation,

* Reprinted by permission from the October, 1962, issue of the *Bulletin of the Atomic Scientists*, published by the Educational Foundation for Nuclear Science, 935 East 60th Street, Chicago, Illinois. This paper is from Vol. 18, pp. 2–6. The author is Director, The Center for Research in Conflict Resolution, University of Michigan, and author of a recent book, *Conflict and Defense: A General Theory*.

we begin to get cities and civilization. Civilization is what happens in cities, and the city is dependent on there being a surplus from the food producer and on some existing organization which can take it away from him. With this food surplus, the political organization feeds kings, priests, armies, architects, and builders, and the city comes into being. Political science in its earliest form is the knowledge of how to take the food surplus away from the food producer without giving him very much in return.

Now I argue that we are in the middle, perhaps not even in the middle, of the second great change in the state of man, which is as drastic and as dramatic, and certainly as large if not larger, as the change from precivilized to civilized society. This I call the change from civilization to postcivilization. These great changes can be thought of as changes of gear in the evolutionary process, resulting in progressive accelerations of the rate of evolutionary change. Man himself represents a large acceleration of the evolutionary process. Whether he evolved from preexisting forms or whether he landed from a space ship and was not able to get back to where he came from is immaterial. Once he had arrived on earth, the process of evolution could go on within the confines of the human nervous system at a greatly accelerated rate. The human mind is the result of an enormous mutation-selection process. Instead of the mutation-selection process being confined, as it were, to the flesh, it can take place within the image and hence, very rapid changes are possible. Man seems to have been slow to exploit this potentiality, but one suspects that even with primitive man, the rate of change in the biosphere was much larger than it had been before, because of the appearance of what de Chardin calls the nöosphere, or sphere of knowledge.

SAVAGERY, CIVILIZATION, AND AFTER

Civilization represents a further acceleration of the rate of change, mainly because one of the products of civilization is history. With the food surplus from agriculture, it becomes possible to feed specialized scribes. With the development of writing, man did not have to depend on the uncertain memories of the aged for records, and a great process of accumulation of social knowledge began. The past could communicate, at last in one direction, with the present, and this enormously increased the possibility and range of enlargements of the human mind.

Out of civilization comes science, a superior way of organizing the evolution of knowledge. We can trace the first beginnings of science almost as far back as the beginning of civilization itself. Beginning about 1650, however, science began to be organized into a community of knowledge, and this led again to an enormous acceleration of the rate of change. The world of 1650 is more remote from us than the world of ancient Egypt or Sumeria would have been from the man of 1650. Already in the United States and Western Europe, and to a lesser degree in the USSR and some other parts of the world, there are the beginnings of postcivilized society—a state of man as different from civilization as civilization is from savagery. What we really mean, therefore, by the anemic term "economic development" is the second great transition in the state of man. It is the movement from civilized to postcivilized society. It is nothing short of a major revolution in the human condition, and it does not represent a mere continuance and development of the old patterns of civilization.

As a dramatic illustration of the magnitude of the change, we can contemplate Indonesia, a country with about the same population and per capita income as the Roman empire at its height. Jakarta is a city about the size of ancient Rome, though perhaps a little less splendid. Indonesia is a good example of a country of high civilization. It is also one of the poorest countries in the world. It is unhappy about its present condition and desperately anxious to break out of it. All this points up the fact that the Roman empire was a desperately poor and underdeveloped society, with a civilization that always existed on a shoestring. The Roman cities always seem to have been within about three weeks of starvation, and even at its height it is doubtful whether the Roman empire ever had less than 75 to 80% of its population in agriculture.

Civilization is a state of society in which techniques are so poor that it takes about 80% of the population to feed the 100%. About 20% of the people can be spared from food producing to build parthenons and cathedrals, to write literature and poetry, and to fight wars. By contrast, the United States today is rapidly reaching the point where all food can be produced by only 10% of the population, and there are still large agricultural surpluses. Agriculture may even be on its way out altogether; within another generation or so we may be able to produce our food in totally different ways. Perhaps both fields and cows are merely relics of civilization, the vestiges of a vanishing age. Even our society, which is at an early stage of postcivilization, can now spare about 90% of the people to produce bathtubs, automobiles, hydrogen bombs, and all the other luxuries and conveniences of life. Western Europe and Japan are coming up behind the United States rapidly. The Russians are advancing toward postcivilization, although by a very different road. At the moment, their ideology is a handicap to them in some fields—especially in agriculture, where they still employ 45% of their population. Even this is better than ancient Rome. And if the Soviets ever discover that superpeasants are a good deal more efficient than collective farms, they might cut away some of the ideology that hangs around their necks, and move even more rapidly toward postcivilized society.

I'm not at all sure what postcivilization will look like; indeed, I suspect there will be several varieties of it. But it will certainly be radically different from the civilized society it is displacing. It will certainly be a worldwide society, if only because of the ease of communication and transportation. I flew last year from Idlewild to Brussels, and on glimpsing the new Brussels airport out of the corner of my eye, I thought for a moment we had come back and landed at Idlewild again. I had for a moment a horrifying vision of a world in which we went faster and faster to places more and more like the places we had left behind, until at the end of the process we might as well have stayed home. For the first time in history there is now a world style, at least in airports, which is a symbol of the coming postcivilization. We see this world style in art, in architecture, in music, in literature, in all fields of life. What in Europe looks like Americanization, in America looks like Japonification. It is simply the creeping onset of postcivilized style.

DISINTEGRATION OF INSTITUTIONS

The great problem of our age, however, is the disintegration of the institutions of civilization under the impact of advancing postcivilization. Agriculture, as we have seen, diminishes until it occupies only a small proportion of the society. The city (in the classical sense) disintegrates. Los Angeles is perhaps the first example of the postcivilization, posturban agglomeration—under no stretch of the imagination could it be called a city. War, too, is an institution in process of disintegration. National defense as a social system has fundamentally broken down on a world scale. The ICBM and the nuclear warhead have made the nation-state as militarily obsolete as the city-state, for in no country now can the armed forces preserve an area of internal peace by pushing violence to the outskirts. Poverty and inequality, too, are tending to disappear, at least on their classical scale. Postcivilized society is an affluent society, and it produces large quantities of goods, even though it may fall rather short on services. It is a society in which the technology almost prohibits great inequalities in consumption. In civilized societies the king or the emperor could live in a Versailles and the peasant in a hovel. In postcivilized society, the proletariat disappears; everybody becomes at least middle-class; and when the product of the economy consists of automobiles, mass-produced clothing, domestic appliances, and prefabricated homes, it is almost impossible for the rich to consume on a scale which is more, let us say, than 10 times that of the poor. There is no sense in having more than 10 automobiles!

Another profound change is in the expectation of life. In civilized society, both birth and death rates about 40 per thousand, and the expectation of life at birth is 25 years. In postcivilized society, the expectation of life at birth rises to at least 70 years, and perhaps more. It may be that we are on the brink of a biologic revolution just as dramatic and far reaching as the discovery of atomic energy, and that we may crack the problem of aging, prolonging human life much beyond its present span. Whether we go forward to Methuselah or not, the mere increase of the average age of death to 70 is a startling and far reaching change. It means, for instance, that in a population which is in equilibrium, the birth and death rates cannot be more than about 14 per thousand. This unquestionably implies a form of conscious birth control, and limitations on the number of children per family. It means also a radical change in the age distribution of the population, with a much larger proportion of the population being older.

Unquestionably there will be many varieties of postcivilization, some more unpleasant than others. It is perfectly possible to paint an anti-utopia which appears universally vulgar, or even universally dull. On the whole, however, I welcome postcivilization, and I have little affection for civilization. In most precivilized societies, the fact that the life of man is for the most part nasty, brutish, and short, does not prevent poets and philosophers from sentimentalizing about the noble savage. We may expect the same kind of sentimentalizing about the noble Romans and civilized survivals like Winston Churchill. On the whole, I will not shed tears over the grave of civilization any more than I do over precivilized society. Postcivilization is a realization of man's potential; its credit balance is large. It gives us at least a chance of a modest utopia, in which slavery, poverty, exploitation, gross inequality, war, and disease—prime costs of civilization—will fall to the vanishing point. Neither the disappearance of the classical city nor the disappearance of the peasant fill me with much sorrow. We may even have culture cities in which vehicular traffic is prohibited, where the rich indulge in the costly luxury of walking, while the masses live scattered about the surface of the earth, commuting occasionally to quasi-automatic factories and offices, and snuggling down with three-dimensional TV at the end of the day.

TRAPS ALONG THE ROAD

Modest as these visions of utopia may be, there is no guarantee that we will realize them. What we have at the moment is a chance to make this second transition—a chance probably unique in the history of this planet. If we fail, the chance will probably not be repeated in this part of the universe. Therefore we must look at the traps which lie along the path of the transition, which might prevent us from making the transition.

The most imminent trap is the trap of war. War is an institution peculiarly characteristic of civilization. Precivilized societies have sporadic feuding and raiding, but they do not generally have permanently organized armed forces, nor develop conquest and empire. An armed force is essentially a mobile city designed to throw things at another mobile or stationary city, with presumably evil intent. If precivilized society cannot afford war, postcivilized society can afford far too much of it, and hence will be forced to get rid of the institution, because it is simply inappropriate to the technologic age. The breakdown in the world social system of national defense really dates from about 1949, when the United States lost its monopoly on nuclear weapons. A system of national defense is only feasible if each nation is stronger at home than its enemies, so that it can preserve a relatively large area of peace within its critical boundaries. Such a system is only possible if the range of the deadly missile is short and if the armed forces of each nation lose power rapidly as they move away from home. The technologic developments of the twentieth century have destroyed these foundations of national defense, and have replaced it with another social system altogether, deterrence.

Deterrence is a social system with properties different from those of national defense, which it has replaced. Under national defense it is possible to use the armed forces; under deterrence it is not—that is, if the deterring forces are ever used, the system will have broken down. Deterrence is like an egg on a golf tee. It is stable for small but not large disturbances. If Humpty Dumpty falls off his wall, not all the king's horses nor all the President's ICBMs' will ever be able to put him back together again. We live in a society with a positive possibility of irretrievable disaster—a possibility which grows every year. This is an uncomfortable society to live in. The armed forces of the world are caught in a mutual technologic process from which we do not seem to be able to escape, which not only destroys their own function, but threatens all the rest of us.

Even if a few of us do crawl out of the fallout shelters, it is by no means clear that we can put the world back together again; for, as I shall show later, the transition of postcivilization depends on the existence of a capital fund of natural resources, which we are busy squandering and will never be able to enjoy again.

THE POPULATION EXPLOSION

In a stable postcivilized society the birth and death rates must be about 14 per thousand, and the average number of children per family cannot much exceed two. We have not developed social institutions which might accomplish this end. So far the only really certain method of controlling population is starvation and misery—the Malthusian spectre still broods over us. For most of the human race at the moment postcivilized techniques of civilized society have produced a crisis of growth which may easily be fatal. In the tropics, with DDT and a few simple public health measures, it is easy to reduce the death rate to nine or 10 per thousand, but the birth rate stays at 40 per thousand. This means in annual increase of population of three % per year, most of it concentrated in the lower age groups. This is illustrated dramatically in places like the West Indies, Ceylon, and Formosa; but thanks to the activity of the World Health Organization, it is taking place rapidly all over the tropical world.

The ultimate Malthusian equilibrium is not the problem; it is the strain put on the society by the rapid population growth, a rate of growth without precedent in history. Perhaps the most important key to the transition to postcivilization is heavy investment in human resources—that is, in education. However, conquest of disease and infant mortality before a corresponding adjustment of the birth rate produces enormous cohorts of children in societies which do not have the resources to educate them. This is an uncomfortable analogy to a hormone which kills plants by making them grow too rapidly. At the moment, the human race is heading for monumental disasters in many parts of the world.

Even in the developed countries population control presents a serious problem. The United States at the moment is increasing in population even more rapidly than India. The time when we thought that a mere increase in income would automatically solve the population problem has gone by. The child has become an object of conspicuous domestic consumption in a spending pattern which goes like this: first car, first child, washer and dryer, second child, deep freeze, third child, second car, fourth child, and so on. We now seem able to afford an average of something like four children per family. Because in a postcivilized society these four children all survive, the population doubles every generation. A hundred years of this and even the United States will be uncomfortably crowded.

A TECHNOLOGY OF SUICIDE

The third trap on the road to postcivilization is the technologic trap. Our present technology is fundamentally suicidal. It is based on the extraction of concentrated deposits of fossil fuels and ores, which are exhaustible. Even at present rates of consumption they will be exhausted in a time span which is not long, even measured against human history, and which is infinitesimally small on the geologic time scale. If the rest of the world advances to American standards of consumption, these resources will disappear almost overnight. From this point of view, economic development is the process of bringing closer the evil day when everything will be gone—all the oil, all the coal, all the ores—and we will have to go back to primitive agriculture and scratching in the woods.

There are indications, however, that suicidal technology is not absolutely necessary, and that a permanent high-level technology is possible. Beginning in the early part of the twentieth century, it is possible to detect an anti-entropic movement in technology. It begins, perhaps, with the Haber process for fixing nitrogen from the air. A development of similar significance is the Dow process for extracting magnesium from the sea. Both these processes take the diffuse and concentrate it, instead of taking the concentrated and diffusing it, as most processes of mining and economic production do. Sir William Crookes in the last years of the nineteenth century predicted that we would all be starving by the middle of the twentieth century because of the exhaustion of Chilean nitrates. Fortunately, this prediction was falsified by the Haber process. These anti-entropic processes foreshadow a technology in which we shall draw all the materials we need from the virtually inexhaustible reservoirs of the sea and air, and draw our energy from controlled fusion—either artificially produced on earth or from the sun. It is clear, however, that a fundamental technologic transition is still to be accomplished.

When we look at possible remedies for our immediate problems, it seems clear that we are all engulfed in a profound and appallingly dangerous misallocation of our intellectual resources. Our chance of solving these problems, therefore, depends on our ability to do something about this. Resources are misallocated because although our major problems are problems of social systems, we persist in regarding them as if they were essentially problems of physical or biologic systems. We persist in regarding the agricultural problem, for instance, as one of crops, whereas it is fundamentally a problem of farmers. We persist in regarding flood control as a problem of the river, even turning it over to army engineers, who treat the river as an enemy. But a flood is no problem to a river; it is a perfectly normal part of its action. A flood is essentially a problem of people and social institutions, of architecture and locating cities.

We regard national defense as a problem of physical systems and hardware, whereas it is essentially also a problem of social systems. Despite the fact that war and peace is the major problem of our age, we are putting practically nothing into peace research; even when we do put money into arms control and disarmament research, we spend $60 million for project Vela, which deals wholly with physical systems, and $150,000 on project Vulcan, which deals with social systems. We are diverting our major intellectual effort into solving problems that have no answers, and putting no effort into the solution of real problems. Unless we can awaken many people to the true nature of the intellectual crisis of our times, and unless we can mobilize our intellectual resources to work on the true problems, I think our chances of making the transition to postcivilization are slim.

If the human race is to survive it will have to change its ways of thinking more in the next 25 years than it has done in the last 25,000. There is hope in the fact that we have far from exhausted the capacity of the extraordinary organism we call man. I once calculated the capacity of the human nervous system in terms of the number of different states it might assume, and found it to be two to the ten billionth power, assuming that each of our ten billion neurons is capable of only two states. This is an extremely large number. It would take 90 years to write it down at the rate of one digit a second. For a standard of comparison, the total number of neutrinos (the smallest known particle), which could be packed into the known astronomical universe (this is the largest physical number I could think of) could easily be written down in three minutes. I find it hard to believe, therefore, that the capacity of the human organism has been exhausted. It has an extraordinary capacity to learn.

Now we need to develop an almost new form of learning. We have to learn from rapidly changing systems. Ordinarily we learn from stable systems. Because the world repeats itself, we learn the "law of repetition." Learning from changing systems is perhaps another step in the acceleration of evolution that we have to take. I have been haunted by the remark (possibly made by Mark Twain) that a cat who jumps on a hot stove never jumps on a cold one. This seems to describe precisely the state we may be in today. We have jumped on a lot of hot stoves and now perhaps onto the cold stove is the only place left to jump. In a rapidly changing system it is desperately easy to learn things which are no longer true. Perhaps the greatest task of applied social science at the moment is to study the conditions under which we learn from rapidly changing systems. If we can discover these conditions, there may still be hope for the human race.

Index

Absenteeism, 170–186
Accidents, motor vehicle, 74–93, 112, 312, 367
  other, 46, 168, 178, 312
Accident prevention, 78
Aerospace medicine, 515–521
Aging, 149–163, 304, 474–480, 610
Agricultural Health, Institute of, 50
Air pollution, 62–73, 116
Alcoholics Anonymous, 189, 604, 660–669
Alcoholism, 187–191, 238, 660–669
American Cancer Society, 379, 389, 711
American Heart Association, 375, 379, 386, 711
American Medical Association, 674, 744, 760
American Public Health Association, 12, 266, 390, 402, 449, 545, 570, 674
Anthropology, 500–501, 570–579
Armed services, 360–373, 610–611
Arteriosclerosis, 675–709
Arthritis, 766

Behavioral sciences, 567–582, 827–837
Bilharziasis, 106
Biostatistics and biostatisticians, 427, 445–450
Blue Cross and Blue Shield, 336, 616–617, 744–745
Brain damage, 199–210, 238–239, 250–251
British National Health Service, 333, 860
Budgeting, 448

Canada, 187, 337, 482–489
Cancer, 111, 142–143, 168, 301, 303, 310, 523, 767
Casefinding, 144, 315, 352–359, 398, 749–758
Cerebral palsy, 199–212
Chemical hazards, 47–48, 64–66
Children, see Youth
Children's Bureau of U.S., 21, 195, 255, 347, 452, 475
Cirrhosis, hepatic, 313
Chronic illness, 110, 140–148, 317, 397–398, 474–480, 542–545, 659
Color additives, 286
Commission on Chronic Illness, 474
Commonwealth Fund, 335
Communication, 583–598
Community structure, 799–809
Congenital malformation, 315, 812–824
Contergan, see Thalidomide
Continuity of care, 197
Costs of illness, 253, 345, 636, 659
Council on Social Work Education, 463

Crash programs, 792–798
Crippled Children's Services, 350, 394–395, 453–455, 614
Crop dusting, 518

Dental health, 317
Dentistry, Public Health, 482–490, 626
Dependency, 146, 415–421, 653
Diabetes mellitus, 143, 314, 755–756, 766
Disability insurance, 623
Divorce, 133
Donora, Pennsylvania, 62, 71
Drug addiction, 614, 835

Education, 33–34, 223, 337, 646
Epidemiology, 74–93, 199–212, 369, 371, 431, 432–445, 533, 675–709, 710–714, 827–837
Epilepsy, 199–212

Families, 127–140, 257, 270–271, 831–833
Family planning, 37–44, 135–139, 871–872
Farms, see Rural Health
Federal Aviation Agency, 515–516
Federal Trade Commission, 282
Filariasis, 106
Fluoridation, 41, 839
Folk medicine, 53–58
Food additives, 285
Food and Drug Administration, 276–287
Food, Drug and Cosmetic Acts, 282–287
Fund–raising, 379–382
Future in Public Health, 299, 479, 529, 629–630, 827–837, 852–866, 866–874

Gastrointestinal disease, 176, 766
Genetics, 305, 531–541
Glaucoma, 143, 317
Government, Federal, 255, 545–546, 646
Gynecologic disease, 176

Health, 360–362
Health Administration, 328
Health agencies, see Voluntary Health Agencies
Health education, 491–505, 506–507
Health examinations, 349, 352–359, 511, 759–782
Health Insurance Plan of New York City, 621
Health personnel, 120, 255, 277, 337, 445, 483–485, 521, 561, 583–598, 626–628, 631, 648–649, 795–797
Health services, 119, 236, 254, 262, 308, 397, 607, 645, 838–851
Hearing acuity, 756

Heart disease, 110, 168, 303, 310, 674–709, 754, 766
Hernia, 766
Hill–Burton Act, see Hospital and Medical Facilities Construction Program
History of medicine and Public Health, 3, 11, 14–22, 281, 291, 333, 428, 432–438, 451, 509, 567–572, 583–590, 684, 735–738, 760–761, 867–869
Home care, 735–746
Hospital and Medical Facilities Construction, (Hill–Burton) Program, 278 335, 649
Hospital councils, 337
Hospitalization, 243, 275
Hospitals, 332–340, 341–342, 343–344
Housekeeping services, 324–325
Housing, 149–163, 260

Iatrogenic disease, 812–824
Immunization, 143, 783–791
Infant mortality, 192–199, 312, 447, 833
Institutions, 400, 559
International health, 100–123, 500–503, 678–681, 715–721, 792–798

Japan, 69

Kaiser Foundation Health Plan, 621

Laboratories, Public Health, 542–547
Land use, 26–27
Legislation, 281–288
Leprosy, 108
Licensure of institutions, 399
Los Angeles County Health Department, 452

Malaria, 104
Marriage, 129–131
Maternal and child health, 322–324
Maternal mortality, 192–199, 237
Meat inspection, 287
Medical care, 275–281, 318, 412–423, 488, 563, 602–635, 635–642
Medicare program, 276
Mental Health, 53–54, 114, 157, 177, 199–212, 235–246, 304, 548–566, 613–614, 724–725, 766, 827–837, 838–851
Mental retardation, 199–212, 247–258
Merchant Marine, 611
Metabolic diseases, 536–537
Migrant workers, 259–267, 612
Migration, 671
Morocco, 792–798
Mortality trends, 110–113, 237, 289, 309–316, 685–693, also see Infant mortality
Multiphasic screening, see Casefinding

National Academy of Sciences, 286, 287
National Association for Mental Health, 385
National Center for Health Statistics, 277
National Council on Alcoholism, 190
National Health Survey, 75, 142, 363
National Institutes of Health, 255, 290–299, 517, 549, 558–559, 711
National Tuberculosis Association, 70, 384
Negro health, 203–205, 689–692
New Mexico, 51
New York City Department of Health, 349–352, 586
Nucleic acids, 305
Nursing homes, 401
Nursing, Public Health, 19, 393, 466–473, 627
Nutrition, 238–239, 402, 681–682, 699–700, 701–702, 715–721, 722–734, 756
    Public Health, 402, 474–481

Obesity, 722–734, 766
Occupational diseases, 49
Occupational health, 45–51, 261, 430, 508–514, 769–782

Parent counseling, 254
Parasitic diseases, 101, 367
Patients counseling, 4–6, 181–183, 341–342, 469, 477
Perception, 491–505
Personnel, see Health personnel
Philanthropy, 375–376
Physicians, 8–10, 120, 146–147, 584–596, 625–626
Poison control, 670–674
Population trends, 23–36, 38, 134–135, 871–872
Posters in Health Education, 506–507
Pregnancy, 43–44, 197, 199–212, 236
Prematurity, 197
Prevention, 236–246, 316, 539, 673
Reading disabilities, 199–212
Preventive Medicine, 360–373, 428–430
Prisoners, 613
Progressive patient care, 343
Psychiatry, Public Health, see Mental Health

Radiologic health and radiation, 99, 117, 166, 522–530, 531
Regional hospital councils, 337
Regionalization, 332–341
Rehabilitation, 254, 300, 317–318, 398, 405, 563, 615, 643–654, 654–660, 660–669, 743–744, 792–798
Research, medical, 279, 289–307, 326, 360–373, 379, 516, 650–652
Respiratory disease, 175, 312, 366

Rheumatic fever, 143
Rheumatic heart disease, 143
Rural health, 45–61, 692–693

Sanitation, 17–18, 261, 429
Saskatchewan, 482
School health, 346–351, 352–359
Scientific management, 509
Sewage treatment, 16–17, 95–97
Smoking, 506–507, 710–714
Social Security Act, 419, 453
Social work, 254, 451–473
Sociology, 571
South Dakota, 50
Space Medicine, *see* Aerospace medicine
Speech disorders, 199–212
Staten Island Marine Hospital, 291
Statistics and statisticians, *see* Biostatistics and biostatisticians
Stream pollution, 93–99, 116
Stress, 170–186, 268–271, 441
Stroke, 312, 317
Suburban areas, 32–36
Suicide, 315
Surgical operations, 178
Syphilis, 105, 756

Thalidomide, 812–824
Tics, 199–212
Trachoma, 107
Triorthocresyl phosphate poisoning, 792–798
Trypanosomiasis, 109
Tuberculosis, 103, 315, 395, 442–444, 614, 755

United Mine Workers of America Welfare and Retirement Fund, 635–642
UNICEF, 100

U.S. Department of Agriculture, 282–287, 335
U.S. Department of Defense—Medicare Program, *see* Medicare program
U.S. Department of Health, Education, and Welfare, 225, 255–256, 282, 422
U.S. Public Health Service, 20, 65, 98, 111, 255, 265, 275–281, 391–399, 475, 527
Uranium, 164–170
Urban health, 11–13, 692–695, 835
Urbanization, 23–36, 834

Venereal disease, 224–234
Veterans, 21, 611–612
Veterans Administration, 276, 549
Virus diseases, 102
Visual acuity, 766
Vocational Rehabilitation Administration, 255
Voluntary health agencies, 374–384, 384–389, 604, 609

Water supply, 16–17, 96–99
Welfare and welfare agencies, 239–240, 378, 390–412
Welfare medical care, 330, 390, 406–410, 414–417, 606–610
Working abroad, 268–271
Workmen's Compensation, 406, 622
World Health Organization, 100–101, 111, 188, 716–719, 793–798

Yaws, 105
YMCA and YWCA, 386–387
Youth, 29–32, 128, 213–224, 224–234, 393, 412–423, 614–615, 668, 714–721
Youth and employment, 213–224

Zoonosis, 47